DENTISTRY
English for Dental Practice
Textbook and Exercise Book

DENTISTRY

English for Dental Practice
Textbook and Exercise Book

Stomatologie
Angličtina pro zubní praxi
učebnice a cvičebnice

IRENA BAUMRUKOVÁ

To order additional copies of this book, contact:
Xlibris LLC
0-800-056-3182
www.xlibrispublishing.co.uk
Orders@xlibrispublishing.co.uk
307189

CONTENTS / OBSAH

PŘEDMLUVA

Předkládaná práce je čítankou odborných textů z nejnovějších originálních pramenů, učebnicí a cvičebnicí lékařské angličtiny v oboru stomatologie a poslouží i jako příručka pro lékaře a zdravotníky, kteří se ve své praxi setkávají s anglicky mluvícími klienty.

Skvělou pomůckou se může stát rovněž pro odborníky a studenty, kteří se chystají pracovat či studovat v zahraničí a také pro lektory lékařské angličtiny, kteří je na tyto pobyty budou připravovat a povedou specializované kurzy na vysokých školách, ve firmách a dalších institucích.

Předpokládá se středoškolská znalost jazyka, ale v podrobných slovnících u každé lekce i na konci učebnice je mnoho zcela základních výrazů, vždy s přepisem výslovnosti, což umožní rychlý start ke zvládnutí bohaté slovní zásoby.

Cennou součástí studijního materiálu je klíč k lekcím, který vedle původních textů ke spojovacím a doplňovacím cvičením obsahuje všechny věty z překladů seřazené podle české abecedy. Kromě snadného nalezení anglického ekvivalentu se dá výborně procvičit překlad zpětný, což umožňuje vyšší stupeň aktivního ovládnutí důležitých sousloví a frází.

Texty v klíči je možno použít jako zdroje pro cvičení porozumění textu, konverzační cvičení, vytváření cvičných prezentací na rozmanitá témata dle potřeb učitelů a jejich studentů

Krátké texty a jednotná struktura lekcí činí učebnici velmi vhodnou zejména pro samostatné studium a vytváření individuálních studijních plánů.

Práce prohlubuje látku probíranou v základní učebnici Medical English in Stomatology I a II a je zde mnoho zajímavých cvičení pro dlouhodobé podrobné studium.

PhD Irena Baumruková
Praha 2011

Připomínky a objednávky zasílejte laskavě na
e mail:irena.baumrukova@seznam.cz
sms: 606765821
Korespondenční adresa:
Jičínská 17
130 00 Praha 3
Česká republika

ÚVOD

Než se pustíme do studia, projděme si obsah kapitol. Překlad pojmů Je
určen učitelům angličtiny a studentům, kteří nejsou stomatology, na svou profesi
se teprve připravují a terminologii oboru budou postupně získávat od svých
odborných pedagogů.

Unit 1

Preventive and Community Dental Practice

The Philosophy of Prevention. Health Promotion. Barriers to Healthy Behaviour. Dental Caries. DMFT Index. Microbiology of Dental Caries. Diet and Dental Caries. Fluoride. Fluorosis. Prevention in Elderly Patients.

Text 1

The Philosophy of Prevention

The **major oral diseases—dental caries, periodontal disease, and oral cancer**—are influenced by **environmental, social, and lifestyle** factors. **Prevention** has traditionally been defined in three s Exercise 1 tages:

- **primary** prevention - steps taken to ensure disease does not occur
- **secondary** prevention - promoting early intervention in those already affected
- **tertiary** prevention - treatment of well- established disease to restore function and avoid further episodes

Measures applied on a population basis include **water fluoridation** and **health-promoting campaigns**. Preventive measures on an individual basis can be applied either by a dental professional (fissure sealants, diet counselling) or by the subject, e.g. tooth brushing.

Health Promotion

The key messages of health education are:

- **reduce the intake of sugar-containing** food and drink, avoid between-meal sugar snacks
- **brush teeth twice daily** with a toothpaste containing fluoride
- **attend** the dentist **regularly**

Barriers to Healthy Behaviour

Dental disease is heavily influenced by **socio-economic and other constraints**. Parents may realise that fresh fruit is preferable to chocolate bars; non-availability or price may preclude its provision. Similarly, sugar-containing foodstuffs are given to children not only when they are hungry but also as a reward or a pacifier.

Dental Caries

Dental caries is a dynamic process involving the exchange of calcium and phosphate ions between tooth structure and saliva (plaque fluid) in the presence of acids produced by the fermentation of carbohydrates by oral microorganisms.

We can distinguish **enamel caries, fissure caries, dentine caries, occult caries, root caries, recurrent caries, secondary caries, rampant caries, nursing bottle caries, and arrested caries**.

Caries can be difficult to diagnose by **clinical examination** alone. Further aids are **radiographic diagnosis, fibre-optic transillumination, electronic caries detector, and dyes** (which enable easier visualisation).

DMFT Index
Decay, missing, filled index is the most widely used method of recording caries experience.
D = decayed
M = missing
F = filled
T = teeth
DMFT applies to permanent teeth. DMFS applies to permanent teeth surfaces.

Exercise 1
1. Define three stages of prevention.
2. What are the key messages of health education?
3. Which are the barriers to healthy behaviour?
4. Talk about different types of dental caries.
5. Which aids used in diagnosis of dental caries do you know?
6. What is DMFT index?

Translation 1
Ústní onemocnění, zubní kazy, onemocnění parodontu, rakovina, faktory prostředí, faktory sociální, životní styl, včasný zásah, obnovit funkci, vyhnout se dalším epizodám, preventivní opatření, fluorizace vody, kampaně propagující zdraví, utěsnění prasklin, dietní poradenství, omezte příjem jídla a pití s obsahem cukru, čistěte si zuby dvakrát denně, navštěvujte pravidelně zubního lékaře, čerstvé ovoce je vhodnější než čokoládové tyčinky, zubní kaz, kaz skloviny, fisurální kaz, kaz zuboviny, skrytý kaz, kaz kořene, recidivující kaz, sekundární kaz, akutní kaz, kaz způsobený dětskou lahvičkou, zastavený zubní kaz, rentgenová diagnóza, prosvícení skleněným optickým vláknem, elektronický detektor kazů, barviva, zuby zkažené, chybějící, vyplněné.

Text 2
Microbiology of Dental Caries
Caries does not develop in germ-free animals. Most important organisms are *Mutans streptococci* and Lactobacillus species. Dental caries will not develop in the absence of dental plaque, and **plaque removal is essential in maintaining periodontal health**. **Dietary control** and use of fluoride are more important in caries prevention than plaque removal itself.

Diet and Dental Caries
There is clear and extensive evidence of the **correlation between the frequency and amount of sugar consumption and the prevalence and severity of dental caries**. **Sticky retentive foods** are more cariogenic than liquid nonretentive

forms, e.g. toffee is more cariogenic than chocolate. The frequency of consumption is crucial. The ultimate message is **'eat less sugar and eat sugar less often'**.

Nonsugar sweeteners are noncariogenic and are useful sugar substitutes, but **use of artificial sweeteners perpetuates the craving for sweet foods**. Their use should be restricted in small children due to possible side effects on the gastrointestinal system.

Sugar-free chewing gum stimulates saliva and **enhances washout** of sugar. **Carbonated beverages** can cause marked loss of tooth structure via **erosion**, an increasing problem in teenagers.

Detersive foodstuffs are of little or **no benefit** in removal of plaque. Effective plaque removal is dependent on tooth brushing. However, carrots, apples, etc. are preferable to high-sugar snacks.

Fluoride
Evidence that fluoride prevents caries:
- caries prevalence is lower in areas **where fluoride is present naturally** in the water supply
- **addition of fluoride to the water supply** is effective in preventing caries
- fluoride supplements in the form of **tablets, drops, salt, and milk** have all been shown to be effective in caries prevention
- fluoride-containing **toothpastes** are effective in preventing caries

Mechanisms for delivering fluoride
- **water fluoridation** has been shown in numerous studies to reduce caries incidence

- **fluoride toothpastes** (restrict the amount of toothpaste used by **children to a pea-sized smear** amount at each brushing, **mint flavours** are preferred to discourage children eating the paste)
- **fluoride drops and tablets** can exert both a systemic and topical effect. Give them **last thing at night** and allow them to **dissolve slowly** in the mouth.

Fluorosis
Fluorosis occurs due to the **excessive intake** of fluoride during the **period of tooth formation**. It ranges from **white flecks to brown stains** in more severe cases. Mild forms diminish with time. Fluorosis can be markedly **improved by etching and polishing**. Fluoride tablets, toothpastes, and mouthwashes should be stored out of the reach of children.

Prevention in Elderly Patients
Care of elderly people will become increasingly important to the dental profession. There are several **factors complicating prevention:**
Plaque control
- **gingival recession, migrated and tilted teeth**
- **partial dentures** increase **plaque retention**
- **poor eyesight** and **reduced dexterity** make tooth brushing difficult
- **polypharmacy** is common in the elderly, some drugs **reduce salivary flow**

Diet
- tendency to **snacking**—cakes and biscuits, the elderly patients are

particularly prone to recurrent
caries and root caries

Denture care

* encourage **removal of dentures at night** and good **denture hygiene**
* emphasize the importance of annual **dental examinations even if edentulous**, because this permits early detection of mucosal disease (e.g. oral cancer)

Exercise 2

1. Give the information about microbiology of dental caries.
2. Talk about diet and dental caries.
3. How can fluoride be used? What is fluorosis?
4. Talk about prevention in elderly patients.

Translation 2

Zubní kaz se nerozvine při nepřítomnosti zubního plaku, kontrola diety a užití fluoridu, odstraňování plaku, konzumace cukru, frekvence, množství, výskyt a závažnost zubních kazů, jezte méně cukru, jezte cukr méně často, sladidla bez cukru udržují touhu po sladkém, náhražky cukru, možné vedlejší účinky na zažívací systém, žvýkačky bez cukru stimulují tvorbu slin, perlivé nápoje způsobují znatelnou ztrátu zubní struktury erozí, dávat přednost mrkvi a jablkům před svačinou s vysokým obsahem cukru, přidávání fluoridu do vody, fluoridové doplňky, tablety, kapky, sůl, mléko, pasty s obsahem fluoridu, účinný v prevenci kazů, omezte množství pasty s fluoridem u dětí, příchuť máty peprné odradí děti od požívání pasty, nechte pomalu rozpustit v ústech, fluoróza

vzniká kvůli nadměrnému příjmu fluoridu, období tvoření zubu, bílé fleky, hnědé skvrny v závažnějších případech, mírné formy se časem zmenší, zlepšit leptáním, leštěním, ukládat mimo dosah dětí, péče o starší lidi, faktory komplikující prevenci, kontrola plaku, ústup dásní, vyviklané a skloněné zuby, částečné protézy, chabý zrak a snížená zručnost, nadměrné užívání léčiv je běžné, některé léky snižují tok slin, náchylní k opakujícím se kazům, kazům kořenů, péče o protézy, vyjímání na noc, dobrá hygiena, každoroční prohlídky u bezzubých pacientů, včasné objevení onemocnění sliznic.

Vocabulary

absence /ˈæb.sᵊnts/ absence, nepřítommnost
acid /ˈæs.ɪd/ kyselina
addition /əˈdɪʃ.ᵊn/ přidání
affect /əˈfekt/ ovlivnit, postihnout
aid /eid/ pomůcka
alone /əˈləʊn/ samotný
amount /əˈmaʊnt/ množství
animal /ˈæn.ɪ.məl/ živočich
annual /ˈæn.ju.əl/ každoroční
applied /əˈplaɪd/ aplikovaný
arrest /əˈrest/ zástava, zachycení
artificial /ˌɑː.tɪˈfɪʃ.ᵊl/ umělý
attend /əˈtend/ navštěvovat
bar /bɑːʳ/ tyčinka
barrier /ˈbær.i.əʳ/ bariéra
behaviour /bɪˈheɪ.vjər/ chování
benefit /ˈben.ɪ.fɪt/ výhoda, příspěvek
beverage /ˈbev.ər.ɪdʒ/ nápoj
biscuit /ˈbɪs.kɪt/ sušenka
brushing /brʌʃ.ɪŋ/ čistění
cake /keɪk/ koláč, dort
calcium /ˈkæl.si.əm/ vápník

promote /prəˈməʊt/ propagovat, podporovat

provision /prəˈvɪʒ.ᵊn/ poskytování

radiographic /ˌreɪ.diˈɒg.rə.fik/ rentgenový

rampant /ˈræm.pᵊnt/ útočný, nekontrolovatelný

reach /riːtʃ/ dosah

realise /ˈrɪə.laɪz/ uvědomovat si

recession /rɪˈseʃ.ᵊn/ ústup

record /rɪˈkɔːd/ zaznamenat

recurrent /rɪˈkʌr.ᵊnt/ opakující se, recidivující

reduce /rɪˈdjuːs/ snížit, napravit, přemoct

regularly /ˈreg.jʊ.lə.li/ pravidelně

removal /rɪˈmuː.vᵊl/ odstranění

restricted /rɪˈstrɪk.tɪd/ omezený

retentive /rɪˈten.tɪv/ nepropouštějící

reward /rɪˈwɔːd/ odměna

root /ruːt/ kořen

saliva /səˈlaɪ.və/ sliny

salivary /səˈlaɪ.vᵊr.i/ slinný

salt /sɒlt/ sůl

secondary /ˈsek.ən.dri/ sekundární (druhotný), závislý-porucha

side /saɪd/ **effect** /ɪˈfekt/ vedlejší účinek

similarly /ˈsɪm.ɪ.lə.li/ podobně

smear /smɪəʳ/ nepatrné množství

snack /snæk/ lehké jídlo, přesnídávka

species /ˈspiː.ʃiːz/ druhy

stage /steɪdʒ/ stupeň, stádium (období)

stain /steɪn/ kaz, vada

step /step/ krok

sticky /ˈstɪk.i/ lepkavý

stimulate /ˈstɪm.jʊ.leɪt/ stimulovat, podněcovat

store /stɔːʳ/ skladovat, zásoba, materiál

streptococcus /ˌstrep.təˈkɒk.əs/ (pl. **streptococci**) streptokok

subject /ˈsʌb.dʒekt/ předmět

substitute /ˈsʌb.stɪ.tjuːt/ nahradit

sugar /ˈʃʊg.əʳ/ cukr

supplement /ˈsʌp.lɪ.mənt/ doplněk

sweetener /ˈswiːt.nəʳ/ umělé sladidlo

systemic /sɪˈstem.ɪk/ systemický, systémový

tablet /ˈtæb.lət/ tabletka

take /teɪk/ vzít, brát

teenager /ˈtiːn.eɪ.dʒəʳ/ -náctiletý

tertiary /ˈtɜː.ʃᵊr.i/ terciálně, v třetí řadě

tilt /tɪlt/ naklonit

toffee /ˈtɒf.i/ karamelový bonbón

topical /ˈtɒp.ɪ.kᵊl/ místní

traditionally /trəˈdɪʃ.ᵊn.ᵊl.i/ tradičně

transillumination /ˌtræn.zɪˈluː.mɪˈneɪ.ʃᵊn/ prosvícení

twice /twaɪs/ dvakrát

ultimate /ˈʌl.tɪ.mət/ základní, konečný

use /juːs/ užívání

via /vaɪə/, /ˈviː.ə/ skrz, pomocí (čeho)

visualisation /ˌvɪʒ.u.ᵊl.aɪˈzeɪ.ʃᵊn/ znázornění (vizuální)

washout /ˈwɒʃ.aʊt/ pohroma

widely /ˈwaɪd.li/ široce

Unit 2

History Taking and Examination

Professionals Complementary to
Dentistry. History. Previous Dental
History, Previous Medical History.
Social History. Examination. Treatment
Planning.

Text 1

Professionals Complementary to Dentistry

A varied group of health-care workers
support dental surgeons.

- **Dental nurse**

Main role is **assisting at the chairside**
but may also undertake **receptionist
and administrative duties**.

- **Dental hygienist**

Role involves patient **education,
scaling, polishing,** and **application
of prophylactic materials** including
fissure sealants. She can administer
local anaesthesia by infiltration.
Dental hygienists must work to the
written prescription of a dentist who
has first examined the patient.

- **Dental therapist**

Dental therapists undertake the same
work as hygienists but can also do
**simple restorations and extract
primary teeth.**

- **Dental technicians**

Dental technicians **construct** all forms
of **fixed and removable prostheses**.

History

The ability to take a good history is an
**essential first step in the diagnosis
and management** of any dental
condition. It is necessary to establish
the **nature of the problem**, e.g.:

- **pain, discomfort,** an **abnormal
feeling**
- an **aesthetic** problem, **altered
function**
- **bleeding or exudate**
- **swelling**
- **halitosis**

Determine:

- **When** was the problem **first noticed**?
- Is it **continuous or intermittent**?
- **How frequently** does it occur?
- Are there any **initiating or
relieving factors**?
- Is the problem **becoming better,
worse, or about the same**?
- **Where** exactly is the problem?

If pain is the main problem, the
following must be established:

- **location** – specific tooth or
generalised
- **initiating or relieving** factors –
hot/cold, worse on **biting**, worse
on **bending forwards**

- **character** – dull, sharp, **throbbing, shooting**
- **severity** – e.g. causing **sleep loss**, **relieved by** mild **analgesics**
- **spread/radiation** – to adjacent structures, referred pain

Remember, **pain thresholds vary** greatly between individuals.

Exercise 1
1. Characterise the roles of professionals complementary to dentistry.
2. Describe principles of history taking.
3. Talk about pain as the main problem.

Translation 1
Role sestry, vzdělávání pacientů, asistovat u křesla, odstraňování zubního kamene, leštění, aplikace profylaktických materiálů, včetně pečetidla fisur, podávat místní anestesii injekčně, pracovat dle písemných pokynů lékaře, vykonávat administrativní a recepční práce, dělat jednoduché náhrady, trhat první zuby, konstruovat pevné a vyjímatelné náhrady, schopnost vytvořit správnou anamnézu, bolest, nepohoda, abnormální pocit, estetický problém, zhoršená funkce, krvácení, výpotek, otok, zápach z úst, obtíž, kde přesně, kdy byla poprvé zaznamenána, je problém stálý nebo přerušovaný, jak často se objevuje, spouštějící nebo ulevující faktory, zlepšuje se, zhoršuje, stejný, bolest v určitém zubu, celková, šíření, vyzařování, teplo, chlad, zhoršující se při kousání, při předklonu, bolest tupá, ostrá, škubavá, vystřelující,

způsobující nespavost, zklidněná mírnými analgetiky, práh bolesti se u jednotlivců velice liší.

Text 2
Previous Dental History, Previous Medical History
Establish:
- **previous episodes** of similar nature
- **regular/irregular attendee**
- when the patient last received dental **treatment**
- **attitude** to dental treatment— **anxious, relaxed**

Knowledge of a **patient's general health** is essential and should be obtained before examination. This part of the history should be **updated routinely** at each patient visit. It is worth asking a general question such as 'Are you generally fit and well?' or 'Are you attending any doctors or clinics or taking any medicines or tablets?'

Social History
It is desirable to establish:
- **patient's age**
- **occupation**
- **marital circumstances**
- **dependants**
- **smoking** habit
- **alcohol consumption**

Relevant questions in a medical history:
1. Do you feel **generally healthy**?
2. Have you had **rheumatic fever**?
3. Have you had **hepatitis or jaundice**?
4. Do you have any heart problems such as **angina, heart murmur,**

replacement valve, or have you suffered a **heart attack?**

5. Do you have **high blood pressure?**

6. Do you suffer from **bronchitis, asthma,** or any other chest condition?

7. Do you have **diabetes?**

8. Do you have **arthritis?**

9. Are you receiving any **tablets, creams, or ointments** from your doctor?

10. Are you using any tablets, creams, ointments, powders, or medicines bought **over the counter** in a pharmacy or shop?

11. Are you taking or have you taken **steroids** in the last two years?

12. Are you **allergic** to any medicines, food, or material?

13. Do you suffer from **epilepsy,** or are you prone to **fainting** attacks?

14. Have you ever **bled excessively** following a cut or tooth extraction?

15. Are you an **expectant mother?**

16. Have you been **hospitalised?** If yes, what for and when?

17. Are you attending any **other hospital clinics or specialists?**

18. Do you **smoke?**

19. **Who** is your **doctor?**

Exercise 2

1. Ask about previous dental history, previous medical history, and social history.

2. Learn by heart relevant questions in a medical history.

Translation 2

Předchozí anamnéza dentální, lékařská, sociální, návštěvy pravidelné, nepravidelné, kdy byl pacient naposledy ošetřen, postoj k ošetření, úzkostný, klidný, obecné otázky, relevantní dotazy v lékařské diagnóze„Jste celkově zdráv a v pořádku?", „Navštěvujete nějaké lékaře či střediska, užíváte nějaké léky či tabletky?", pacientův věk, povolání, okolnosti manželství, vyživované osoby, návyk kouření, požívání alkoholu, „Cítíte se celkově zdráv? ", „Měl jste někdy revmatickou horečku? "„Měl jste někdy zánět jater nebo žloutenku? ", „Máte nějaké problémy se srdcem jako je srdeční angína, srdeční šelest, náhrada chlopně, utrpěl jste někdy srdeční záchvat? ", „Máte vysoký krevní tlak? ", „Trpíte zánětem průdušek, astmatem, nebo jinými hrudními obtížemi? ", „Máte cukrovku?", „Máte zánět kloubů? ", „Dostáváte nějaké tabletky, krémy, masti od Vašeho lékaře? ", „Používáte nějaké tabletky, krémy, masti, prášky, nebo léky koupené bez receptu v lékárně či obchodě?", „Berete nebo jste v posledních dvou letech bral steroidy? ", „Jste alergický na nějaké léky, potraviny, látky? ", „Trpíte epilepsií, jste náchylný k záchvatům mdloby? "„Krvácel jste někdy nadměrně po říznutí či vytržení zubu? ", „Jste nastávající matka? Jste těhotná? ", „Byl jste někdy hospitalizován? Pokud ano, z jakého důvodu a kdy? ", „Navštěvujete jinou nemocnici, kliniku či specialisty? "„Kdo je Vaším lékařem? "

Text 3

Examination

Extraoral examination, **intraoral** examination, **diagnosis, treatment planning**

Examination essentially begins when patients enter the surgery:
Do they **look fit and well**? Are they **relaxed or apprehensive**?

Look for:

- general **appearance** of the patient
- **swellings** of the face and neck
- **skeletal pattern**
- **lip competence**
- TMJ (**temporomandibular joint**) problems

Palpate:

- **lymph nodes**
- **TMJ** problems
- **muscles of mastication**

Note:

- condition of **soft tissues**
- teeth **present, missing, unerupted**
- **general state** of the dentition
- **oral hygiene** status
- **presence and site** of **restorations and carious lesions**
- presence and age of **dentures**
- **not carious** tooth surface loss
- **periodontal** condition

Diagnosis

Special tests and investigations: **radiographs, sensitivity tests, study models, biopsy**

Treatment Planning

The purpose of treatment planning is to provide a work schedule.
The following **principles** apply:

- **relieve pain**
- **extract** teeth of hopeless prognosis
- provide **preventive advice**
- **improve periodontal** condition
- **restore** carious teeth
- more advanced treatment procedures (**endodontics, crowns, bridges, partial dentures**)

- **recall** maintenance

Factors influencing treatment include:

Patient-related factors:

- complicating **medical history**
- patient **anxiety**
- good **oral hygiene** and adherence to preventive advice is of prime importance
- inability/unwillingness to maintain adequate standards of **plaque control**
- inability to **afford time** required for proposed treatment

Dentist-related factors:

- ability of dentist
- access to specialist services

Cost-related factors

- treatment available may depend on what patient can afford
- availability of planned procedures under the **health-care system or insurance scheme** covering the patient's treatment

---

Exercise 3

1. Give the main principles of examination, diagnosis, and treatment planning.
2. What do you have to look for, palpate, note?
3. What do you know about special tests and investigations?
4. Talk about treatment planning and factors influencing treatment.

Translation 3

Vyšetření vně úst, v ústech, diagnóza, plán léčby, sledujte celkový vzhled pacienta, otoky na obličeji a krku, celistvost rtů, prohmatejte lymfatické uzliny, temporo-mandibulární oblast, žvýkací svaly, zaznamenejte stav měkkých tkání, přítomné, chybějící a neprořezané zuby, celkový stav chrupu, stav ústní hygieny, přítomnost a umístění oprav a kazů, přítomnost a stáří protéz, stav parodontu, rentgenové snímky, testy citlivosti, studijní modely, biopsie, plán léčby, zásada, zmírnit bolest, vytrhnout zuby s beznadějnou prognózou, endodoncie, korunky, můstky, částečné protézy, poskytnout poradenství o prevenci, zlepšit stav parodontu, opravit zkažené zuby, faktory ovlivňující léčbu, komplikující lékařská anamnéza, úzkost pacienta, neschopnost či neochota udržovat adekvátní úroveň kontroly plaku, faktory týkající se nákladů, co si pacient může dovolit, dostupnost plánovaných postupů v rámci systému zdravotnické péče nebo systému pojištění, který kryje pacientovu léčbu.

Vocabulary

ability /ə'bɪl.ɪ.ti/ schopnost, dovednost

abnormal /æb'nɔː.məl/ abnormální

access /'æk.ses/ přístup

adequate /'æd.ə.kwət/ adekvátní, přiměřený

adherence /əd'hɪə.rənts/ dodržování

adjacent /ə'dʒeɪ.sənt/ přiléhající, vedlejší, hraničící

administer /əd'mɪn.ɪ.stəʳ/ podávat

administrative /əd'mɪn.ɪ.strə.tɪv/ administrativní

afford /ə'fɔːd/ dovolit si, poskytovat, přinášet

allergic /ə'lɜː.dʒɪk/ alergický, přecitlivělý

alter /'ɒl.təʳ/ změnit

anaesthesia /ˌæn.əs'θiː.zi.ə/ anestezie, znecitlivění

analgesic /ˌæn.əl'dʒiː.zɪk/ analgetikum

angina pectoris /æn,dʒaɪ.nə'pek.tə.rɪs/ angina pectoris

anxiety /æŋ'zaɪ.ə.ti/ úzkost

anxious /'æŋk.ʃəs/ úzkostný

appearance /ə'pɪə.rənts/ zjev, objevení (se), vzhled

application /ˌæp.lɪ'keɪ.ʃən/ aplikace, užití

apply /ə'plaɪ/ aplikovat

apprehensive /ˌæp.rɪ'hent.sɪv/ uvědomující si, mající obavy

arthritis /ɑː'θraɪ.tɪs/ artritida, zánět kloubů

assist /ə'sɪst/ asistovat, pomáhat

asthma /'æs.mə/ astma, dušnost

attack /ə'tæk/ záchvat

attend /ə'tend/ navštívit, ošetřovat

attitude /'æt.ɪ.tjuːd/ postoj

availability /ə,veɪ.lə'bɪl.ɪ.ti/ dostupnost

available /ə'veɪ.lə.bl̩/ dostupný, dosažitelný, k dispozici

become /bɪ'kʌm/ **better** /'bet.ər/ zlepšit se

become /bɪ'kʌm/ stát se

become /bɪ'kʌm/ **worse** /wɜːs/ zhoršit

bend /bend/ ohnout se

biopsy /'baɪ.ɒp.si/ biopsie

biting /baɪ.tɪŋ/ kousání

bleeding /'bliː.dɪŋ/ krvácení, krvácející

blood /blʌd/ **pressure** /'preʃ.ər/ krevní tlak

bridge /brɪdʒ/ můstek

bronchitis /brɒŋ'kaɪ.tɪs/ bronchitida, zánět průdušek

carious /'keər.i.əs/ kariézní, kazivý, zkažený zub

cause /kɔːz/ způsobit, zapříčinit

character /'kær.ɪk.təʳ/ charakter, vlastnosti

chest /tʃest/ hrudník

circumstance /ˈsɜː.kəm.stɑːnƭs/ okolnost

complementary /ˌkɒm.plɪˈmen.tər.i/ pomocný, doplňující

condition /kənˈdɪʃ.ən/ stav

consumption /kənˈsʌmp.ʃən/ spotřeba

continuous /kənˈtɪn.ju.əs/ nepřetržitý

cost /kɒst/ finanční náklady

covering /ˈkʌv.ər.ɪŋ/ pokrytí

cream /kriːm/ krém, pasta

crown /kraʊn/ korunka

cut /kʌt/ říznutí

dental /ˈden.tᵊl/ zubní

dentition /denˈtɪʃ.ən/ dentice

denture/ˈden.tʃə/ zubní protéza

depend /dɪˈpend/ záviset

dependant /dɪˈpen.dᵊnt/ závislá osoba, rodinný příslušník

desirable /dɪˈzaɪə.rə.bl̩/ vhodné, žádoucí

determine /dɪˈtɜː.mɪn/ určit, vymezit, rozhodnout

diabetes /ˌdaɪəˈbiː.tiːz/ úplavice cukrová, cukrovka

diagnosis /ˌdaɪ.əgˈnəʊ.sɪs/ diagnóza, určení

discomfort /dɪˈskʌmp.fət/ nepohoda

dull /dʌl/ tupý

duty /ˈdjuː.ti/ povinnost

education /ˌed.jʊˈkeɪ.ʃᵊn/ instruktáž, školení

endodontics /ˌen.dəˈdɒn.tɪks/ endodoncie, nauka o onemocnění zubní dřeně a kořenového kanálku

epilepsy /ˈep.ɪ.lep.si/ epilepsie

episode /ˈep.ɪ.səʊd/ příhoda, záchvat

essential /ɪˈsen.ƭʃᵊl/ podstatný, základní

establish /ɪˈstæb.lɪʃ/ ustanovit

exactly /ɪgˈzækƭ.li/ přesně, úplně, doslovně

examination /ɪgˌzæm.ɪˈneɪ.ʃᵊn/ vyšetření

examine /ɪgˈzæm.ɪn/ vyšetřovat

excessively /ekˈses.ɪv.li/ nadměrně, nepřiměřeně

expectant /ɪkˈspek.tᵊnt/ mother / ˈmʌð.ər/ nastávající matka

extract /ɪkˈstrækt/ vytrhnout

extraction /ɪkˈstræk.ʃən/ extrakce, vytržení

extraoral /ˌek.strəˈɔː.rəl/ mimo ústa

exudate /eks.juːdeɪt/ exsudát, zánětlivá tekutina, výpotek

fainting /feɪnt.ɪŋ/ mdloba

feel /fiːl/ cítit, hmatat

feeling /ˈfiː.lɪŋ/ pocit, hmat, mínění, nálada

fever /ˈfiː.vəʳ/ horečka

fissure /ˈfɪʃ.əʳ/ fisura, prasklina

fit /fɪt/ and well /wel/ v dobrém zdravotním stavu

fixed /fɪkst/ fixovaný, upevněný

food /fuːd/ jídlo, potrava

forwards /ˈfɔː.wədz/ směrem kupředu

frequently /ˈfriː.kwənt.li/ často

function /ˈfʌŋk.ʃᵊn/ funkce

generalized /ˈdʒen.ər.ə.laɪzd/ celkový, všeobecný

generally /ˈdʒen.ə r.əl.i/ obecně

halitosis /ˌhæl.ɪˈtəʊ.sɪs/ halitóza, páchnoucí dech

health /helθ/ care /keəʳ/ system /ˈsɪs. təm/ systém zdravotní péče

healthy /ˈhel.θi/ zdravý

heart /hɑːt/ attack /əˈtæk/ srdeční záchvat

hepatitis /ˌhep.əˈtaɪ.tɪs/ hepatitis, zánět jater

history /ˈhɪs.tᵊr.i/ anamnéza

hopeless /ˈhəʊ.pləs/ beznadějný

hygienist /haɪˈdʒiː.nɪst/ hygienista

importance /ɪmˈpɔː.tənƭs/ důležitost

improve /ɪmˈpruːv/ zlepšit, zdokonalit

inability /ˌɪn.əˈbɪl.ɪ.ti/ neschopnost, nezpůsobilost

individual /ˌɪn.dɪˈvɪd.ju.əl/ jednotlivec

infiltration /ˌɪn.fɪlˈtreɪ.ʃ°n/ infilfrace

influence /ˈɪn.flu.ənts/ ovlivnit

initiate /ɪˈnɪʃ.i.eɪt/ iniciovat, zahájit, uvést

insurance /ɪnˈʃɔː.rənts/ pojištění, pojistka

intermittent /ˌɪn.təˈmɪt.ənt/ občasný, vracející se

intraoral /ɪn.trəˈɔː.rəl/ uvnitř úst

investigation /ɪnˌves.tɪˈgeɪ.ʃ°n/ vyšetření

involve /ɪnˈvɒlv/ zahrnovat, vyžadovat

irregular /ɪˈreg.jə.ləʳ/ nepravidelný

jaundice /ˈdʒɔːn.dɪs/ žloutenka

knowledge /ˈnɒl.ɪdʒ/ znalost, vědomosti

lesion /ˈliː.ʒ°n/ zranění, porucha, postižené místo

lip /lɪp/ **competence** /ˈkɒm.pɪ.tənts/ celistvost rtu

location /ləʊˈkeɪ.ʃən/ lokace, umístění

look /lʊk/ **for** /fɔːʳ/ pátrat po

loss /lɒs/ ztráta

lymph /lɪmpf/ **node** /nəʊd/ lymfatická uzlina

maintain /meɪnˈteɪn/ udržet, zachovat

maintenance /ˈmeɪn.tɪ.nənts/ udržování

management /ˈmæn.ɪdʒ.mənt/ péče, vedení, ředitelství

marital /ˈmær.ɪ.t°l/ **circumstance** /ˈsɜː.kəm.staːnts/ manželská situace

mastication /ˌmæs.tɪˈkeɪ.ʃ°n/ mastikace, žvýkání

medical /ˈmed.ɪ.k°l/ lékařský

medicine /ˈmed.ɪ.sən/ lék

mild /maɪld/ slabý, mírný

missing /ˈmɪs.ɪŋ/ chybějící

model /ˈmɒd.°l/ model

murmur /ˈmɜː.məʳ/ šelest

muscle /ˈmʌs.l̩/ sval, svalový

nature /ˈneɪ.tʃəʳ/ povaha

notice /ˈnəʊ.tɪs/ zaznamenat

nurse /nɜːs/ zdravotní sestra, ošetřovatelka

obtain /əbˈteɪn/ obdržet

occupation /ˌɒk.jʊˈpeɪ.ʃən/ zaměstnání, povolání, obsazení

ointment /ˈɔɪnt.mənt/ mazání, mast

over /ˈəʊ.vəʳ/ **the counter** /ˈkaʊn.təʳ/ přes pult, bez receptu lékaře

palpate /ˈpæl.peɪt/ prohmatávat

partial /ˈpaː.ʃ°l/ **dentures** /ˈden.tʃəz/ částečné protézy

periodontal /ˌper.ɪ.əˈdɒn.tl̩/ periodontální

pharmacy /ˈfaː.mə.si/ lékárna, lékárnický

planning /ˈplæn.ɪŋ/ plánování

polish /ˈpɒl.ɪʃ/ leštit

powder /ˈpaʊ.dəʳ/ prášek, pudr, posypat

prescription /prɪˈskrɪp.ʃ°n/ předpis

present /ˈprez.°nt/ přítomný

preventive /prɪˈven.tɪv/ ochranný, předběžný, ochranné opatření

previous /ˈpriː.vi.əs/ předchozí, předešlý

primary /ˈpraɪ.mə.ri/ primární, začáteční

prime /praɪm/ prvotní, hlavní

principle /ˈprɪn.sɪ.pl̩/ zásada, metoda, postup

prognosis /prɒgˈnəʊ.sɪs/ prognóza

prone /prəʊn/ náchylný, šikmý, ležící na břiše

prophylactic /ˌprɒf.ɪˈlæk.tɪk/ profylaktický, preventivní

propose /prəˈpəʊz/ navrhnout, nabídnout

prosthesis /ˈprɒs.θiː.sɪs/ (pl.
prostheses) protézy
purpose /ˈpɜː.pəs/ účel, záměr, mít v
úmyslu
radiation /ˌreɪ.diˈeɪ.ʃᵊn/ záření,
ozařovací, emise
radiograph /reɪ.di.ə.grɑːf/
rentgenovat, rentgenový snímek
recall /rɪˈkɔːl/ vzpomenout, znovu
zavolat, přivést k vědomí
receive /rɪˈsiːv/ obdržet
refer /rɪˈfɜːr/ uvést, uvádět
regular /ˈreg.jʊ.ləʳ/ pravidelný
related /rɪˈleɪ.tɪd/ vztahující se k,
spojený
relaxed /rɪˈlækst/ uvolněný,
relaxovaný
relevant /ˈrel.ə.vᵊnt/ relevantní,
příslušný
relieve /rɪˈliːv/ pain /peɪn/ ulevit bolesti
removable /rɪˈmuː.və.bl̩/ pohyblivý
replacement /rɪˈpleɪs.mənt/
nahrazení, výměna (vadné součásti),
vrácení
restoration/ˌres.tᵊrˈeɪ.ʃᵊn/ obnovení,
zotavení, uzdravení
restore /rɪˈstɔːʳ/ obnovit, uzdravit,
opravit
rheumatic /ruːˈmæt.ɪk/ fever /ˈfiː.vəʳ/
revmatická horečka
routinely /ruːˈtiːn.li/ rutinně, běžně
same /seɪm/ stejný
scale /skeɪl/ odstraňovat zubní kámen
schedule /ˈʃed.juːl/ rozvrh,
naplánovat, tabulka, cedule
scheme /skiːm/ nákres, plán, projekt,
program
sealant /ˈsiː.lənt/ pečetidlo
sensitivity /ˌsenᵗ.sɪˈtɪv.ɪ.ti/ senzitivita,
citlivost, vnímavost
severity /sɪˈver.ɪ.ti/ vážnost, útrapy,
potíže

sharp /ʃɑːp/ ostrý
shooting /ˈʃuː.tɪŋ/ vystřelující
simple /ˈsɪm.pl̩/ jednoduchý
site /saɪt/ místo
skeletal /ˈskel.ɪ.tᵊl/ pattern /ˈpæt.ən/
kosterní typ
sleep /sliːp/ loss /lɒs/ nespavost
smoking /ˈsməʊ.kɪŋ/ kouření
spread /spred/ rozšířit
state /steɪt/ stav
status /ˈsteɪ.təs/ status (stav), životní
úroveň, společenské postavení
step /step/ krok
study /ˈstʌd.i/ studijní
suffer /ˈsʌf.əʳ/ trpět, utrpět
surface /ˈsɜː.fɪs/ povrch
surgeon /ˈsɜː.dʒᵊn/ chirurg
swelling /ˈswel.ɪŋ/ otok, edém
tablet /ˈtæb.lət/ tabletka
take /teɪk/ brát
temporomandibular /ˌtem.
pər.ə.mænˈdɪ.bjʊ.ləʳ/ joint /dʒɔɪnt/
temporo-mandibulární kloub
therapist /ˈθer.ə.pɪst/ terapeut
threshold /ˈθreʃ.h aʊld/ práh, mez
citlivosti
throb /θrɒb/ tepat
tooth /tuːθ/ extraction /ɪkˈstræk.ʃən/
vytrhnutí zubu
treatment /ˈtriːt.mənt/ ošetření,
zacházení (s), léčebný postup,
pohoštění
undertake /ˌʌn.dəˈteɪk/ podniknout
unerupted /ʌn.ɪrˈʌp.tᵊd/ neprořezaný
unwillingness /ʌnˈwɪl.ɪŋ.nəs/
neochota
update /ʌpˈdeɪt/ aktualizovat
valve /vælv/ chlopeň
worse /wɜːs/ horší
worth /wɜːθ/ mít cenu, za něco stát
written /ˈrɪt.ᵊn/ psaný

Unit 3

Text 1

Advanced Imaging Techniques
Digital imaging uses conventional
X-ray machines, but the film
is replaced by either a sensor
containing a charged couple device
or a photostimulable phosphor plate.
The **image receptors convert the
information received into digital
form**. The digital data is stored on a
computer and **converted into a grey
scale image** which is **displayed** on a
monitor.

Conventional Tomography
Cross-sectional slices of the maxilla
and mandible are produced using
conventional tomography. The
machines look similar to panoramic
units but have a greater range of
movement, allowing slices to be
made through the jaws **in almost any
position**. Used for **implant planning**
and for assessing the buccolingual
extension of **pathology** and the
position of impacted teeth.

Computer Tomography (CT)
An X-ray tube passes in a circle around
the body and a series of detectors
measure the blocking of the beam
at each point. A computer then gives
a value to each unit of tissue within
that slice, and from this it constructs
a picture of what structures must lie
within that section of the body. CT
shows **both soft tissues and bone** but
does not demonstrate soft-tissue lesions
as well as magnetic resonance imaging.
It is particularly useful for **assessing
serious midfacial trauma or disease
involving bone**.

Magnetic Resonance Imaging (MRI)
This involves placing the patient
**into a strong magnetic field and
then applying a pulse of radio
waves**. The frequency of these
waves is chosen specifically so that
the abundant **hydrogen protons in
body fluid take up energy from
the signal**. The protons then **emit a
radio signal**, which is picked up and
processed by a computer. Several
different images of each slice through
the patient are produced. MRI gives

good soft-tissue detail and is excellent for **tumour staging** and for the **assessment of intracranial disease**. MRI is not good for imaging bone and is **contraindicated in patients with ferromagnetic surgical clips, pacemakers, cochlear implants, and in the first three months of pregnancy**.

Ultrasonography

This technique involves scanning the patient with a transducer that emits **high-frequency sound waves** and then **detects the waves reflected from various interfaces** within the tissue. The time taken for the waves to be reflected back allows the machine to **calculate the depth of the structures** that reflect them, and from this a **picture is created**. Ultrasound is excellent for the assessment of **superficial soft-tissue structures, such as salivary glands, lymph nodes, and the thyroid**.

Exercise 1

Describe the main principles and the use of:

conventional tomography
computer tomography (CT)
magnetic resonance imaging (MRI)
ultrasonography

Translation 1

Plánování implantátů, zhodnocení rozsahu patologie tváří a jazyka, pokročilé techniky zobrazování, digitální zobrazování, konvenční rentgenové přístroje, senzor, fosforová destička citlivá na světlo, receptory obrazu, převést získanou informaci do digitální formy, konvenční tomografie, tenké plátky znázorněné na průřezu, digitální údaje uložené v počítači, škálový obraz ukazující se na monitoru, přístroje vypadají podobně jako panoramatické jednotky, mají větší rozsah pohybu, umožňují vytvářet průřezy čelistmi téměř v jakékoli poloze, počítačová tomografie, zhodnocení závažného traumatu střední části obličeje nebo onemocnění zahrnujícího kost, trubice rentgenu prochází v kruhu kolem těla, řada detektorů měří v každém bodu blokování paprsku, CT ukazuje jak měkké tkáně tak kost, zobrazování pomocí magnetické resonance, umístit pacienta do silného magnetického pole, použít ráz radiových vln, vybrat frekvenci, protony vodíku v tělesné tekutině převezmou energii ze signálu, protony vydávají radiový signál, který je zachycen a zpracován počítačem, předvedení tumoru, zhodnocení nitrolebečního onemocnění, kontraindikován u pacientů s feromagnetickými chirurgickými svorkami, srdečními stimulátory, kochleárními implantáty a v prvních třech měsících těhotenství, zobrazování pomocí ultrazvuku, skenování pacienta čidlem, které vydává vysokofrekvenční zvukové vlny, zjišťuje vlny odražené od různých styčných ploch uvnitř tkání, spočítat hloubku částí a vytvořit obraz, povrchové měkké části jako slinné žlázy, lymfatické uzliny a štítná žláza.

Vocabulary

abundant /əˈbʌn.dənt/ početný, hojný
any /ˈen.i/ libovolný
apex /ˈeɪ.peks/ **(pl. apices)** vrchol, hrot

apply /əˈplaɪ/ aplikovat

around /əˈraʊnd/ okolo

block /blɒk/ blokovat

blur /blɜːr/ znejasnit

blurred /blɜːd/ rozmazaný

body /ˈbɒd.i/ fluid /ˈfluː.ɪd/ tělní tekutina

buccolingual /ˌbʌk.əˈlɪŋ.gwəl/ bukolingvální, týkající se tváří a jazyka

calculate /ˈkæl.kjʊ.leɪt/ počítat, zamýšlet

charge /tʃɑːdʒ/ účtovat si

check /tʃek/ kontrolovat, zkontrolovat, kontrola

choclear /kɒk.lɪ.ə/ kochleární, hlemýžďovitý

circle /ˈsɜː.kl̩/ kruh

clip /klɪp/ svorka, ruční nůžky

computer /kəmˈpjuː.təʳ/ tomography /təˈmɒ.grə.fɪ/ počítačová tomografie

contraindicate /ˌkɒn.trə.ˈɪn.dɪ.keɪt/ kontraindikovat

conventional /kənˈven.ʃən.əl/ tradiční

convert /kənˈvɜːt/ přeměnit

couple /ˈkʌp.l̩/ dvojice, spojený, připojit

create /kriˈeɪt/ vytvořit

cross-section /ˌkrɒsˈsek.ʃən/ příčný řez, průřez

demonstrate /ˈdem.ən.streɪt/ ukázat, dokázat

depth /depθ/ hloubka, tloušťka

detector /dɪˈtek.təʳ/ snímač, čidlo, detekční přístroj

device /dɪˈvaɪs/ zařízení, prostředek

digital /ˈdɪdʒ.ɪ.təl/ digitální

emit /ɪˈmɪt/ vydávat, vysílat

energy /ˈen.ə.dʒi/ energie, schopnost

excellent /ˈek.səl.ənt/ vynikající

ferromagnetic /ˌfer.ə.mægˈnet.ɪk/ feromagnetický

fluid /ˈfluː.ɪd/ tekutina

frequency /ˈfriː.kwənt.si/ časté opakování, četnost (výskytu jevu v čase)

grey /greɪ/ šedivý

high-/haɪ/ frequency /ˈfriː.kwənt.si/ vysokofrekvenční

hydrogen /ˈhaɪ.drɪ.dʒən/ vodík

image /ˈɪm.ɪdʒ/ zobrazení

imaging /ɪˈmɪdʒ.ɪŋ/ zobrazování

implant /ɪmˈplɑːnt/ implantát

investigation /ɪnˌves.tɪˈgeɪ.ʃən/ vyšetřování

lymph /lɪmpf/ node /nəʊd/ lymfatická uzlina

magnetic /mægˈnet.ɪk/ field /fiːld/ magnetické pole

magnetic /mægˈnet.ɪk/ resonance /ˈrez.ən.ənts/ imaging /ɪˈmɪdʒ.ɪŋ/ zobrazování magnetickou rezonancí

movement /ˈmuːv.mənt/ pohyb

pacemaker /ˈpeɪsˌmeɪ.kəʳ/ srdeční stimulátor

panoramic /ˌpæn.ərˈæm.ɪk/ celkový, panoramatický

pass /pɑːs/ projít, překonat

phosphor /ˈfɒs.fəʳ/ luminofor

photo /ˈfəʊ.təʊ/ foto

photostimulable /ˈfəʊ.təʊ.ˈstɪm.jʊ.lə.bl̩/ reagující na světlo

pick /pɪk/ up /ʌp/ zvednout

planning /ˈplæn.ɪŋ/ plánování

plate /pleɪt/ destička

processed /ˈprəʊ.sest/ zpracovaný

proton /ˈprəʊ.tɒn/ proton

pulse /pʌls/ impulz

radio /ˈreɪ.di.əʊ/ rádio-

range /reɪndʒ/ rozsah

receptor /rɪˈsep.təʳ/ příjemce, čidlo

reflect /rɪˈflekt/ odrážet, reflektovat

salivary /səˈlaɪ.vər.i/ gland /glænd/ slinná žláza

scale /skeɪl/ škála (stupnice)

scan /skæn/ skenovat, postupně snímat (po řádcích)

section /ˈsek.ʃ°n/ část, úsek

sensor /ˈsent.sə^r/ snímač

series /ˈsɪə.riːz/ sada, sled, skupina

serious /ˈsɪə.ri.əs/ opravdový (vážný)

slice /slaɪs/ seškrábnout, krájet na plátky

soft /sɒft/ tissue /ˈtɪʃ.uː/, /ˈtɪs.juː/ měkká tkáň

sound /saʊnd/ zvuk

staging /ˈsteɪ.dʒɪŋ/ představení, rozdělování do stupňů

strong /strɒŋ/ silný (mocný), silně

superficial /ˌsuː.pəˈfɪʃ.°l/ povrchový

surgical /ˈsɜː.dʒɪ.k°l/ chirurgický

take /teɪk/ up /ʌp/ zvednout, nabrat, nasát, upevnit

transducer /trænzˈdjuː.sə^r/ snímač, čidlo

tumour /ˈtjuː.mə^r/ tumor, nádor

ultrasonography /ˌʌl.trəˈsɒn.ˈnɒg.rə.fi/ nauka o ultrazvuku

ultrasound /ˈʌl.trə.saʊnd/ ultrazvukový, sonogram

wave /weɪv/ vlna

Unit 4

Psychological Aspects of Dental Care

Introduction. Social and Psychological Influences on Dental Care. Communication.

Text 1

Introduction

Above all else the practice of dentistry involves **working with people,** and an understanding of how **social and psychological factors** impact on oral health is important. The aetiology of many dental diseases is influenced greatly by **behavioural and lifestyle** factors. An appreciation of psychological factors enables the practitioner to:

- **communicate** more effectively
- **understand** causes of **anxiety**
- understand the **nature of pain**
- **motivate patients** and influence behaviour change

Social and Psychological Influences on Dental Care

Oral health has been defined as a standard of **health of the oral and related tissues** which enables an individual to eat, speak, and socialise without active disease, discomfort, or embarrassment and which contributes to general well-being.

Not everyone who has disease will seek professional care, and so there is a difference between the need for dental treatment and the demand for it.

The **decision to attend a dentist** will be influenced by many factors:

- **value** placed on **oral health** by patient
- **perceived ability to influence** oral health
- worsening of symptoms – patients may accept intermittent pain and seek care only when **pain becomes constant or intolerable**
- **perceived seriousness** of a disease may encourage or discourage attendance
- **access to dentist** – influenced by location of the office and availability of public transport
- disruption of daily life – attendance may involve having to **take time off work, arrange a babysitter**, etc.
- **financial cost** may be a barrier
- advice from family and friends can have **positive or negative influences**
- in common with health in general, oral health is influenced markedly by **social class** and is related to **income, education, living, and working conditions**

Communication

Successful dental practice requires the development of a **relationship between dentist and patient.** The ability to communicate effectively is an essential skill and is necessary when:

- **eliciting a history** from a patient
- **explaining proposed treatment**
- managing anxious patients— **reducing anxiety** requires skilled communication
- **encouraging behaviour change**

Factors inhibiting good communication include:

- difference in **social class** between dentist and patient
- **priorities** of the clinician may differ from those of the patient
- **supine dentistry** places the patient in a passive position
- **technical language** is not understood by patients
- patients may have their own concept of a particular problem and be **reluctant to accept** the correct explanation
- **time pressures** may lead to information being presented too quickly for the patient to understand
- **anxiety** hinders ability to absorb information

Nonverbal communication is also very important.

This applies to the **postures, gestures, and expressions** of the clinician but also to the patient's reaction. It is the dentist's responsibility to communicate effectively with members of the practice staff as well (dental nurse, hygienist, receptionist, and technician).

Exercise 1

1. How can good appreciation of psychological factors help the practitioner?
2. Which factors influence the decision to attend a dentist?
3. When is effective communication necessary?

Translation 1

Praxe zubního lékařství zahrnuje práci s lidmi, etiologie je ovlivněna chováním a životním stylem, rozumět příčinám úzkosti, pochopit povahu bolesti, motivovat pacienty a ovlivnit změnu chování, sociální a psychologické vlivy na dentální péči, zdraví úst, normální stav tkání úst a okolních tkání, umožňuje jedinci jíst, mluvit a společensky žít, nemoc, nepohoda či překážka, přispívat k celkovému pocitu zdraví, rozhodnutí navštívit zubního lékaře, možnost zdraví úst ovlivnit, zhoršení symptomů, akceptovat občasnou bolest, vyhledávat péči až když se bolest stane stálou nebo nesnesitelnou, předpokládaná závažnost onemocnění, povzbudit nebo odradit od návštěvy, umístění ordinace, dostupnost veřejné dopravy, vzít si volno z práce, zařídit hlídání dítěte, finanční náklady mohou být překážkou, příjmy, vzdělání, životní a pracovní podmínky, schopnost efektivně komunikovat, získávání anamnézy pacienta, vysvětlování navrhované léčby, zvládání úzkostných pacientů, povzbuzení ke změně chování, priority se mohou lišit, pacienti nerozumí technickým výrazům, časová tíseň, informace předávané příliš rychle, úzkost brání schopnosti informace vstřebat, postoje, gestikulace a výraz lékaře, reakce pacienta, komunikovat efektivně se členy personálu, zubní zdravotní sestra, hygienista, recepční, technik.

Vocabulary

ability /ə'bɪl.ɪ.ti/ schopnost, dovednost

above /ə'bʌv/ **all** /ɔːl/ především

absorb /əb'zɔːb/ vstřebat

accept /ək'sept/ akceptovat, přijmout, připustit

advice /'æd.vɜːs/ rada, oznámení

aetiology /ˌiː.ti'ɒl.ə.dʒi/ etiologie, nauka o původu a příčinách

anxiety /æŋ'zaɪ.ə.ti/ úzkost

anxious /'æŋk.ʃəs/ úzkostný

appreciation /əˌpriː.ʃi'eɪ.ʃən/ ocenění, pochvala, zhodnocení

attend /ə'tend/ navštěvovat, ošetřovat (nemocné), mít službu

attendance /ə'ten.dənts/ návštěvnost

availability /əˌveɪ.lə'bɪl.ɪ.ti/ dostupnost, vhodnost, vybavenost

babysitter /'beɪ.bi.sɪt.ər/ pečovatelka (k dítěti)

barrier /'bær.i.ər/ bariéra, zábrana, překážka

behaviour /bɪ'heɪ.vjər/ chování, jednání, způsob práce

behavioural /bɪ'heɪ.vjə.rəl/ týkající se chování

cause /kɔːz/ příčina

change /tʃeɪndʒ/ změna

clinician /klɪ'nɪʃ.ən/ klinický lékař

communicate /kə'mjuː.nɪ.keɪt/ komunikovat

concept /'kɒn.sept/ představa

condition /kən'dɪʃ.ən/ podmínka

constant /'kɒn.stənt/ stálý

contribute /kən'trɪb.juːt/ přispívat

correct /kə'rekt/ správný, přesný

cost /kɒst/ finanční náklady

decision /dɪ'sɪʒ.ən/ rozhodnutí, nález

demand /dɪ'mɑːnd/ poptávka

dentist /'den.tɪst/ zubní lékař

dentistry /'den.tɪ.stri/ zubní lékařství

differ /'dɪf.ər/ lišit se, neshodovat se, nesouhlasit

difference /'dɪf.ər.ənts/ rozdílnost

discomfort /dɪ'skʌmp.fət/ nepohodlí, nevolnost, obtěžovat

discourage /dɪ'skʌr.ɪdʒ/ odradit

disease /dɪ'ziːz/ onemocnění

disruption /dɪs'rʌp.ʃən/ přerušení, porucha, protržení

education /ˌed.jʊ'keɪ.ʃən/ vzdělání

effectively /ɪ'fek.tɪv.li/ účinně

elicit /ɪ'lɪs.ɪt/ vyžadovat, vyvolat (reakci), získat, dosáhnout

embarrassment /ɪm'bær.ə.smənt/ rozpaky, nedostatek (vada), potíže

enable /ɪ'neɪ.bl̩/ umožnit, dát možnost, uzpůsobit

encourage /ɪn'kʌr.ɪdʒ/ povzbuzovat, dodat odvahu, doporučovat

essential /ɪ'sen.tʃəl/ základní, podstatná věc, výtažkový

explanation /ˌek.splə'neɪ.ʃən/ vysvětlení

expression /ɪk'spreʃ.ən/ výraz tváře, vyjádření, vytlačení

general /'dʒen.ər.əl/ celkový

gesture /'dʒes.tʃər/ gesto, posuněk, ukázat

greatly /'greɪt.li/ velmi, z velké části

hinder /'hɪn.dər/ bránit, být překážkou, zadní

history /'hɪs.tər.i/ anamnéza

hygienist /haɪ'dʒiː.nɪst/ hygienista

impact /'ɪm.pækt/ vliv, výsledek, dopadat, natlačit

income /'ɪn.kʌm/ příjem

influence /'ɪn.flu.ənts/ vliv, ovlivňovat, působit

inhibit /ɪnˈhɪb.ɪt/ inhibovat, bránit (překážet), zakázat, zpomalovat

intermittent /ˌɪn.təˈmɪt.ənt/ přerušovaný, nestálý

intolerable /ɪnˈtɒl.ər.ə.bl̩/ netolerovatelný, nesnesitelný, nesnášenlivý

introduction /ˌɪn.trəˈdʌk.ʃən/ úvod, zavedení

lifestyle /ˈlaɪf.staɪl/ životní styl

limit /ˈlɪm.ɪt/ limit, vymezit, krajní hranice

living /ˈlɪv.ɪŋ/ životní, žijící

location /ləʊˈkeɪ.ʃən/ lokace, umístění, poloha

manage /ˈmæn.ɪdʒ/ zvládnout, řídit

markedly /ˈmɑː.kɪd.li/ značně, zjevně, nápadně

marrow /ˈmær.əʊ/ kostní dřeň

motivate /ˈməʊ.tɪ.veɪt/ motivovat

nature /ˈneɪ.tʃər/ povaha, přirozená vlastnost, charakter

need /niːd/ potřeba

negative/ˈneg.ə.tɪv/ negativní

nonverbal /ˌnɒnˈvɜː.bəl/ neverbální, mimoslovní

nurse /nɜːs/ zdravotní sestra, ošetřovat, kojit

pain /peɪn/ bolest, námaha

particular /pəˈtɪk.jʊ.lər/ zvláštní

perceive /pəˈsiːv/ vnímat, uvědomit si, pochopit

positive /ˈpɒz.ə.tɪv/ pozitivní

posture /ˈpɒs.tʃər/ pozice, postoj

practitioner /prækˈtɪʃ.ən.ər/ praktický lékař

pressure /ˈpreʃ.ər/ tlak

priority /praɪˈɒr.ɪ.ti/ prvenství, přednost, důležitá věc

receptionist /rɪˈsep.ʃən.ɪst/ recepční

related /rɪˈleɪ.tɪd/ vztahující se k

relationship /rɪˈleɪ.ʃən.ʃɪp/ souvislost (vztah), příbuznost, vzájemný poměr

reluctant /rɪˈlʌk.tənt/ neochotný, váhavý

require /rɪˈkwaɪər/ vyžadovat

responsibility /rɪˌspɒn.sɪˈbɪl.ɪ.ti/ zodpovědnost, spolehlivost

seek /siːk/ vyhledávat, požadovat, pátrat

seriousness /ˈsɪə.ri.ə.snəs/ vážnost, závažnost, nebezpečnost

skill /skɪl/ schopnost, dovednost

socialise /ˈsəʊ.ʃəl.aɪz/ socializovat, stýkat se (společensky)

standard /ˈstæn.dəd/ úroveň

supine /ˈsuː.paɪn/ ležící naznak, ležící tváří vzhůru, klidný

take /teɪk/ time /taɪm/ využít času

technical /ˈtek.nɪ.kəl/ technický

technician /tekˈnɪʃ.ən/ technik

time /taɪm/ off /ɒf/ work /wɜːk/ volno z práce

tissue /ˈtɪʃ.uː/, /ˈtɪs.juː/ tkáň

value /ˈvæl.juː/ cena, hodnota, ohodnotit, význam

well-being /ˌwelˈbiː.ɪŋ/ dobré zdraví

worsen /ˈwɜː.sən/ zhoršit se, poškodit, pokazit se

Unit 5

Paediatric Dentistry

Behaviour Change. Maintaining Change, Relapse. Anxiety. Pain. Organising Treatment for Children. Managing Behaviour in Children. Traumatic Injuries. Maintenance of the Operating Field. Children with Special Needs.

Text 1

Behaviour Change

Before behaviour can be changed, patients must:

- **want** to change
- **believe** they **can change**
- believe change will have the **desired effect**
- have the **knowledge and skills** to permit change

However, simply providing information (e.g. brush your teeth twice daily) is frequently insufficient. In providing information it is necessary to ask:

- Do the patients **know how to brush**?
- **How frequently** do they brush?

Then **provide an explanation** of why change is necessary. Written information (**a leaflet**) may be helpful, but information overload should be avoided. Changes should be introduced gradually. **Targets** for behaviour change should be **achievable, realistic, important to the patient, measurable, positive, time related, and specific**.

Maintaining Change, Relapse

Maintenance of behaviour change is difficult. The ultimate aim is to **integrate positive behaviour into patient's everyday lifestyles**. Behaviour change is cyclical in nature with patients frequently experiencing **relapses and setbacks** before achieving their goal.

Anxiety

There are many possible causes of anxiety. **Principal factors** include **fear of pain, uncertainty, previous experience, and preparedness**. Questionnaires are available which can be used to measure anxiety.

Be honest and **do not make unrealistic promises**. Explain that the procedure may be slightly uncomfortable. If a patient looks anxious, ask what is worrying them and take time to discuss and explain.

Factors which may help alleviate anxiety include:

- friendly and understanding **attitude of the dental team**

- welcoming **environment**
- communication during treatment
  - **warn patients** before **reclining chair, blowing air** from 3-in-1 syringe, etc.
- decrease vulnerability – instructions such as 'raise your hand if you want me to stop' help **patients feel they have some control**

Pain

There is a difference between **pain sensation and pain behaviour.** Anxious patients are much more likely to experience pain, and in turn **pain is likely to increase anxiety.** Pain may be experienced **during treatment or as a consequence** of treatment.

Pain is a common symptom of dental disease. Pain leads many patients to seek care. Fear of pain may prevent patients from seeking treatment. Pain is influenced by higher centres in the CNS. Pain is a highly personal experience. Reaction to pain is influenced by **cultural and emotional factors.**

Psychological approaches to pain control

Techniques available include:

- distraction by **shifting the patient's attention**
- provision of **audiotapes, pictures on the ceiling** of the surgery
- effective **communication**
- in some patients **hypnosis** can be useful

Exercise 1

1. Describe the aims of behavioural change, maintaining the change, relapse.
2. Talk about possible causes of anxiety and factors which may help to alleviate it.
3. Characterise pain and psychological approaches to pain control.

Translation 1

Změna chování, věřit, že změna bude mít žádaný účinek, mít znalosti a dovednosti dovolující změnu, poskytnutí informace je často nedostatečné.

Vědí pacienti jak zuby čistit? Jak často si je čistí?, písemné pokyny (letáček) mohou být užitečné, vyhnout se přemíře informací, cíle změny chování by měly být: dosažitelné, realistické, pro pacienta důležité, měřitelné, pozitivní, časově vymezené, přesně stanovené, udržení změny, opětné zhoršení, konečným cílem je integrovat pozitivní chování do pacientova každodenního životního stylu, příčiny úzkosti, strach z bolesti, nejistota, předchozí zkušenosti, připravenost, zmírnit úzkost, přátelský a chápavý postoj, příjemné prostředí, varujte pacienta než skloníte křeslo, pustíte vzduch ze stříkačky,"zvedněte ruku pokud si budete přát, abych přestal", procedura možná bude trochu nepříjemná, věnujte dost času rozhovoru a vysvětlování, bolest je běžným symptomem, vede pacienty k vyhledání péče, strach z bolesti může zabránit pacientům vyhledat ošetření, reakce na bolest je ovlivněna kulturními a emočními faktory, zvládnutí bolesti, rozptýlení, odvrácení pacientovy pozornosti, zvukové nahrávky, obrázky na stropě účinná komunikace, u některých pacientů může být užitečná hypnóza.

Text 2
Organising Treatment for Children
A planned atraumatic introduction is necessary to provide children with the appropriate skills to cope with dental treatment:

- provide **a positive introduction** to dentistry
- provide child with the **skills necessary to accept dental treatment**
- institute good **preventive practice**
- provide any necessary **restorative care**

Practical points:
- for maximum benefit children **should spit, not rinse, after brushing**
- under 7 years, children **lack sufficient manual dexterity** to brush their teeth effectively
- young children should **be supervised** when brushing to ensure effective brushing and limit amount of toothpaste consumed
- keep preventive **messages simple**

Remember:
- **attention span** is short, plan treatment accordingly
- call child by his or her **correct name**
- children are very sensitive to environment and **nonverbal communication,** so smile!
- child-friendly environment is important (**posters, toys,** etc.)
- ensure **parents understand** their role in the process

Managing Behaviour in Children
The child's attitude and behaviour will be influenced by many factors:
- **age, maturity, personality**
- **attitude of parents**
- **previous medical experience**
- previous **dental experience**
- **attitude of dental staff**
- **environs** of surgery
- whether (s)he has a **dental problem**

Tell-show-do is one of the simplest methods.
Basic **principles:**
- tell child what you are going to do, use simple language
- demonstrate
- then do

Modelling
The child learns by watching others. It is important that the patient can relate to and **identify with the model.** Dental procedures require complex behaviours that need to be learned. **Stickers, badges, and praise** act as positive reinforcers. Behaviour management techniques may not always work with extremely anxious patients.

Exercise 2
1. How would you organise treatment for children?
2. Which are the factors influencing the child's attitude and behaviour?
3. Explain tell -show-do method and modelling.

Translation 2
Dětské zubní lékařství, netraumatizující přijetí, dovednosti nezbytné pro přijetí zubního ošetření, zavést dobrou prevenci, poskytnout nutnou opravnou

péči, maximální účinek, po čistění vyplivnout, nikoli vypláchnout, postrádat dostatečnou manuální zručnost, malé děti by měly být pod dohledem, omezit množství spolknuté pasty, jednoduché pokyny pro prevenci, rozsah pozornosti je malý, děti jsou velmi citlivé na prostředí a neverbální komunikaci, oslovujte dítě jeho správným jménem, usmívejte se, dětem přátelské prostředí, plakáty, hračky, postoje dítěte a jeho chování jsou ovlivněny mnoha faktory, věk, zralost, osobnost, ovládání chování u dětí, praktické otázky, předchozí zkušenost s lékaři, se zubními lékaři, přístup personálu, prostředí ordinace, přístup rodičů, řekněte dítěti co se chystáte udělat, předveďte, potom proveďte, vytváření vzorů – dítě se učí pozorováním ostatních, nálepky, odznaky a pochvala působí pozitivní posílení.

Text 3

Traumatic Injuries

Trauma to children's teeth is a common occurrence and one of the true emergencies likely to present in dental practice. In any patient presenting with **dental trauma**, the **possibility of more serious underlying injury** (e.g. **concussion**) should be considered. Aetiology is related to the age; **common causes** include:

- toddlers – **trips and falls**
- older children – **bicycle accidents**
- teenagers – **contact sports, fights, alcohol**

Classification of trauma

- **fractures** (enamel, dentine, pulp, root)
- **concussion** (tooth traumatised but not loosened)
- **subluxation** (tooth loosened in the pocket but not displaced)
- **extrusion** (tooth displaced in occlusal direction)
- **intrusion** (tooth displaced apically into socket)
- **lateral displacement** (tooth pushed laterally, buccally, or palatally)
- **avulsion** (tooth totally displaced from the socket)

Maintenance of the Operating Field

Adequate **isolation of the tooth** during the operative procedures can be achieved by **retractors, saliva ejectors**, high- and low-volume **aspirators, cotton-wool rolls, absorbent pads**, and **rubber dam**.

Objectives of treatment

Immediate

- **reassurance** of patient and parent
- **relieve of pain**
- **protection of pulp**
- **suture** of soft tissue lacerations
- **stabilisation** of fractured or mobile teeth

Intermediate

- **pulp** therapy
- semipermanent **restoration**

Long-term

- **crown**
- **replacement** of lost teeth
- **orthodontic** therapy
- removable/fixed **prosthodontics**

Children with Special Needs

Special needs describe a wide range of conditions which result in patients requiring **extra attention or special facilities** in order to attain and maintain oral health. Various definitions of

handicap and disability have been described. They can be usefully classified as:

- **learning disability** – can be **congenital** (Down's syndrome) or **acquired** (e.g. as a result of **brain damage** pre-, peri-, or postnatally)
- **physical** disability – includes cerebral palsy, spina bifida, muscular dystrophy
- **sensory** disability – **blindness, deafness**
- **medically compromised** – patients with underlying medical condition, e.g. cardiac disorders, haemophilia

Prevention should include:

- **dietary advice** to parents
- **fluoride** supplements
- appropriate arrangements for **oral hygiene**

Exercise 3

1. What are the most common causes of traumatic injuries?
2. Give classification of trauma.
3. Which instruments are used to maintain the operating field?
4. Describe objectives of treatment.
5. Talk about children with special needs.

Translation 3

Poranění úrazem, běžný výskyt, jeden z opravdu naléhavých případů, obvyklé příčiny zahrnují: batolata – zakopnutí a pády, starší děti – nehody na kole, dospívající – kontaktní sporty, rvačky, alkohol, klasifikace úrazu, zlomeniny (sklovina, zubovina, dřeň, kořen), pohmoždění (zub je poraněný, ale není uvolněný), neúplné vyvrácení (zub je rozviklán v chobotu, ale není odstraněný), vyčnívání (zub je posunutý ve směru kousání), vtlačení (zub je posunutý v chobotu směrem ke kořenovému hrotu), posunutí do strany (zub je zatlačen do strany, směrem k tváři či směrem k patru), odtržení (zub je úplně odstraněn z chobotu), udržování operačního pole, izolace zubu během operačních postupů, retraktor, odsavač slin, vysoko- a nízko-objemový odsávací přístroj, vatové svitky, absorpční tampony, gumová blána, zvážit možnost závažnějšího základního poranění (např. otřes mozku), léčebné cíle, cíle okamžité, uklidnění pacienta a rodiče, úleva od bolesti, ochrana dřeně, sešití lacerací měkké tkáně, zpevnění zlomených a pohyblivých zubů, cíle střednědobé, léčba dřeně, polo-trvalé náhrady, cíle dlouhodobé, korunky, náhrada ztracených zubů, ortodontická léčba, snímatelná pevná protéza, děti se zvláštními potřebami, vyžadovat zvláštní ošetření či speciální vybavení, dosáhnout a udržet ústní zdraví, neschopnost učení vrozená (Downův syndrom), získaná (např. jako důsledek poškození mozku před porodem, při porodu či po porodu), fyzické poškození zahrnuje mozkovou obrnu, zadní rozštěp páteře, svalovou dystrofii, smyslové poškození, slepota, hluchota, zdravotně oslabení, srdeční poruchy, hemofilie, dietní doporučení určené rodičům, fluoridové doplňky, vhodná opatření pro dentální hygienu.

Vocabulary

absorbent /əbˈzɔː.bənt/ pad /pæd/ absorbční tampon

accept /ək'sept/ akceptovat, přijmout, připustit

accident /'æk.sɪ.dənt/ nehoda, úraz, havárie

according /ə'kɔː.dɪŋ/ podle

achievable /ə'tʃiː.və.bļ/ dosažitelný, proveditelný

achieve /ə'tʃiːv/ dosáhnout

acquire /ə'kwaɪəʳ/ získat

amount /ə'maʊnt/ množství

anxiety /æŋ'zaɪ.ə.ti/ úzkost

anxious /'æŋk.ʃəs/ úzkostný

apical /'eɪ.pɪ.kəl/ apikální, ležící v okolí hrotu

approach /ə'prəʊtʃ/ přístup, blížit se, cesta, kontakt

appropriate /ə'prəʊ.pri.ət/ přiměřený, náležitý, vhodný

aspirator /,æs.pɪ'reɪ.təʳ/ odsavač slin, krve

atraumatic /'eɪ.trɔːˈmæt.ɪk/ nezraňující

attain /ə'teɪn/ dosáhnout, docílit

attention /ə'ten.tʃən/ span /spæn/ rozsah pozornosti

attention /ə'ten.tʃən/ pozornost, ošetření, výstraha, pozor!

audio /'ɔː.di.əʊ/ tape /teɪp/ magnetofonová páska

avulsion /æ'val.ʃ°n/ avulse, odtržení

badge /bædʒ/ odznak

behavioural /bɪ'heɪ.vjə.rəl/ týkající se chování

benefit /'ben.ɪ.fɪt/ výhoda

blindness /'blaɪnd.nəs/ slepota

blow /bləʊ/ air /eəʳ/ vhánět vzduch

brain /breɪn/ mozek, rozum

bucca /bʌk.ə/ (pl. buccae /bʌk.siː/) tvář

care /keəʳ/ péče, dohled, pozornost, mít zájem, ošetřovat

cause /kɔːz/ příčina

ceiling /'siː.lɪŋ/ strop

classification /,klæs.ɪ.fɪ'keɪ.ʃ°n/ klasifikace, třídění

common /'kɒm.ən/ běžný, společný

compromise /'kɒm.prə.maɪz/ oslabit

concussion /kən'kʌʃ.ən/ otřes, pohmoždění

condition /kən'dɪʃ.ən/ okolnost

congenital /kən'dʒen.ɪ.t°l/ vrozený

consequence /'kɒnt.sɪ.kwənts/ následek, závažnost, závěr

consider /kən'sɪd.əʳ/ zvážit, vzít do úvahy

consume /kən'sjuːm/ zkonzumovat, spotřebovat

cope /kəʊp/ zvládnout, stačit

correct /kə'rekt/ správný, přesný

cotton /'kɒt.°n/ wool /wʊl/ roll /rəʊl/ svitek vaty

crown /kraʊn/ korunka

damage /'dæm.ɪdʒ/ poškození

deafness /'def.nəs/ hluchota

decrease /dɪ'kriːs/ snížení, snížit se, být na ústupu

demonstrate /'dem.ən.streɪt/ předvádět, vyložit (názorně)

dentine /'den.tiːn/ dentin, zubovina

desired /dɪ'zaɪəd/ požadovaný

dexterity /dek'ster.ə.ti/ obratnost, zručnost

dietary /'daɪ.ə.tər.i/ dietní

direction /daɪ'rek.ʃ°n/ směr, vedení

displaced /dɪ'spleɪst/ odstraněný, posunutý

displacement /dɪ'spleɪs.mənt/ posunutí, vytlačení

distraction /dɪ'stræk.ʃən/ rozptýlení, rozrušení, napravení zlomeniny tahem

dystrophy /dɪs.trə.fi/ dystrofie

effective /ɪ'fek.tɪv/ účinný

effectively /ɪ'fek.tɪv.li/ efektivně

emotional /ɪˈməʊ.ʃ°n.°l/ vzrušivý, citový, dojemný

enamel /ɪˈnæm.°l/ sklovina

ensure /ɪnˈʃɔːʳ/ zajistit, postarat se

environment /ɪnˈvaɪə.rən.mənt/ prostředí

environs /ɪnˈvaɪə.rənz/ prostředí

experience /ɪkˈspɪə.ri.°nts/ zkušenost, pocítit, prožitek, zkušenost, praxe

extremely /ɪkˈstriːm.li/ extrémně

extrusion /ɪkˈstruː.ʒ°n/ extruze, vysunutí, vypuzení

facility /fəˈsɪl.ɪ.ti/ zařízení, vybavení

fall /fɔːl/ pád

fear /fɪəʳ/ obava

fight /faɪt/ bojovat, rvačka

fixed /fɪkst/ fixovaný, upevněný

frequently /ˈfriː.kwənt.li/ mnohdy, opakovaně

haemophilia /ˌhiː.məˈfɪl.i.ə/ hemofilie, dědičná krvácivost

high- /haɪ/ volume /ˈvɒl.juːm/ vysoko-objemový

honest /ˈɒn.ɪst/ poctivý, otevřený, řádný

hypnosis /hɪpˈnəʊ.sɪs/ zhypnotizování, hypnotický stav

identify /aɪˈden.tɪ.faɪ/ určit

in /ɪn/ turn /tɜːn/ střídavě

influence /ˈɪn.flu.ənts/ vliv, ovlivňovat, působit

injury /ˈɪn.dʒ°r.i/ poranění

insufficient /ˌɪn.səˈfɪʃ.ənt/ nedostatečný

integrate /ˈɪn.tɪ.greɪt/ začlenit, tvořit nedílný celek, doplnit

intermediate /ˌɪn.təˈmiː.di.ət/ střední, prostřední

introduction /ˌɪn.trəˈdʌk.ʃ°n/ úvod, zavedení

intrusion /ɪnˈtruː.ʒ°n/ intruze, pronikání, vstup

isolation /ˌaɪ.s°l.eɪ.ʃ°n/ izolace, oddělování, osamocení

laceration /ˌlæs.°rˈeɪ.ʃ°n/ lacerace, tržná rána

lack /læk/ postrádat, nedostatek

lateral /ˈlæt.r°l/ laterální, postranní, vedlejší

leaflet /ˈliː.flət/ leták (propagační), prospekt

learning /ˈlɜː.nɪŋ/ disability /ˌdɪs.əˈbɪl.ɪ.ti/ porucha učení

likely /ˈlaɪ.kli/ pravděpodobný

limit /ˈlɪm.ɪt/ limit, vymezit, krajní hranice

loosen /ˈluː.s°n/ uvolnit, vyviklat

low /ləʊ/ -volume /ˈvɒl.juːm/ nízko-objemový

maintain /meɪnˈteɪn/ udržovat

manual /ˈmæn.ju.əl/ ruční (konaný rukama), příručka, rukojeť

maturity /məˈtjʊə.rɪ.ti/ zralost, vyspělost

measurable /ˈmeʒ.ər.ə.bl̩/ měřitelný

message /ˈmes.ɪdʒ/ sdělení

mobile /ˈməʊ.baɪl/ mobilní, pohyblivý

modelling /ˈmɒd.əl.ɪŋ/ modelový, modelování

occurrence /əˈkʌr.°nts/ výskyt

orthodontics /ˌɔː.θəʊˈdɒn.tɪks/ úprava skusu

overload /ˈəʊ.və.ləʊd/ přetížení, přílišný náklad, zahltit

palatal /ˈpæ.lə.tl̩/ předopatrový

perinatal /ˌper.ɪˈneɪ.tl̩/ kolem porodu, do 10 dní po porodu

poster /ˈpəʊ.stəʳ/ plakát

praise /preɪz/ chválit, pochvala

prenatal /ˌpriːˈneɪ.tl̩/ prenatální, předporodní

preparedness /prɪˈpeəd.nəs/ pohotovost (připravenost)

present /ˈprez.°nt/ přítomný

preventive /prɪˈven.tɪv/ ochranný, předběžný

previous /ˈpriː.vi.əs/ před, předchozí, dosavadní, překotný

principle /ˈprɪnt.sɪ.pl̩/ princip, zásada

prosthodontics /ˌprɒs.θəˈdɒnt.ɪks/ protézy, specializace na zubní náhrady

protection /prəˈtek.ʃən/ ochrana, ochranný

pulp /pʌlp/ dřeň, dužnina, vláknina

push /pʊʃ/ tlačit

questionnaire /ˌkwes.tʃəˈneəʳ/ dotazník

raise /reɪz/ zvednout, zvýšení, zřídit

reassurance /ˌriː.əˈʃɔː.rənts/ opětovné ujištění, útěcha

reclining /rɪˈklaɪ.nɪŋ/ chair /tʃeəʳ/ sklápěcí křeslo

reinforce /ˌriː.ɪnˈfɔːs/ posílit, zesílit, zpevnit

relapse /rɪˈlæps/ úpadek, dostat recidivu

related /rɪˈleɪ.tɪd/ mající vztah

relieve /rɪˈliːv/ ulehčit, zmírňovat

removable /rɪˈmuː.və.bl̩/ odstranitelný, snímatelný

replacement /rɪˈpleɪs.mənt/ nahrazení, protéza

restorative /rɪˈstɒr.ə.tɪv/ posilňující, obnovující

retractor /rɪˈtræk.təʳ/ retraktor, hák na rány, držák

rinse /rɪnts/ vypláchnout

root /ruːt/ kořen

rubber /ˈrʌb.əʳ/ dam /dæm/ gumová blána

saliva /səˈlaɪ.və/ ejector /ɪːˈdʒekt.əʳ/ ejektor, vývěva, odsavač slin

seek /siːk/ vyhledávat, požadovat, pátrat

semipermanent /sem.i.ˈpɜː.mə.nənt/ semipermanentní, polotrvalý

sensation /senˈseɪ.ʃən/ pocit, vjem

sensitive /ˈsent.sɪ.tɪv/ vnímavý, choulostivý

sensory /ˈsent.sər.i/ disability /ˌdɪs.əˈbɪl.ɪ.ti/ smyslové postižení

setback /ˈset.bæk/ zhoršení situace, zhoršení zdravotního stavu, neúspěch

shifting /ˈʃɪf.tɪŋ/ přesouvání, posunování, přeřaďování

simple /ˈsɪm.pl̩/ jednoduchý

skill /skɪl/ schopnost, dovednost

slightly /ˈslaɪt.li/ mírně, trochu, slabě

socket /ˈsɒk.ɪt/ zubní lůžko, zdířka

soft /sɒft/ tissue /ˈtɪʃ.uː/, /ˈtɪs.juː/ měkká tkáň

spina bifida /ˌspaɪ.nəˈbɪf.ɪ.də/ zadní rozštěp páteře, obratle

spiral /ˈspaɪə.rəl/ točit se

spit /spɪt/ plivat, odplivnout

stabilization /ˌsteɪ.bɪ.laɪˈzeɪ.ʃən/ stabilizace (ustálení)

staff /stɑːf/ zaměstnanci, vybavit personálem

sticker /ˈstɪk.əʳ/ štítek, cedulka

subluxation /ˌsʌb.lʌkˈseɪ.ʃən/ subluxace, neúplné vykloubení

sufficient /səˈfɪʃ.ənt/ dostatečný

supervise /ˈsuː.pə.vaɪz/ dohlížet

supplement /ˈsʌp.lɪ.mənt/ doplněk

suture /ˈsuː.tʃəʳ/ sutura, sešití (stehy)

syringe /sɪˈrɪndʒ/ vstříknout, injekční

take /teɪk/ time /taɪm/ dát si na čas

target /ˈtɑː.gɪt/ cíl, terč, zamířit, plán

technique /tekˈniːk/ pracovní postup, metoda

time /taɪm/ related /rɪˈleɪ.tɪd/ vztahující se k času

toddler /ˈtɒd.ləʳ/ batole

toy /tɔɪ/ hračka

trauma /ˈtrɔː.mə/ úraz

traumatize /ˈtrɔː.mə.taɪz/ traumatizovat

uncertainty /ʌnˈsɜːtᵊn.ti/ nejistota, nespolehlivost

uncomfortable /ʌnˈkʌmp f.tə.bl̩/ diskomfortní, nepříjemný

underlying /ˌʌn.dəˈlaɪ.ɪŋ/ základní

vulnerability /ˌvʌl.nər.əˈbɪl.ɪ.ti/ zranitelnost, náchylnost

warn /wɔːn/ varovat

watch /wɒtʃ/ sledovat (zrakem), hlídat, dávat pozor

welcoming /ˈwel.kəm.ɪŋ/ přívětivý

well-being /ˌwelˈbiː.ɪŋ/ blaho, prospěch

youngster /ˈjʌŋk.stə/ výrostek

Unit 6

General Medicine of Relevance to Dentistry

History Taking. Cardiovascular System. Respiratory System. Gastrointestinal System. Haematological System. Renal Disease. Endocrine Disorders. Locomotor System Disease. Neurological Disorders. Psychiatric Disorders. Dermatology. Immune System Disorders.

Text 1

History Taking

The art of history taking is central to good medical and dental practice. Past medical and drug history and systemic inquiry are essential elements.

Past **medical history** should cover the following:

- **hospital** admissions and **operative procedures**
- **medications** taken currently and in the past
- **illnesses** (including **arthritis**, **heart failure**, **hypertension**, **asthma**, **bleeding disorders**, myocardial **infarction**, **angina**, **pacemakers**, **rheumatic fever**, **stroke**, **epilepsy**, **diabetes** mellitus, **renal** disease, **hepatic** disease, especially hepatitis).

- **HIV** exposure

Exercise 1

Which items should past medical and drug history cover?

Translation 1

Všeobecná medicína ve vztahu ke stomatologii, určení anamnézy, lékařská a léková anamnéza, přijetí do nemocnice, operace, léky užívané v současnosti a minulosti, nemoci, zánět kloubů, srdeční selhání, hypertenze, astma, poruchy s krvácením, infarkt myokardu, srdeční angína, stimulátory, revmatická horečka, mrtvice, epilepsie, cukrovka, choroby ledvin, onemocnění jater, zánět jater.

Text 2

A full review will include the following:

1. **general** – weight loss or gain, anorexia, energy level, fevers, and night sweats
2. **dermatological** – hair or nail changes, scaling, dryness, pigmentation, jaundice, itching, lesions, biopsy
3. **haematological** – bruising, bleeding, nodes, lumps, anaemia
4. **endocrine** – goitre, hot/cold intolerance, voice changes,

hair pattern, increased thirst, increased production of urine, development of breasts and sexual characteristics

5. **neurological** – headache, fainting, nausea, vomiting, vertigo, dizziness, pains, loss of smell, taste, or vision, muscle weakness or wasting, change in sensation, loss of sensation, loss of coordination, tremors, seizures, spectacles, double vision, blind spots, tunnel vision, pain, swelling, redness or dryness of the eyes, decreased hearing, ringing in the ears

6. **respiratory** – epistaxis, rhinorrhoea, cough, sputum production, dyspnoea, wheezing, cyanosis, pleuritic pain

---

Exercise 2

Which conditions will a full review include?

Translation 2

Úplný přehled bude zahrnovat následující, obecné údaje, váhový úbytek či přibývání na váze, anorexie, hladina energie, horečky a noční pocení, dermatologické, změny týkající se vlasů a nehtů, olupování kůže, suchost, pigmentace, zažloutnutí, svědění, poranění, biopsie, hematologické, zhmožděniny, krvácení, uzliny, bulky, anémie, endokrinní, struma, nesnášenlivost tepla/chladu, změny hlasu, struktury vlasů, zvýšená žízeň, zvýšená tvorba moči, vývoj prsů a pohlavních znaků, neurologické, bolest hlavy, mdloby, nevolnost, zvracení, závratě, bolesti,

ztráta čichu, chuti nebo zraku, svalová slabost, nebo ochabování, změny pocitů, ztráta smyslového vnímání, ztráta koordinace, třes, záchvaty, brýle, dvojité vidění, slepé skvrny, tunelové vidění, bolest, otok, začervenání, suchost očí, snížené slyšení, zvonění v uších, údaje o dýchání, epistaxe (krvácení z nosu), rinorea (vodnatý výtok z nosu), kašel, vytváření hlenu, dyspnoe (dušnost), sípání, cyanóza (promodrání kůže), bolesti pohrudnice.

Text 3

A full review will also include the following:

1. **cardiovascular** – palpitations, chest pain radiations, number of pillows used, hypertension, cyanosis, haemoptysis (coughing up blood), oedema, varicose veins and phlebitis, congenital or acquired cardiac anomalies, murmurs, exercise tolerance

2. **gastrointestinal** – appetite, food tolerance, flatulence, indigestion, abdominal pain, nausea, vomiting, vomiting blood, constipation or diarrhoea, stool colour, consistency and quality, mucus, haemorrhoids, hepatitis and jaundice, alcohol abuse, oral, mucosal, and dental problems

3. **genitourinary** – urinary frequency, hesitancy, changes in stream, difficulties starting or stopping stream, urinary tract infections, impotence, sexually transmitted diseases

4. **obstetric/gynaecology** – complications of pregnancy, abortion or miscarriages,

menstrual history, premenstrual syndrome, dysmenorrhoea, menorrhagia, date of last menstrual period, menopause, postmenopausal bleeding

5. **musculoskeletal** – fractures, arthritis, joint pain and swelling, muscle pain and weakness, limitation of movement and deformity

6. **psychiatric** – mood and appearance, anxiety, depression, and personality disorders, insomnia, early morning wakening, hallucinations, delusions

---

Exercise 3

Which conditions will a full review include?

Translation 3

Kardiovaskulární systém, palpitace (bušení), vyzařování, bolesti na hrudi, počet používaných polštářů, hypertenze, cyanóza, hemoptýza (vykašlávání krve), edém (otok), křečové žíly a flebitida (zánět žil), vrozené či získané srdeční anomálie, šelesty, tolerance tělesné námahy, gastrointestinální systém, chuť k jídlu, snášenlivost potravin, flatulence (nadýmání), špatné trávení, bolest břicha, nevolnost, zvracení, zvracení krve, zácpa či průjem, barva stolice, konzistence a vlastnosti, hlen, hemeroidy, zánět jater a žloutenka, zneužívání alkoholu, problémy v ústech, na sliznici a se zuby, pohlavní a vylučovací systém, frekvence močení, prodlévání, změny v proudu, obtíže při zahájení a zastavení, infekce močového

traktu, impotence, sexuálně přenosné nemoci, porodnictví/gynekologie, komplikace v těhotenství, potrat a spontánní potrat, průběh menstruace, před menstruační syndrom, dysmenorea (bolestivá menstruace), menoragie (silné menstruační krvácení), datum posledních měsíčků, menopauza, krvácení po menopauze, svalový a kosterní systém, zlomeniny, artritida, bolest a otok kloubů, bolest a slabost svalů, omezení hybnosti a deformita, psychiatrické okolnosti, nálada a vzhled, úzkost, deprese, poruchy osobnosti, nespavost, časné probouzení, halucinace, bludy.

Text 4

Diseases and Disorders I
Cardiovascular System:
ischaemic **heart disease**, cardiac failure, **hypertension**, cardiac murmurs

Respiratory System:
asthma, infections and chronic obstructive **pulmonary disease**, **bronchial carcinoma,** cystic fibrosis

Gastrointestinal System
Oral manifestations may be primary (a direct extension of the disease process into the mouth, e.g. lip swelling in Crohn's disease) or secondary (an indirect effect of the disease process, e.g. sialosis in anorexia nervosa).

*   **dysphagia** (difficulty in swallowing)
*   **gastric acid reflux** – may cause oesophagitis and heartburn. Predisposing factors include hiatus hernia, **pregnancy, obesity,** and **smoking.** Reflux may also be habitual, e.g. **bulimia nervosa.**

- gastric **carcinoma**
- peptic **ulceration** – divided into two main groups: gastric and duodenal
- **coeliac disease** – characterised by diarrhoea, steatorrhoea, weight loss, and failure to thrive normally in children
- **irritable bowel syndrome** – a common disorder, symptoms of altered bowel habit, abdominal pain and bloating. A diet deficient in fibre is important in the causation, and **psychological factors** are frequently evident.
- **Crohn's disease** – a chronic inflammation affecting any part of GI tract. The terminal ileum and proximal colon are the most commonly affected sites.
- **ulcerative colitis** – a chronic inflammatory disease of the colon. **Chronic blood loss**, causing iron deficiency, may lead to secondary oral manifestations such as recurrent **aphthous stomatitis**.
- **colonic cancer** – it may manifest, prior to overt abdominal signs, as an iron deficiency state with resultant oral mucosal problems such as recurrent aphthous stomatitis.
- **hepatic disease** (acute viral hepatitis, chronic hepatitis, chronic liver disease) – clearly **blood-borne viral infections** are of great concern to the dental professions. **Jaundice** is the main sign of liver disease and is best seen as **yellow discolouration of the sclera**. The skin and oral mucous membranes may also be involved.
- **pancreatic disease** – inflammation of the pancreas may be either acute or chronic.

Exercise 4

Give information about the diseases and disorders of:
1. Cardiovascular system
2. Respiratory system
3. Gastrointestinal system

Translation 4

Srdečně cévní systém, ischemická choroba srdeční, srdeční selhání, hypertenze, srdeční šelest, respirační systém, astma, infekce, chronické obstrukční onemocnění plic, bronchiální karcinom, cystická fibróza, gastrointestinální systém, ústní projevy, primární, sekundární, otok rtu při Crohnově nemoci, slinění při anorexii, dysfagie (obtížné polykání), zpětný tok žaludečních kyselin, ezofagitida (zánět jícnu), pálení žáhy, predisponujícími faktory jsou výhřez v otvoru jícnu, těhotenství, obezita, kouření, reflux návykový, bulimie, žaludeční karcinom (rakovinný nádor), peptický vřed, žaludeční, dvanáctníkový, celiakie, průjem, steatorea (tuková stolice), úbytek váhy a u dětí nemožnost správně prospívat, syndrom dráždivého střeva, symptomy zhoršeného stavu střev, bolesti břicha, nadmutí břicha, strava chudá na vlákninu, psychologické faktory, Crohnova choroba, chronický zánět, vředovitá kolitida, chronické zánětlivé onemocnění tlustého střeva, chronická ztráta krve, způsobující nedostatek železa, druhotné ústní projevy, opakující se aftózní stomatitida, rakovina tlustého střeva, nedostatek železa s výslednými problémy ústní sliznice, jaterní onemocnění, akutní virový zánět jater, chronický zánět jater, chronická jaterní choroba, krví přenášené virové infekce jsou velmi důležité pro zubní obory, žloutenka, žluté zbarvení skléry (oční bělimy), kůže a sliznice úst, onemocnění slinivky, zánět pankreatu, akutní, chronický.

Text 5

Diseases and Disorders II
Haematological System

- **anaemia** is defined as a haemoglobin concentration less than the reference range for that age and gender of patient
- **bleeding disorders** include blood vessel defects, platelet defects (qualitative and quantitative), and coagulation cascade defects (hereditary and acquired)

Renal Disease

- **infections** can be either **pyelonephritis** (affecting the kidney) or **cystitis** (affecting the bladder). They are common in women, with 50% experiencing symptoms of a urinary tract infection at some point of their lifetime. Symptoms include frequency, urgency, dysuria (pain on micturition), and incontinence or retention.
- **chronic renal failure** causes increased levels of circulating urea (uraemia) as a result of progressive kidney damage. May be due to diabetes, hypertension, glomerulonephritis, pyelonephritis, reflux, or connective tissue

disorders. Symptoms include polyuria, nocturia, anorexia, vomiting, and itchiness of the skin.

Endocrine Disorders

- **diabetes mellitus** - persistent hyperglycaemia due to deficiency (Type 1) or reduced effectiveness (Type 2) of insulin. Routine dentistry should be performed soon after mealtimes (breakfast or lunch) with the patient on usual drug/diet regimens.
- **thyroid and parathyroid disease** – hyperthyroidism, hypothyroidism, hyperparathyroidism, hypoparathyroidism.
- **pituitary and adrenal gland disorders** – the anterior pituitary secretes FSH, LH, GH, prolactin, ACTH, and THS; the posterior pituitary secretes ADH and oxytocin
- **pregnancy** and **menopause** – pregnancy may lead to worsening of **gingivitis** and development of inflammatory **epulides**. It is a time to avoid radiographs, general anaesthesia, and drugs (except if essential). Menopause is a time of great physiological and psychological change. Psychogenic **orofacial pain syndromes** such as burning mouth syndrome are relatively common at this time.

Exercise 5

Give information about the diseases and disorders of:
1. Haematological system

2. Renal disease
3. Endocrine disorders

Translation 5
Krevní systém, anémie, koncentrace hemoglobinu, udávaný rozsah, věk a pohlaví pacienta, poruchy krvácení, defekty krevních cév, defekty krevních destiček, defekty koagulace (dědičné a získané), onemocnění ledvin, infekce, pyelonefritida (postihující ledvinu), cystitida (postihující močový měchýř), symptomy, časté močení, nutkání, dysurie (bolest při močení) a inkontinence, zadržování, chronické selhání ledvin, zvýšená hladina obíhající močoviny (urémie), postupující poškození ledvin, cukrovka, hypertenze, glomerulonefritida (zánět ledvin spojený se zánětem glomerulů), pyelonefritida (současný zánět ledvinné pánvičky a ledviny), symptomy, polyurie (nadměrné močení), nokturie (noční močení), anorexie, zvracení a svědivost kůže, endokrinní poruchy, hyperglykemie (zvýšené množství cukru v krvi) kvůli nedostatku (Typ 1) nebo sníženému účinku (Typ 2) insulinu, rutinní dentální ošetření by měla být prováděna krátce po jídle, onemocnění štítné žlázy a příštitných tělísek, zvýšená činnost štítné žlázy, snížená činnost štítné žlázy, zvýšená činnost příštitných tělísek, snížená činnost příštitných tělísek, poruchy hypofýzy (podvěsek mozkový) a poruchy žlázy nadledvin, těhotenství, zhoršení zánětu dásní, rozvoj zánětlivých nádorků dásně, vyhýbat se rentgenu, celkové anestézii a lékům, pokud nejsou nezbytné, menopauza je obdobím velké fyziologické a psychologické proměny, syndromy bolesti úst a obličeje psychického původu, syndrom pálení v ústech jsou v této době relativně běžné.

Text 6
Diseases and Disorders III
Locomotor System Disease
* **developmental** bone disease
* **metabolic** bone disease (e.g. **osteoporosis**, defined as a reduction in bone mass). Features are bone pain, backache, and fractures of vertebrae, distal radius, and neck of femur. Women are predominantly affected. Causes include postmenopausal, endocrine, nutritional, and iatrogenic.
* **joint disease** (e.g. **osteoarthritis**) is a common age-related disease of joints. It is characterised by pain and stiffness, particularly of weight-bearing joints.
* **rheumatoid arthritis** is a chronic inflammatory, destructive, and deforming polyarthropathy with extra-articular systemic manifestations. It is characterised by the presence of circulating autoantibodies (rheumatoid factor).

The systemic manifestations include:
* **anorexia, malaise, lethargy, myalgia**
* **vasculitic** lesions (e.g. nail bed infarcts)
* **pancarditis** and **lung** lesions
* **anaemia**
* **neuropathies**
* **Sjögren's syndrome**

Neurological Disorders

Examination of the nervous system is a complex and time-consuming process best left to physicians trained in that area. However, knowledge of the cranial nerves may be useful in discriminating organic disease from the psychosomatic.

- **palsy** and **neuropathy** – many systemic diseases can cause palsies and neuropathies
- **headache** and **migraine** – three common headaches dominate clinical practice: migraine, mixed headache, and tension headache. Local organic disease excluded, the patient should be seen by a physician with an interest in headache.
- **epilepsy** – may be classified according to seizure type: **partial** (partial seizures) and **generalised** (absence seizures)
- **multiple sclerosis** – an inflammatory, demyelinating disorder affecting any part of CNS in a variable and unpredictable manner
- **Parkinson's disease** – caused by degeneration of neurons in the CNS with resultant tremor, rigidity, bradykinesia, and disturbed postural reflexes
- **chronic fatigue syndrome** – previously called postviral syndrome. This condition is a complex disorder characterised by lassitude.

Exercise 6

Talk about
1. The locomotor system disease
2. The systemic diseases
3. Neurological disorders

Translation 6

Onemocnění pohybového ústrojí, onemocnění vývoje kosti, metabolické onemocnění kosti (např. osteoporóza, definovaná jako snížení hmoty kosti), charakteristickými rysy jsou bolest kosti, bolest zad, zlomeniny obratlů, zlomeniny periferní kosti vřetenní a krčku kosti stehenní, příčinami jsou stavy po menopauze, endokrinní, výživové a iatrogenní (lékařem vyvolané), onemocnění kloubů (např. osteoartritida) je běžnou nemocí kloubů související s věkem, bolest a ztuhlost, zejména kloubů nesoucích váhu, revmatická artritida je chronické, zánětlivé, ničící a deformující onemocnění více kloubů s mimo-kloubními systémovými projevy, přítomnost cirkulujících antigenů, působících proti vlastnímu organismu (revmatický faktor), projevy systémové (týkající se těla jako celku), anorexie, malátnost, letargie, myalgie (bolest svalů), cévní léze (např. infarkt nehtových lůžek), pankarditida (zánět všech vrstev srdeční stěny) a poranění plic, neuropatie (onemocnění nervů), nervové poruchy, vyšetření nervového systému je složitý a časově náročný proces, znalost lebečních nervů může být užitečná při rozlišení onemocnění organického od psychosomatického, ochrnutí a neuropatie, migréna, smíšená bolest hlavy a bolest hlavy spojená s tlakem, epilepsie, klasifikována dle typu záchvatu, částečná (částečné záchvaty) a celková (záchvaty s bezvědomím), roztroušená skleróza, zánětlivá porucha s demyelinizací (zničení myelinu v nervových vláknech), Parkinsonova nemoc, způsobená degenerací neuronů v CNS, třes, ztuhlost, bradykineze (extrémní zpomalení pohybu) a porušené postojové reflexy, syndrom chronické únavy, složitá porucha, charakteristická malátností.

Text 7

Diseases and Disorders IV

Psychiatric Disorders

Personality disorders, **neuroses**, and **psychoses** are all part of the broad spectrum of psychiatric disorders. The possibility of such disorders being part of the aetiology of certain conditions (e.g. **chronic orofacial pain disorders**) must be borne in mind. The role of the dental professional in chronic orofacial pain disorders is to exclude contributory dental disease (such as pulpitis) and be supportive and understanding of contributing psychiatric disease.

When local dental disease has been excluded, the patient should be referred to a physician with an interest in such disorders—preferably at a combined oral medicine/psychiatry clinic. Unnecessary and prolonged treatment must be resisted since this will only add to the patient's problem.

Dermatology

The facial and perioral manifestations of skin conditions, such as **psoriasis** and **dermatitis**, should be dealt with by a general practitioner or dermatologist, as should skin manifestations of systemic diseases.

Immune System Disorders

Immune system disorders may be the result of many aetiologies, but all are characterised by increased susceptibility to infection.

- **congenital** (primary) immunodeficiency
- **acquired** (secondary) immunodeficiency—related to diseases or immunosuppressive therapy.

The major entity today is, of course, **HIV and AIDS**, but there are many others, including leukaemia and lymphomas, malnutrition, rheumatoid arthritis, chronic active hepatitis, diabetes mellitus, Down's syndrome, tuberculosis, and numerous viral infections.

Immunosuppresive therapy is now extremely common and may be used in the management of connective tissue disorders, dermatological diseases, mucosal diseases, and following organ transplant surgery (e.g. heart, lung, kidney, liver, pancreas). The problems associated with these conditions are many (e.g. likelihood of infection, bleeding diathesis, steroid prophylaxis), and management of dental and oral diseases is best suited to specialist units.

Exercise 7

1. Discuss psychiatric disorders as a part of the aetiology of certain conditions.
2. Which immune system disorders do you know?

Translation 7

Psychiatrické poruchy, poruchy osobnosti, neurózy a psychózy, součást etiologie určitých stavů (např. chronické bolesti úst a obličeje), vyloučit přispívající dentální onemocnění (jako třeba zánět zubní dřeně), dát podporu a porozumění, pacient by měl být převeden k lékaři, zabývajícímu se těmito poruchami, odmítnout ošetření, které není nezbytné a dlouho trvající ošetření, dermatologie, obličejové a periorální (kolem úst) projevy stavů kůže jako je lupénka a dermatitida (zánět kůže), poruchy imunitního systému, zvýšená náchylnost k infekci, imunitní nedostatečnost vrozená (primární), získaná (sekundární), související s nemocemi nebo terapií, která potlačuje imunitu, hlavní skutečností je HIV a AIDS, leukémie a lymfomy (maligní tumor lymfatické tkáně), špatná výživa, revmatická artritida, chronická aktivní hepatitida, léčba, která má imunosupresivní účinky (snížení schopnosti organismu reagovat na cizí látky) je nyní velice běžná, léčba poruch pojivové tkáně, kožní onemocnění, onemocnění sliznice, po chirurgických transplantacích (např. srdce/plíce, ledviny, jater, slinivky), pravděpodobnost infekce, dispozice ke krvácení, profylaxe steroidy.

Vocabulary

abdominal /æbˈdɒm.ɪ.nəl/ břišní
abortion /əˈbɔː.ʃən/ interrupce
abuse /əˈbjuːz/ zneužívání
acid /ˈæs.ɪd/ kyselina
acquire /əˈkwaɪəʳ/ získat
add /æd/ přidávat
admission /ədˈmɪʃ.ən/ přijetí
adrenal /əˈdriː.nəl/ týkající se nadledviny

aetiology /ˌiː.tiˈɒl.ə.dʒi/ etiologie, nauka o původu a příčinách
anaemia /əˈniː.mi.ə/ chudokrevnost
anaesthesia /ˌæn.əsˈθiː.zi.ə/ znecitlivění
angina /ænˌdʒaɪ.nə/ angína
anomaly /əˈnɒm.ə.li/ odchylka
anorexia /æn.əˌrek.si.ə/ chorobné nechutenství
anxiety /æŋˈzaɪ.ə.ti/ pocit úzkosti
aphthous /ˈæf.θəs/ aftózní
appearance /əˈpɪə.rənts/ vzhled, objevení se
appetite /ˈæp.ɪ.taɪt/ chuť k jídlu
arthritis /ɑːˈθraɪ.tɪs/ zánět kloubů
asthma /ˈæs.mə/ astma
autoantibody /ɔː.təʊ.ˈæn.ti.bɒd.i/ vlastní protilátka
avoid /əˈvɔɪd/ vyvarovat se
biopsy /ˈbaɪ.ɒp.si/ biopsie
bladder /ˈblæd.əʳ/ měchýř
bleeding /ˈbliː.dɪŋ/ krvácení
blind /blaɪnd/ **spot** /spɒt/ slepé místo na sítnici; bolavé místo (přen.)
bloating /ˈbləʊ.tɪŋ/ nadmutí břicha
blood /blʌd/ krev
bowels /ˈbaʊ.əlz/ vnitřnosti
bradykinesia /ˌbræ.di.kiˈniːzɪ.ə/ bradykineze, extrémní zpomalení pohybu
breast /brest/ hruď, prsa
bronchial /ˈbrɒŋ.ki.əl/ průduškový
bruising /ˈbruː.zɪŋ/ podlitina, odřeniny
bulimia /bʊˌlɪm.i.ə/ chorobná chuť k jídlu
cancer /ˈkænt.səʳ/ rakovina
carcinoma /kɑː.sɪˈnəʊ.mə/ rakovinný nádor
cardiac /ˈkɑː.di.æk/ srdeční
cardiovascular /ˌkɑː.di.əʊˈvæs.kjʊ.ləʳ/ kardiovaskulární

cascade /kæsˈkeɪd/ seřazení za sebou, kaskáda

causation /kɔːˈzeɪ.ʃən/ příčina

cerebral palsy /ˌser.ə.brəlˈpɔːl.zi/ mozková obrna

coagulation /kəʊˈæg.jʊ.leɪ.ʃ°n/ koagulace, srážení

coeliac disease /ˈsiː.li.æk.dɪˌziːz/ celiakie, břišní onemocnění

colitis /kəʊ ˈlaɪ.təs/ zánět tlustého střeva

colon /ˈkəʊ.lɒn/ tlusté střevo

concentration /ˌkɒnʃ.sənˈtreɪ.ʃ°n/ soustřeďování

congenital /kənˈdʒen.ɪ.t°l/ vrozený

connective tissue /kəˌnek.tɪvˈtɪʃ.uː/ pojivová tkáň

consistency /kənˈsɪs.t°nʃ.si/ konzistence, tuhost

constipation /ˌkɒnʃ.stɪˈpeɪ.ʃən/ zácpa

contribute /kənˈtrɪb.juːt/ přispívat

coordination /kəʊˌɔː.dɪˈneɪ.ʃən/ koordinace, uvedení v soulad

cough /kɒf/ kašel

cranial /ˈkreɪ.ni.əl/ **nerve** /nɜːv/ lebeční nerv

currently /ˈkʌr.ənt.li/ aktuálně, v současné době

cyanosis /ˈsʌɪəˈnəʊ.sɪs/ cyanóza, zmodrání kůže a sliznic

cystic fibrosis /ˌsɪs.tɪk.faɪˈbrəʊ.sɪs/ cystická fibróza, fibrotické onemocnění slinivky

cystitis /sɪˈstaɪ.tɪs/ cystitida, zánět močového měchýře

deficiency /dɪˈfɪʃ.ənʃ.si/ nedostatek

deficient /dɪˈfɪʃ.ant/ deficitní, nedostatečný

deform /dɪˈfɔːm/ deformovat, změnit tvar

deformity /dɪˈfɔː.mɪ.ti/ deformita, znetvoření

degeneration /dɪˌdʒen.əˈreɪ.ʃən/ degenerace, rozklad

delusion /dɪˈluː.ʒən/ halucinace, klam

demyelination /dɪˈmaɪ.ə.li.naɪˈzeɪ.ʃən/ demyelinizace, zničení myelinu

depression /dɪˈpreʃ.ən/ deprese, sklíčenost

dermatitis /ˌdɜː.məˈtaɪ.təs/ dermatitida, zánět kůže

dermatology /ˌdɜː.məˈtɒl.ə.dʒi/ dermatologie, kožní lékařství

destructive /dɪˈstrʌk.tɪv/ destruktivní, zhoubný

developmental /dɪˌvel.əpˈmen.t°l/ vývojový

diabetes /ˌdaɪəˈbiː.tiːz/ cukrovka

diarrhoea /ˌdaɪ.əˈriː.ə/ diarea (průjem)

diathesis /ˌdaɪˈæ.θiː.sɪs/ diatéza, dispozice

direct /daɪˈrekt/ přímý

discoloration /dɪˌskʌl.əˈreɪ.ʃən/ změna barvy zubů

discriminate /dɪˈskrɪm.ɪ.neɪt/ rozlišovat

disease /dɪˈziːz/ onemocnění

disorder /dɪˈsɔː.dəʳ/ porucha (zdraví)

distal /dɪ.stəl/ vzdálený, zadní (zuby)

dizziness /ˈdɪz.ɪ.nəs/ závrať, mrákotný stav

double /ˈdʌb.l̩/ dvojitý

Down's syndrome /ˈdaʊnzˌsɪn.drəʊm/ Downova choroba

dryness /draɪ.nəs/ suchost

due /djuː/ **to** /tʊ/ následkem, kvůli

duodenal /ˌdjuː.əʊ ˈdiː.nəl/ duodenální, dvanáctníkový

dysmenorrhoea /ˌdɪs.me.nəˈriː.ə/ dysmenorea, bolestivá menstruace

dysphagia /dɪˈsfeɪ.dʒiə/ dysfagie, porucha polykání

dyspnoea /dɪs.pniː.ə/ dyspnoe, dušnost

dysuria /dɪs.ˈju.ə.ri.ə/ dysurie, obtíž při močení

effect /ɪˈfekt/ účinek, výsledek

effectiveness /ɪˈfek.tɪv.nəs/ účinnost, působení

endocrine /ˈen.də.kr*a* ɪn/ endokrinní, s vnitřním vyměšováním

epilepsy /ˈep.ɪ.lep.si/ epilepsie

epistaxis /ˌe.pɪ.ˈstæk.sɪs/ epistaxe, krvácení z nosu

epulis /eˈpjuː.lɪs/ **(pl. epulides** / eˈpjuː.lɪ.diːz/) epulis, nádorek dásně v okolí zubního krčku

essential /ɪˈsen.t ʃəl/ základní, hlavní, nepostradatelný

examination /ɪgˌzæm.ɪˈneɪ.ʃ°n/ prohlídka, vyšetření

exclude /ɪkˈskluːd/ vyloučit

exercise /ˈek.sə.saɪz/ cvičení, používání

exposure /ɪkˈspəʊ.ʒəʳ/ vystavení

extension /ɪkˈsten.t ʃən/ rozšíření

extra- /ˈek.strə/ **articular** /ˈa.ːtɪ.kjʊ.ləʳ/ mimo-kloubní

failure /ˈfeɪ.ljəʳ/ selhání, porucha

faint /feɪnt/ omdlít, mdloba

fatigue /fəˈtiːg/ únava, vyčerpání

feature /ˈfiː.tʃəʳ/ charakteristická vlastnost

femur /ˈfiː.məʳ/ femur, stehenní kost

fibre /ˈfaɪ.bəʳ/ vlákno

flatulence /ˈflæt.jʊ.lən*t* s/ flatulence, plynatost

fracture /ˈfræk.t ʃ°r/ fraktura, zlomenina

frequency /ˈfriː.kwən*t*.si/ časté opakování

gastric /ˈgæs.trɪk/ gastrický, žaludeční

gastrointestinal /ˌgæs.trəʊˌɪn.tesˈtaɪ.n°l/ gastrointestinální, týkající se žaludku a střeva

gender /ˈdʒen.dəʳ/ pohlaví

general /ˈdʒen.°r.°l/ hlavní, všeobecný, celkový

generalized /ˈdʒen.ər.ə.laɪzd/ obecný, zobecněný, celkový

genitourinary /ˌdʒen.ɪ.təʊˈjʊə.rɪn.ri/ genitourinární, močopohlavní

gingivitis /ˌdʒɪn.dʒɪˈvaɪ.tɪs/ gingividita, zánět sliznice dásní

gland /glænd/ žláza

glomerulonephritis / glɒˈme.ru.lə.nəfˈraɪ.tɪs/ glomeluronefritida, zánět ledvin, spojený se zánětem glomerulů

goitre /ˈgɔɪ.təʳ/ struma, vole

gynaecology /ˌgaɪ.nəˈkɒl.ə.dʒi/ gynekologie, ženské lékařství

habitual /həˈbɪtʃ.u.əl/ habituální, navyklý, častý, notorický

haematological /ˌhiː.mə.təˈlɒdʒ.ɪ.kəl/ zabývající se studiem krve a tkání

haemoglobin /ˌhiː.məˈgləʊ.bɪn/ hemoglobin

haemoptysis /hiːˈmɒ.ptɪ.sɪs/ hemoptýza, vykašlávání krve

haemorrhoids /ˈhem.°r.ɔɪdz/ hemeroidy

hallucination /həˌluː.sɪˈneɪ.ʃ°n/ halucinace, přelud

headache /ˈhed.eɪk/ bolest hlavy

hearing /ˈhɪə.rɪŋ/ sluch, schopnost slyšet

heart /haːt/ srdce, srdeční

heartburn /ˈhaːt.bɜːn/ pálení žáhy

hepatic /hepˈæt.ɪk/ jaterní

hepatitis /ˌhep.əˈtaɪ.tɪs/ hepatitida, zánět jater

hereditary /həˈred.ɪ.tri/ dědičný, vrozený

hernia /ˈhɜː.ni.ə/ hernie (kýla)

hesitancy /ˈhez.ɪ.t°n*t*.si/ váhavost, rozkolísanost

hiatus /haɪˈeɪ.təs/ mezera, otvor

hyperglycaemia /ˌhaɪ.pə.glaɪˈsiː.mi.ə/ hyperglykémie, zvýšené množství glukózy v krvi

hypertension /ˌhaɪ.pəˈten.tʃ°n/ zvýšený tlak

hyperthyroidism /ˌhaɪ.pə.ˈθaɪə.rɔɪdɪ.z°m/ hypertyroidismus, zvýšená činnost štítné žlázy

hypothyroidism /ˌhaɪ.pəʊ.ˈθaɪə.rɔɪdɪ.z°m/ hypotyreóza, snížená činnost štítné žlázy

iatrogenic /aɪˌætrəˈdʒen.ɪk/ iatrogenní, lékařem vyvolaný

ileum /ˈɪl.i.əm/ kyčelník

immune /ɪˈmjuːn/ imunní, odolný, bezpečný před něčím

immunodeficiency /ˌɪm.jʊ.nəʊ.dɪˈfɪʃ.°nt.si/ imunodeficience, deficit imunity

immunosuppression /ˌɪm.jə.nəʊ.səˈpreʃ.°n/ imunosuprese, snížení schopnosti organismu reagovat na cizí látky

increase /ɪnˈkriːs/ zvýšit, zvětšování

indigestion /ˌɪn.dɪ.dʒes.tʃ°n/ porucha trávení, zažívací potíže

indirect /ˌɪn.daɪˈrekt/ nepřímý, vedlejší

inflammation /ˌɪn.fləˈmeɪ.ʃ°n/ zápal, zánět

inflammatory /ɪnˈflæm.ə.tər.i/ zánětlivý

inquiry /ɪnˈkwaɪə.ri/ dotaz, vyšetřování

insomnia /ɪnˈsɒm.ni.ə/ insomnie, nespavost

insulin /ˈɪn.sjʊ.lɪn/ inzulín

intolerance /ɪnˈtɒl.°r.°nts/ nesnášenlivost

iron /aɪən/ železo

irritable /ˈɪr.ɪ.tə.bl̩/ podrážděný, přecitlivělý

ischaemic /ɪsˈkiː.mɪk/ ischemický, nedokrvený

itchiness /ˈɪtʃ.ɪ.nəs/ svědění

itching /ˈɪtʃ.ɪŋ/ svědivý

jaundice /ˈdʒɔːn.dɪs/ žloutenka

joint /dʒɔɪnt/ místo připojení, kloub

kidney /ˈkɪd.ni/ ledvina

knowledge /ˈnɒl.ɪdʒ/ znalost, vědomost

lassitude /ˈlæs.ɪ.tjuːd/ malátnost, únava

lesion /ˈliː.ʒ°n/ poranění, poškození, porucha

lethargy /ˈləθ.ə.dʒɪ/ letargie, strnulost, netečnost

leukaemia /luːˈkiː.mi.ə/ leukémie

likelihood /ˈlaɪ.kli.hʊd/ pravděpodobnost, možnost

limitation /ˌlɪm.ɪˈteɪ.ʃ°n/ limitace, omezení, nedostatek, vada

liver /ˈlɪv.ə'/ játra

locomotor /ˌləʊ.kəˈməʊ.tə'/ lokomotorický, pohybový

lump /lʌmp/ boule (na těle), opuchlina

lung /lʌŋ/ plíce (jedna)

lymphoma /lɪmpˈfəʊ.mə/ lymfom, maligní tumor lymfatické tkáně

major /ˈmeɪ.dʒə'/ velký, významnější, závažný, převážný

malaise /mælˈeɪz/ nevolnost, malátnost

malnutrition /ˌmæl.njuːˈtrɪ.ʃən/ nesprávná výživa, podvýživa

management /ˈmæn.ɪdʒ.mənt/ péče, vedení, snaha o zvládnutí

manifestation /ˌmæn.ɪ.fesˈteɪ.ʃən/ manifestace, projev, objevení

manner /ˈmæn.ə'/ způsob, chování, metoda

menopause /ˈmen.ə.pɔːz/ menopauza, klimakterium

menorrhagia /ˌmen.əˈreɪ.dʒɪ.ə/ menoragie, silné menstruační krvácení

menstrual /ˈmen.strəl/ menstruační

micturition /ˌmɪkt.juəˈrɪʃ.ᵊn/ močení

migraine /ˈmiː.greɪn/, /ˈmaɪ/ migréna, silná bolest hlavy

miscarriage /ˈmɪsˌkær.ɪdʒ/ potrat, umělé přerušení těhotenství

mood /muːd/ nálada, kondice

movement /ˈmuːv.mənt/ pohyb, postup, vyprázdnění střev

mucosal /ˌmjuːˈkəʊ.sl/ mukózní, slizniční

mucous membrane /ˌmjuː.kəsˈmem.breɪn/ sliznice

multiple /ˈmʌl.tɪ.pl̩/ **sclerosis** / skləˈrəʊ.sɪs/ multiplex, roztroušená skleróza

murmur /ˈmɜː.məʳ/ šelest, šeptat

muscle /ˈmʌs.l̩/ sval

musculoskeletal /ˈmʌs.kjʊ.ləˈskel.ɪ.tᵊl/ muskuloskeletální, skládající se ze svalů a kostí

myalgia /mʌɪˈæl.dʒɪ.ə/ myalgie, svalová bolest

myocardial /ˌmaɪ.əˈkɑː.diəl/ **infarction** /inˈfaːk.ʃᵊn/ infarkt myokardu

nausea /ˈnɔː.zi.ə/ pocit nevolnosti, nucení ke zvracení

neurological /ˌnjʊə.rəˈlɒdʒ.ɪ.kᵊl/ neurologický

neuron /ˈnjʊə.rɒn/ neuron, nervová buňka

neuropathy /ˌnjʊəˈrɒ.pə.θi/ neuropatie, onemocnění nervů

neurosis /njʊəˈrəʊ.sɪs/ **(pl. neuroses)** neuróza

nocturia /nɒkˈtjʊ.ə.rɪ.ə/ nokturie, noční močení

node /nəʊd/ uzel, uzlina, otok

nutritional /njuːˈtrɪʃ.ᵊn.ᵊl/ nutriční, výživový

obesity /əʊˈbiː.sɪ.ti/ obezita, otylost

obstetric /ɒbˈstet.rɪk/ porodnický, spojený s porodem

obstructive /əbˈstrʌk.tɪv/ obstruktivní, ucpávající

oedema /ɪˈdiː.mə/ edém, otok

oesophagitis /ˌiːsɒ.fəˈdʒaɪ.tɪs/ ezofagitida, zánět jícnu

oral /ˈɔː.rəl/ orální, ústní

orofacial /ˌəʊ.rəˈfeɪ.ʃᵊl/ orofaciální, týkající se úst a obličeje

osteoarthritis /ˌɒs.ti.əʊ.ɑːˈθraɪ.tɪs/ osteoartritida, zánět kostních kloubů

osteoporosis /ˌɒs.ti.əʊ.pəˈrəʊ.sɪs/ osteoporóza, prořídnutí kostí

pacemaker /ˈpeɪsˌmeɪ.kəʳ/ srdeční stimulátor

pain /peɪn/ bolest, námaha

palpitations /ˌpæl.pɪˈteɪ.ʃᵊnz/ palpitace, bušení (srdce ap.)

pancarditis /ˌpæn.kɑːˈdaɪ.tɪs/ pankarditida, zánět všech vrstev srdeční stěny

pancreas /ˈpæŋ.kri.əs/ pankreas, slinivka břišní

pancreatic /ˌpæŋ.kriˈæt.ɪk/ pankreatický, slinivkový

parathyroid gland / ˌpær.əˈθaɪə.rɔɪdˌglænd/ příštitná žláza

partial /ˈpɑː.ʃᵊl/ částečný, dílčí, neúplný

perioral /ˌper.ɪˈɔː.rəl/ umístěný kolem úst

persistent /pəˈsɪs.tᵊnt/ stálý, neústupný, dlouhotrvající

personality /ˌpɜː.sᵊnˈæl.ə.ti/ **disorder** / dɪˈsɔː.dəʳ/ porucha osobnosti

phlebitis /flɪˈbaɪ.tɪs/ flebitida, zánět žil

physician /fɪˈzɪʃ.ən/ ošetřující lékař, lékařský

pigmentation /ˌpɪg.mənˈteɪ.ʃᵊn/ zbarvení

pillow /ˈpɪl.əʊ/ polštář, položit na polštář

pituitary gland /pɪˈtjuː.ɪ.tªr.iˌglænd/ hypofýza, podvěsek mozkový

platelet /ˈpleɪt.lət/ destička, krevní destička

pleuritic /pluə.rət.ɪk/ nemocný zánětem pohrudnice

polyarthropathy /ˌpɒl.ɪ.ɑːˈθrəp.ə.θi/ současný zánět několika kloubů

polyuria /ˌpɒl.ɪ.ˈjuə.rɪə/ polyurie, nadměrné močení

postmenopausal /ˌpəʊstˈmen.ə.ˈpɔː.zªl/ pomenopauzální

postural /pɒs.tjʊ.ə.rəl/ posturální, postojový

practitioner /præk.ˈtɪʃ.ªn.ªr/ praktický lékař, odborník

predisposition /ˌpriː.dɪ.spəˈzɪʃ.ªn/ predispozice, náchylnost, sklon

pregnancy /ˈpreg.nənt.si/ těhotenství

premenstrual /priː.ˈmen.strəl/ syndrome /ˈsɪn.drəʊ m/ předmenstruační syndrom

presence /ˈprez.ªnt s/ přítomnost (osoby, věci ap.), zevnějšek

primary /ˈpraɪ.mə.ri/ primární, první, základní

procedure /prəˈsiː.dʒəʳ/ procedura (postup), průběh

process /ˈprəʊ.ses/ proces, postup, průběh

production /prəˈdʌk.ʃªn/ produkce, tvorba

prophylaxis /ˌprɒf.ɪˈlæk.sɪs/ profylaxe, prevence

proximal /prɒˈk.sɪ.məl/ proximální, bližší trupu, hlavě, středu

psoriasis /səˈraɪə.sɪs/ psoriáza, lupénka

psychiatric /ˌsaɪ.kiˈæt.rɪk/ psychiatrický, duševní

psychogenic /ˈsaɪ.kəˌdʒə.nɪk/ psychogenní, mentálního původu

psychological /ˌsaɪ.kªlˈɒdʒ.ɪ.kªl/ duševní

psychosis /saɪˈkəʊ.sɪs/ psychóza, porucha myšlení a jednání s následným rozpadem osobnosti

psychosomatic /ˌsaɪ.kəʊ.səˈmæt.ɪk/ psychosomatický, týkající se vztahu těla a mysli

pulmonary /ˈpʊl.mə.nə.ri/ pulmonární, plicní

pulpitis /pʌlˈpaɪ.tɪs/ pulpitida, zánět zubní dřeně

pyelonephritis /ˌpaɪ.ə.lə.neˈfraɪ.tɪs/ pyelonefritida, současný zánět ledvinné pánvičky a ledviny

qualitative /ˈkwɒl.ɪ.tə.tɪv/ kvalitativní, jakostní

quantitative /ˈkwɒn.tɪ.tə.tɪv/ kvantitativní (mnohostní)

radiation /ˌreɪ.diˈeɪ.ʃªn/ radiace, záření, vyzařování

radiograph /reɪ.di.ə.grɑːf/ rentgenový snímek

radius /ˈreɪ.di.əs/ radius, kost vřetenní, okruh, poloměr

recurrent /rɪˈkʌr.ªnt/ opakující se, recidivující

reduce /rɪˈdjuːs/ snížit, napravit, přemoct

refer /rɪˈfɜːr/ týkat se, odvolávat se, vztahovat se, poukázat

reflex /ˈriː.fleks/ reflex, výraz, odraz, přemítání

reflux /riː.flʌks/ reflux, zpětné proudění

regimen /ˈredʒ.ɪ.mən/ režim, životospráva

renal /ˈriː.nªl/ renální, ledvinový

respiratory /rɪˈspɪr.ə.tri/ respirační, dýchací

retention /rɪ'ten.tʃᵊn/ zácpa, zadržení, paměť

review /rɪ'vjuː/ prohlédnout, zhodnotit, konfrontovat, přehled

rheumatic /ruː'mæt.ɪk/ **fever** /'fiː.vəʳ/ revmatická horečka

rheumatoid arthritis /ˌruː.mə.tɔɪd. ɑː'θraɪ.tɪs/ kloubní revmatismus

rhinorrhoea /ˌraɪ.nə'ri.ə/ rinorea, vodnatý výtok z nosu

rigidity /rɪ'dʒɪd.ɪ.ti/ tuhost, strnulost, tvrdost

routine /ruː'tiːn/ pravidelný postup, běžná praxe, obvyklý, rutinní

scale /skeɪl/ váha (na vážení), zubní kámen, škála (stupnice)

sclera /'sklɪə.rə/ skléra, oční bělmo

secondary /'sek.ən.dri/ sekundární (druhotný), závislý-porucha

seizure /'siː.ʒəʳ/ uchopení, záchvat (nemoci), záchvatový

sensation /sen'seɪ.ʃᵊn/ pocit, cit, smyslové vnímání

sexual /'sek.sjʊəl/ **characteristic** /ˌkær.ɪk.tə'rɪs.tɪk/ pohlavní znak

sexually /'sek.sjʊə.li/ pohlavně

sialosis /ˌsaɪə'ləʊ.sɪs/ salivace, slinění

spectacles /'spek.tɪ.kl̩ z/ brýle (dioptrické)

sputum /'spjuː.təm/ sputum, výměšek dýchacího ústrojí

steatorrhoea /ˌstɪ.ə.tə'riː.ə/ steatorea, tuková stolice

steroid /'ste.rɔɪd/, /'stɪər.ɔɪd/ steroid, organická látka, např. hormony pohlavní nebo kůry nadledvin

stiffness /'stɪf.nəs/ strnulost, ztuhnutí

stomatitis /ˌstəʊ.mə'taɪ.tɪs/ stomatitida, zánět sliznice ústní dutiny

stool /stuːl/ sedačka, stolice (vyprazdňování střev)

stream /striːm/ běh, chod, příval, dělit, plynout

stroke /strəʊk/ úder, mrtvice, bití (pulsu), rána

stroke /strəʊk/ pohladit

supportive /sə'pɔː.tɪv/ **surgery** /'sɜː.dʒᵊr.i/ podpůrný chirurgický zákrok

susceptibility /sə,sep.tɪ'bɪl.ɪ.ti/ susceptibilita, náchylnost, citlivost

sweat /swet/ potit se, pot

swelling /'swel.ɪŋ/ otok, nádor, boule

syndrome /'sɪn.drəʊ m/ syndrom, příznak

systemic /sɪ'stem.ɪk/ systémový

taste /teɪst/ chuť, chutnat, záliba

tension /'tenʧ.ʃᵊn/ tenze, napínání (tahem), tlak

terminal /'tɜː.mɪ.nəl/ termínový, mezní, konečný, smrtelný

therapy /'θer.ə.pi/ terapie, léčba

thrive /θraɪv/ prospívat (dobře růst), dařit se

thyroid (gland) /'θaɪə.rɔɪd,glænd/ štítná žláza

time-consuming /'taɪm.kən,sjuː.mɪŋ/ časově náročný

tolerance /'tɒl.ᵊr.ᵊnʧ s/ tolerance (dovolená úchylka), snášenlivost, odolnost

transmit /trænz'mɪt/ přenášet, rozšířit

transplant /træn'splɑːnt/ transplantovat, transplantace, transplantovaný orgán

tremor /'trem.əʳ/ strach, třes, chvění

tuberculosis /tjuːˌbɜːkjʊ'ləʊ.sɪs/ tuberkulóza

tunnel /'tʌn.ᵊl/ tunel, nálevka, trychtýř, chodba

ulceration /ˌʌl.sᵊr'eɪ.ʃᵊn/ ulcerace, tvoření vředů, vředovitost

ulcerative /ˈʌl.sər.ə.tɪv/ **colitis** / kəʊ ˈlaɪ.təs/ ulcerativní kolitida (zánět tlustého střeva)

understanding /ˌʌn.dəˈstæn.dɪŋ/ pochopení (porozumění), rozum (inteligence), dohoda (vzájemná)

unpredictable /ˌʌn.prɪˈdɪk.tə.bl̩/ nepředvídatelný, neočekávaný

uraemia /jʊəˈriː.mi.ə/ uremie, chronické selhání činnosti ledvin

urea /jʊəˈriː.ə/ močovina

urgency /ˈɜː.dʒᵊnʧ.si/ nutná potřeba, nutnost (naléhavost)

urine /ˈjʊə.rɪn/ moč, močový

variable /ˈveə.ri.ə.bl̩/ variabilní (proměnlivý), nestálý, kolísavý

varicose vein /ˌvær.ɪ.kəʊ sˈveɪn/ varikózní žíla (křečová)

vasculitis /ˌvæs.kjʊˈlaɪ.tɪs/ vaskulitida, zánět cév

vertebra /ˈvɜː.tɪ.brə/ obratel, páteř

vertigo /ˈvɜː.tɪ.gəʊ/ závrať

vessel /ˈves.ᵊl/ céva, prázdná nádoba

vision /ˈvɪʒ.ᵊn/ vidění, zrak (pohled), zorný

voice /vɔɪs/ hlas, hlasový, vyjádřit (názor, mínění)

vomit /ˈvɒm.ɪt/ zvracet, zvracení

waken /ˈweɪ.kən/ probouzet se

wasting /ˈweɪst.ɪŋ/ zhoubný, ničivý, plýtvání

weakness /ˈwiːk.nəs/ slabá stránka, slabá odolnost, vada

weight /weɪt/ **loss** /lɒs/ úbytek váhy

weight /weɪt/ **bearing** /ˈbeə.rɪŋ/ nesoucí váhu

wheeze /wiːz/ sípat

worsening /ˈwɜː.sən.ɪŋ/ zhoršující se

Unit 7

Emergencies in Dental Practice. Medical Emergencies and Drugs

Team Care. Emergency Equipment and Drugs. Fainting. Acute Chest Pain. Cardiorespiratory Arrest. Anaphylactic Shock. Epilepsy. Asthma. Inhaled Foreign Bodies. Cerebrovascular Accidents (stroke). Types of Emergency, Resuscitation, and First Aid, Drug Therapy.

Text 1

Team Care

The concept of team care is essential in dealing with emergencies confidently and competently in the dental surgery. The dental team (surgeon, nurse, hygienist, receptionist, technician) should practise emergency procedures regularly and develop predetermined roles (e.g. opening emergency kit, telephoning for help).

Emergency Equipment and Drugs
Emergency equipment
- **portable defibrillator** (incorporating ECG printout)
- portable **oxygen delivery system**
- **Ambu bag** (self- inflating with valve and mask)
- cropharyngeal airways

- cricothyroid puncture needles
- high-volume **aspiration** with suction catheters
- disposable **syringes**
- **needles and butterflies**
- **tourniquet, sphygmomanometer,** and **stethoscope**
- venous access **cannulae**
- **IV infusion** sets
- sticks for rapid assessment of **blood sugar** levels

Emergency drugs
- **oxygen**
- **nitrous oxide**
- **epinephrine** (adrenaline) injection
- **hydrocortisone** injection
- **antihistamine** injections and tablets
- diazepam emulsion
- flumazenil injection
- **glucose** for injection and powder for oral use
- glucagon injection
- atropine sulphate injection
- salbutamol inhaler
- glyceryl trinitrate aerosol spray
- colloid solution for infusion

Exercise 1

List the necessary emergency equipment and drugs.

Translation 1
Koncepce týmové péče, procvičovat
pravidelně záchranné postupy,
nezbytný pro spolehlivé a kompetentní
zvládání naléhavých případů,
lékař, sestra, hygienista, recepční,
technik, předem určené úlohy,
otvírání pohotovostních lékárniček,
telefonování pro pomoc, vybavení
a léky pro první pomoc, přenosný
defibrilátor (s možností záznamu
EKG), přenosný kyslíkový přístroj,
ambu vak, samo-nafukovací s ventilem
a maskou, orofaryngeální průchody,
krikotyreoidní punkční jehly, jehly
pro koniopunkci, vysoko-objemové
odsávání se sacími katétry, stříkačky
na jedno použití, jehly a motýlky,
škrtidlo, přístroj na měření tepu a
krevních plynů, stetoskop, kanyly
na venózní přístup (venózní kanyly),
sety na intravenózní infuse, tyčinky
na rychlé určení úrovně cukru
v krvi, indikátorové tyčinky do
glukometru, kyslík, oxid dusný (rajský
plyn), injekce adrenalinu, injekce
hydrokortisonu, antihistaminika -
injekce a tablety, emulze diazepamu,
glukóza injekční a prášek pro
ústní užití, injekce glukagonu,
inhalátor salbutamolu, aerosol sprej
nitroglycerinu, koloidní roztok pro
infuze.

Text 2
Fainting
Dentistry predisposes to fainting due
to fear, pain, unusual sights and smells,
anxiety, fatigue, and fasting.
Symptoms and signs
- **light-headed** feeling
- **warm, sweaty** feeling
- **pallor**
- **skin cool and moist** to touch
- **bradycardia**
- loss of consciousness and **collapse** with resultant rapid, full pulse

Management
- lie patient flat with **head bellow heart**
- determine bradycardia by **taking pulse at major vessel**
- **loosen clothing** and open windows
- establish verbal **encouragement** of patient and administer **glucose**
- delay dental treatment unless urgent

Acute Chest Pain
Symptoms and signs
- severe **crushing retrosternal pain**
- **radiations** to arm, neck, or jaw
- myocardial **infarction** likely if pain is accompanied by **breathlessness**, **nausea**, **vomiting**, loss of consciousness, weak/ **irregular pulse**, **hypotension**

Management
- give patient's own medication
- wait 3 minutes and repeat if necessary, then assume MI
- send for **medical assistance** by 112
- do not lie flat as it increases feelings of breathlessness and panic
- administer nitrous oxide and oxygen as **pain relief**
- obtain **venous access** in case CPR is required
- establish verbal **encouragement** of patient
- administer oral **aspirin** (one tablet) as antiplatelet agent
- **urgent transfer** to hospital

Cardiorespiratory Arrest

Signs

- **loss of consciousness**
- **absence of central arterial pulses**
- **absence of breath** sounds/chest movement

Management

- **assess responsiveness** by gently shaking the patient and shouting 'Are you all right?'
- send for help and get helper to **summon medical assistance** by dialling 112
- **lie patient flat** on the floor on his or her back
- open the airway with a gentle **head tilt and chin lift**
- **look, listen, and feel for** normal **breathing**
- if the patient is not breathing or the attempts are weak, give **two slow, effective rescue breaths**
- check for **signs of a circulation at the carotid** pulse (take no longer than 10 seconds to do this)
- if there is evidence of a circulation, continue rescue breaths until the patient is able to breathe unaided
- if there is **no evidence** of a circulation, **start chest compressions** at a **rate 100 per minute; after 15 compressions, give two effective breaths** and continue compressions and breaths in a **ratio 15:2**
- the same regimen should be used for one and two-rescuer resuscitation
- the patient should be turned to the **recovery position** when he or she shows evidence of recovery; otherwise continue resuscitation

until help arrives and takes over or you become exhausted

Exercise 2

Write short notes about: fainting, acute chest pain, cardiorespiratory arrest.

Translation 2

Mdloby kvůli strachu, bolesti, nezvyklé podívané, pachům, úzkosti, slabosti, hladovění, pocit závrati, pocit horka, pocení, nadměrná bledost, pokožka na dotek chladná a vlhká, bradykardie, ztráta vědomí a zhroucení s následným rychlým a silným pulsem, položte pacienta rovně, hlava je níže než srdce, změřte puls na hlavní cévě, rozhodněte, zda jde o bradykardii, uvolněte oděv a otevřete okna, zahajte slovní povzbuzování pacienta a podejte glukózu, odložte ošetření úst, není-li naléhavé, náhlá bolest na hrudi, krutá drtivá bolest za hrudní kostí, vyzařování do paže, krku nebo čelisti, infarkt myokardu, bolest doprovázena dušností, nevolností, zvracením, ztrátou vědomí, slabý, nepravidelný puls, snížený tlak, podejte pacientovi jeho vlastní léky, nepokládejte pacienta dolů, zvyšuje to pocity dušnosti a paniky, podejte ústy jednu tabletu aspirinu proti srážlivosti krve, naléhavý převoz do nemocnice, zástava srdeční a dechová, ztráta vědomí, absence pulsu na hlavních tepnách, absence zvuků dechu a pohybů hrudníku, zatřeste lehce pacientem a zavolejte "Jste v pořádku?", pošlete pro pomoc, položte pacienta na podlahu rovně na záda, otevřete dýchací cesty jemným zakloněním hlavy a vytáhnutím čelisti, pátrejte zrakem, sluchem a hmatem po normálním dýchání, pacient nedýchá, poskytněte dva pomalé, účinné záchranné vdechy, kontrolujte známky cirkulace na pulsu karotidy, pokračujte se záchrannými vdechy, dokud pacient není schopen dýchat bez pomoci, známky cirkulace chybí, zahajte stlačování hrudníku v rytmu 100 za minutu, po 15 stlačeních dejte dva účinné vdechy a pokračujte ve stlačování a dýchání v poměru 15:2, známky zotavení, uložit do stabilizované polohy.

Text 3
Anaphylactic Shock
Symptoms and signs:
* **facial flushing**
* **itching** of the skin
* **paraesthesia**, particularly of the extremities, face, and lips
* **oedema**
* **wheezing**
* **abdominal pain**, nausea, and vomiting
* **panic** with loss of consciousness
* facial flushing is replaced by **pallor** and then by **cyanosis**
* **skin** becomes **cold and clammy**
* **pulse** is **weak** (often impalpable) and **rapid**
* **blood pressure is low** and often unrecordable

Management
* lay patient flat and **raise the legs**
* if cardiorespiratory arrest occurs proceed with **CPR**
* **urgent transfer** to hospital

Epilepsy
Stress, fasting, hypoglycaemia, and fainting can all cause a fit in the

surgery. **Seizures** are often preceded by an **aura**, followed rapidly by **loss of consciousness** and a rigid, extended body (**tonic phase**) and jerking or flailing movements (**clonic phase**). Postictal **drowsiness** and the desire to sleep follow. Most fits last less than 5 minutes and require no intervention except **protecting the patient from self-inflicted damage**.

Asthma
Asthma may be predisposed to by **anxiety**. The underlying problem is that of respiratory tract hyperactivity with resultant bronchospasm.
Symptoms and signs:
* **breathlessness**
* **wheezing**
* **panic** and fear
* if severe, inability to speak

Inhaled Foreign Bodies
If simple **coughing** does not dislodge the offending article, give up to **five sharp slaps** between the shoulder blades.
If this is unsuccessful, the **Heimlich manoeuvre** should be performed: the patient is **encircled by your arms from behind** at the level of the lower border of the **rib cage** and a sudden **forceful squeeze** is exerted by pulling your arms together with the hands directed **upwards** towards the chest. With small children, swinging the patient around by the legs may be sufficient to dislodge the article.

Cerebrovascular Accidents (stroke)
Cerebrovascular accidents are uncommon dental emergencies.

Management:
- maintain the airway
- urgent transfer to hospital

Exercise 3

Write short notes about anaphylactic shock, epilepsy, asthma, and inhaled foreign bodies at the dental practice.

Translation 3

Anafylaktický šok, zrudnutí obličeje, svědění pokožky, poruchy citlivosti, zejména na končetinách, obličeji a rtech, otok, sípání, bolest břicha, nevolnost, zvracení, panika se ztrátou vědomí, nadměrná bledost, promodrání, chladná, vlhce lepkavá pokožka, puls je slabý, nehmatný, rychlý, krevní tlak nízký, nelze zaznamenat, položte pacienta na záda a zvedněte mu nohy, srdeční a dechová zástava, kardiopulmonární resuscitace, epilepsie, stres, hladovění, hypoglykémie, mdloba mohou způsobit záchvat v ordinaci, záchvaty jsou často předcházeny aurou, ztráta vědomí, tělo ztuhlé a napjaté (tonická fáze), pohyby trhavé nebo ochromené (klonická fáze), po záchvatu ospalost a touha spát, většina záchvatů netrvá déle než 5 minut a nevyžaduje jiný zásah než ochranu pacienta před sebepoškozením, astma, základním problémem je nadměrná aktivita respiračního traktu s výsledným bronchiálním spasmem, dušnost, sípání, panika, strach, neschopnost mluvit, vdechnutí cizího tělíska, kašlání neodstraní obtěžující předmět, dejte až pět ostrých plesknutí mezi lopatky, provést Heimlichův manévr, zezadu obemkněte pacienta rukama, dolní

hranice hrudního koše, ruce míří nahoru směrem k hrudníku, náhlé prudké stlačení, cerebrovaskulární příhody, mrtvice, v dentální praxi neobvyklé, udržet dýchací cesty, naléhavý převoz do nemocnice.

Text 4

Types of Emergency, Resuscitation, and First Aid, Drug Therapy

A simple faint

Patients appear **pale with clammy skin,** they suddenly **collapse,** and their **pulse is weak but rapid.** It is caused by **a lack of oxygenated blood to the brain**, especially when the patient is fearful or anxious of the onset of a painful episode. Treatment is therefore aimed at improving the circulation of oxygenated blood to the brain. **Undo tight neck clothing,** keep the **patient lying down, and raise their legs.** Ensure the patient has a supply of fresh air, or even give oxygen therapy. Monitor the pulse, and reassure the patient as they recover.

A grand mal epileptic fit

This is the most severe form of epilepsy and is caused by **abnormal electrical impulses in the brain.** The patient may appear vacant or report a **visible or olfactory aura.** Sudden **loss of consciousness** will occur, accompanied by jerking movements. The patient may lose continence. Recovery is slow, and the patient is often confused afterwards. Management is based on ensuring that the **patient does not injure themselves during the fit,** but under no circumstances should an attempt be made to insert any kind of mouth prop—not only could this compromise the patient's airway but the first-aider is likely to get their own fingers bitten. **Maintain the patient's airway**, and give oxygen therapy if necessary. Unless the patient is an undiagnosed epileptic, allow the patient to go home with an escort once they have made a full recovery. If they are undiagnosed, ensure the patient is escorted to a hospital.

Respiratory arrest

Respiratory arrest is due to loss of a patent airway; in the dental surgery this is most likely to be due to **obstruction with a foreign body**. The patient will cough uncontrollably, their face will become congested, and consciousness will be lost. When respiration ceases, the lips will appear blue.

The situation is **life-threatening and speed is required** to avoid a fatality. In the dental surgery, use the high-speed **suction apparatus** to clear any obvious oral blockage. Grasp and pull the **tongue forwards** if it has fallen into the throat. Open the patient's airway by **lifting the neck up while tilting the head back**— respiration may often commence spontaneously at this point. If not, begin **mouth-to-mask ventilations with oxygen therapy. Call for help.** Under no circumstances leave the patient unattended. Ensure the patient is transferred to a hospital if there is no obvious cause or if recovery is not complete following the clearing of any obstruction.

Severe chest pain

If the **pain is of sudden onset and severe**, it should be assumed that the cause is either **angina or a heart attack** (myocardial infarction, MI). Angina is the likeliest cause if the pain occurs immediately after exertion; it is due to a poor oxygenated blood supply to the heart muscle itself. Tell the patient they must **sit down and rest**. Place a **glyceryl trinitirate** (GTN) tablet under their tongue, or administer an oral spray of the same (one or the other should be kept at the practice with other emergency drugs), and give **oxygen therapy**.

As angina sufferers often suffer a heart attack, ensure they are **taken to a hospital** for investigation and coronary care. **Myocardial infarction** occurs following a sudden loss of oxygenated blood to the heart muscle, with death of that part of the heart muscle. The **pain is not relieved by rest** and usually lasts for more than 30 minutes.

The **situation is life-threatening**, as **heart failure or cardiac arrhythmias** may develop. Summon **emergency help** immediately.

Keep the **patient sitting upright**, and reassure them. Give oxygen therapy. The latest information suggest that an **aspirin** given at this point may prevent heart failure ensuing. However, the patient may be vomiting, so administration may not be possible. Ensure the patient is **taken to a hospital by ambulance for coronary care** and investigation.

Exercise 4

How should the following emergencies be dealt with?

- A simple faint
- A grand mal epileptic fit
- Respiratory arrest
- Severe chest pain

Translation 4

Pacient se zdá bledý, náhle kolabuje, puls je slabý, rychlý, pacient má strach, je úzkostný, zlepšení oběhu, rozvázat těsný oděv u krku, zásoba čerstvého vzduchu, léčba kyslíkem, uklidňovat pacienta když se zotaví, velký epileptický záchvat, abnormální elektrické impulsy v mozku, pacient se zdá netečný, zraková, čichová aura (předzvěst), náhlá ztráta vědomí, možná inkontinence, neporanit se během záchvatu, nevkládat žádnou podporu, poškodit dýchací cesty pacienta nebo si nechat pokousat prsty, zotavit se úplně, jít domů s doprovodem, zástava dechu kvůli ucpání cizím tělískem, kašlat nezvladatelně, překrvený obličej, dojde ke ztrátě vědomí, dýchání ustává, modré rty, život ohrožující situace, vyčistit zjevnou překážku v ústech, přístroj na vysoko-rychlostní odsávání, uchopte a vytáhněte jazyk dopředu, pokud zapadl do hrdla, často dýchání může začít samovolně, nenechávejte pacienta bez dozoru za žádných okolností, krutá bolest na hrudi s náhlým nástupem, předpokládaná příčina je buď angína pectoris nebo srdeční záchvat, bolest nastává ihned po námaze, sednout si a odpočinout, dát tabletku pod jazyk, podat ústní sprej, infarkt myokardu, následující po náhlé ztrátě okysličené krve v srdečním svalu s odumřením příslušné části, bolest není zmírněna odpočinkem,

trvá víc než 30 minut, srdeční selhání, srdeční arytmie, nechte pacienta sedět zpříma, dejte aspirin, kyslíkovou terapii, vzít pacienta do nemocnice sanitkou.

Text 5

Basic first-aid procedures

1. **Check a pulse**

A pulse can be felt wherever an artery travels across bone. Usual points of taking a pulse are the carotid pulse in the neck and the radial pulse in the wrist. It should be taken **using fingers, not a thumb**, as your own pulse can be felt in the thumb.

Carotid pulse: find the muscle which lies on either side of the trachea in the neck, slide the fingers up towards the mandible along this muscle, and the pulse should be felt about halfway up the muscle.

Radial pulse: turn the patient's wrist up then place your first three fingers (touching a flat) below the base of their thumb so that your third finger is at their wrist. Exert a little pressure, and the pulse should be felt under your middle finger.

2. **Clear and open an airway**

Clear the airway by hooking a **finger around the oral cavity** and **removing any debris**, or by using a portable or mains-operated **suction unit**.

Open the airway by **lying the casualty on their back**, placing one hand firmly under their neck for support, then placing the flat of the other hand on the patient's forehead and pushing down so their **head is tilted right back**—the airway opens naturally in this position. Hold the head in this position; otherwise, it will tend to slump forwards and close the airway.

3.   **Stop venous bleeding**
Venous bleeding is bleeding **under low pressure** from a vein. It will gush from a wound and is dark red in colour. The best method of stopping venous bleeding is to **apply direct pressure** to the bleeding site, with the fingers if necessary, but **ideally with a sterile pad** to reduce the risk of infection. If a **large wound** is involved, physically **hold the edges of the wound together** to allow clotting to occur naturally. If the **bleeding point is on a limb, elevate the limb** above the level of the heart so that blood flow is reduced.

4.   **Do mouth-to-mask ventilation**
Mouth-to-mask ventilation is required following respiratory arrest. First clear the airway of any obstructions. **Open the airway** by lifting the patient's head with a hand placed under their neck and pushing down onto the forehead with the palm of the other hand. **Blow into the mask through the valve**, at a rate of 20 breaths a minute for patients in respiratory arrest. If full cardiopulmonary resuscitation (CPR) is being administered, the latest recommended **CPR ratio with chest compressions** should be given—i.e. **30 chest compressions at a rate of 100 per minute to 2 breaths.**

First-aid requirements

All staff must be trained in basic first aid on an annual basis, and there should be a nominated and named first-aider in the practice.
A first-aid kit must be available, containing a selection of sterile dressings, pads, plasters, and disposable sachets of sterile saline, as a minimum.
An emergency drugs kit and oxygen cylinder must also be held in stock, with all items present within their shelf-life dates.
An accident book must be available, to fully record all accidents involving staff, patients, and visitors to the practice.
All staff should be comfortable with providing reassurance and **help to a casualty until paramedics arrive, including the skills to maintain life** if necessary.

'Doctor ABC'
Pronounced 'Doctor ABC', this **abbreviation** is used as an aide-memoire **during an emergency situation** by those who have minimal opportunity to practise their first-aid skills in real life, such as dental staff. It **sets out the sequence** in which the first-aider should **approach, assess, and help** the casualty in order to give the best chance of maintaining life until advanced help arrives.
Dangers – area around the casualty should be assessed for any dangers to the first-aider, such as **chemical spillages and electrical supplies**, before approaching the casualty.
Responsiveness – level of alertness of the casualty should be determined by **calling to them and gently shaking them.** This determines if they are

fully conscious, semiconscious and possibly disorientated, or unconscious and unresponsive. At this point the first-aider should **shout for help if there is no response** from the casualty. **Airway** – should be visibly checked for **blockages** (vomit, pieces of fractured tooth, or other debris) which **should be removed**, ideally using suction equipment; the casualty's head should then be tilted back and supported to **maintain an open airway**.

Breathing – signs of spontaneous breathing should be checked: look to **see if the chest rises, listen for breath sounds,** and **feel for any breath by placing the cheek close to the casualty's nose and mouth**. If breathing is abnormal or absent after 10 seconds, call the emergency services.

Circulation – the first-aider should begin **external heart massage** by performing 30 chest compressions at the rate of 100 per minute—effectively **squeezing the heart between the sternum and the spine** and maintaining a blood flow around the body but most importantly to the brain—followed by 2 ventilations, either using a mask or the mouth-to-mouth technique. This sequence should be **continued until the patient revives, the first-aider is exhausted, or help arrives.**

Exercise 5

1. The following are all basic first-aid procedures. How would you:
   - Check a pulse
   - Clear and open an airway
   - Stop venous bleeding

   - Do mouth-to-mask ventilation
2. List the basic first-aid requirements that should be held by all dental practices.
3. Briefly describe the use of the abbreviation DRABC when dealing with a medical emergency.

Translation 5

Základní postupy první pomoci, kontrolovat puls, puls na karotidě, na krku, radiální puls, na zápěstí, použít prsty, ne palec, vykonat malý tlak, cítit puls pod prostředníčkem, vyčistit, a otevřít dýchací cesty, odstranit zbytky, ruční odsávací jednotka, položení postiženého na záda, hlava je zakloněna dozadu, dýchací cesty se otevřou přirozeně, zastavit žilní krvácení, vytékání z rány, použít přímý tlak na místo krvácení, sterilní čtverec, pokud jde o velkou ránu, přidržte okraje rány k sobě, zvednout končetinu, omezit tok krve, dýchání pomocí masky, foukat do masky přes ventil rychlostí 20 dechů za minutu, v případě zástavy dechu, u kardiopulmonární resuscitace 30 stlačení s rychlostí 100 za minutu po 2 vdechnutích, požadavky na první pomoc, lékárna první pomoci, sterilní obvazy, čtverce, náplasti, sáčky s fyziologickým roztokem na jedno použití, souprava léků pro naléhavé případy, kyslíkový přístroj, všechny věci v platné době použití, zaznamenat všechny nehody, udržet naživu, zkratka doktor ABC, stanovit pořadí, přístup, zhodnocení, pomoc, nebezpečí, rozlití chemických látek, elektřina, reakce, při vědomí úplně, napolo, možná dezorientovaný, v bezvědomí, bez reakce, dýchací cesty, zkontrolovat zrakem překážky (zvratky, kousky zlomeného zubu a jiné zbytky), dýchání, podívat se, zda se hruď zvedá, poslouchat zvuky dechu, pocítit přiložením tváře blízko úst a nosu postiženého, dýchání abnormální, chybí, po 10 vteřinách, volejte pohotovostní službu, cirkulace, zahájit vnější masáž srdce, zmáčknutí srdce mezi hrudní kostí a páteří.

Text 6

1. **Scald from autoclave steam**
A scald is a **wet burn that causes rapid and painful blistering** of the exposed area. The casualty should be removed from steam or hot liquid source immediately. The scalded area should be **immersed in cold water** for a minimum of 10 minutes to cool the tissues down and reduce the amount of blistering that occurs.

All jewellery (including rings) **should be removed** from the affected area **before swelling occurs**; otherwise, these items will constrict the tissues. **Clothing should not be removed as it may be stuck to the skin** and removing it may cause further tissue damage. The area should **be covered with a nonadhesive dressing**; medical attention should be sought if the scalded area is extensive.

The incident should be recorded in the accident book, and a risk assessment of the event should be carried out to determine how it occurred and how to prevent recurrences.

2. **Faint in the dental reception area**

The patient will have either slumped in their chair or have fallen to the floor. The patient **should be placed onto the floor with their legs higher than their head, to improve blood flow to the brain**. Help should be summoned, and **onlookers cleared away** to maintain the patient's dignity, as sometimes incontinence occurs. Tight neck clothing should be loosened, and ventilation to the reception area improved.

The patient should be reassured as they regain consciousness and recover. A glucose drink or glucose tablet should be provided on recovery to **raise their blood glucose** levels.

The practice should ensure the patient has an escort home. The incident should be recorded in the accident book and on the patient's record card.

3. **Clean needlestick injury**
A clean needlestick injury indicates that there is **no risk of cross-infection** to the injured person. The area should **be run under a cold tap to encourage haemostasis**. Once achieved, the area should be thoroughly **dried and antiseptic cream** applied over it. The area should then be covered with a **waterproof plaster**. No clinical work should be carried out without **wearing gloves**.

The **incident should be recorded** in the accident book, and a risk assessment of the event carried out to determine how it happened and how to prevent further occurrences.

4. **Eye injury from a speck of amalgam**

All dental treatment should be stopped immediately. The **affected eye should be irrigated with copious amounts of saline**, using the disposable sachets of sterile saline **from the first-aid kit**. Medicated drops should not be put into the eye. If the speck of amalgam is successfully removed, staff should **ensure the casualty's vision is unaffected** and continue with treatment if possible, ensuring that everyone is wearing safety glasses. **If removal is unsuccessful, an eye pad should be placed** over affected eye and the **patient removed to a hospital** for further treatment. In any case, the incident should be recorded in the accident book, and a risk assessment carried out to determine how the incident happened and how to prevent recurrences.

Exercise 6
Briefly describe the first-aid treatment that should be carried out for the following emergencies:
• Scald from autoclave steam
• Faint in the dental reception area
• Clean needlestick injury
• Eye injury from a speck of amalgam

Translation 6
Opaření parou z autoklávu nebo horkou tekutinou, rychlé, bolestivé vytvoření puchýřů, ponořit do studené vody nejméně na 10 minut, odstranit šperky než nastane otok, oblečení může být přichycené ke kůži, poškození tkáně, pokrýt nepřilnavým obvazem, vyhledat lékařskou pomoc, zabránit opakovanému výskytu, mdloba,

zhroutit se na židli, upadnout na zem, zavolat pomoc, odstranit přihlížející, zachovat pacientovu důstojnost, poranění čistou jehlou, žádné riziko přenosu, dát pod studenou vodu, osušit, použít antiseptický krém, krýt nepromokavou náplastí, poranění oka úlomkem amalgámu, okamžitě zastavit zubní ošetření, vypláchnout postižené oko velkým množstvím fyziologického roztoku, použít sáčky z lékárničky první pomoci, odstranit zrnko, ujistit se, že vidění postiženého není zasaženo, nosit rukavice, bezpečnostní brýle.

Text 7
Symptoms and signs of the most common medical emergencies
The signs will be what the first-aider sees, whereas the symptoms are what the casualty actually feels during the emergency.

Anaphylactic shock
Anaphylactic shock occurs when a casualty has a severe allergic reaction to an allergen.
Signs – within minutes of exposure to the allergen, **skin flushing and facial swelling** occur, followed by **pallor and then cyanosis** as breathing becomes more difficult due to throat constriction. Sudden hypotension causes **collapse, loss of consciousness,** and **possible cardiac arrest** if untreated.
Symptoms – **paraesthesia and tingling** of the extremities, **difficulty in breathing.**

Epileptic fit
Epileptic fits can either be mild (petit mal) or severe (grand mal).

Signs

Mild – casualty appears to be **daydreaming and inattentive**, eyes may be unfocused and staring, may become unconscious briefly but are rarely confused on recovery.

Severe – **sudden loss of consciousness, with muscle rigidity followed by jerking movements** (known as tonic-clonic seizures), incontinence often occurs, casualty may be confused during recovery.

Symptoms (mild or severe) – casualty can experience **an aura** (such as a certain smell) before the fit begins; they are **rarely aware of their surroundings during the fit**. Those suffering from a severe fit are often disorientated and confused during recovery.

Simple faint

A simple faint occurs when there is a temporary reduction in oxygenated blood flow to the brain.

Signs – **skin pallor and clamminess**, especially on the brow and upper lip, followed by a **brief loss of consciousness**. The **pulse will be weak and thready**, and the casualty may yawn repeatedly before collapsing.

Symptoms – casualty will **feel unwell and light-headed**, followed by **dizziness and tunnel vision** just before they **lose consciousness**. When a faint occurs, the casualty **should be placed supine with their legs higher than their head** to improve blood flow to the brain. Tight neck **clothing should be loosened** or removed and **good ventilation provided** to the area. Oxygen can be provided, but recovery is usually rapid. A **glucose** drink or

tablet should be given to raise the casualty's blood glucose levels.

Cardiac arrest

Cardiac arrest occurs when the casualty has collapsed and **no central pulse is present**. The first-aid principles described by the abbreviation DRABC would have been followed to determine that cardiac arrest had occurred, as given bellow:

- **Dangers** – would assess for any external causes of the emergency, such as **electrocution or inhalation of poisonous vapours**.
- **Responsiveness** – would gently shake and call to the casualty to **determine their level of consciousness** and would shout for help to **raise the alarm**.
- **Airway** – would be checked for an **obstruction, clearing** it as necessary with suction equipment if possible, or a finger sweep if equipment was not at hand, then **the head would be tilted back and the chin lifted** to open and maintain the airway.
- **Breathing** – would **look, listen, and feel for breath sounds** for 10 seconds while **observing the chest movement**. The **emergency services** (112) would be called if breathing was abnormal or absent.
- **Circulation** – **the base of the sternum** would be identified and 30 **cardiac compressions** performed over this site at a rate of 100 per minute—to compress the heart between the spine and the sternum and effectively **maintain blood flow to the major organs and brain**—followed

76

by 2 **ventilations** using a mask or ideally an Ambu bag or the mouth-to-mouth technique.

The **carotid pulse would be checked every minute**, and **CPR continued** until the patient revived, the first-aider exhausted, or help arrived. CPR is extremely tiring to administer. But the **ventilations and chest compressions would be efficiently carried out** in compliance with the latest recommendations—30 chest compressions at a rate of 100 per minute followed by 2 breaths— between all trained first-aiders present, **with no breaks**, until the patient revived, the first-aiders were exhausted, or help arrived.

Three drugs that should be kept in the emergency drug box:
- Adrenaline 1:1, 000 – to be given intramuscularly during anaphylactic shock
- GTN spray – to be used orally during a suspected angina attack
- Salbutamol inhaler – to be used orally during an asthma attack

Exercise 7
1. Describe the signs and symptoms of the following medical emergencies:
- Anaphylactic shock
- Epileptic fit
- Simple faint
2. Explain the action to be taken in the event of a simple faint.
3. Describe in detail the first-aid action you would take in the event of a cardiac arrest.

4. List three drugs that should be kept in the emergency drug box of all dental practices, indicating the emergency they should be used for.

Translation 7

Znaky, to co vidíme, symptomy, to co postižený pociťuje, anafylaktický šok nastává jako závažná reakce na alergen, zčervenání kůže, otok obličeje, bledost, cyanóza, kolaps, ztráta vědomí, srdeční zástava, změněná citlivost, mravenčení končetin, obtíže s dýcháním, epileptický záchvat, mírný, denní snění, nepozorný, oči nezaostřené, zírající, krátce v bezvědomí, zřídka zmatený při zotavení, epileptický záchvat, závažný, náhlá ztráta vědomí, svalová ztuhlost, trhavé pohyby, tonicko-klonické záchvaty, inkontinence, zmatený během zotavování, mdloba, dočasné omezení toku okysličené krve do mozku, bledost a lepkavost kůže, na oboří a horním rtu, krátká ztráta vědomí, puls slabý, nitkovitý, před zhroucením opakovaně zívat, cítit nevolnost, lehká závrať, závrať, tunelové vidění, rychlé zotavení, poskytnout kyslík, nápoj s glukózou či tabletku, zástava srdce, kolaps, není puls, vnější příčiny, úraz elektrickým proudem, nadýchání jedovatých výparů, určit úroveň vědomí, volat o pomoc, vyvolat poplach, dýchací cesty, vyčistit prstem, když odsávací zařízení není po ruce, hlava zakloněná, brada zvednutá, dýchání, dívat se, poslouchat zvuky dechu, procítit, pozorovat pohyb hrudníku, cirkulace, udržet tok krve do hlavních orgánů a mozku ventilace, ambu-vak, technika z úst do úst, kontrolovat puls na karotidě každou minutu, pokračovat CPR bez přestávek, dokud pacient není oživen, zachránce vyčerpán, nebo nepřijede pomoc, léky uložené v pohotovostní lékárničce, adrenalin, k podání do svalu během anafylaktického šoku, GTN sprej k použití ústně při podezření na záchvat angíny pectoris, inhalátor salbutamolu k ústnímu použití během astmatického záchvatu.

Text 8

Types of Emergency, Resuscitation, and First Aid, Drug Therapy
Study the following information and answer questions in exercise 5.

- The five **signs of acute inflammation** are

heat, swelling, redness, pain, and loss of function.

- **Medical emergencies and their treatment:**

Treatment	Medical emergency
Oxygen	faint; cardiac arrest; angina attack; anaphylaxis; epileptic fit; steroid crisis; hypoglycaemia
Epinephrine (adrenaline)	anaphylaxis; cardiac attack
GTN spray	angina attack
Aspirin	suspected myocardial infarction
Glucagon	unconscious hypoglycaemia

- **The sequence of events during cardiopulmonary resuscitation** (CPR): Dangers, Responsiveness, Airway, Breathing, Circulation
- In the event of someone having **an epileptic fit** you should remove

any dangerous objects from the area.

- Study the table bellow giving **signs and symptoms** of the most urgent medical emergencies:

Emergency	Signs	Symptoms
Angina attack	irregular pulse, shallow breathing, distressed	crushing chest pain, breathlessness, nausea
Faint	Pale and clammy, and thready pulse, loss of consciousness	light-headed, dizzy, weak tunnel vision, nauseous,
Epileptic fit	loss of consciousness, tonic-clonic seizure, incontinence	aura before fit, confusion during recovery
Anaphylactic shock	Flushing and swelling of face/neck, low blood pressure, breathing difficulties, collapse	tingling of extremities, acute breathing difficulties

- A **sphygmomanometer** can be used to measure a patient's blood pressure.
- **Hypoglycaemia** is a condition that may occur in diabetes.
- The first action to take in the event of **inoculation injury** is to squeeze the wound.
- These are the drugs that should be kept in the **emergency drugs box**. They would be used for the following medical emergencies:

Drug	Emergency
Epinephrine (adrenaline)	used for cardiac arrest and anaphylaxis

Aspirin	used for suspected myocardial infarction
Diazepam	used for severe epileptic fits (status epilepticus)
GTN spray or tablet	used for angina attack
Salbutamol inhaler	used for asthma attack
Glucagon	used for hypoglycaemia when the patient has become unconscious
Glucose	used for faints and conscious hypoglycaemia
Hydrocortisone	used for steroid crisis and anaphylaxis
Chlorphenamine	used for anaphylaxis

• Think about the **possible cause** for each of the following events in the dental surgery:

Event	Cause
Burn	naked flame, touching hot equipment or instrument, fire
Poisoning	ingestion of any poisonous substance or liquid
Scald	autoclave steam
Choking	inhalation of any foreign object or debris

• The first-aid treatment that should be given to a patient suffering **an angina attack** is oxygen therapy, GTN tablet or spray, and reassurance.

Exercise 8

1. Which are the signs of acute inflammation?
2. State a medical emergency that each of the following may be used for: oxygen, adrenaline, GTN spray, aspirin, glucagons.
3. Complete the right sequence of events during cardiopulmonary resuscitation (CPR).
4. What should the first-aider do in the event of someone having an epileptic fit?
5. Give the signs and symptoms of the following medical emergencies: angina attack, faint, epileptic fit, anaphylactic shock.
6. Which can be used to measure a patient's blood pressure?
7. When can hypoglycaemia occur?
8. What is the first action to take in the event of inoculation injury?
9. List the drugs that should be kept in the emergency drugs box, and state the medical emergency they would be used for.
10. Give one possible cause for each of the following events in the dental surgery: burn, poisoning, scald, choking.
11. What is the first-aid treatment that should be given to a patient suffering an angina attack?

Exercise 9 / Homework

The sentences have been divided into separate halves. Match the half-sentences in column A with the half-sentences in column B to make sentences which are complete and correct.

A
1. A salbutamol inhaler is an emergency drug kept for patients who suffer from asthma and acts by . . .
2. Atenolol is a drug that many patients take for hypertension and is important when the patient undergoes dental treatment because . . .
3. Patients taking oral contraceptives should be warned of the risk

79

involved in pregnancy when prescribed . . .

4. Patients allergic to penicillin can safely be prescribed . . .

5. Lidocaine is present at most dental surgeries as a local anaesthetic and also as . . .

6. Ibuprofen is . . .

7. Patients whose lips go blue are suffering from respiratory arrest and should be treated by . . .

8. Patients taking steroids should carry a medical warning because . . .

9. Chlorhexidine is a . . .

10. Blue compressed-gas canisters contain . . .

11. A patient suffering from diabetes requires appointments timed . . .

12. Aclovir is an antiviral drug, which can be prescribed especially for . . .

13. Long-term aspirin therapy must be taken by patients to avoid stroke and care should be taken when these patients are to have . . .

14. The likeliest emergency to be seen in the dental surgery is a simple faint, which can be diagnosed by . . .

15. Anaphylaxis is . . .

B

a) *by removing any blockage, providing a patent airway and giving oxygen therapy immediately.*

b) *indicates an underlying cardiovascular problem.*

c) *herpes labialis (cold sores).*

d) *they are likely to collapse if the treatment is stopped suddenly for any reason.*

e) *a nonsteroidal anti-inflammatory drug (NSAID) with analgesic properties.*

f) *dilating the bronchioles and allowing sufficient oxygen to enter the lungs.*

g) *minor oral surgery or extractions.*

h) *disinfectant.*

i) *nitrous oxide.*

j) *not to interfere with their normal meal times, nor should they be kept waiting if at all possible.*

k) *a severe allergic reaction to an allergen.*

l) *antibiotics by the dentist.*

m) *the sudden collapse of the patient, who will be pale, cold, and clammy, and whose pulse will be weak but rapid.*

n) *erythromycin as an alternative.*

o) *an emergency drug to prevent cardiac arrhythmias.*

Exercise 10 / Homework

The sentences have been divided into separate halves. Match the half-sentences in column A with the half-sentences in column B to make sentences which are complete and correct.

A

1. GTN stands for glyceryl trinitrate and is an emergency drug required . . .

2. Patients with reactionary haemorrhage should . . .

3. Metronidazole is an antibiotic, and is the drug of choice when treating . . .

4. Nystatin is used to treat oral candidiasis (thrush), which often occurs . . .

5. Felypressin is a vasoconstrictor and is usually reserved . . .
6. An injury sustained from steam is called a scald and should . . .
7. A petit mal is . . .
8. Patients with a history of rheumatic fever require antibiotics cover for all invasive dental treatment because . . .
9. Patients suffering from chickenpox are infected with . . .
10. The likeliest patients to suffer from osteoporosis are postmenopausal women, and the condition has an effect on dental treatment, in that they are . . .
11. A haemostatic drug is one that . . .
12. The quickest route for a drug to take effect is . . .
13. The shelf life of a drug is . . .
14. Diazepam is a . . .
15. Glucagon is an emergency drug used for . . .

B

a) *when a patient suffers an angina attack to prevent the precipitation of a heart attack.*
b) *be treated by immersing the scalded area under cold water immediately.*
c) *be sat upright with a bite pack in situ until the dentist arrives.*
d) *causes blood flow to stop.*
e) *in fully or partially edentate patients.*
f) *acute ulcerative gingivitis.*
g) *for patients who cannot be given adrenaline-containing local anaesthetics.*
h) *a mild form of an epileptic fit.*
i) *reversing hypoglycaemia.*

j) *more likely to experience jaw fracture.*
k) *bacteria from the mouth which enter the blood will pass to the heart and cause endocarditis.*
l) *by being injected intravenously.*
m) *a sedative prescribed to anxious patients.*
n) *the length of time after its manufacture that is considered in date and safe to use.*
o) *herpes varicella virus.*

Exercise 11 / Homework

Fill in the missing words. Choose the correct ones.

1. Drugs used to kill _____ causing infection are called disinfectants. Antiviral agents kill _____, whereas antifungal agents act on _____. _____ are used to prevent viral infections before they occur, rather than treating a viral infection once it has occurred.	Vaccinations, bacteria, viruses, fungi
2. Patients given penicillin when allergic to it can suffer from anaphylaxis. Anaphylactic shock occurs when the body overreacts to being exposed to an_____, producing a massive allergic reaction. Its sudden onset and severity can prove _____. Epilepsy is a disorder of the _____, involving the electrical stimuli that are initiated there, and a faint is loss of brain _____ due to the lack of oxygenated blood to the brain.	consciousness, brain, fatal, allergen

3. Analgesics are drugs used to relieve pain. _____ are the drugs of choice for fighting bacterial infections. Antiviral agents are used to treat viral infections, although viruses are quite unsusceptible to ____ _____ generally. Anti-inflammatory agents, e.g. _____ ___ _____, are used to control inflammation; steroids, such as _____, are powerful anti-inflammatory drugs but, generally, are not the first-line drugs of choice.	drug therapy, ibuprofen and aspirin, cortisone, Antibiotics
4. The vasoconstrictor used in the majority of dental local anaesthetics is _____. A vasoconstrictor reduces the ____ of blood vessels in the immediate vicinity of its use, thus _____ bleeding and preventing its rapid removal from the area by the bloodstream.	size, Adrenaline, controlling
5. Midazolam is the drug commonly used in dentistry to produce sedation. Midazolam is the safest and most commonly used _____ _____ in dentistry, used to produce a steady _____ state in the anxious patient so that all types of dental treatment can be carried out. It has no anaesthetic, analgesic, or anti-inflammatory _____.	properties, sedative, intravenous tranquilliser
6. All the following analgesics may be recommended to a patient postextraction: paracetamol, ibuprofen, and codeine, except aspirin.	extraction socket, heart disease, analgesic

Besides having _____ and anti-inflammatory properties, aspirin also reduces the stickiness of platelets and thus allows unhindered blood flow. This is a very useful side effect in the management of ____ _____ but can be disastrous when an open wound is present, such as an _____ _____.	
7. A common antiviral drug used in dentistry is _____. Acyclovir (Zovirax) is the treatment of choice for herpes labialis, or ____ _____, which are caused by the herpes simplex virus. As they are highly _____, their treatment is of paramount importance to dental personnel.	cold sores, contagious, acyclovir
8. The gaseous mixture used to produce _____ analgesia is nitrous oxide and oxygen. Halothane is an anaesthetic agent used to maintain _____ anaesthesia once it has been induced and has no place in the provision of relative analgesia. As with any _____ _____ for direct inhalation, oxygen must always be provided to avoid hypoxia (____ __ _____), which can lead to brain damage or even death.	Relative, lack of oxygen, gaseous mixture, general
9. In case of _____ _____ during an emergency at the dental practice, the following is a necessity: portable, _____ suction equipment. The easiest and most effective way of _____	Manual, clearing, lifesaver, electrical failure

an airway is by high-speed suction. All dental practices are equipped with suction devices, but all are dependent on an electricity supply. A portable, manual suction device is therefore a possible _____ in times of power cuts.	
10. A sphygmomanometer is used to measure blood pressure. This is a cuffed device connected to a mercury pressure gauge which is wrapped around the patient's _____ ___ and filled with air. The air is slowly let out and the _____ at which the pulse is _____ heard (systolic) and ____ heard (diastolic) with a _____ over the brachial artery are recorded. A normal _____ _____ blood pressure should be in the region of 120/80 mmHg.	stethoscope, healthy adult's, pressures, upper arm, first, last
11. _____ is a medical emergency that may occur and is due to low glucose levels in the blood. This condition is seen in patients who have been _____, as well as in diabetics who have missed their_____ _____. If not treated promptly, the patient could slip into a ____. The conscious patient should be given a glucose tablet or drink. Unconscious patients require an intravenous injection of _____ — this must never be given by staff, only by the dentist.	Fasting, insulin injections, coma, glucagons, Hypoglycaemia
12. The correct term for a cardiac arrest is _____ _____.	Angina, embolism, oxygenated, hypoxia, myocardial infarction

This is the sudden loss of _____ blood to the heart muscle, causing the heart to stop (arrest). _____ is the pain, felt by patients with heart disease upon exertion or stress, due to poor flow of oxygenated blood to the heart. _____ is a low level of oxygen in the blood and tissues, and an _____ is an arterial blockage due to material or air in the bloodstream.	
13. A patient who has fainted will exhibit the following: weak pulse and clammy complexion. Although the pulse is weak it is quite often _____, whereas breathing is normal. ____ _____ are only evident when the patient's respiration is poor or absent. _____ _____ are usually a diagnostic sign of an epileptic fit.	blue lips, Muscle spasms, rapid
14. An epileptic who has a grand mal fit at the practice should be treated thus: left where they are until the fit has passed. Attempting to ____ the patient during a fit could well be dangerous for the patient as well as the first-aiders and should only ever be necessary when their life is in danger, for example by _____ or _____. Under no circumstances should restraint be attempted, nor the insertion of a _____ _____. Besides the improbability of inserting it, the patient could be _____ whilst a foreign body is inserted into their mouth, or the first-aider could be _____ seriously	Tongue guard, choked, hurting, electrocution, bitten, move, drowning

during the attempt. However, if possible, a space should be cleared around the patient to avoid the possibility of them _____ themselves whilst fitting, and onlookers should be moved away.	
15. To determine that cardiac arrest has occurred, the following will be noted: grey pallor, no pulse, no chest movements There will be no pulse if cardiac arrest has occurred, as the heart will have stopped _____. Blue lips _____ that poorly oxygenated blood is being _____ by the heart, as in _____ arrest, whereas a purple face and gasping motions indicate _____ in a conscious patient.	choking, indicate, pumped, respiratory, beating
16. The following conditions require the use of nonadrenaline local anaesthetics during dental treatment: hypertension, hyperthyroidism, depression An increased _____ _____ brought about by the administration of adrenaline during local anaesthesia could be _____ to patients suffering from hypertension or hyperthyroidism, bringing about their _____. Patients suffering from depression are usually prescribed antidepressant drugs, many of whose actions are _____ by adrenaline, especially tricyclic antidepressants.	collapse, altered, heart rate, catastrophic
17. All of the following are the correct actions to take in the event of	Glucose drink, loosening, fall,

a simple faint: loosen tight neck clothing, maintain the airway, give a glucose drink, except keep the casualty sitting upright. A simple faint occurs when there is a temporary reduction in oxygenated blood flow to the brain, and recovery is rapid once the _____ blood flow is restored. Casualties usually become unconscious and _____ to the ground so that the cranial blood flow begins to improve naturally. It can be improved further by _____ the casualties' legs above their head level so that the blood in their legs can also flow to the brain. Keeping the casualty sitting upright will _____ the time that oxygenated blood flow is reduced to the brain and is the worst action that can be taken in the event of a simple faint. _____ tight neck clothing to aid respiration and maintaining the _____ are both routine actions to take in medical emergencies. Many simple faints are triggered by low blood glucose levels, so giving a _____ _____ on recovery will help the overall situation.	raising, prolong, airway, cranial
18. The following emergency drugs may be required in the event of anaphylaxis: oxygen, _____, antihistamine. Anaphylaxis is a rapid state of collapse caused by the body's overreaction (allergic reaction) to an allergen, and in dental practice the likeliest event is an allergic reaction to _____ and its derivatives. The casualty	Release, heart function, drop, shock, oxygen, penicillin, adrenaline

experiences a sudden _____ in blood pressure due to vasodilation that may be severe enough to cause _____ and cardiac arrest, so adrenaline is required to stimulate the _____ _____. Bronchospasm and breathing difficulties also occur, so _____ is required to help maintain an oxygenated blood flow, and antihistamines are drugs that act to reduce histamine _____ by the body during the allergic response.	
19. Aspirin may be given in the event of the following emergency situation: suspected _____ _____ Aspirin is principally an analgesic (pain killer), but it also acts to prevent _____ _____. During myocardial infarction (MI) one of the coronary arteries supplying the heart itself becomes blocked by a blood clot (thrombus), causing a sudden loss of oxygenated blood to this area of the heart muscle. Administration of aspirin when an MI is suspected helps to _____ clot formation and therefore reduces the risk of _____ before the casualty can be removed to a hospital. Aspirin has no antiepileptic effects. If given during ____ _____, bleeding it will actually worsen the situation by allowing further bleeding to occur, as it will following a needlestick injury.	postoperative, prevent, death, myocardial infarction, blood clotting
20. Flumazenil is an emergency drug that must be stocked by those carrying out intravenous sedation.	conscious sedation, reverse, emergency drugs, antidote

Flumazenil is the _____ drug for midazolam, which is the intravenous agent used to produce _____ _____ in dental practice. As only some dental practices and hospital dental departments offer this technique to anxious patients, it need only be kept in their _____ _____ kits and is then available to _____ the effects of intravenous sedation in an emergency situation. Flumazenil has no effect on nitrous oxide gas, which is the sedative agent used in relative analgesia.	
21. In the event of a scald injury, the following first-aid treatment should be carried out: run under cold water. A scald injury is a wet burn due to exposure to _____ and causes rapid and painful _____ of the exposed area. First-aid treatment should be aimed at limiting the extent and severity of the blistering by quickly _____ the area following the injury, and this is best achieved by running the affected area under or immersing in cold water. The use of hot water will cause more blistering, and the blisters will be torn open when _____ _____ are removed. _____ the blisters will expose the delicate tissues underneath to infection, so they should always be left to ____ themselves.	sticking plasters, bursting, cooling, steam, blistering, heal
22. Venous bleeding can be determined by its blue/ purple colour. _____ _____ is that which is deoxygenated and is travelling back to	Capillary bleeding, spurt, venous blood, arterial blood, gush

85

the heart in the veins to be transported to the lungs for reoxygenating. It is characteristically blue/purple in colour, and as it is under low pressure from the heart, it tends to ____ steadily rather than _____ rhythmically. Conversely, highly oxygenated _____ _____ is bright red in colour and tends to spurt due to the pressure it is under as it leaves the heart. Venous bleeding requires direct pressure to the area to stop the blood flow, whereas _____ _____ slows and stops itself as the blood is exposed to the atmosphere and clotting occurs.	

23. Care should be taken during extractions in elderly women because of the increased risk of jaw fracture. Both men and women become more likely to develop _____ as they age, but it especially occurs in women after the _____ as the reduced amount of _____ hormone allows the bones to thin and become _____. They are therefore more likely to experience bone fractures, including to the jaws, during extractions. This patient group has no more tendencies to bleed, faint, or react to local anaesthetic than any other, unless they are taking long-term aspirin, in which case they will be more _____ to bleeding after minor oral surgery.	Brittle, menopause, oestrogen, osteoporosis, prone
24. Following electrocution, the casualty's heart may go into both fibrillation and asystole.	fibrillation, disrupt, rhythmically, asystole, right atrium, electrocution

_____ occurs when an external electrical current passes through the body. The heart beats _____ due to the controlled, internal generation and passage of a small electrical current over its surface, starting at the _____ _____. Any large, external source of electricity can _____ this internal process and cause the heartbeat to become arrhythmic and erratic (_____), or to stop completely (_____).	

Solution to Exercise 9
1f, 2b, 3l, 4n, 5o, 6e, 7a, 8d, 9h, 10i, 11j, 12c, 13g, 14m, 15k

Solution to Exercise 10
1a, 2c, 3f, 4e, 5g, 6b, 7h, 8k, 9o, 10j, 11d, 12l, 13n, 14m, 15i

Vocabulary
abbreviation /əˌbriː.viˈeɪ.ʃən/ zkratka
abdominal /æbˈdɒm.ɪ.nəl/ břišní
absence /ˈæb.sᵊnts/ nepřítomnost, nedostatek
access /ˈæk.ses/ přístup, vstup
accident /ˈæk.sɪ.dᵊnt/ nehoda
administer /ədˈmɪn.ɪ.stəʳ/ podat lék
adrenaline /əˈdren.əl.ɪn/ adrenalin
advanced /ədˈvɑːnʧst/ pokročilý
afterwards /ˈɑːf.tə.wədz/ potom
agent /ˈeɪ.dʒənt/ agens, činitel, zprostředkovatel
aide-memoire /eɪd.ˈmem.wɑːʳ/ mnemotechnická pomůcka
aim /eɪm/ zaměřit
air /eəʳ/ **passage** /ˈpæs.ɪdʒ/ dýchací cesta
airway /ˈeə.weɪ/ dýchací cesty

alertness /əˈlɜːt.nəs/ bdělost

allergen /ˈæl.ə.dʒən/ alergen

allergic /əˈlɜː.dʒɪk/ alergický

alternative /ɒlˈtɜː.nə.tɪv/ alternativa, druhá možnost

although /ɔːlˈðəʊ/ ačkoli

Ambu bag /æm.bjʊ.bæg/ ambu vak

amount /əˈmaʊnt/ množství

anaphylactic /ˌæn.ə.fɪˈlæk.tɪk/ shock /ʃɒk/ anafylaktický šok

angina pectoris /ænˌdʒaɪ.nəˈpek.tə.rɪs/ angina pectoris

annual /ˈæn.ju.əl/ roční

antihistamine /æn.ti.ˈhɪs.tə.miːn/ protihistaminový prostředek

antiplatelet /æn.ti.ˈpleɪt.lət/ proti srážení krve

antidote /ˈæn.ti.dəʊt/ protilátka

antifungal /ˌæn.ti.ˈfʌŋ.gəl/ protiplísňový

anti-inflammatory /ˌæn.ti.ɪnˈflæm.ə.tri/ protizánětlivý

antiviral /ˌæn.ti.ˈvaɪ.rəl/ protivirový prostředek

anxiety /æŋˈzaɪ.ə.ti/ úzkost

apparatus /ˌæp.əˈreɪ.təs/ přístroj

applied /əˈplaɪd/ aplikovaný, použitý

appointment /əˈpɔɪnt.mənt/ setkání, schůzka

approach /əˈprəʊtʃ/ přístup

arm /ɑːm/ ruka, rukáv, opěradlo

around /əˈraʊnd/ okolo

arrest /əˈrest/ zástava

arrhythmia /æˈriθ.mɪ.ə/ arytmie

arrhythmic /æˈrɪθ.mɪk/ arytmický

arrive /əˈraɪv/ přijet, dosáhnout

artefact /ˈɑː.tɪ.fækt/ artefakt, výtvor

arterial /ɑːˈtɪə.ri.əl/ tepenný

aspiration /ˌæs.pɪˈreɪ.ʃən/ odsávání

assess /əˈses/ zhodnotit, určit

assessment /əˈses.mənt/ posouzení

assistance /əˈsɪs.tənts/ podpora, pomoc

assume /əˈsjuːm/ předpokládat, domnívat se

asystole /ə.sis.təli/ asystola

at /ət/ a /ə/ rate /reɪt/ rychlostí

atropine /æt.rəp.ɪn/ sulphate / sʌl.feɪt/ atropinsíran

attack /əˈtæk/ záchvat

attempt /əˈtempt/ pokus, pokoušet se

attention /əˈten.tʃ°n/ pozornost, ošetření

aura /ˈɔː.rə/ předzvěst

autoclave /ˈɔː.təʊ.kleɪv/ autokláv

available /əˈveɪ.lə.bļ/ dostupný

back /bæk/ zpět, záda, opěradlo

bacterial /bækˈtɪə.ri.°l/ bakteriální

basic /ˈbeɪ.sɪk/ základní

beating /ˈbiː.tɪŋ/ tlukot

behind /bɪˈhaɪnd/ za, vzadu

below /bɪˈləʊ/ níže, dolů

between /bɪˈtwiːn/ mezi

bite /baɪt/ pack /pæk/ skusový tampon

bitten /ˈbɪt.ən/ kousnutý

blistering /ˈblɪs.tər.ɪŋ/ vytvoření puchýřů

blockage /ˈblɒk.ɪdʒ/ blokáda, ucpání

blood /blʌd/ pressure /ˈpreʃ.ər/ krevní tlak

blood /blʌd/ clotting /klɒt.ɪŋ/ srážení krve

bloodstream /ˈblʌd.striːm/ krevní řečiště

blow /bləʊ/ úder, rána

body /ˈbɒd.i/ tělo, těleso

border /bɔː.dəʳ/ okraj, hrana

brachial /breɪk.ɪ.əl/ brachiální, pažní

bradycardia /ˌbræd.ɪ.ˈkɑː.di.ə/ bradykardie, zpomalená srdeční činnost

break /breɪk/ přerušení

breath /breθ/ dech, vdechnutí

breathing /ˈbriː.ðɪŋ/ dýchání

breathless /'breθ.ləs/ bez dechu, udýchaný

briefly /'briː.fli/ krátce

bring /brɪŋ/ about /ə'baʊt/ způsobit

brittle /'brɪt.l̩/ křehký

bronchospasm /'brɒŋ.kə.spæz.ᵊm/ bronchospasmus, křeč průdušek

brow /braʊ/ obočí, čelo

burst /bɜːst/ protrhnout

butterfly /'bʌt.ə.flaɪ/ motýlek, škrticí klapka

candidiasis /ˌkæn.di'daɪ.ə.sɪs/ kandidóza

canister /'kæn.ɪ.stəʳ/ kanystr

cannula /'kæn.jʊ.lə/ (pl. cannulae) kanyla, dutá jehla, trubička

cardiorespiratory / kɑː.di.əʊ.rɪ'spɪr.ə.tri/ arrest / ə'rest/ zástava srdeční a dechová

carotid /kə‚rɒt.ɪd/ karotida

carotid /kə‚rɒt.ɪd/ pulse /pʌls/ puls na karotidě

casualty /'kæʒ.ju.əl.ti/ oběť, postižený, zraněný

catheter /'kæθ.ɪ.təʳ/ katétr, cévka

cause /kɔːz/ příčina

cease /siːs/ ustat, zastavit se

central /'sen.trəl/ ústřední

central /'sen.trəl/ ústřední, nejdůležitější

cerebrovascular /ˌser.ɪ.brə'væs.kjʊ. ləʳ/ accident /'æk.sɪ.dᵊnt/ mozková cévní příhoda

check /tʃek/ zkontrolovat, kontrola

chemical /'kem.ɪ.kᵊl/ chemická látka

chest /tʃest/ compression /kəm'preʃ.ᵊn/ stlačení hrudníku

chest /tʃest/ hrudník

chickenpox/'tʃɪk.ɪn.pɒks/ plané neštovice, varicella

chin /tʃɪn/ brada

choice /tʃɔɪs/ výběr

choke /tʃəʊk/ dusit se, přestat dýchat

circulation /ˌsɜː.kjʊ'leɪ.ʃᵊn/ cirkulace, oběh

clamminess /'klæm.ɪ.nəs/ vlhká lepkavost

clammy /'klæm.i/ chladný a lepkavý, vlhce lepkavý

clear /klɪəʳ/ away /ə'weɪ/ odstranit

clearing /'klɪə.rɪŋ/ odstranění

clonic /klɒn.ik/ klonický, škubavý

clothing/'kləʊ.ðɪŋ/ oděv, oblečení

cold /kəʊld/ chlad, studený, nachlazení

cold /kəʊld/ sore /sɔːʳ/ opar

collapse /kə'læps/ kolaps, zhroucení (přen., zhroutit se

colloid /kɒl.ɒ.id/ koloid, druh roztoku homogenní, želatinový, rosolovitý

commence /kə'menₜs/ zahájit

competently /'kɒm.pɪ.tənt.li/ schopně

complexion /kəm'plek.ʃᵊn/ pleť, pokožka

compliance /kəm'plaɪ.ənₜs/ shoda, souhlas

compress /kəm'pres/ stlačit

compression /kəm'preʃ.ən/ komprese, stisk, stlačení, zhuštění

compromise /'kɒm.prə.maɪz/ vydat v nebezpečí

concept /'kɒn.sept/ návrh (koncept), způsob, provedení

condition /kən'dɪʃ.ᵊn/ stav

confidently /'kɒn.fɪ.dənt.li/ jistě

confused /kən'fjuːzd/ zmatený

congested /kən'dʒes.tɪd/ překrvený

conscious /'kɒn.tʃəs/ při vědomí

consciousness /'kɒn.tʃə.snəs/ vědomí

constrict /kən'strɪkt/ stisknout, tisknout

contagious /kən'teɪ.dʒəs/ nakažlivý

continence /'kɒn.tɪ.nənt/ schopnost udržet moč

continue /kən'tɪn.juː/ pokračovat, vytrvat

contraceptive /ˌkɒn.trəˈsep.tɪv/ antikoncepce

cool /kuːl/ down /daʊn/ ochladit

cool /kuːl/ chladný, klidný

cooling /ˈkuː.lɪŋ/ ochlazení

copious /ˈkəʊ.pi.əs/ hojný

cough /kɒf/ kašel

cover /ˈkʌv.əʳ/up /ʌp/ zakrýt, skrýt

covered /kʌv.əd/ pokrytý

CPR /ˌsiː.piːˈɑːʳ/ cardiopulmonary / ˌkɑː.di.əˈpʌl.mə.nə.ri/ resuscitation /rɪˌsʌs.ɪˈteɪ.ʃᵊn/ kardiopulmonární resuscitace

cranial /ˈkreɪ.ni.əl/ lebeční

cricothyroid /ˌkraɪ.kəˈθaɪə.rɔɪd/ krikotyreoidní, týkající se spoje chrupavky prstencové a štítné

cross /krɒs/ bite /baɪt/ zkřížený skus

cross-infection /krɒs.ɪnˈfek.ʃᵊn/ šíření infekce

crushing /ˈkrʌʃ.ɪŋ/ drtivý, zdrcující

cuff /kʌf/ opatřit manžetou

cyanosis /ˈsaɪəˈnəʊ.sɪs/ cyanóza, promodrání

cylinder /ˈsɪl.ɪn.dəʳ/ válec

damage /ˈdæm.ɪdʒ/ poškození

danger /ˈdeɪn.dʒəʳ/ nebezpečí

dangerous /ˈdeɪn.dʒᵊr.əs/ nebezpečný

daydreaming /ˈdeɪ.driːm/ snění

deal /dɪəl/ jednat, zacházet

debris /ˈdeb.riː/, /ˈdeɪ.briː/ úlomky

defibrillator /ˌdiːˈfɪb.rɪ.leɪ.tər/ defibrilátor

delay /dɪˈleɪ/ zdržet, zpoždění, odkládat

delicate /ˈdel.ɪ.kət/ jemný

dental /ˈden.tᵊl/ zubní

derivative /dɪˈrɪv.ə.tɪv/ derivát, odvozenina

desire /dɪˈzaɪəʳ/ přát si, přání

device /dɪˈvaɪs/ zařízení, vybavení

dial /ˈdaɪ.əl/ vytočit (telefonní číslo)

diameter /daɪˈæm.ɪ.təʳ/ průměr

diastolic /ˌdaɪ.əˈstɒ.lɪk/ diastolický

diazepam /ˌdaɪˈæz.ə.pəm/ diazepam, sedativum, valium

dignity /ˈdɪg.nɪ.ti/ důstojnost

dilate /daɪˈleɪt/ rozšiřovat

direct /dɑ ɪˈrekt/ přímý, řídit, dohlížet, nasměrovat

disastrous /dɪˈzɑː.strəs/ katastrofální

disinfectant/ˌdɪs.ɪnˈfek.tᵊnt/ definfekční látky

dislodge /dɪˈslɒdʒ/ vypudit, vyplavit

disorder /dɪˈsɔː.dəʳ/ porucha

disorientated /dɪˈsɔː.ri.ən.tɪd/ dezorientovaný

disposable /dɪˈspəʊ.zə.bļ / k dispozici, na jedno použití

disrupt /dɪsˈrʌpt/ přerušit

dizziness /ˈdɪz.ɪ.nəs/ závrať

dressing /ˈdres.ɪŋ/ obvaz

drop /drɒp/ kapka

drowning /ˈdraʊn.ɪŋ/ tonutí

drowsiness /ˈdraʊ.zɪ.nəs/ ospalost, mátožnost

drug /drʌg/ lék

ECG /ˌiː.siːˈdʒiː/ electrocardiogram /ɪˌlek.trəˈkɑː.di.ə.græm/ elektrokardiogram (EKG)

edentate /əˈden.teɪt/ bezzubý

edge /edʒ/ okraj

effective /ɪˈfek.tɪv/ efektivní (skutečný), účinný

either /ˈaɪ.ðəʳ/ buď

electrical /ɪˈlek.trɪ.kᵊl/ current / ˈkʌr.ᵊnt/ elektrický proud

electrical /ɪˈlek.trɪ.kᵊl/ failure/ˈfeɪ.ljəʳ/ porucha elektřiny

electricity /ɪˌlekˈtrɪs.ɪ.ti/ supply / səˈplaɪ/ zásobování elektřinou

electrocution /ɪˌlek.trəˈkjuː.ʃən/ úraz, smrt způsobená elektřinou

elevate /ˈel.ɪ.veɪt/ zvednout

emergency /ɪˈmɜː.dʒən*t*.si/ **kit** /kɪt/ souprava první pomoci

emulsion /ɪˈmʌl.ʃən/ emulze, emulzní

encircle /ɪnˈsɜː.kl̩/ obemknout, obklopit, obejít kolem

encourage /ɪnˈkʌr.ɪdʒ/ povzbudit

encouragement /ɪnˈkʌr.ɪdʒ.mənt/ povzbuzení, dodání odvahy

endocarditis /ˌen.dəˈkɑː.ˈdai.tis/ endokarditida, zánět srdeční nitroblány

ensuing /ɪnˈsjuː.ɪŋ/ nastávající, vyplývající

epinephrine /ˌep.ɪ.ˈnef.riːn/ epinefrin, adrenalin

equipment /ɪˈkwɪp.mənt/ vybavení, zařízení

erratic /ɪˈræt.ɪk/ nestálý, neurčitý, bludný

escort /ɪˈskɔːt/ doprovodit

establish /ɪˈstæb.lɪʃ/ ustanovit, zavést, uvést do chodu

evidence /ˈev.ɪ.dən*t*s/ důkaz (očividný), dokázat, jistota

evident /ˈev.ɪ.dənt/ zjevný

exert /ɪgˈzɜːt/ snažit se, vynaložit úsilí, vyvolávat

exertion /ɪgˈzɜː.ʃən/ úsilí, vypětí

exhausted /ɪgˈzɔː.stɪd/ vyčerpaný

extended /ɪkˈsten.dɪd/ v extenzi, natažený, rozšířený

extent /ɪkˈstent/ rozsah, objem

external /ɪkˈstɜː.nəl/ vnější

extraction /ɪkˈstræk.ʃən/ extrakce, vytržení

extremity /ɪkˈstrem.ɪ.ti/ končetina

eye /aɪ/ oko

face /feɪs/ obličej, čelit (čemu)

facial /ˈfeɪ.ʃəl/ **flushing** /flʌʃ.ɪŋ/ nával horka v obličeji

failure /ˈfeɪ.ljəʳ/ selhání

fainting /feɪnt.ɪŋ/ mdloba

fall /fɔːl/ padnout

fast /fɑːst/ hladovět

fasting /fɑːst.ɪŋ/ hladovění

fatal /ˈfeɪ.təl/ fatální, smrtelný

fatality /fəˈtæl.ə.ti/ smrtelný úraz

fatigue /fəˈtiːg/ slabost, schvácenost

fear /fɪəʳ/ strach

fearful /ˈfɪə.fəl/ bojácný

feel /fiːl/ hmatat, cítit, pocítit

feeling /ˈfiː.lɪŋ/ pocit

fibrillation /ˌfaɪ.brɪˈleɪ.ʃən/ fibrilace

fight /faɪt/ rvačka

fighting /ˈfaɪ.tɪŋ/ rvačka

finger /ˈfɪŋ.gəʳ/ prst na ruce

first-aid /ˈfɜːst.eɪd/ **kit** /kɪt/ lékárnička první pomoci

fit /fɪt/ v kondici

fit /fɪt/ hodit se, vhodný, padnout (oděv)

fit /fɪt/ záchvat, nával

flail /fleɪl/ ochromený, klinkající se

flat /flæt/ plochý, rovný

flow /fləʊ/ tok

flush /flʌʃ/ proud (vody), vypláchnout, zrudnout

follow /ˈfɒl.əʊ/ následovat

forceful /ˈfɔːs.fəl/ mocný, prudký

forehead /ˈfɒr.ɪd/, /ˈfɔː.hed/ čelo

foreign /ˈfɒr.ən/ **body** /ˈbɒd.i/ cizí tělísko

forwards /ˈfɔː.wədz/ směrem dopředu

fungus /ˈfʌŋ.gəs/ **(pl. fungi)** houba, plíseň

further /ˈfɜː.ðəʳ/ dále

gas /gæs/ plyn

gaseous /ˈgeɪ.si.əs/ plynný

gasp /gɑːsp/ těžce dýchat, popadat dech

gently /ˈdʒent.li/ jemně, mírně

give /gɪv/ dát, podat

glove /glʌv/ rukavice

glucagon /gluː.kəg.ən/ glukagon, peptidový hormon, tvořený ve slinivce břišní glucose /ˈgluː.kəʊs/ glukóza, hroznový cukr

glyceryl /ˈglɪs.ə.rɪl/ trinitrate / traɪˈnaɪ.treɪt/ glyceriltrinitrát, nitroglycerin

grand mal /ˈgrɑːnd.ˈmæl/ velký epileptický záchvat

grasp /grɑːsp/ popadat

grey /greɪ/ šedý

guard /gɑːd/ chránit, bránit

gush /gʌʃ/ téci proudem, řinout se

haemostasis /ˌhiːməˈste.sɪs/ hemostáza, zástava krvácení

halfway /ˌhɑːfˈweɪ/ půl cesty

head /hed/ hlava, hlavní

heal /hiːl/ hojit, léčit

heart /hɑːt/ attack /əˈtæk/ srdeční záchvat

heart /hɑːt/ massage /ˈmæs.ɑːdʒ/ masáž srdce

Heimlich manoeuvre /ˈhaɪm.lɪk. məˈnuː.vəʳ/ Heimlichův manévr

herpes /ˈhɜː.piːz/ opar

high /haɪ/ vysoký

high-speed /ˌhaɪˈspiːd/ handpiece / hænd.piːs/ vysokoobrátkový násadec

high-speed /ˌhaɪˈspiːd/ vysoko-rychlostní

hook /hʊk/ ohnout, zahnout

hurt /hɜːt/ bolet, poranit

hydrocortisone /haɪ.drəʊˈkɔː. tɪ.zəʊn/ hydrocortison

hygienist /haɪˈdʒiː.nɪst/ hygienik

hyperactivity /haɪ.pəʳ.ækˈtɪv.ɪ.ti/ nadměrná aktivita

hypertension /ˌhaɪ.pəˈten.tʃ°n/ hypertenze, vysoký krevní tlak

hyperthyroidism /ˌhaɪ.pə.ˈθaɪə.rɔɪdɪ. z°m/ hypertyroidismus, zvýšená činnost štítné žlázy

hypoglycaemia /ˌhaɪ.pəʊ.glaɪˈsiː.mi.ə/ hypoglykémie

hypoxia /haɪˈpɒk.sɪ.ə/ hypoxie, nedostatečné zásobení krve kyslíkem

immerse /ɪˈmɜːs/ ponořit se

impalpable /ɪmˈpæl.pə.bl̩/ nepalpovatelný, nepostižitelný (nehmatatelný)

improbability /ɪmˌprɒb.əˈbɪl.ɪ.ti/ nepravděpodobnost

improve /ɪmˈpruːv/ zlepšit se

inability /ˌɪn.əˈbɪl.ɪ.ti/ neschopnost, nemožnost

inattentive /ˌɪn.əˈten.tɪv/ nepozorný

incident /ˈɪnt.sɪ.d°nt/ nehoda, událost

incontinence /ɪnˈkɒn.tɪ.nənts/ inkontinence, neschopnost udržet moč či stolici

infusion /ɪnˈfjuː.ʒ°n/ infuze, nalévání, nálev

inhalation /ˌɪn.hə ˈleɪ.ʃ°n/ vdechování

inhale /ɪnˈheɪl/ inhalovat (vdechovat)

inhaler /ɪnˈheɪ.ləʳ/ inhalátor

initiate /ɪˈnɪʃ.i.eɪt/ zahájit

injection /ɪnˈdʒek.ʃ°n/ injekce

injury /ˈɪn.dʒər.i/ poranění

insert /ɪnˈsɜːt/ vložit

insertion /ɪnˈsɜː.ʃ°n/ vložení

interfere /ˌɪn.təˈfɪəʳ/ zasahovat, ovlivnit

intervention /ˌɪn.təˈven.ʃ°n/ intervence, zakročení, zásah

intravenously /ˌɪn.trəˈviː.nə.sli/ intravenózně, do žil

invasive /ɪnˈveɪ.sɪv/ invazivní, agresivní

involve /ɪnˈvɒlv/ postihovat, zahrnovat

irrigate /ˈɪr.ɪ.geɪt/ zavlažovat

itching /ˈɪtʃ.ɪŋ/ svědění

IV /ˌaɪˈviː/, intravenous /ˌɪn.trəˈviː.nəs/ intravenózní, nitrožilní

jaw /dʒɔː/ čelist, dáseň

jerk /dʒɜːk/ trhnout, škubnutí, tik

jewellery /ˈdʒuː.°l.ri/ šperky

labia /ˈleɪ.bɪə/ rty

lack /læk/ postrádat

lay /leɪ/ položit

leg /leg/ noha, nohavice

length /leŋkθ/ délka

level /ˈlev.ᵊl/ hladina, úroveň

lie /laɪ/ ležet

lifesaver /ˈlaɪfˌseɪ.vəʳ/ životní záchrana

life-threatening /ˈlaɪfˌθret.ᵊn.ɪŋ/ život ohrožující

lift /lɪft/ zvednout, zvednutí

light-headed /ˌlaɪtˈhed.ɪd/ mající závrať, zmámený

limb /lɪm/ končetina

limited /ˈlɪm.ɪ.tɪd/ omezený

lip /lɪp/ ret

liquid /ˈlɪk.wɪd/ tekutina

listen /ˈlɪs.ᵊn/ poslouchat, sledovat, poslech

look /lʊk/ dívat se, vyhledat, vypadat, vzhled

loosen /ˈluː.sᵊn/ uvolnit, rozvázat

loss /lɒs/ of /əv/ consciousness / ˈkɒn.tʃə.snəs/ ztráta vědomí

mains-operated /meɪnz.ˈɒp.ər.eɪt.ɪd/ ručně ovládaný

maintain /meɪnˈteɪn/ the airway / ˈeə.weɪ/ udržovat, podporovat dýchací cesty

maintain /meɪnˈteɪn/ life /laɪf/ uchovat při životě

major /ˈmeɪ.dʒəʳ/ vessel /ˈves.ᵊl/ velká céva

management /ˈmæn.ɪdʒ.mənt/ zvládnutí, řízení

mandible /ˈmæn.dɪ.bᵊl/ dolní čelist

manual /ˈmæn.ju.əl/ ruční

mask /mɑːsk/ maska

massive /ˈmæs.ɪv/ masivní

medical /ˈmed.ɪ.kəl/ lékařský

medicated /ˈmed.ɪ.keɪ.tɪd/ léčebný

medication /ˌmed.ɪˈkeɪ.ʃᵊn/ léčba, lék

menopause /ˈmen.ə.pɔːz/ menopauza

middle /ˈmɪd.l̩/ finger /ˈfɪŋ.gəʳ/ prostředníček

mild /maɪld/ mírný

minor /ˈmaɪ.nəʳ/ menší

miss /mɪs/ zmeškat

moist /mɔɪst/ mokrý, vlhký (vzduch)

motion /ˈməʊ.ʃᵊn/ pohyb

mouth /maʊθ/ seal /siːl/ uzavření, obemknutí úst

mouth-to-mouth /maʊθ/ z úst do úst

movement /ˈmuːv.mənt/ pohyb, pohybový

myocardial /ˌmaɪ.əˈkɑː.diəl/ infarction /inˈfɑːk.ʃᵊn/ infarkt myokardu

myocardial /ˌmaɪ.əˈkɑː.diəl/ infarction /inˈfɑːk.ʃᵊn/ infarkt myokardu

name /neɪm/ jmenovat se

naturally /ˈnætʃ.ər.əl.i/ přirozeně

nausea /ˈnɔː.zi.ə/ nausea, nevolnost

necessary /ˈnes.ə.ser.i/ nutný

neck /nek/ krk, hrdlo, límec

needle /ˈniː.dl̩/ jehla, sešívat

needle /ˈniː.dl̩/ stick /stɪk/ bodnutí jehlou

nitrous oxide /ˌnaɪ.trəsˈɒk.saɪd/ kysličník dusný, rajský plyn

nominate /ˈnɒm.ɪ.neɪt/ jmenovat, navrhnout

nonadhesive /ˌnɒn.ədˈhiː.sɪv/ nepřilnavý

nurse /nɜːs/ sestra, ošetřovatelka

obstruction /əbˈstrʌk.ʃən/ překážka

obtain /əbˈteɪn/ získat, dostat (obdržet)

obvious /ˈɒb.vi.əs/ zjevný

occur /əˈkɜːʳ/ objevit se, nastat

oedema /ɪˈdiː.mə/ edém, otok

oestrogen /ˈiː.strəʊ.dʒᵊn/ estrogen, ženský pohlavní hormon

offending /əˈfen.dɪŋ/ obtížný, zraňující

olfactory /ɒlˈfæk.tᵊr.i/ čichový

onlooker /ˈɒn.lʊk.əʳ/ přihlížející

onset /ˈɒn.set/ nástup, začátek

orally /ˈɔː.rə.li/ ústně

oropharyngeal /ˌəʊ.rəˈfær.ɪ.ŋˈdʒɪ.əl/ orofaryngeální, týkající se úst a hltanu

osteoporosis /ˌɒs.ti.əʊ.pəˈrəʊ.sɪs/ osteoporóza, prořídnutí kostí

overall /ˌəʊ.vəˈrɔːl/ celkový

overload /ˈəʊ.və.ləʊd/ přetížení, zahlcení

overreaction /ˌəʊ.və.riˈæk.ʃᵊn/ nadměrná reakce

oxygen /ˈɒk.sɪ.dʒən/ delivery / dɪˈlɪv.ər.i/ podávání kyslíku

oxygen /ˈɒk.sɪ.dʒən/ kyslík

pad /pæd/ čtverec, polštářek

pain /peɪn/ bolest, námaha

pale /peɪl/ bledý

pallor /ˈpæl.əʳ/ bledost, zsinalost

palm /pɑːm/ dlaň

panic /ˈpæn.ɪk/ panický strach, zděšení

paraesthesia /ˌpær.əsˈθiː.sɪ.ə/ parestezie, změněná citlivost

paramedic /ˌpær.əˈmed.ɪk/ zdravotník, záchranář

paramount /ˈpær.ə.maʊnt/ velice důležitý

pass /pɑːs/ through /θruː/ procházet

patent /ˈpeɪ.tənt/ průchodný

patient /ˈpeɪ.ʃᵊnt/ pacient

personnel /ˌpɜː.sᵊnˈel/ personál

petit mal /ˌpəˈtiːˈmæl/ malý epileptický záchvat

plaster /ˈplɑː.stəʳ/ náplast

platelet /ˈpleɪt.lət/ destička

poisonous /ˈpɔɪ.zᵊn.əs/ vapour / ˈveɪ.pəʳ/ jedovatý výpar

portable /ˈpɔː.tə.bl̩/ přenosný, příruční

post /pəʊst/ crown /kraʊn/ čepová korunka

postmenopausal / pəʊstˌmen.əˈpɔː.zəl/ po menopauze

postoperation /pəʊst.ɒp.ᵊrˈeɪ.ʃᵊn/ (post-op) pooperačně

postictal /ˈpəʊstˈɪkt.ᵊl/ následně po prodělaném záchvatu

powder /ˈpaʊ.dəʳ/ prášek

power /paʊəʳ/ cut /kʌt/ výpadek elektřiny

practice /ˈpræk.tɪs/ procvičovat

precede /prɪˈsiːd/ předcházet, předstihnout

precipitation /prɪˌsɪp.ɪˈteɪ.ʃᵊn/ precipitace, urychlení

predispose /ˌpriː.dɪˈspəʊz/ predisponovat, učinit náchylným

pregnancy /ˈpreg.nənt.si/ těhotenství

principle /ˈprɪnt.sɪ.pl̩/ zásada

printout /ˈprɪnt.aʊt/ výtisk, výpis

problem /ˈprɒb.ləm/ problém

procedure /prəˈsiː.dʒəʳ/ procedura, postup

proceed /prəʊˈsiːd/ postupovat, probíhat, provést

prolong /prəˈlɒŋ/ prodloužit

promptly /ˈprɒmp t.li/ promptně, rychle

prone /prəʊn/ náchylný

pronounce /prəˈnaʊnt s/ vyslovovat

prop /prɒp/ podpěra

property /ˈprɒp.ə.ti/ vlastnost

protect /prəˈtekt/ chránit, ochrana

prove /pruːv/ dokázat

pull /pʊl/ táhnout, trhat (i s kořenem), zmítat

pulse /pʌls/ puls

puncture /ˈpʌŋk.tʃəʳ/ punkce, vpich, otvor

purple /ˈpɜː.pl̩/ fialový

push /pʊʃ/ tlačit

radial /ˈreɪ.di.əl/ radiální
radiation /ˌreɪ.diˈeɪ.ʃ³n/ záření
raise /reɪz/ zvýšit, zvednout
rapid /ˈræp.ɪd/ rychlý, prudký
rate /reɪt/ rychlost
ratio /ˈreɪ.ʃi.əʊ/ podíl, vztah, vzájemný poměr
reason /ˈriː.z³n/ důvod
reassurance /ˌriː.əˈʃɔː.rənt s/ ujištění, uklidňování
reassure /ˌriː.əˈʃɔːʳ/ uklidňovat
receptionist /rɪˈsep.ʃ³n.ɪst/ sestra (u příjmu pacientů)
recommended /ˌrek.əˈmen.dɪd/ doporučený
record /rɪˈkɔːd/ zaznamenat
recovery /rɪˈkʌv.°r.i/ **position** /pəˈzɪʃ.³n/ zotavovací poloha, stabilizovaná poloha
recurrence /rɪˈkʌr.°nt s/ návrat, opětovný výskyt
reduction /rɪˈdʌk.ʃ³n/ snížení
regain /rɪˈgeɪn/ znovu získat
regimen /ˈredʒ.ɪ.mən/ režim
region /ˈriː.dʒ³n/ oblast
release /rɪˈliːs/ uvolnit
relief /rɪˈliːf/ úleva
relieve /rɪˈliːv/ ulevit, zmírnit
repeat /rɪˈpiːt/ opakovat, opakovaný, zažít znovu
repeatedly /rɪˈpiː.tɪd.li/ opakovaně
require /rɪˈkwaɪəʳ/ vyžadovat
requirement /rɪˈkwaɪə.mənt/ požadavek
rescue /ˈres.kjuː/ záchrana, záchranný, zachránit
rescuer /ˈres.kjuː.əʳ/ zachránce, záchranář, záchranný přístroj
respiratory /rɪˈspɪr.ə.tri/ dýchací
respiratory rɪˈspɪr.ə.tri/ **arrest** /əˈrest/ zástava dechu

responsiveness /rɪˈspɒnt.sɪv.nəs/ schopnost reagovat na podněty, vnímavost
restore /rɪˈstɔːʳ/ obnovit
restraint /rɪˈstreɪnt/ omezování, bránění
resultant /rɪˈzʌl.t³nt/ z toho vyplývající (výsledný)
resuscitation /rɪˌsʌs.ɪˈteɪ.ʃ³n/ resuscitace, kříšení, oživení
retrosternal /ˌret.rəˈstɔː.n³l/ retrosternální, umístěný za hrudní kostí
reverse /rɪˈvɜːs/ obrácený
revive /rɪˈvaɪv/ oživit
rheumatic /ruːˈmæt.ɪk/ **fever** /ˈfiː.vəʳ/ revmatická horečka
rib /rɪb/ **cage** /keɪdʒ/ hrudní koš
rigid /ˈrɪdʒ.ɪd/ rigidní, strnulý (neohebný)
rigidity /rɪˈdʒɪd.ɪ.ti/ ztuhlost
ring /rɪŋ/ prsten
route /ruːt/ cesta
run /rʌn/ **under** /ˈʌn.dəʳ/ **cold** /kəʊld/ **tap** /tæp/ nechat pod studenou tekoucí vodou
sachet /ˈsæʃ.eɪ/ sáček
safely /ˈseɪ.fli/ bezpečně
safety /ˈseɪf.ti/ **glasses** /glɑː.sɪz/ ochranné brýle
saline /ˈseɪ.laɪn/ fyziologický roztok
scald /skɔːld/ opařenina
sedative /ˈsed.ə.tɪv/ uklidňující
seizure /ˈsiː.ʒəʳ/ záchvat (nemoci), uchopení
self-inflicted /ˌself.ɪnˈflɪk.tɪd/ sebeporanění, sebepoškození
semi-/sem.i-/ polo-
sequence /ˈsiː.kwənt s/ pořadí, následnost
set /set/ sada (souprava), stanovený
set /set/ určit, stanovit, nastavit

severe /sɪ'vɪərʳ/ závažný

shake /ʃeɪk/ třást, otřes (otřesení), potřesení (též hlavou)

sharp /ʃɑːp/ prudký (nápor), ostrý (dobře řezající)

shelf life /ʃelf.laɪf/ záruční doba

shoulder /'ʃəʊl.dərʳ/ blade /bleɪd/ lopatka (rameno)

shout /ʃaʊt/ volat, křičet

shouting /'ʃaʊ.tɪŋ/ zvolání, zavolání, křik

side effect /saɪd.ɪ'fekt/ vedlejší účinek

sight /saɪt/ pohled, podívaná, uvidět

sign /saɪn/ znak, znamení, podpis

simple /'sɪm.pl̩/ jednoduchý, prostý

site /saɪt/ místo

situs /saɪ.təs/ místo, poloha

skill /skɪl/ dovednost

skin /skɪn/ kůže (pokožka), pokrýt se kůží (zahojit se)

slap /slæp/ plácnout, plesknutí

slide /slaɪd/ sklouznout, sjet

slip /slɪp/ sklouznout, upadnout

slow /sləʊ/ pomalý, zvolna

slump /slʌmp/ pokles, propadnout, sesunout

smell /smel/ čich, cítit (čichem), být cítit

socket /'sɒk.ɪt/ jamka, zubní lůžko, zásuvka

solution /sə'luː.ʃən/ řešení, roztok, rozpuštění

sound /saʊnd/ zvuk, znít, zdravý

source /sɔːs/ zdroj

space /speɪs/ prostor

spasm /'spæz.ᵊm/ křeč

speck /spek/ zrníčko

speed /spiːd/ rychlost

sphygmomanometer /sfɪg.məʊ.mæn'ɒm.ɪ.tərʳ/ sfygmomanometr, tlakoměr

spillage /'spɪl.ɪdʒ/ rozlité (rozsypané) množství

spine /spaɪn/ páteř

spontaneous /spɒn'teɪ.ni.əs/ spontánní, samovolný

spontaneously /spɒn'teɪ.ni.ə.sli/ samovolně

spurt /spɜːt/ tryskat

squeeze /skwiːz/ mačkat, protlačit, stisknout, stisknutí, stlačit, vymačkat

stare /steərʳ/ zírat

steadily /'sted.ɪ.li/ neustále, pevně

steady /'sted.i/ trvalý, pevný

steam /stiːm/ pára

sternum /'stɜː.nəm/ sternum, hrudní kost

stethoscope /'steθ.ə.skəʊp/ stetoskop, fonendoskop

stick /stɪk/ tyčinka

stickiness /'stɪk.ɪ.nəs/ soudržnost, lepivost

sticking plaster /'stɪk.ɪŋ‚plɑː.stərʳ/ lepicí náplast

stress /stres/ stres, nepohoda, tlak

stroke /strəʊk/ mrtvice

stuck /stʌk/ přilepen

suction /'sʌk.ʃən/ odsávání, nasávání (vzduchu)

sudden /'sʌd.ᵊn/ náhlý

suffer /'sʌf.əʳ/ utrpět

sufferer /'sʌf.ᵊr.əʳr/ trpící

sufficient /sə'fɪʃ.ᵊnt/ dostatečný, přiměřený

sulphate /'sʌl.feɪt/ sulfát, síran, kyselina sírová

summon /'sʌm.ən/ zavolat, přivolat

supine /'suː.paɪn/ ležící naznak, tváří vzhůru

surgeon /'sɜː.dʒᵊn/ praktický lékař, chirurg

surgery /'sɜː.dʒᵊr.i/ ordinace, ošetřovna, chirurgický zákrok

surroundings /sə'raʊn.dɪŋz/ okolí

suspected /sə'spek.tɪd/ suspektní, podezřelý

sustained /sə'steɪnd/ utrpěný, vytrvalý

sweaty /'swet.i/ propocený, opocený

sweep /swiːp/ odstranit, vymést

swelling /'swel.ɪŋ/ otok

swing /swɪŋ/ rozkývat, houpat

symptom /'sɪmp.təm/ symptom

system /'sɪs.təm/ systém

systolic /sɪs.tɒl.ɪk/ systolický

take /teɪk/ **pulse** /pʌls/ měřit puls

take /teɪk/ **over**/'əʊ.vəʳ/ převzetí, přijmout

tear /teəʳ/ roztrhnout

technician /tek'nɪʃ.ᵊn/ technik

temporary/'tem.pər.ər.i/ dočasný

tend /tend/ **to** /tʊ/ mít sklon k

tendency /'ten.dənt.si/ tendence

thin /θɪn/ nepatrný

thready /θred.i/ **pulse** /pʌls/ nitkovitý tep

throat /θrəʊt/ hrdlo

thrombus /θrɒm.bəs/ thrombus, sraženina

thrush /θrʌʃ/ moučnivka

thumb /θʌm/ palec na ruce

tight /taɪt/ těsný

tilt /tɪlt/ nachýlit (naklonit)

tingling /ˌtɪŋ.lɪŋ/ mravenčení

tiring /'taɪə.rɪŋ/ únavný, vyčerpávající

tissue/'tɪʃ.uː/, /'tɪs.juː/ tkáň

together /tə'geð.əʳ/ proti sobě, pohromadě

tongue /tʌŋ/ jazyk

tonic /'tɒn.ɪk/ **phase** /feɪz/ tonický, napjatý

top /tɒp/ navršit, navýšit

touch /tʌtʃ/ dotýkat se, dotek

tourniquet /'tʊə.nɪ.keɪ/ škrtidlo

towards /tə'wɔːdz/ směrem k

trachea /trə'kiː.ə/ trachea, průdušnice

tract /trækt/ trakt

traction /'træk.ʃᵊn/ trakce, náprava tahem

tranquilliser /'træŋ.kwɪ.laɪ.zəʳ/ uklidňující prostředek

transfer /'træns.fɜːʳ/ převoz

treatment /'triːt.mənt/ léčba

trigger /'trɪg.əʳ/ spustit, začít

tunnel /'tʌn.ᵊl/ tunel

ulcerative /'ʌl.sᵊr.ə.tɪv/ vředový

unaffected /ˌʌn.ə'fek.tɪd/ nedotčený, neovlivněný

unaided /ˌʌn'eɪ.dɪd/ bez pomoci

unattended /ˌʌn.ə'ten.dɪd/ bez pomoci

uncommon /ʌn'kɒm.ən/ neobvyklý, neobyčejný

unconscious /ʌn'kɒn.tʃəs/ bezvědomý

uncontrollably /ˌʌn.kən'trəʊ.lə.bli/ nekontrolovatelně

underlying/ˌʌn.də'laɪ.ɪŋ/ základní, vespod ležící

underneath /ˌʌn.də'niːθ/ pod

undo /ʌn'duː/ rozvázat

unfocused /ʌn.'fəʊ.kəst/ nezaostřený

unhindered /ˌʌn'hɪn.dəd/ nenarazivší na překážku

unit /'juː.nɪt/ jednotka

unrecordable /ˌʌn.rɪ'kɔːd.ə.bl̩/ nezaznamenatelný

unresponsive /ˌʌn.rɪ'spɒnt.sɪv/ bez reakce

unsuccessful /ˌʌn.sək'ses.fᵊl/ neúspěšný, nepodařený (nezdařilý)

unsusceptible /ˌʌn.sə'sep.tɪ.bl̩/ necitlivý, nevnímavý

unusual /ʌn'juː.ʒu.əl/ pozoruhodný (neobvyklý), mimořádný

unwell /ʌn'wel/ nedobře

upright /'ʌp.raɪt/ **position** /pə'zɪʃ.ᵊn/ vzpřímená poloha

upwards /'ʌp.wədz/ nahoru

urgent /'ɜː.dʒᵊnt/ nutný (naléhavý)

vacant /'veɪ.kᵊnt/ prázdný

valve /vælv/ chlopeň

varicella /ˌvæ.rɪˈsel.ə/ varicella, plané neštovice

vasodilation /ˌveɪ.zə.daɪˈlə.teɪ.ʃ°n/ vazodilatace, rozšíření cév

venous /ˈviː.nəs/ žilní

ventilation /ˌven.tɪˈleɪ.ʃ°n/ vdech

verbal /ˈvɜː.bəl/ slovní

vicinity /vɪˈsɪn.ɪ.ti/ těsná blízkost

viral /ˈvaɪə.rəl/ virový

visible /ˈvɪz.ɪ.bl̩/ viditelný

vision /ˈvɪʒ.°n/ zrak

volume /ˈvɒl.juːm/ objem

vomit /ˈvɒm.ɪt/ zvracet, zvracení

warn /wɔːn/ varovat

waterproof /ˈwɔː.tə.pruːf/ nepromokavý

weak /wiːk/ slabý

wear /weəʳ/ mít na sobě, obléknout

wet /wet/ mokrý

wheeze /wiːz/ sípat

whereas /weəˈræz/ zatímco, kdežto

wherever /weəˈrev.əʳ/ kdekoli

worsen /ˈwɜː.sən/ zhoršit

wound /wuːnd/ rána

wrapped /ræpt/ zabalený

wrist /rɪst/ zápěstí

yawn /jɔːn/ zívat

Unit 8

Analgesia, Sedation, and General Anaesthesia

Drug Prescribing and Therapeutics. Analgesics and Nonsteroidal Anti-inflammatory Drugs: Aspirin, Ibuprofen, Paracetamol, Opioids, Codeine. Antibiotics. Anxiolytics and Hypnotics. Topical Agents. Analgesia, Sedation, and General Anaesthesia. Local Anaesthesia. Sedation. Intravenous (IV) Sedation. General Anaesthesia. Drug Prescribing. Local Anaesthesia, Sedation Techniques, Hazards of the Procedures. Infiltration Technique. Nerve Block Technique. Intraligamentary Technique. Intraosseous Technique. Postanaesthetic Advice. Use of Aspirating Equipment. No Adrenaline. Intraligamentary Injection. Intravenous Sedation. Outpatient GA Extraction. Advice on Local Anaesthesia.

Text 1

Drug Prescribing and Therapeutics
Prescription writing

- **name** and **address** of patient
- **age** of patient
- total **number of days** of treatment
- the **generic name** of the drug, its **form** and **strength**

- **instruction as to how and when** drug is to be taken, written with no abbreviations
- delete any space remaining on the form
- **date** and prescriber's **signature**

Warnings to patients

- Always take the drug at the **recommended time** and **finish the** prescribed **course**.
- If any **untoward reaction** occurs (e.g. skin rash or severe diarrhoea), stop drug and contact prescriber immediately.
- Patients should be informed of known **side effects or interactions**.
- Medicines should be kept safely **out of the reach of children** and the use of child-safe containers is essential. When no longer needed, medicines should be disposed of by **returning** them to the local **pharmacist**, not discarded where children may find and swallow them.

Patients at particular risk:

Children – doses should be appropriately reduced by age or body weight.

Elderly – elderly people may show exaggerated reactions to drugs. Polypharmacy is common; possible interactions should be identified. Patients often get confused about which drugs are to be taken at which times. Try to avoid adding to their confusion.

Pregnancy - only prescribe when absolutely essential.

Breast feeding - some drugs pass into the milk and are thereby ingested by the baby. This is potentially dangerous.

Liver disease - many drugs are metabolised through the liver. Impaired liver function may affect the breakdown of drugs. Certain drugs may further damage the organ.

Kidney disease - as many drugs are excreted through the kidney, impaired function may lead to:

- increased drug levels in the plasma
- rising sensitivity to certain drugs
- poor tolerance to side effects.

Analgesics and Nonsteroidal Anti-inflammatory Drugs: Aspirin, Ibuprofen, Paracetamol, Opioids, Codeine

The way in which analgesics are prescribed may have a significant bearing on the success of their action. 'Just take aspirin if you have any pain' is not likely to induce confidence in patients whereas explanation of the positive qualities of the drug in the particular patient's context may well result in more benefit.

Antibiotics

An antibiotic is a substance which causes the death of or prevents successful replication of microorganisms. A **bactericidal drug** kills sensitive organisms. A **bacteriostatic drug** prevents successful reproduction. **Narrow spectrum** antibiotics have a limited range of effect, normally against Gram-positive bacteria. **Broad spectrum** antibiotics normally have activity against Gram-positive and Gram-negative bacteria and sometimes mycoplasma.

Bacterial resistance to antibiotics - an increasing problem worldwide is that some microorganisms are acquiring multiresistance. Shorter courses (for 2–3 days) should be considered as this reduces the chances of a resistant form emerging.

Use of antibiotics in dentistry can be considered under two headings:

- **prophylactic** use (e.g. the prevention of infection)
- **therapeutic** treatment of existing infection

Commonly used antibiotics are **penicillin, erythromycin, and ampicillin.**

Anxiolytics and Hypnotics

Anxiolytics are drugs which **reduce anxiety, tension, or fear. Hypnotics** are drugs which **induce sleep**. The benzodiazepines are by far the most common group of drugs used in this context.

Dental uses: **premedication, muscle relaxation, intravenous sedation, anticonvulsant.**

Unwanted effects:

- **overdosage** is considered less dangerous than with other sedative or hypnotic drugs. **Respiration** may be depressed, and **hypotension** may occur.

- **sedative effects** such as **drowsiness** and **ataxia** (particularly in elderly people) are well recognised.
- **dependence** - both physical and psychological dependence occur on prolonged use. Together these may cause severe **anxiety, nervousness, and tremor on withdrawal**. There is no dental indication for long-term prescription.

Topical Agents

Various agents are available for topical use in the mouth. **Chlorhexidine** adheres to tooth enamel, pellicle, and plaque. It causes changes in bacterial cell permeability. As a mouthwash it can cause dramatic fall in bacterial count in saliva.

Dental uses:
- dental **mouthwash**
- **irrigant**
- toothpaste **gel**
- oral **spray**

Exercise 1

1. Talk about prescription writing and warnings to patients.
2. What do we mean by the term 'patients at particular risk'?
3. Give the names of some analgesics and nonsteroidal anti-inflammatory drugs.
4. Think about the use of antibiotics in dentistry.
5. Describe unwanted effects of anxiolytics and hypnotics.
6. Which types of topical agents do you know?

Translation 1

Předepisování léku, psaní receptu, jméno a adresa, věk pacienta, celkový počet dnů léčby, generické jméno léku, forma a síla, pokyny jak a kdy se má lék brát, žádné zkratky, smazat volný prostor na formuláři, datum a podpis, varování pro pacienty, brát lék v doporučený čas a dokončit předepsanou dobu léčby, nepříznivá reakce, vyrážka kůže, závažný průjem, známé vedlejší účinky, interakce, ukládat léky bezpečně z dosahu dětí, pacienti obzvláště ohrožení, děti, dávky zmenšené dle věku nebo tělesné váhy, starší lidé, nadměrné reakce na léky, nadměrné užívání léků je běžné, identifikovat možné vzájemné působení, těhotenství, předepisovat pouze léky nezbytně nutné, kojení, některé léky přecházejí do mléka, což může být nebezpečné pro dítě, jaterní onemocnění, určité léky mohou dále poškodit orgán, zhoršená funkce jater může ovlivnit rozkládáni léků, onemocnění ledvin, mnohé léky jsou vylučovány ledvinami, ledviny, špatná funkce, zvýšená hladina léků v plazmě, rostoucí citlivost na určité léky, špatná snášenlivost vedlejších účinků, analgetika a nesteroidní protizánětlivé léky, vysvětlit pozitivní vlastnosti léku ve vztahu k pacientovi, antibiotika působí odumření mikroorganismu, baktericidní lék ničí citlivé organismy, bakteriostatický lék brání úspěšnému rozmnožení bakterií, odolnost baktérií na antibiotika je vzrůstající problém na celém světě, použití antibiotik v zubním lékařství, profylaktické, prevence infekce, léčebné, ošetření existující infekce, anxiolitika snižují úzkost, napětí či strach, hypnotika navozují spánek, benzodiazepiny, nejběžnější skupinou léků, premedikace, uvolnění svalů, nitrožilní sedace, antikonvulzívum, nežádoucí účinky předávkování, potlačené dýchání, hypotenze, uklidňující účinky, ospalost, ataxie, zejména u starších, závislost jak fyzická, tak psychická při dlouhodobém užívání, při vysazení závažná úzkost, nervozita, třes, místní užití v ústech, chlorhexidin přilne k zubní sklovině, povlaku a plaku, působí dramatický pokles počtu baktérií ve slinách, ústní voda, výplach, gel, ústní sprej.

Text 2
Analgesia, Sedation, and General Anaesthesia
Local Anaesthesia

Local anaesthetic agents block conduction of nerve impulses reversibly and may be administered:

* **topically**
* by **infiltration**
* by **regional block**
* by **intraligament injection**

Practical aspects

Local anaesthetics are the most commonly used drugs in dental practice. They provide a **reversible interruption** to the transmission **of nerve impulses**, particularly in response to **pain** but also to **touch, pressure,** and **thermal stimulation**. They are generally very safe and allow most dental procedures to be carried out without recourse to general anaesthesia.

Uses can be listed as follows:

* comfort during **operative dental procedures**
* **diagnostic**, e.g. differentiation between pain arising from upper or lower tooth
* reduction of bleeding for **periodontal or oral surgery**
* reduction of arrhythmias during surgical manipulation under **general anaesthesia**
* reduction of the depth of general anaesthesia
* immediate **postoperative analgesia** after oral or maxillofacial procedures
* reduces need for postoperative opiates
* pain control in **chronic facial pain**
* long-acting locals may have a role in certain cases

Sedation
Conscious sedation

Many patients have understandable **anxiety** when undergoing dental treatment. The sympathetic and reassuring practitioner has a major role in the successful management of such patients. There remains, however, a number of patients who need **additional help**, which can be achieved by a number of ways:

* **oral premedication**
* **inhalation** sedation
* **intravenous** sedation
* **hypnotherapy**

Sedation is a technique in which the use of a drug or drugs produces a state of **depression of the central nervous system** enabling treatment to be carried out but during which **communication can be maintained** and the modification of the patient's state of mind is such that the patient will **respond to command** throughout the period of sedation. Techniques used should carry a margin of safety wide enough to render unintended loss of consciousness unlikely.

Inhalation sedation
The technique most used is that of **nitrous oxide inhalation** administered **with oxygen**.

Subjective sensory disturbances
Although mainly subjective, some of the following features may be felt by the patient:
- **tingling** sensation (pins and needles) in fingers, toes, lips, and tongue
- **tinnitus** (ringing noise in ears)

Sensory disturbances observed by the operator
- **lethargy** – delay or slowing of reaction to request
- **mild intoxication**

Patients should be able to understand and respond to request by the operator at all times.

Intravenous (IV) Sedation
Intravenous sedation produces no analgesia; therefore, **careful local anaesthetic technique** is important. The technique is normally safe, but a small number of patients may exhibit **hypotension or respiratory depression or both**. It is important that this is recognised and **treated promptly**. Patients should be escorted home, should not drive a motor vehicle or use complicated domestic appliances until the following day.

General Anaesthesia
Dental patients will, from time to time, require general anaesthesia (GA) to allow necessary treatment to be carried out. General anaesthetic agents cause a reversible disorganisation of the functioning brain such that a **state of unconsciousness** is produced. This allows dental or oral surgical procedures to be performed:
- **without pain**
- without **awareness**
- without **movement**
- without excessive **bleeding**
- without detriment to central nervous system function on recovery

Contraindications to outpatient GA:
- medically unfit particularly with **cardiovascular or respiratory problems**
- recent exposure to **infectious fevers**
- **medication** which may interact
- **not starved** (at least 4 hours without food or drink is essential)
- **unaccompanied**
- **no valid consent**
- severe **alcohol or drug abuse** problems
- **pregnancy**
- **trismus** (would require inpatient facilities with fibre-optic technique for intubation)

Exercise 2

1. How may local anaesthetic agents be administered?
2. Give the list of uses of local anaesthetics.
3. What is sedation? How does it work?
4. Talk about sensory disturbances.
5. Why is careful local anaesthetic technique important?
6. How does general anaesthesia help to perform dental or oral surgical procedures?
7. Describe contraindications to outpatient GA.

Translation 2

Místní anestetika, být podán místně, infiltrací, do regionálního bloku, injekcí do vaziva, nejběžněji používané léky, přerušit přenos nervových impulsů, reakce na bolest, dotek, tlak a stimulaci teplem, pohodlí během operačních procedur, odlišení mezi bolestí pocházející z horních či dolních zubů, snížení krvácení, snížení hloubky celkové anestézie, kontrola bolesti u chronické bolestivosti, uklidnění při vědomí, pochopitelná úzkost, uklidňovat pacienta, potřebovat další pomoc, orální premedikace, inhalace, intravenózní sedace, potlačení centrálního nervového systému, udržovat komunikaci během ošetření, pacient bude reagovat na pokyn, vdechování oxidu dusíku podávaného s kyslíkem, smyslové poruchy, pocit mravenčení v prstech nohou a rukou, rtů, jazyka, hučení, zvonění v uších, letargie, zpoždění či zpomalení reakce na požadavek, mírná intoxikace, intravenózní uklidnění, technika je bezpečná, malé množství pacientů může projevovat snížený tlak, deprese dýchání, pacienti by měli mít doprovod domů, neměli by řídit motorové vozidlo či používat složité domácí přístroje, celková anestesie, je vytvořen stav bezvědomí, dentální a chirurgické procedury jsou vykonávány bez bolesti, uvědomění, pohybu, nadměrného krvácení, poškození funkce centrálního nervového systému při zotavení, kontraindikace celkové anestézie u ambulantních pacientů, kardiovaskulární a respirační problémy, nedávná expozice infekcím, léky, které se mohou vzájemně ovlivňovat, hladovět alespoň čtyři hodiny je nezbytně nutné, bez doprovodu, není platný souhlas, závažné problémy, zneužívání alkoholu a drog, těhotenství, skřípání zuby by vyžadovalo vybavení lůžkového zařízení.

Text 3
Local Anaesthesia, Sedation Techniques, Hazards of the Procedures

Local anaesthetic techniques
Infiltration Technique
Used to anesthetise all upper teeth, all lower incisors, and all gingivae. It acts by **depositing local anaesthetic solution at nerve endings** lying just beneath the alveolar bone surface. Anaesthetic solution **soaks through pores in the bone surface**. It can be given **painlessly** if a warmed solution is injected slowly. A narrow-bore needle is used. Surrounding soft tissues will be seen to blanch as solution is injected.

Nerve Block Technique

Used to anaesthetise all lower teeth and can be used to anaesthetise upper second and third molars. Acts by **anaesthetising the main nerve trunk** before it enters the bone through the various foramina. Several teeth can be anaesthetised with one injection, if necessary.

Specific injections are:

- **inferior** dental nerve block, with needle tip next to the mandibular foramen—requires a longer and wider bore needle as several muscles have to be penetrated
- **posterior superior** dental nerve block distal to the maxillary tuberosity
- **mental** nerve block between the roots of the lower premolars—this is the end branch of the inferior dental nerve as it exits the body of the mandible through the mental foramen

There is a need to use an **aspirating technique to ensure that the nearby blood vessels are not penetrated**. Inferior dental nerve block is usually a little sore for the patient due to the amount of soft tissues that have to be penetrated.

Intraligamentary Technique

Used to help anaesthetise individual teeth where routine techniques have not provided adequate operative anaesthesia. Also used as an alternative for deciduous tooth anaesthesia. **Except for the gingivae surrounding the actual tooth, no soft-tissue anaesthesia is produced. Special local anaesthetic syringes and cartridges** are required to deposit the solution as it has to be forcibly injected into the periodontal ligament space and quite often the cartridge shatters. Normal narrow-bore needles are used. Unless given very slowly, it can be a painful injection to have.

Intraosseous Technique

Intraosseous technique is a relatively new technique which can be used for all lower teeth in preference to an inferior dental nerve block. The mental foramen region should be avoided. **Administered by infiltrating the buccal papilla then drilling a hole through the compact bone** of the alveolar process, which is exactly the diameter of the special needles provided.

The anaesthetic **solution is then deposited directly around the roots of the chosen tooth**, with no soft-tissue anaesthesia being produced. It is an exacting technique but gives **excellent results** and less painful for the patient than an inferior dental nerve block.

Postanaesthetic Advice

The effects will last for several hours from their onset, so beware of traumatising the soft tissues. This can be avoided by **not attempting to eat or drink hot fluids until the effects have completely worn off.** The area will feel completely numb and swollen until the solution begins to wear off, with no control of the surrounding soft tissues. **A pins-and-needles tingling sensation** will herald the wearing off of the anaesthetic. If an inferior dental nerve block has been given, then opening the mouth may cause tenderness for a day or so. If an intraligamentary injection has been given, then the surrounding gingivae may be sore for a day or so.

Exercise 3
1. Name and discuss four types of local anaesthetic technique used in dentistry.
2. What advice should be given to a patient who has received a local anaesthetic?

Translation 3

Techniky místní anestézie, technika infiltrace, uložení roztoku anestetika do nervových ukončení, ležících pod povrchem dásňové kosti, dát bezbolestně, vpíchnout pomalu zahřátý roztok, jehla s úzkým kalibrem, okolní měkké tkáně viditelně zblednou, technika zablokování nervu, znecitlivění hlavního nervového kmene než vstoupí do kosti různými otvory, technika aspirace zajistí, že sousední krevní cévy nejsou proniknuty, technika do vaziva, pomáhá znecitlivět jednotlivé zuby, dásně obklopující aktuální zub, speciální stříkačky a náplně pro místní anestézii, technika do kosti, roztok anestetika je uložen přímo kolem kořenů vybraného zubu, vynikající výsledky, méně bolestivé, účinky budou trvat několik hodin, vyvarovat se zraňování měkkých tkání, horkých tekutin, oblast se bude zdát necitlivá a oteklá, dokud roztok nezačne vyprchávat, pocit mravenčení, otvírání úst může způsobit citlivost, dásně mohou být bolestivé.

Text 4

Use of Aspirating Equipment

These items of equipment should be used whenever an inferior dental nerve block local anaesthetic injection is to be given. Their use could also be argued for whenever several other local anaesthetic injections are given intraorally.

Their use is indicated for administering a local anaesthetic **when the site of the needle tip will lie close to large blood vessels,** as in the case of nerve block injections where **the nerve to be anaesthetised lies within a neurovascular bundle**. There is a risk of the local anaesthetic solution being inadvertently **deposited into a blood vessel, with possibly disastrous consequences,** especially when the solution contains adrenaline as a vasoconstrictor. The **solution would be carried to the heart via the circulatory system,** where the anaesthetic and the vasoconstrictor could act directly to produce **cardiac stimulation and arrhythmias**. This can be avoided by using a **special anaesthetic syringe and cartridge** which, once the needle tip has been positioned, can be **pressed without depositing any of the solution in a blood vessel**. If a blood vessel has been penetrated, **blood will flow back** into the anaesthetic cartridge and be **spotted by the dentist**. The needle tip can then be repositioned and the **aspirating technique repeated** until blood is not aspired. The anaesthetic solution can then be injected safely.

No Adrenaline

Adrenaline is a **heart stimulant as well as a vasoconstrictor,** and it also potentiates the effects of certain drugs. Its use in local anaesthesia is therefore **contraindicated** in certain patients, specifically:

- all patients with **heart disease**
- all patients with **hypertension**
- all **elderly** patients
- all **diabetic** patients
- all patients with **hyperthyroidism**
- all patients taking **drugs for depression**
- all patients taking **drugs for hypertension**
- all patients with **complicated medical histories** where several different drugs are being taken.

Patients falling into any of these categories can be given local anaesthetic solutions containing **another vasoconstrictor or can be given plain local anaesthetics** that do not contain a vasoconstrictor. The anaesthetic effects of the plain types of solution wear off more quickly, but at least the patient has not been put at risk for the sake of undergoing dental treatment.

Intraligamentary Injection

This is an injection technique where local anaesthetic is deposited **directly into the periodontal ligament of a tooth**. It is used to gain better anaesthesia of a tooth that has received the usual injection types first—nerve block infiltration—but which **is still sensitive** to stimulation.

This can happen in patients with **anatomical variations** to the norm, where nerve block injections do not appear to be close enough to the nerve to produce sound local anaesthesia.

It can also happen when a tooth is suffering from **irreversible pulpitis** and becomes hypersensitive to stimuli, requiring more anaesthesia than usual to allow the dentist to work painlessly. The technique is also used by some dentists to provide local anaesthesia of **deciduous teeth**, as no soft-tissue effects are experienced by the patient, which often makes anaesthetic administration more acceptable to them. It can also be given to a specific tooth to allow root planing to be carried out, again with **no unwanted soft-tissue effects** being produced.

Exercise 4

When should the following be used in dentistry, and why:

- aspirating local anaesthetic syringe and cartridge
- local anaesthetic cartridge containing no adrenaline
- intraligamentary injection.

Translation 4

Použití vybavení pro aspiraci, podání místního anestetika, místo hrotu jehly leží blízko velkých krevních cév nebo uvnitř neurovaskulárního svazku, riziko vpíchnutí roztoku místního anestetika do krevní cévy, být přenesen k srdci oběhovým systémem, srdeční stimulace, arytmie, hrot jehly může být znovu umístěn a aspirace opakována, dokud krev už není nasávána, roztok anestetika může být pak vpíchnut bezpečně, použití adrenalinu je kontraindikováno u pacientů se srdečním onemocněním, hypertenzí, starších pacientů, diabetiků, pacientů se zvýšenou činností štítné žlázy, pacientů, kteří užívají léky proti depresi, pacientů s komplikovanou lékařskou anamnézou, přímo do periodontálního vaziva u zubu, který je dosud citlivý na stimulaci, u pacientů s anatomickým odchylkami od normy, zánět dřeně, zub je nadměrně citlivý, místní anestézie mléčných zubů, podání anestetik je pro pacienty přijatelnější, umožnit vyhlazení stěn kořene bez nežádoucích účinků na měkké tkáně.

Text 5

Intravenous Sedation
Preoperative instructions

- Come with a **responsible adult to escort** you to and from the dental surgery.
- Eat **a light meal about three hours before** the procedure.
- **Do not drink alcohol for 24 hours before** the procedure.
- **Take your normal medications** as usual, unless the dentist has instructed otherwise.
- **Do not wear tight clothing** on arms.
- **Do not wear nail varnish**.
- **Wear flat shoes** as you will be unsteady on your feet postoperatively.
- Make suitable **arrangements for private transport home** and have an adult escort for the remainder of the day.

Postoperative instructions

- **Do not attempt to drive or operate machinery or electrical appliances** until the following day. This includes household appliances such as cookers and fires.
- Normal **postoperative instructions will be given to your escort** if extractions or surgical procedures have been performed.
- If possible, **go to bed on arriving home**, as the effects of the drug will be present for several hours postoperatively.
- **Do not drink alcohol for 24 hours after** the procedure.

Outpatient GA Extraction
Preoperative instructions

- **Do not drink for 6 hours preoperatively**.
- Make sure a **responsible adult escorts** you to and from the anaesthetic centre.
- **Do not wear restrictive clothing** around the neck.
- **Complete and up-to-date medical history form**.
- **Declare any recent experience of general anaesthesia**.
- **Report any respiratory tract infections** before attending—this includes the common cold.

Postoperative instructions

- **Do not drink alcohol** until the following day at the earliest.
- **Do not drive a vehicle or operate machinery** until the following day, including household electrical appliances.
- **Keep the bite pack in place at least 30 minutes**.
- **Do not drink hot liquids or use mouthwashes** for the remainder of the day.

- Arrange to be **escorted home** by a responsible adult with private transport.
- **Follow the advice** issued on taking **painkillers** and about postoperative **haemorrhage**.

Advice on Local Anaesthesia
Preoperative instructions
- Administration involves an **intraoral injection**; the dentist can use a topical anaesthetic beforehand if requested.
- Inform the dentist of **any change in medical history** before the local anaesthetic is administered.
- **Have a light snack a few hours before**; otherwise, you may become nauseous.
- **Report any previous adverse reactions to local anaesthesia** to the dentist beforehand.
- The sensation of local anaesthesia is of a **profound numbness** of the surrounding soft tissues within a minute of the injection being given.
- The area will **feel swollen**.

Postoperative instructions
- The effects will last for approximately **2 hours after administration.**
- **A pins-and-needles sensation** will be felt as the anaesthetic wears off (paraesthesia).
- **Do not try to eat or drink hot fluids** until the effects have worn off completely, as they may traumatise the soft tissues.
- **The mouth may be sore from opening** for a day after an inferior dental nerve block.

- Any intraligamentary injection may cause **soreness in the gums** of the affected tooth for a day afterwards.

Exercise 5

What preoperative and postoperative instructions would the dental nurse give to a patient who:
- is having treatment provided under intravenous sedation
- is being sent for an outpatient general anaesthetic extraction
- is requesting advice on local anaesthesia

Translation 5

Intravenózní sedace, poučení před operací a po operaci, přijďte se zodpovědným dospělým, aby Vás doprovodil do ordinace a domů, snězte lehké jídlo asi tři hodiny před procedurou, nepijte alkohol 24 hodin před procedurou a po proceduře, vezměte léky jako obvykle, pokud lékař nenařídil jinak, neoblékejte si oblečení těsné na pažích, nepoužívejte lak na nehty, obujte si boty bez podpatku, zajistěte si vhodně soukromou dopravu domů, nepokoušejte se řídit nebo obsluhovat stroje či elektrická zařízení do následujícího dne, po příjezdu domů jděte do postele, účinky léku budou přítomny několik hodin po operaci, ambulantní extrakce v celkové anestézii, nepijte 6 hodin před operací, neoblékejte si oblečení těsné kolem krku, vyplňte a aktualizujte formulář pro anamnézu, oznamte jakoukoli nedávnou celkovou anestézii, nahlaste jakékoli infekce dýchacího traktu, včetně běžného nachlazení, ponechte tampon na místě skusu alespoň 30 minut, nepoužívejte ústní vody po zbytek dne, řiďte se radami o braní léků proti bolesti, rady o místní anestézii, podání zahrnuje injekci v ústech, na požádání může lékař použít předtím místní anestetikum, několik hodin předem si dejte lehkou přesnídávku, jinak vám může být špatně od žaludku, nahlaste předem jakékoli předchozí nežádoucí reakce na lokální anestézii lékaři, pocit hlubokého znecitlivění okolních měkkých tkání, oblast se cítí jako oteklá, účinky budou trvat přibližně 2 hodiny po podání, pocit pichlavosti, nejezte ani nepijte horké tekutiny, injekce do vaziva může způsobit bolestivost dásní postiženého zubu během následujícího dne.

Exercise 6 / Homework

The sentences have been divided into separate halves. Match the half-sentences in column A with the half-sentences in column B to make sentences which are complete and correct.

A

1. Local analgesia is used in dentistry to . . .
2. The four types of injection given dentally are . . .
3. The vasoconstrictor used dentally, besides adrenaline, is . . .
4. With needle-bore sizes, the higher the gauge number, the . . .
5. If the anaesthetic solution is inadvertently injected into a blood vessel, the patient may feel . . .
6. Some anaesthetic cartridges do not contain a vasoconstrictor, and these are useful for . . .
7. Injection into a blood vessel can be avoided by using an . . .
8. Anaesthesia of the *anterior superior dental and long . . .*
9. When anaesthesia of the whole of one side of the mandible is required, the needle tip must be placed . . .
10. An infiltration anaesthetic injection acts by *the . . .*
11. The following nerves require anaesthetising before a lower molar tooth can be painlessly extracted . . .
12. A throat pack is used to . . .

B

a) *palpitations and light-headed.*
b) *the local anaesthetic solution filtering through the compact bone of the alveolar ridge to anaesthetise the nerve endings around the root apex.*
c) *nerve block, infiltration, intraligamentary, and intraosseous.*
d) *smaller the bore size.*
e) *Octapressin but should be used with caution in pregnant patients.*
f) *patients with complicated medical histories, especially the elderly.*
g) *anterior superior dental and long sphenopalatine nerves.*
h) *very close to the mandibular foramen.*
i) *the inferior dental nerve, the lingual nerve, and the long buccal nerve.*
j) *allow all dental treatment to be carried out painlessly.*
k) *seal off the pharynx in order to prevent inhalation or ingestion of debris during general anaesthesia.*
l) *aspirating technique of injection.*

Exercise 7 / Homework

The sentences have been divided into separate halves. Match the half-sentences in column A with the half-sentences in column B to make sentences which are complete and correct.

A

1. Relative analgesia machines all have a flush button which is used . . .
2. When dental treatment other than simple extractions is to be carried out under general anaesthesia, the patient is intubated . . .
3. Inhalation sedation uses . . .
4. Besides altering consciousness, nitrous oxide has . . .
5. Oxygen therapy may be required during intravenous sedation because . . .
6. Midazolam is the drug used to . . .
7. A pulse oximeter is used to . . .
8. Patients undergoing sedation should not wear nail varnish because . . .
9. A suitably trained dental nurse can act as . . .
10. A sedated patient should maintain . . .
11. Following sedation, patients should be escorted home . . .
12. All postoperative instructions should be given *to* . . .

B

a) *guarantee a patent airway.*
b) *the drug used usually slows the respiration rate and blood oxygenation may drop.*
c) *by a responsible adult, who will stay with the patient for the rest of the day.*
d) *nitrous oxide and oxygen so that the patient is sedated but conscious.*
e) *produce intravenous sedation and its antidote is flumazenil.*
f) *to the patient's escort in written form and explained fully to the escort when patients have been sedated.*
g) *a monitor during intravenous sedation.*
h) *consciousness and verbal contact throughout the procedure.*
i) *as a safety device to flush 100% oxygen through the machine and into the patient, especially if an emergency arises.*
j) *analgesic property, which makes it especially useful for needle phobics.*
k) *the pulse oximeter finger probe will not function correctly, if at all, through nail varnish.*
l) *monitor the blood oxygenation and pulse rate and quality of a sedated or anaesthetised patient.*

Exercise 8 / Homework

Fill in the missing words. Choose the correct ones.

1. Local analgesia is the local loss of pain sensation. Analgesia strictly means '___ __ ___' and is the correct term to describe the effect of routine local dental anaesthesia. Anaesthesia is the loss of sensation, and patients can vouch for the ability to still feel _____ and _____ during dental treatment when they have been given a _____ anaesthetic injection.	local, pressure, touch, loss of pain

2. A dental infiltration type injection affects the nerve endings in the immediate area. Anaesthetising the main nerve trunk, or the full trigeminal nerve division, is the technique of _____ _____, which is used especially in dentistry to block the _____ dental nerve. Any injection given within 1 centimetre of a tooth will anaesthetise the _____ soft tissues too, due to the close _____ of the nerves involved.	surrounding, inferior, proximity, nerve blocking
3. An intraligamentary injection is placed around the periodontal _____ of the tooth. This type of injection is especially useful in cases where a routine anaesthetic technique has failed to provide sufficient analgesia of the tooth being _____ __ and can therefore be given as an adjunct in these situations. It is exclusive to dentistry. Local anaesthetic agents can be _____ in root canals, but no special technique is involved, whereas anaesthetic injection into the TMJ ligaments is _____.	operated on, unknown, deposited, ligament
4. An aspirating technique is used in some dental anaesthesia to prevent injection into local _____ _____. Once the needle is __ ____, slight pressure is exerted onto the rubber bung of the cartridge	intravenously, blood vessels, in situ, repositioned, flowback

and then eased off. Although no anaesthetic solution is deposited, a _____ of blood will occur into the cartridge if a blood vessel has been penetrated. The needle can then be _____ to prevent the dangerous consequences of injecting the cartridge contents, effectively, _____. An electric-shock-type sensation is felt when the needle tip touches the nerve trunk itself but does no damage. The minimal trauma of the needle passing through muscles to be positioned correctly is unavoidable and self-healing.

5. Vasoconstrictors are required in local anaesthesia to narrow the blood vessels to maintain the anaesthesia. Vasoconstrictors act by _____ the diameter of the blood vessels so that local blood flow is _____. This prevents the anaesthetic agent from being carried away from the area in the bloodstream and thus _____ its effect. By the same action they reduce blood loss following _____, a desirable effect as copious bleeding after extraction tends to increase the chances of postoperative _____, such as localised infection. _____ the blood vessels would dissipate the agent more quickly and reduce its time of action.	complications, reduced, prolongs, extraction, narrowing, widening

6. Patients who should not be given local anaesthesia containing adrenaline include those taking tricyclic antidepressants. Adrenaline acts to stimulate the heart and increase the heartbeat, so those suffering from _____ (low blood pressure) would suffer no ill effects. There is a theoretical risk of _____ contractions being induced in pregnant women following the _____ of the vasoconstrictor Octapressin, but no such effect has been reported with adrenaline. Tricyclic (and other) antidepressants often have cardiac ____-_____ and these can be dangerously potentiated by drugs such as adrenaline, with the possible consequences of precipitating a ____-_____.	heart attack, uterine, administration, side effects, hypotension
7. The normal _____ of adrenaline present in a 2.2 ml local anaesthetic cartridge is 1:80,000. Higher _____ would be dangerous due to the action of adrenaline on the _____ system, whereas lower doses would be _____.	ineffective, cardiovascular, concentration, doses
8. The oxygen and nitrous oxide cylinders used for relative analgesia are black with white shoulder and blue.	Oxygen, colour code, consequences, importance

The _____ of knowing this universal _____ _____ system for medical gas cylinders cannot be stressed too highly. Imagine the _____ if the code is not known and nitrous oxide is administered instead of _____— certain brain damage, if not death, for the patient.	
9. During intravenous sedation, the patient should be relaxed but conscious and _____. The ___ of sedation is to remove the patient's _____ of the dental procedure so that it can be carried out without concern to the patient. If any loss of _____ is produced, then the patient is being induced into the realm of general anaesthesia, with all its hazards and for which the normal sedation surgery is not _____.	Cooperative, equipped, consciousness, anxiety, aim
10. The onset of intravenous sedation is marked by ptosis and _____ _____. Partial drooping of the _____, or ptosis, is the classic indication of the required _____ of relaxation to be achieved so that dental treatment can be carried out without _____ for the patient. At this point the speech is usually slurred too. Consciousness ____ __ maintained throughout the procedure, and if the patient is snoring, they have usually _____ _____ and should be _____ immediately.	alarm, eyelid, fallen asleep, slurred speech, must be, degree, roused

11. Inhalation sedation is also known as relative analgesia. Again, a relaxed state is the aim but with the use of a _____ _____ of nitrous oxide, oxygen, and air, as opposed to the use of _____ _____. As nitrous oxide is a potent painkiller, or analgesic, the procedure is often referred to as _____ _____ (in contrast to local analgesia). Hypnotherapy produces an altered state of awareness to the patient's surroundings and is usually achieved by mental suggestion without the use of the drugs. As with intravenous sedation, inhalation sedation should ____ _____ the patient's level of consciousness.	intravenous agents, relative analgesia, not alter, gaseous mixture
12. Whilst monitoring a sedated patient, the dental nurse must observe and check the pulse and respiration rates of the patient. Instruments should be ready _____ the procedure begins, as with any dental treatment. The distraction of _____ ___ instruments and _____ __ dental notes during the procedure can only detract from the necessary ____ ___ the patient and is unacceptable. There is no reason for the blood pressure to be monitored throughout the procedure, although it should be read and recorded before the _____ begins.	sedation, writing up, searching for, care for, before

13. Besides the routine first aid and emergency equipment that should be present in all dental surgeries, those undertaking sedation must also have a pulse oximeter. This reads the pulse and _____ _____ of the blood through a _____ _____ and alerts the team to any _____ changes in the patient's condition. An oxygen supply should be _____ in all dental practices. A defibrillator is only necessary in those providing _____ anaesthesia.	available, oxygen saturation, unwanted, finger probe, general

Solution to Exercise 6
1j, 2c, 3e, 4d, 5a, 6f, 7l, 8g, 9h, 10b, 11i, 12k

Solution to Exercise 7
1i, 2a, 3d, 4j, 5b, 6e, 7l, 8k, 9g, 10h, 11c, 12f

Vocabulary
abbreviation /əˌbriː.viˈeɪ.ʃən/ zkratka
ability /əˈbɪl.ɪ.ti/ schopnost
absolutely /ˌæb.səˈluːt.li/ absolutně, naprosto
abuse /əˈbjuːz/ zneužívání, zneužít
acceptable /əkˈsept.ə.bl̩/ přijatelný
achieve /əˈtʃiːv/ dosáhnout, uspět
acquire /əˈkwaɪəʳ/ získat
action /ˈæk.ʃən/ postup, působení
additional /əˈdɪʃ.ən.əl/ dodatečný, doplňkový
adhere /ədˈhɪəʳ/ držet se, lepit se na
adjunct /ˈædʒ.ʌŋk t/ doplněk
administer /ədˈmɪn.ɪ.stəʳ/ podávat lék

adrenaline /ə'dren.əl.ɪn/ adrenalin, epinefrin

adverse /'æd.vɜːs/ nepříznivý

advertising /'æd.və.taɪ.zɪŋ/ inzerát

advice /əd'vaɪs/ rada

affected /ə'fek.tɪd/ zasažený

afterwards /'ɑːf.tə.wədz/ potom

agent /'eɪ.dʒənt/ činitel, prostředek

alert /ə'lɜːt/ varovat

allow /ə'laʊ/ dovolit, poskytovat

alter /'ɒl.tə^r/ změnit se

alveolar /ˌæl.vi'əʊ.lə^r/ dásňový

ampicillin /əm'pəs.ɪ.lɪn/ ampicilin

analgesic /ˌæn.əl'dʒiː.zɪk/ analgetikum

anesthetise /ə'niːs.θə.taɪz/ dát narkózu, umrtvit

antibiotics /ˌæn.ti.baɪ'ɒt.ɪk/ antibiotika

anticonvulsant /ˌæn.ti.kən'vʌl.s°nt/ antikonvulzívum, protikřečový

antidote /'æn.ti.dəʊt/ protilátka

anti-inflammatory /ˌæn.ti.ɪn'flæm.ə.tri/ protizánětlivý

anxiety /æŋ'zaɪ.ə.ti/ úzkost

anxiolytic /ˌænks'.aɪəl.ɪ.tɪk/ anxiolytikum, lék proti úzkosti

appear /ə'pɪə^r/ zdát se

appearance /ə'pɪə.rənts/ vzhled

appliance /ə'plaɪ.ənts/ přístroj, spotřebič

appropriate /ə'prəʊ.pri.ət/ vhodný

argue /'ɑːg.juː/ for /fɔːr/ obhajovat

arise /ə'raɪz/ vyskytnout se, vyskytnout se, nastat, vzniknout

arrangement /ə'reɪndʒ.mənt/ opatření, uspořádání

arrhythmia /æ'rɪθ.mɪ.ə/ arytmie

aspect /'æs.pekt/ hledisko, poloha, vzhled

aspirate /'æs.pɪ.reɪt/ nasávat

aspirin /'æs.pɪ.rɪn/ aspirin

ataxia /ə'tæk.sɪ.ə/ ataxie, ztráta kontroly volních pohybů

attempt /ə'tempt/ pokus

attend /ə'tend/ navštěvovat

available /ə'veɪ.lə.bļ/ dostupný, k dispozici

avoid /ə'vɔɪd/ vyhnout se

awareness /ə'weə.nəs/ uvědomění, připravenost

bacterial /bæk'tɪə.ri.əl/ bakteriální

bactericidal /bæk,tɪə.ri.saɪdl/ baktericidní, zabíjející bakterie

bacteriostatic /bæk,tɪə.ri.ə'stæt.ɪk/ bakteriostatický, bránící množení

bearing /'beə.rɪŋ/ nosný, ložisko

beat /biːt/ bít

beforehand /bɪ'fɔː.hænd/ předem

benefit /'ben.ɪ.fɪt/ prospěch, pomoc

benzodiazepine /ben.'zəʊ.daɪ.æ.sə,paɪn/ benzodiazepin

beware /bɪ'weə^r/ dát si pozor, varovat se

bite /baɪt/ kousat, kousnutí

blanch /blɑːntʃ/ zblednout

block /blɒk/ blokovat

body /'bɒd.i/ weight /weɪt/ tělesná váha

bore /bɔːr/ kalibr, vývrt

branch /brɑːntʃ/ rozvětvení

break down /'breɪk.daʊn/ rozbít

breastfeeding /'brest,fiːd.ɪŋ/ kojení

broad /brɔːd/ široký, obsáhlý

bundle /'bʌn.dļ/ svazek

bung /bʌŋ/ čep, zátka

button /'bʌt.°n/ tlačítko

cancellation /ˌkænt.səl'eɪ.ʃən/ zrušení

careful /'keə.fəl/ pečlivý, opatrný

carry /'kær.i/ away /ə'weɪ/ nést pryč

carry /'kær.i/ out /aʊt/ vykonat

cartridge /'kɑː.trɪdʒ/ náplň

case /keɪs/ případ, důvod, věc

cause /kɔːz/ způsobit, být příčinou

caution /'kɔː.ʃ°n/ opatrnost

cell /sel/ buňka

chance /tʃɑːnʦs/ šance, možnost

chlorhexidine /ˌklɒː.hek.sɪˈdiːn/ chlorhexidin

chosen /ˈtʃəʊ.zᵊn/ (inf. choose) vybraný

chronic /ˈkrɒn.ɪk/ vleklý, trvalý

close /kləʊz/ blízký

code /kəʊd/ kód

codeine /ˈkəʊ.diːn/ kodein

comfort /ˈkʌm.fət/ pohodlí, uklidnění

command /kəˈmɑːnd/ příkaz, nařídit

common /ˈkɒm.ən/ běžný, častý

compact /kəmˈpækt/ pevný, hustý

complete /kəmˈpliːt/ dokončený

complicated /ˈkɒm.plɪ.keɪ.tɪd/ složitý

concern /kənˈsɜːn/ znepokojení

condition /kənˈdɪʃ.ən/ stav

conduction /kənˈdʌk.ʃən/ vedení, přenos

confidence /ˈkɒn.fɪ.dənʦs/ důvěra, spolehnutí

confused /kənˈfjuːzd/ zmatený, nejasný

conscious /ˈkɒn.ʧəs/ při vědomí, uvědomělý

consciousness /ˈkɒn.ʧə.snəs/ vědomí

consent /kənˈsent/ souhlas, shoda

consequence /ˈkɒnʧ.sɪ.kwənʦs/ následek

container /kənˈteɪ.nəʳ/ obal, schránka

content /ˈkɒn.tent/ obsah

context /ˈkɒn.tekst/ souvislost

contraindicate /ˌkɒn.trə.ˈɪn.dɪ.keɪt/ kontraindikovat

contraindication / ˈkɒn.trə.ˌɪnd.ɪ.ˈkeɪʃᵊn/ kontraindikace

cooker /ˈkʊk.əʳ/ sporák

cooperative /kəʊˈɒp.ᵊr.ə.tɪv/ spolupracující

copious /ˈkəʊ.pi.əs/ hojný

count /kaʊnt/ počet, spočítat

course /kɔːs/ průběh, kúra (léčebná)

cylinder /ˈsɪl.ɪn.dəʳ/ tlaková láhev

damage /ˈdæm.ɪdʒ/ poškození

dangerous /ˈdeɪn.dʒər.əs/ nebezpečný

debris /ˈdeb.riː/, /ˈdeɪ.briː/ úlomky, pozůstatky

deciduous /dɪˈsɪd.ju.əs/ dočasný, mléčný

declare /dɪˈkleəʳ/ prohlašovat

defibrillator /ˌdiːˈfɪb.rɪ.leɪ.tər/ defibrilátor

delay /dɪˈleɪ/ zpoždění

delete /dɪˈliːt/ vymazat, vynechat

dependence /dɪˈpen.dᵊnts/ závislost, vztah

deposit /dɪˈpɒz.ɪt/ uložit

depressed /dɪˈprest/ skleslý, stlačený, snížený

depression /dɪˈpreʃ.ən/ deprese, potlačení

depth /depθ/ hloubka, tloušťka

desirable /dɪˈzaɪə.rə.bļ/ žádoucí

detract /dɪˈtrækt/ odvést pozornost

detriment /ˈdet.rɪ.mənt/ neprospěch, poškození

diameter /daɪˈæm.ɪ.təʳ/ průměr (kružnice)

differentiation /ˌdɪf.ər.en.t ʃiˈeɪ.ʃən/ rozlišování, rozdílnost

disastrous /dɪˈzɑː.strəs/ katastrofální

discard /dɪˈskɑːd/ vyřadit, vyřazení

disorganization /dɪˌsɔː.gə.naɪˈzeɪ.ʃᵊn/ rozpad, rozklad, nepořádek

dispose /dɪˈspəʊz/ uspořádat, použít, likvidovat

dissipate /ˈdɪs.ɪ.peɪt/ rozptýlit se

distal /dɪs.təl/ distální, vzdálený

distraction /dɪˈstræk.ʃən/ rozptýlení

disturbance /dɪˈstɜː.bənʦs/ nesprávnost funkce, porušení, rozrušení

division /dɪˈvɪʒ.ᵊn/ dělení

domestic /dəˈmes.tɪk/ domácí, používaný v domácnosti

dose /dəʊs/ dávka (zpravidla léku),
   dávkovat
drill /drɪl/ vrtat
droop /druːp/ sklesnout
drop /drɒp/ klesnout
drowsiness /ˈdraʊ.zɪ.nəs/ ospalost
ease /iːz/ **off** /ɒf/ odstranit
effect /ɪˈfekt/ účinek
elderly /ˈel.dəl.i/ postarší, vyššího věku
emerge /ɪˈmɜːdʒ/ objevit se (náhle),
   vyjít najevo
enable /ɪˈneɪ.bl̩/ umožnit, učinit
   schopným
enamel /ɪˈnæm.əl/ sklovina (zubní)
ending /ˈen.dɪŋ/ zakončení
equipped /ɪˈkwɪpt/ vybavený
erythromycin /əˌrɪθ.rəˈmaɪ.sɪn/
   erytromycin
escort /ɪˈskɔːt/ doprovázet, odvést
essential /ɪˈsen.tʃəl/ podstatný, důležitý
exacting /ɪɡˈzæk.tɪŋ/ náročný
exaggerate /ɪɡˈzædʒ.ə.reɪt/ přehánět,
   zveličovat
excessive /ekˈses.ɪv/ nadměrný
exclusive /ɪkˈskluː.sɪv/ vylučující
excrete /ɪkˈskriːt/ vylučovat
exert /ɪɡˈzɜːt/ použít
exhibit /ɪɡˈzɪb.ɪt/ ukázka, projevit
experience /ɪkˈspɪə.ri.ənts/ ucítit
exposure /ɪkˈspəʊ.ʒəʳ/ vystavení
eyelid /ˈaɪ.lɪd/ oční víčko
fail /feɪl/ selhat
fall /fɔːl/ **asleep** /əˈsliːp/ usnout
fall /fɔːl/ **into** /ˈɪn.tuː/ spadat do
fall /fɔːl/ pád, padat
fear /fɪəʳ/ strach
feature /ˈfiː.tʃəʳ/ charakteristický rys
feel /fiːl/ cítit
fever /ˈfiː.vəʳ/ horečka
fibre optic /ˈfaɪ.bə.ˈɒp.tɪk/ optické
   vlákno
filter /ˈfɪl.təʳ/ infiltrovat

finger /ˈfɪŋ.ɡəʳ/ prst, ohmatat
finish /ˈfɪn.ɪʃ/ skončit, dokončit, závěr
fire /faɪəʳ/ oheň
flat /flæt/ plochý
flow /fləʊ/ tok
flush /flʌʃ/ přítok
following /ˈfɒl.əʊ.ɪŋ/ následující
for /fɔːʳ/ **the sake** /seɪk/ kvůli, v zájmu
foramen /fəˈreɪ.mən/ **(pl. foramina)**
   otvor, průchod
forcibly /ˈfɔː.sɪ.bli/ násilně
form /fɔːm/ forma, formulář, podoba
function /ˈfʌŋk.ʃən/ funkce, fungovat
gain /ɡeɪn/ získat
general /ˈdʒen.ər.əl/ **anaesthesia** /
   ˌæn.əsˈθiː.zi.ə/ celková anestézie,
   narkóza
generic /dʒəˈner.ɪk/ všeobecný,
   druhový (označující druh)
gingiva /ˌdʒɪn.dʒaɪ.və/ **(pl. gingivae)**
   dáseň
gram /ɡræm/ **negative** /ˈneg.ə.tɪv/
   gram negativní
gram /ɡræm/ **positive** /ˈpɒz.ə.tɪv/
   gram pozitivní
guarantee /ˌɡær.ənˈtiː/ zaručit
gum /ɡʌm/ dáseň
happen /ˈhæp.ən/ stát se
hazard /ˈhæz.əd/ riziko
heading /ˈhed.ɪŋ/ záhlaví, hledisko,
   přední část
herald /ˈher.əld/ ohlašovat
hole /həʊl/ dírka
household /ˈhaʊs.həʊld/ domácnost
hypertension /ˌhaɪ.pəˈten.tʃən/
   vysoký tlak
hyperthyroidism /ˌ
   haɪ.pə.ˈθaɪə.rɔɪdɪ.zəm/
   hypertyroidismus, zvýšená činnost
   štítné žlázy
hypnotherapy /ˌhɪp.nəʊ ˈθer.ə.pi/
   hypnoterapie, léčení spánkem

hypnotic /hɪpˈnɒt.ɪk/ uspávající, lék navozující spánek

hypotension /ˌhaɪ.pəʊˈten.tʃ°n/ nízký tlak

ibuprofen /ˌaɪ.bjuːˈprəʊ.fen/ ibuprofen

identify /aɪˈden.tɪ.faɪ/ identifikovat, ztotožňovat se

ill /ɪl/ **effect** /ɪˈfekt/ škodlivý následek

immediate /ɪˈmiː.di.ət/ okamžitý, bezprostřední

impaired /ɪmˈpeəd/ zhoršený, poškozený

impulse /ˈɪm.pʌls/ podnět, náraz

in situ /ˌɪnˈsɪt.juː/ na původním místě

inadvertent /ˌɪn.ədˈvɜː.t°nt/ nepozorný, nedbalý

increase /ɪnˈkriːs/ zvýšit

indication /ˌɪn.dɪˈkeɪ.ʃ°n/ indikace, údaj, označení

induce /ɪnˈdjuːs/ navodit

ineffective /ˌɪn.ɪˈfek.tɪv/ neúčinný

infectious /ɪnˈfek.ʃəs/ nakažlivý, přenosný

inferior /ɪnˈfɪə.ri.əʳ/ spodní

infiltration /ˌɪn.fɪlˈtreɪ.ʃ°n/ infiltrace, pronikání, prosakování

ingestion /ɪnˈdʒes.tʃ°n/ přijímání potravy

inhalation /ˌɪn.hə'leɪ.ʃ°n/ inhalace

instead /ɪnˈsted/ **of** /əv/ namísto

instruction /ɪnˈstrʌk.ʃ°n/ pokyn, návod, směrnice

interact /ˌɪn.tə'rækt/ reagovat vzájemně, vzájemně na sebe působit

interaction /ˌɪn.tə'ræk.ʃ°n/ spolupůsobení, vzájemná součinnost

interruption /ˌɪn.tə'rʌp.ʃ°n/ přerušení, překážka

intoxication /ɪnˌtɒk.sɪˈkeɪ.ʃ°n/ intoxikace, omámení

intraligament /ɪn.trə.ˈlɪg.ə.mənt/ do vaziva

intraorally /ˌɪn.trə.ˈɔː.rə.li/ intraorálně

intraosseous /ˌɪn.trəˈɒs.i.əs/ intraoseální, nitrokostní, ležící uvnitř kosti

intravenous /ˌɪn.trəˈviː.nəs/ intravenózní, nitrožilní

intubation /ˌɪŋ.tjʊˈbeɪ.ʃ°n/ intubace, zavedení rourky do průdušnice

irreversible /ˌɪr.ɪˈvɜː.sɪ.bl̩/ nevratný

irrigation /ˌɪr.ɪˈgeɪ.ʃ°n/ nálev, výplach

lethargy /ˈleθ.ə.dʒɪ/ letargie, strnulost, netečnost

level /ˈlev.°l/ úroveň

ligament /ˈlɪg.ə.mənt/ vazivo

light /laɪt/ lehký

light-headed /ˌlaɪt'hed.ɪd/ zmámený, mající závrať

limited /ˈlɪm.ɪ.tɪd/ omezený

lingual /ˈlɪŋ.gw°l/ jazykový

lip /lɪp/ ret

liquid /ˈlɪk.wɪd/ tekutina

long-acting /lɒŋ.ˈæk.tɪŋ/ dlouhodobě působící

loss /lɒs/ ztráta

machinery /məˈʃiː.nə.ri/ strojové vybavení

maintain /meɪnˈteɪn/ uchovat, udržet

major /ˈmeɪ.dʒəʳ/ velký, důležitý

manipulation /məˌnɪp.jʊˈleɪ.ʃ°n/ zpracování, obsluha

margin /ˈmɑː.dʒɪn/ okraj, lemování

marked /mɑːkt/ označený

maxillofacial /ˌmæk.sɪ.lə'feɪ.ʃ°l/ maxilofaciální, týkající se horní čelisti a tváře

meal /mɪəl/ jídlo (denní)

medical /ˈmed.ɪ.k°l/ **history** /ˈhɪs.tər.i/ lékařská anamnéza medication /ˌmed.ɪˈkeɪ.ʃᵊn/ léky, léčení

mental /ˈmen.tl̩/ duševní, psychický

metabolise /məˈtæb.ᵊl.aɪz/ metabolizovat

microorganism /maɪ.krəʊ.ˈɔː.gən.ɪ.zᵊm/ mikroorganismus, mikrob

mild /maɪld/ mírný, klidný

mind /maɪnd/ mysl, vadit, paměť

modification /ˌmɒd.ɪ.fɪˈkeɪ.ʃᵊn/ přizpůsobení, obměna

mouthwash /ˈmaʊθ.wɒʃ/ ústní voda

movement /ˈmuːv.mənt/ pohyb

mycoplasma /maɪ.kəˈplæz.mə/ mykoplazma

nail /neɪl/ varnish /ˈvɑː.nɪʃ/ lak na nehty

narrow /ˈnær.əʊ/ úzký, zužovat se

nauseous /ˈnɔː.zi.əs/ působící zvedání žaludku

nearby /ˌnɪəˈbaɪ/ blízký, sousední

needle /ˈniː.dl̩/ jehla

nerve /nɜːv/ block /blɒk/ nervový blok

nerve /nɜːv/ trunk /trʌŋk/ nervový kmen

nervousness /ˈnɜː.və.snəs/ nervozita, nervóza

neurovascular /ˌnjʊə.rəʊˈvæs.kjʊ.ləʳ/ neurovaskulární

nitrous oxide /ˌnaɪ.trəsˈɒk.saɪd/ kysličník dusný, rajský plyn

noise /nɔɪz/ hluk, zvuk, poruchy

note /nəʊt/ poznámka

numb /nʌm/ necitlivý

numbness /ˈnʌm.nəs/ znecitlivění

observe /əbˈzɜːv/ sledovat

onset /ˈɒn.set/ příchod (počátek, nástup)

operate /ˈɒp.ᵊr.eɪt/ operovat, obsluhovat (stroj ap.)

opiate /ˈəʊ.pi.ət/ opiát, narkotický lék

opioid /əʊ.ˈpiː.ɒɪd/ opiát

opposed /əˈpəʊzd/ protikladný

otherwise /ˈʌð.ə.waɪz/ jinak, nebo

outpatient /ˈaʊt.peɪ.ʃᵊnt/ ambulantní pacient

over /ˈəʊ.vəʳ/ dosage /ˈdəʊ.sɪdʒ/ předávkování

oximeter /ˌɒk.sɪ.miː.təʳ/ oximetr

oxygen /ˈɒk.sɪ.dʒən/ kyslík

oxygenation /ˌɒk.sɪ.dʒəˈneɪ.ʃᵊn/ oxygenace, okysličení

pack /pæk/ balíček

painkiller /ˈpeɪnˌkɪl.əʳ/ lék proti bolesti

painlessly /ˈpeɪn.lə.sli/ bezbolestně

palpitations /ˌpæl.pɪˈteɪ.ʃᵊnz/ palpitace, bušení srdce

papilla /pəˈpɪl.ə/ (pl. papillae) bradavka, papila

paracetamol /ˌpær.əˈsiː.tə.mɒl/ paracetamol

paraesthesia /ˌpær.əsˈθiː.sɪ.ə/ parestezie, změněná citlivost

partial /ˈpɑː.ʃᵊl/ částečný

particular /pəˈtɪk.jʊ.ləʳ/ zvláštní

pass /pɑːs/ projít, podat

pellicle /pel.ɪ.kl̩/ povlak

penetrate /ˈpen.ɪ.treɪt/ proniknout

penicillin /ˌpen.əˈsɪl.ɪn/ penicilin

perform /pəˈfɔːm/ vykonat, fungovat

period /ˈpɪə.ri.əd/ doba, období

permeability /ˌpɜː.mi.əˈbɪl.ɪ.ti/ permeabilita, propustnost

pharmacy /ˈfɑː.mə.si/ farmacie, lékárnička

pharynx /ˈfær.ɪŋks/ farynx, hltan

phobic /ˈfəʊ.bɪk/ panický

pins /pɪns/ and needles /ˈniː.dlz̩/ brnění (mravenčení)

plain /pleɪn/ jednoduchý

plaque /plɑːk/ plak, zubní kámen

plasma /ˈplæz.mə/ plazma

polypharmacy /pɒl.ɪ.ˈfɑː.mə.si/ nadměrné užívání léčiv

poor /pɔːʳ/ slabý

pore /pɔːʳ/ pór

position /pəˈzɪʃ.ᵊn/ umístit

posterior /pɒsˈtɪə.ri.əʳ/ pozdější, zadní část

postoperative /ˌpəʊstˈɒp.ᵊr.ə.tɪv/ pooperační

potent /ˈpəʊ.tᵊnt/ silně účinný

potentially /pəʊ ˈten.tʃᵊl.i/ potenciálně

potentiate /pəʊ ˈten.tʃi.eɪt/ znásobit, umocnit

practitioner /prækˈtɪʃ.ᵊn.əʳ/ praktický lékař

precipitate /prɪˈsɪp.ɪ.teɪt/ urychlovat

preference /ˈpref.ᵊr.ᵊnts/ přednost (priorita)

pregnancy /ˈpreg.nənt.si/ těhotenství

pregnant /ˈpreg.nənt/ gravidní (těhotná)

premolar /ˌpriːˈməʊ.ləʳ/ třenový zub

preoperative /priː.ˈɒp.ᵊr.ə.tɪv/ předoperační

prescribe /prɪˈskraɪb/ předepisovat, naordinovat

prescription /prɪˈskrɪp.ʃᵊn/ lékařský předpis

pressed /prest/ stlačený

pressure /ˈpreʃ.əʳ/ tlak

previous /ˈpriː.vi.əs/ předchozí

profound /prəˈfaʊnd/ hluboký (důkladný)

prolong /prəˈlɒŋ/ prodloužit

prolonged /prəˈlɒŋd/ dlouhodobý, prodloužený

promptly /ˈprɒmpt.li/ okamžitě, rychle

prophylactic /ˌprɒf.ɪˈlæk.tɪk/ preventivní

proximity /prɒkˈsɪm.ɪ.ti/ těsná blízkost

ptosis /təu.sɪs/ ptóza, sklesnutí orgánu

pulpitis /pʌlˈpaɪ.tɪs/ pulpitida, zánět zubní dřeně

range /reɪndʒ/ rozsah, roztřídit, seřadit

rate /reɪt/ poměr, rychlost

reach /riːtʃ/ dosáhnout, rozpětí

realm /relm/ doména, oblast

reassuring /ˌriː.əˈʃɔː.rɪŋ/ uklidňování

recent /ˈriː.sᵊnt/ současný, poslední (nedávný)

recognise /ˈrek.əg.naɪz/ rozpoznat, připustit, uznat

recourse /rɪˈkɔːs/ pomoc, východisko, přístup

recovery /rɪˈkʌv.ᵊr.i/ zotavení, uzdravení

reduce /rɪˈdjuːs/ zmenšit

reduction /rɪˈdʌk.ʃᵊn/ zmenšení, omezení, zmírnění

regional /ˈriː.dʒᵊn.ᵊl/ týkající se dané oblasti, ohraničený

relative /ˈrel.ə.tɪv/ poměrný, nikoli absolutní

relaxed /rɪˈlækst/ uvolněný

remain /rɪˈmeɪn/ zbývat (zůstat)

remainder /rɪˈmeɪn.dəʳ/ zbytek

remaining /rɪˈmeɪ.nɪŋ/ zbývající

render /ˈren.dəʳ/ poskytovat

repeat /rɪˈpiːt/ opakovat

replication /ˌrep.lɪˈkeɪ.ʃᵊn/ replikace, reprodukce stejným způsobem

report /rɪˈpɔːt/ ohlásit, oznámit

reposition /rɪ.pəˈzɪʃ.ən/ přemístit

request /rɪˈkwest/ požádání, prosba, žádat

require /rɪˈkwaɪəʳ/ požadovat

resistance /rɪˈzɪs.tᵊnts/ odpor

respiratory /rɪˈspɪr.ə.tri/ dýchací

respond /rɪˈspɒnd/ reagovat (odpovídat)

response /rɪˈspɒnts/ reakce

responsible /rɪˈspɒnt.sɪ.bl̩/ odpovědný

restrictive /rɪˈstrɪk.tɪv/ omezující

result /rɪˈzʌlt/ být následkem, mít za následek

reversible /rɪˈvɜː.sə.bl̩/ reverzibilní, vratný

ridge /rɪdʒ/ hřbet, rýha, okraj

ring /rɪŋ/ zvonit

rise /raɪz/ vzestup, zdvihat se (stoupat)

root /ruːt/ planing /pleɪn.ɪŋ/ vyhlazení stěn kořene

rouse /raʊz/ vzbudit

rubber /ˈrʌb.əʳ/ guma

safe /seɪf/ bezpečný, důvěryhodný

safety /ˈseɪf.ti/ device /dɪˈvaɪs/ bezpečnostní zařízení

saturation /ˌsæt.jʊˈreɪ.ʃᵊn/ saturace (nasycení)

seal /siːl/ off /ɒf/ zablokovat, zatarasit

search /sɜːtʃ/ for /fɔːʳ/ hledat

sedate /sɪˈdeɪt/ zklidnit

sedation /sɪˈdeɪ.ʃᵊn/ uklidňující lék, utišení

sedative /ˈsed.ə.tɪv/ bolesti utišující lék, uklidňující

self-healing /self.ˈhiː.lɪŋ/ samoregenerační

sensitivity /ˌsent.sɪˈtɪv.ɪ.ti/ citlivost, vnímavost

sensory /ˈsent.sᵊr.i/ disability /ˌdɪs.əˈbɪl.ɪ.ti/ smyslové postižení

shatter /ˈʃæt.əʳ/ roztříštit se

side /saɪd/ effect /ɪˈfekt/ vedlejší účinek

signature /ˈsɪg.nɪ.tʃəʳ/ podpis, podepsání

significant /sɪgˈnɪf.ɪ.kənt/ významný

site /saɪt/ poloha, umístění

slight /slaɪt/ nepatrný, mírný

slow /sləʊ/ zpomalit

slurred /slɜːʳd/ nezřetelný

snore /snɔːʳ/ chrápat

soak /səʊk/ vsáknout se

sore /sɔːʳ/ bolavý

soreness /ˈsɔː.nəs/ bolestivost

sound /saʊnd/ pořádný, seriózní

space /speɪs/ místo (volné)

sphenopalatine /ˌsfiː.n.əˈpæl.ə.taɪn/ sfenopalatální, týkající se kosti klínové a patrové

spotted /ˈspɒt.ɪd/ spatřený

starved /stɑːvd/ hladový

state /steɪt/ stav

stimulant /ˈstɪm.jʊ.lənt/ povzbuzující prostředek

stimulation /ˌstɪm.jʊˈleɪ.ʃᵊn/ podnět, povzbuzení

strength /streŋθ/ síla (moc), stabilita, silná stránka

subjective /ˈsʌb.dʒek.tɪv/ subjektivní (osobní)

substance /ˈsʌb.stᵊn/ s/ látka

suffer /ˈsʌf.əʳ/ from /frɒm/ trpět něčím

sufficient /səˈfɪʃ.ᵊnt/ dostatečný

suggestion /səˈdʒes.tʃᵊn/ sugesce (vnuknutí)

suicidal /ˌsuː.ɪˈsaɪ.dᵊl/ idea /aɪˈdɪə/ sebevražedná myšlenka

suitable /ˈsjuː.tə.bl̩/ vhodný

supply /səˈplaɪ/ zásoba, dodání

surrounding /səˈraʊn.dɪŋ/ okolní, sousední tkáň

swollen /ˈswəʊ.lən/ oteklý

sympathetic /ˌsɪm.pəˈθet.ɪk/ sympatický, účastný (soucitný)

syringe /sɪˈrɪndʒ/ injekční stříkačka

tenderness /ˈten.də.nəs/ bolestivost, citlivost (na dotek)

tension /ˈten.ʃᵊn/ napětí

therapeutic /ˌθer.əˈpjuː.tɪk/ terapeutický (léčebný), lék

therefore /ˈðeə.fɔːʳ/ proto tedy, tudíž

thermal /ˈθɜː.məl/ tepelný

throat /θrəʊt/ hrdlo

throughout /θruːˈaʊt/ celkový

thus /ðʌs/ takto, tudíž

tight /taɪt/ těsný

tingle /ˈtɪŋ.gl̩/ zvonit (v uších), brnět (v těle), tetelit se (chvět se) tinnitus /'tɪn.ɪ.təs/ tinitus, hučení v ušich

tip /tɪp/ hrot

toe /təʊ/ prst (na noze)

tolerance /'tɒl.ᵉr.ᵊnts/ snášenlivost

tongue /tʌŋ/ jazyk

topical /'tɒp.ɪ.kᵊl/ místní, aktuální (soudobý)

touch /tʌtʃ/ dotek, hmat

trained /treɪnd/ vyškolený

transmission /trænz'mɪʃ.ᵊn/ transmise (převod), zaslání, odevzdání

traumatize /'trɔː.mə.taɪz/ traumatizovat, poranit

tremor /'trem.əʳ/ třes, chvění

trigeminal /'traɪ'dʒem.ɪ.nᵊl/ nerve / nɜːv/ trojklaný nerv

trismus /'trɪz.məs/ trizmus, křeč žvýkacího svalstva

trochlear /trə.kli.ə/ horní sval oční

try /traɪ/ pokusit se, zkoušet, zkusit

tuberosity /'tjuː.bə'rɒs.ə.ti/ hrbol na kosti

unacceptable /ˌʌn.ək'sep.tə.bl̩/ nepřijatelný

unaccompanied /ˌʌn.ə'kʌm.pᵊn.id/ samotný, nedoprovázený

unavoidable /ˌʌn.ə'vɔɪ.də.bl̩/ nevyhnutelný

unconsciousness /ʌn'kɒn.tʃə.snəs/ bezvědomí, mdloby

undergo /ˌʌn.də'gəʊ/ podstoupit

understandable /ˌʌn.də'stæn.də.bl̩/ pochopitelný

undertake /ˌʌn.də'teɪk/ provést, ujmout se

unfit /ʌn'fɪt/ neschopný (čeho), nezpůsobilý

unintended /ˌʌn.ɪn'ten.dɪd/ neúmyslný, nezamýšlený

unknown /ʌn'nəʊn/ neznámý

unlikely /ʌn'laɪ.kli/ nepravděpodobný

unwanted /ʌn'wɒn.tɪd/ nežádoucí

upper /'ʌp.əʳ/ horní

use /juːs/ užití, funkce, praxe

uterine /'juː.tᵊr.aɪn/ děložní

valid /'væl.ɪd/ platný, oprávněný

variation /ˌveə.ri'eɪ.ʃᵊn/ odchylka

vasoconstrictor /ˌveɪz.ə.kən'strɪkt.əʳ/ vazokonstrikční látka, vyvolávající smrštění cévy

vehicle /'viː.ɪ.kl̩/ dopravní prostředek

vouch /vaʊtʃ/ for /fɔːʳ/ zaručit

warm /wɔːm/ nahřát

warning /'wɔː.nɪŋ/ upozornění

wear /weəʳ/ off /ɒf/ mizet (ztrácet se)

weight /weɪt/ váha

whereas /weə'ræz/ kdežto (zatímco naopak)

whilst /waɪlst/ zatímco

wide /waɪd/ široký

widen /'waɪ.dᵊn/ rozšířit

withdrawal /wɪð'drɔː.ᵊl/ stažení (ústup), odnětí, vysazení

worldwide /wɜːld.waɪd/ světový, celosvětově

write /raɪt/ up /ʌp/ dokončit (dopsat)

Unit 9

Oral Medicine

Oral Infection. Local and Systemic Factors Predisposing to Candidal Infection. Potentially Malignant Lesions and Conditions. Oral Cancer. Salivary Gland Disorders. Sjögren's Syndrome. Ocular Symptoms. Oral Symptoms. Aetiological Factors in Oral Dysaesthesia. Atypical Facial Pain. Trigeminal Neuralgia. Periodic Migrainous Neuralgia (cluster headache). HIV Infection and AIDS.

Text 1

Oral Infection

Bacterial infection

A wide variety of bacterial infections may have oral lesions although, with the exception of dental caries and periodontal disease, they are all relatively uncommon (tuberculosis, gonorrhoea, syphilis).

Fungal infections

The oral mucosa may be affected by a variety of fungal diseases. With the exception of candidosis, all are uncommon.

Local and Systemic Factors Predisposing to Candidal Infection

Local factors:
- **trauma**
- **denture** wearing
- **poor denture hygiene**
- **xerostomia**

Systemic factors:
- **radiotherapy**
- **antibiotic** therapy
- **corticosteroid** therapy
- extremes of life—**infancy** and **old age**
- **diabetes** mellitus
- **nutritional deficiency** (iron, folate, and vitamin B12)
- **immunosuppression**
- cigarette **smoking**
- **high carbohydrate diet**

Viral infection

A wide range of viruses are responsible for causing oral lesions. These include:
- **herpes simplex** types 1 and 2
- herpes **zoster**
- **human papilloma** viruses

Recurrent herpetic infection

Approximately 30% of patients subsequently develop recurrent infections. The virus **lies dormant** and is reactivated by a variety of **precipitating factors** including:
- **trauma**
- exposure to **sunlight**

- **stress**
- **menstruation**
- **immunosupression**

Recurrence is heralded by a **prodromal burning** or **prickling** sensation in the area followed by the formation of small **vesicles** which enlarge and then rupture. Lesions then **crust** over and **heal spontaneously.**

Recurrent oral ulceration

Ulceration is defined as breaking in the continuity of an epithelial lining.

Causes:

- **traumatic** (mechanical, chemical, thermal, radiation)
- **idiopathic** (recurrent aphthous stomatitis)
- **infection** (viral, bacterial, fungal)
- associated with **systemic disease** (haematological disorders, Crohn's disease, ulcerative colitis)
- associated with **dermatological** diseases (lichen planus, vesiculobullous disorders)
- **neoplastic** (squamous cell carcinoma and other tumours)
- **drug induced** (cytotoxic agents)

Exercise 1

1. Which bacterial infections may have oral lesions?
2. What is candidosis?
3. Describe local and systemic factors predisposing to candidal infection.
4. Which viral infections do you know?
5. Talk about recurrent herpetic infection (precipitating factors, sensations, healing).
6. What do you know about the causes of recurrent oral ulceration?

Translation 1

Ústní infekce, zubní kazy, nemoci parodontu, poměrně neobvyklé (tuberkulóza, kapavka, syfilis), ústní sliznice mohou být zasaženy rozmanitými plísňovými chorobami, kandidóza, místní a systemické faktory předcházející infekci kandidózy, místní faktory, úraz, nošení protéz, chabá hygiena protéz, xerostomie, systemické faktory, radioterapie, léčba antibiotiky, léčba kortikosteroidy, dětství, stáří, cukrovka, nedostatky ve výživě, potlačení imunity, kouření cigaret, výživa s vysokou spotřebou uhlovodanů, viry způsobující ústní poranění, opar rtu, pásový opar, lidské papilom viry, opakované herpetické infekce, virus setrvává v klidovém stadium a je reaktivován rozmanitými urychlujícími faktory, zranění, vystavení slunečnímu světlu, stress, menstruace, potlačení imunity, pocit pálení, píchání, vytvoření malých puchýřků, které se zvětšují a pak prasknou, strupy, samovolně se hojí, opakující se tvoření vředů v ústech, vředovatění, porušení celistvosti epitelové výstelky, úrazové (mechanické, chemické, tepelné, zářením), idiopatické, nezávisle vzniklé (opakovaná aftózní stomatitida), infekce (virové, bakteriální, plísňové), systemické onemocnění (krevní onemocnění, Crohnova choroba, vředová kolitida – zánět tlustého střeva), kožní choroby (lišej, poruchy s tvořením puchýřků a puchýřů), novotvary (karcinom – rakovinný nádor plochých buněk a jiné tumory), způsobené léky, cytotoxické činitele (škodlivé pro buňky).

Text 2
Potentially Malignant Lesions and Conditions

A lesion can be regarded as potentially malignant if it is associated with a significantly **increased risk of cancer**. However, it must be stressed that **most oral cancers arise de novo** with no recognisable preceding premalignant state. Unfortunately, it is not possible to predict behaviour of an individual lesion although some clinical and histological features are associated with an increased risk of malignant transformation.

Oral Cancer
Aetiological factors:

- **tobacco** – all forms of smoking tobacco (cigarettes, cigars, and pipe smoking) are associated with an increased risk of oral cancer. The use of snuff and chewing tobacco also increases the risk.
- **alcohol** – increased risk in association with alcohol consumption. Alcohol acts synergistically with tobacco and multiplies the risk of oral cancer.
- **diet and nutrition** – increased risk of oesophageal and oropharyngeal tumours in patients with primary sideropenic anaemia.
- **ultraviolet light** – important risk factor for carcinoma of the lip.
- **chronic candida infection** - considered to be a premalignant condition.
- **chronic trauma** – mechanical trauma from ill-fitting dentures and a poorly maintained dentition as well as poor oral hygiene.

Salivary Gland Disorders
Xerostomia – possible causes:

- **psychogenic** (anxiety, depression, hypochondria)
- **drug-induced** (atropine, antihypertensive agents, antihistamines)
- **postirradiation**
- **dehydration** (e.g. diabetes mellitus, renal failure, fluid loss)
- **HIV salivary gland disease**

Sjögren's Syndrome – chronic inflammatory disease with probable autoimmune basis. Oral complications include:

- increased incidence of dental **caries**
- predisposition to oral **candidosis**
- ascending bacterial **sialadenitis**
- an increased incidence of **lymphoma**

Exercise 2

1. Write a few notes about oral cancer and individual aetiological factors.
2. Describe possible causes of xerostomia.
3. Which are the oral complications of Sjögren's syndrome?

Translation 2

Potenciálně maligní poškození a stavy, významně zvýšené riziko rakoviny, rakovina úst většinou vzniká nově, bez poznatelných předcházejících před- rakovinných stavů, klinické a histologické rysy, spojeny se zvýšeným rizikem maligních přeměn, etiologické (příčinné) faktory rakoviny, tabák, kouření cigaret, doutníků, dýmky, šňupání a žvýkání tabáku, alkohol, zvýšené riziko v souvislosti s požíváním alkoholu, zvyšuje a znásobuje účinek tabáku, strava a výživa, zvýšené riziko nádorů jícnu a nosohltanu u pacientů s prvotní anémií z nedostatku železa, ultrafialové záření, důležitý rizikový faktor karcinomu rtu, chronická infekce kandidy je považována za před-rakovinný stav, chronické trauma, mechanické trauma ze špatně upevněných protéz, špatně udržovaný chrup, chabá ústní hygiena, poruchy slinné žlázy, xerostomie (suchost úst), možné příčiny, psychogenní, úzkost, deprese, hypochondrie, způsobený léky, atropin, léky proti vysokému tlaku, antihistaminika, po ozáření, dehydratace (např. cukrovka, selhání ledvin, ztráta tekutin), onemocnění slinné žlázy při HIV, Sjögrenův syndrom, chronické zánětlivé onemocnění pravděpodobně na autoimunitním základě, zvýšený výskyt zubních kazů, náchylnost ke kandidóze, rostoucí bakteriální sialoadenitida (zánět slinné žlázy), zvýšený výskyt lymfonu (maligní nádor lymfatické tkáně).

Text 3

Ocular Symptoms—a positive response to at least one of the following questions:

- Have you had daily, persistent, troublesome **dry eyes** for at least 3 months?
- Do you have a recurrent **sensation of sand or gravel** in the eyes?
- Do you use **tear substitutes** more than 3 times daily?

Oral Symptoms—a positive response to at least one of the following questions:

- Have you had a daily feeling of a **dry mouth** for more than 3 days?
- Have you had recurrently or persistently **swollen salivary glands** as an adult?
- Do you frequently drink **liquids to aid swallowing** dry food?

Aetiological Factors in Oral Dysaesthesia:

- **nutritional deficiencies** (iron, folate, and vitamin B12, vitamin B1, and B6)
- undiagnosed or **poorly controlled diabetes** mellitus
- **denture** factors (inadequate tongue space, unstable dentures, inadequate freeway space, hypersensitivity to acrylic monomer)
- **mucosal infections** (candidosis)
- **xerostomia**
- **parafunctional activity** (tongue thrusting, clenching, bruxism)
- **psychological** factors (anxiety, depression, cancerphobia)
- **drugs**
- **allergy** (denture based materials, food additives)

Atypical Facial Pain

It is a poorly defined term describing a condition characterised by **continuous, deep, diffuse pain** of variable intensity and severity with **no obvious organic pathology** in the affected area. While the pain is generally not sufficiently severe to disturb sleep, patients may report **early morning wakening**.

Essentially it means a diagnosis of exclusion. Atypical odontalgia is considered to be a variant of atypical facial pain. Predominantly affects females in the fourth or fifth decade of life.

Trigeminal Neuralgia
Pain is often described as **like an electric shock, lancinating, stabbing, or piercing** in nature. Some patients describe **a trigger zone** which may be either extraoral or intraoral. Thus patients may **avoid washing or shaving** a particular area on the face for fear of precipitating an attack of pain.

Periodic Migrainous Neuralgia (cluster headache)
It is characterised by **unilateral pain** predominantly affecting the **ocular, frontal, and temporal** regions. Males are more commonly affected. Pain occurs in discrete bouts, each lasting 30–90 minutes, and is often sufficiently severe to **waken** patient. Episodes are often accompanied by **rhinorrhoea, lacrimation, and conjunctival infection**. Some patients report that alcohol may be a precipitant. Episodes occur **in bouts** which can last for several days or weeks and then be followed by variable period of **remission**.

HIV Infection and AIDS
Oral lesions occur commonly in HIV-seropositive patients. In general they are not specific to HIV infection and simply reflect the immunocompromised state. Thus many of the oral lesions occur in patients who are immunosuppressed for other reasons. The prevalence of oral lesions among HIV-seropositive patients is dramatically **reduced by highly active antiretroviral therapy.**

Exercise 3
1. How will you ask a patient to get information about ocular symptoms?
2. How will you ask a patient to get information about oral symptoms?
3. Describe aetiological factors in oral dysaesthesia.
4. Give the symptoms of atypical facial pain.
5. Describe trigeminal neuralgia.
6. Characterise periodic migrainous neuralgia.
7. Talk about the prevalence of oral lesions among HIV-seropositive patients.

Translation 3
Oční symptomy, suché oči, každý den, trvale, nepříjemně, po dobu nejméně 3 měsíců, pocit písku nebo štěrku v očích, užívat léky zvlhčující oči více než třikrát denně, ústní symptomy, každodenní pocit suchých úst po dobu delší 3 dnů, opakovaně nebo stále oteklé slinné žlázy, pít často tekutiny na pomoc při polykání suché potravy, příčinné faktory při ústní dyzestezii (abnormální pocity na kůži jako pálení, píchání, svědění), nedostatky ve výživě, nediagnostikovaná či špatně léčená cukrovka, faktory spojené s protézou, nedostatek prostoru pro jazyk, nestabilní protézy, nedostatek volného místa, přecitlivělost, infekce

sliznice, kandidóza, nefunkční činnosti, vystrkování jazyka, svírání, skřípání zuby, psychologické faktory, úzkost, deprese, zveličený strach z rakoviny, alergie, materiály protéz, přídavky do jídla, bolest v obličeji, syndrom pálení v ústech, postihující ústní měkké tkáně, nepřítomnost klinicky prokázaného onemocnění sliznice, atypická bolest obličeje, nepřetržitá, hluboká, difuzní bolest proměnlivé intenzity a závažnosti, bez zjevné organické patologie v postižené oblasti, bolest obecně není dostatečně silná, aby rušila spánek, pacienti mohou hlásit časné ranní probouzení, postihuje ženy mezi 40 a 50 lety, atypická bolest zubů považována za variantu atypické bolesti obličeje, bolest trojklanného nervu, bolest je často popisována jako podobná elektrickému šoku, povahou řezavá, bodavá, pronikavá, pacienti odmítají umývání a holení určitého místa na obličeji ze strachu z vyvolání záchvatu bolesti, periodická migrenózní neuralgie (bolest hlavy podobná migréně), bolest jednostranná, převážně zasahující oblast očí, čela a spánků, muži jsou postiženi častěji, bolest dostatečně vážná, aby pacienta vzbudila, epizody často doprovází rinorea, slzení a infekce spojivek, záchvaty, mohou trvat několik dnů i týdnů, následovány různě dlouhou dobou remise (vymizení příznaků), ústní poranění se objevuje běžně u HIV-séropozitivních pacientů, odráží stav zhoršené imunity, výskyt se snižuje vysoce účinnou anti-retrovirální léčbou.

Vocabulary

accompany /əˈkʌm.pə.ni/ provázet, spojovat

acrylic /əˈkrɪl.ɪk/ akrylový, pryskyřičný

active /ˈæk.tɪv/ účinný, působivý, účinný

additive /ˈæd.ɪ.tɪv/ aditivní, přísada, dodatkový

adult /ˈæd.ʌlt/ dospělý člověk

aetiological /ˌiː.ti.ɒlˈə.dʒi.kəl/ etiologický, podle příčiny

aid /eɪd/ pomoc, pomáhat, podpora, zařízení

antiretroviral /æn.ti̩ˌret.rəʊ ˈvaɪə.rəl/ proti-retrovirový

approximately /əˈprɒk.sɪ.mət.li/ přibližně, zhruba

arise /əˈraɪz/ nastat, vyskytnout se, vystoupit, být důsledkem

ascend /əˈsend/ stoupat, nastoupit (přen.), dostat se

associate /əˈsəʊ.si.eɪt/ asociovat, spojovat, spolupracovník

autoimmune /ˌɔː.təʊ.ɪˈmjuːn/ autoimunní

basis /ˈbeɪ.sɪs/ báze, základ, podstata

behaviour /bɪˈheɪ.vjər/ jednání (chování), způsob práce, reakce

bout /baʊt/ záchvat, perioda

break /breɪk/ přerušení, přestávka, zlámat, porušit

bruxism /ˈbruːk.sɪ.zəm/ bruxismus, skřípání zuby

cancerphobia /ˈkænt.səˑˈfəʊ.bi.ə/ chorobný strach z rakoviny

candidosis /ˈkæn.dɪ.dəʊ.sɪs/ kandidóza, infekce způsobená některými druhy Candidy

caries /ˈkeə.riːz/ zubní kaz

chew /tʃuː/ žvýkat, rozmělnit

clench /klentʃ/ sevřít, zatnout, pevně uchopit

cluster /ˈklʌs.təʳ/ shluk, hrozen, nahromadit se

conjunctiva /ˌkɒn.dʒʌŋkˈtaɪ.və/ oční spojivka

consumption /kənˈsʌmp.ʃən/ spotřeba, strávení, opotřebování (člověka), zničení

continuity /ˌkɒn.tɪˈnjuː.ɪ.ti/ kontinuita, nepřetržitost, souvislost, neprůchodnost

continuous /kənˈtɪn.ju.əs/ plynulý, neustálý, pravidelný

corticosteroid /ˈkɔː.tɪkɒˈster.ɔɪd/ kortikosteroid

crust /krʌst/ kůra, strup, povlak, usazenina

cytotoxic /saɪ.təˈtɒk.sɪk/ cytotoxický, škodlivý pro buňky

decade /ˈdek.eɪd/ dekáda, desetiletí, desítka

deep /diːp/ hluboký, hlubina, ponořený

dehydration /ˌdiː.haɪˈdreɪ.ʃən/ odvodnění, vysychání

dentition /denˈtɪʃ.ən/ dentice, chrup

denture /ˈden.tʃə/ zubní protéza

diagnosis /ˌdaɪ.əgˈnəʊ.sɪs/ rozpoznání (choroby), určení, popsání

diffuse /dɪˈfjuːs/ rozptýlený, neohraničený, rozšířit se, pronikat

discrete /dɪˈskriːt/ diskrétní, jednotlivý, oddělený, samostatný

disturb /dɪˈstɜːb/ rušit, porušit, působit poruchy

dormant /ˈdɔː.mənt/ dormantní, spící, skrytý, latentní (možnosti)

dysaesthesia /dɪs.æs.ˈθiː.sɪ.ə/ dysestézie, porucha citlivosti

enlarge /ɪnˈlɑːdʒ/ zvětšit, rozšířit se, vzmáhat se

episode /ˈep.ɪ.səʊd/ příhoda, záchvat, vedlejší děj

epithelial /e.pɪˈθiː.li.əl/ epitelový, výstelkový

essentially /ɪˈsen.tʃ°l.i/ v podstatě, nezbytně, zásadně

facial /ˈfeɪ.ʃ°l/ faciální, obličejový, lícní

female /ˈfiː.meɪl/ ženský, žena, pro ženy

folate /ˈfəʊ.leɪt/ folát, sůl kyseliny listové

formation /fɔːˈmeɪ.ʃən/ utváření, sestava, nástup, vznik

freeway /ˈfriː.weɪ/ komunikace, volný prostor

frontal /ˈfrʌn.təl/ frontální, přední, čelní

fungal /ˈfʌŋ.gəl/ týkající se hub, plísňový

gonorrhoea /ˌgɒn.əˈriː.ə/ gonorea, kapavka

gravel /ˈgræv.°l/ štěrk, močové kamínky, písek v moči

heal /hiːl/ hojit, léčit se, zahojit se

herald /ˈher.°ld/ ohlašovat, hlasatel

herpes /ˈhɜː.piːz/ herpes, opar

herpetic /hɜːˈpe.tik/ týkající se oparu

histological /ˌhɪ.stəˈlɒdʒ.ɪ.k°l/ histologický, tkáňový

human /ˈhjuː.mən/ člověk, lidský

hygiene /ˈhaɪ.dʒiːn/ hygiena, zdravověda

hypersensitivity /ˈhaɪ.pə.sen.sɪˈtɪv.ɪ.ti/ hypersensitivita, nadměrná citlivost

hypochondria /ˌhaɪ.pəʊ ˈkɒn.dri.ə/ hypochondrie

idiopathic /ˈɪdiəˈpæθɪk/ idiopatický, samostatný

immunocompromised /ɪˈmjuː.nəˈkɒm.prə.maɪ.zd/ se sníženou imunitou

immunosuppression /
ˌɪm.jə.nəʊ.sə'preʃ.ᵊn/
imunosuprese, snížení schopnosti
organismu reagovat na cizí látky

inadequate /ɪ'næd.ɪ.kwət/
nepřiměřený, neschopný, chybný,
mentálně opožděný

incidence /'ɪnt.sɪ.dənts/ dopad,
výskyt, rozsah působení

induced /in.dju:st/ indukovaný,
přivozený

infancy /'ɪn.fənt.si/ dětství, počátek

infection /ɪn'fek.ʃᵊn/ nákaza,
nakažlivost, infekční nemoc

intensity /ɪn'tent.sɪ.ti/ intenzita, síla,
hustota

irradiation /ɪˌreɪ.di'eɪ.ʃᵊn/ iradiace,
ozáření, osvětlení

lacrimation /læk.rɪ'məɪ.ʃᵊn/ slzení

lancinate /'laːn.sɪ.nəɪt/ řezat

lichen /'laɪ.kən/ planus /pleɪ.nəs/ lišej

lining /'laɪ.nɪŋ/ výstelka

liquid /'lɪk.wɪd/ kapalina, tekutý,
průzračný

local /'ləʊ.kᵊl/ místní

maintain /meɪn'teɪn/ udržovat,
podporovat, pokračovat, živit se

male /meɪl/ muž, mužský

malignant /mə'lɪg.nənt/ maligní,
zhoubný, zákeřný

mechanical /mə'kæn.ɪ.kᵊl/
mechanický, bezděčný

menstruation /ˌmen.stru'eɪ.ʃᵊn/
menstruace

migrainous /maɪ.grə.nəs/ migrénový,
týkající se migrény

monomer /mɒn.ə.məʳ/ monomer

multiply /'mʌl.tɪ.plaɪ/ násobit,
rozmnožovat se, vícenásobný

neoplastic /'niːə'plæs.tɪk/
neoplastický, nově vytvořený

neuralgia /njʊə'ræl.dʒə/ neuralgie,
ostrá nervová bolest

obvious /'ɒb.vi.əs/ zřejmý,
samozřejmý, nápadný

occur /ə'kɜːr/ vyskytovat se, nastat,
přihodit se

ocular /'ɒk.jʊ.lər/ oční, zrakový,
očividný

odontalgia /ˌəʊ.dɒn'tæl.dʒɪə/ bolest
zubů

oesophageal /ɪːˌsɒf.ə.'dʒɪ.əl/ jícnový

opacity /əʊ'pæs.ə.ti/ neprůhlednost,
temnost, matnost

oropharyngeal /ˌəʊ.rə'fær.ɪ.ŋ'dʒɪ.əl/
orofaryngeální, týkající se úst a hltanu

papilloma /ˌpæp.ɪ.'ləʊ.mə/ papilom,
nezhoubný epitelový nádor

parafunction /ˌpær.ə'fʌnk.ʃᵊn/
parafunkce, poškozená funkce

particular /pə'tɪk.jʊ.ləʳ/ specifický
(určitý), jednotlivý, přesný,
podrobnost

pathology /pə'θɒl.ə.dʒi/ patologie
(obor), stav způsobující onemocnění

periodontal /ˌper.ɪ.ə'dɒn.tl/
periodontální

piercing /'pɪə.sɪŋ/ ostrý (pronikavý),
bodavý, propichování těla kroužky

positive /'pɒz.ə.tɪv/ kladný, jasný,
nesporný, prokázaný

preceding /prɪ'siː.dɪŋ/ předcházející,
předešlý

precipitant /prɪˌsɪp.ɪ.'tənt/ překotný,
spěšný, srážecí činidlo

predict /prɪ'dɪkt/ předpovídat, tvrdit

predisposition /ˌpriː.dɪ.spə'zɪʃ.ᵊn/
predispozice, náchylnost, předpoklad

predominantly /prɪ'dɒm.ɪ.nənt.li/
převážně, hlavně

premalignant /ˌpre.mə'lig.nənt/ před
rakovinný

prevalence /ˈprev.ᵊl.ənt s/ prevalence, převládání, převaha, častý výskyt

prickle /ˈprɪk.l̩/ osten, bodání, brnění, svrbění

prodromal /prɒ.drə.ml/ prodromální, předzvěstný

radiotherapy /ˌreɪ.di.əʊˈθer.ə.pi/ radioterapie, léčba ozařováním

reactivate /riˈæk.tɪ.veɪt/ reaktivovat, znovu aktivovat, oživit

recognizable /ˈrek.əg.naɪ.zə.bl̩/ rozeznatelný, poznatelný

recurrence /rɪˈkʌr.ᵊnt s/ rekurence, návrat, opětovný výskyt

reflect /rɪˈflekt/ odrážet, vyjadřovat, zrcadlit (se)

region /ˈriː.dʒᵊn/ oblast (též správní), část, rozsah

remission /rɪˈmɪʃ.ᵊn/ remise, dočasné vymizení projevů nemoci, úleva

responsible /rɪˈspɒnt.sɪ.bl̩/ odpovědný, významný, rozvážný

rupture /ˈrʌp.tʃəʳ/ ruptura, protržení, zlomení, kýla, výhřez

sand /sænd/ písek

seropositive /ˌsɪ.ə.rəˈpɒz.ə.tɪv/ séropozitivní, obsahující sérové protilátky

severity /sɪˈver.ɪ.ti/ krutost, vážnost, útrapy

shaving /ˈʃeɪ.vɪŋ/ holení

sialadenitis /ˈsɑɪəlˌædəˈnʌɪ.tis/ sialoadenitida, zánět slinné žlázy

sideropenia /ˌsɪd.ə.rə.ˈpiː.nɪ.ə/ sideropenie, nedostatek železa v krvi

significantly /sɪgˈnɪf.ɪ.kənt.li/ významně, závažně

snuff /snʌf/ šňupat (tabák), čichat, nadýchnutí nosem

space /speɪs/ prostor, prázdné místo, vzdálenost

spontaneously /spɒnˈteɪ.ni.ə.sli/ spontánně, samovolně

squamous /skweɪ.məs/ cell /sel/ plochá (dlaždicová) buňka

stabbing /ˈstæb.ɪŋ/ bodnutí, očkovat vpichem, cukavý

state /steɪt/ status, stav, okolnosti, prohlásit

subsequently /ˈsʌb.sɪ.kwənt.li/ následovně, postupně, později

substitute /ˈsʌb.stɪ.tjuːt/ nahradit, zastupovat, náhražka

sufficiently /səˈfɪʃ.ᵊnt.li/ dostatečně

sunlight /ˈsʌn.laɪt/ sluneční světlo

swallow /ˈswɒl.əʊ/ polykat, pozřít, hlt

swollen /ˈswəʊ.lən/ oteklý, zduřený

synergistic /ˌsɪn.ə.ˈdʒi.stik/ synergistický, souhlasně působící

syphilis /ˈsɪf.ɪ.lɪs/ syfilis (příjice)

tear /tɪəʳ/ slza, trhat, trhlina

temporal /ˈtem.pər.əl/ temporální, skráňový (na spáncích), přechodný

thermal /ˈθɜː.məl/ termální, tepelný

thrust /θrʌst/ úder, probodnout, cpát

tongue /tʌŋ/ jazyk, špice

transformation /ˌtræns.fəˈmeɪ.ʃᵊn/ transformace (přeměna), přechod

trauma /ˈtrɔː.mə/, /ˈtraʊ-/ trauma, úraz

traumatic /trɔːˈmæt.ɪk/, /traʊ-/ traumatický, úrazový

trigeminal /ˈtraɪˈdʒem.ɪ.nᵊl/ trigeminální, trojklaný

trigger /ˈtrɪg.əʳ/ spustit (náhle uvolnit), spouštěč

troublesome /ˈtrʌb.l̩.sᵊm/ obtížný, komplikující situaci, otravný (nepříjemný)

tumour /ˈtjuː.məʳ/ tumor, nádor

ultraviolet /ˌʌl.trəˈvaɪə.lət/ ultrafialový (UV)

unilateral /ˌjuː.nɪˈlæt.ᵊr.ᵊl/
unilaterální, pouze na jedné straně
unstable /ʌnˈsteɪ.bl̩/ nestabilní,
proměnlivý (nestálý)
variant /ˈveə.ri.ənt/ variantní, lišící se,
proměnný
variety /vəˈraɪə.ti/ varianta,
rozmanitost, mnohotvárnost, druh
vesicle /ˈvesɪkl/ váček, dutina, puchýřek
vesiculobullous /ve.ˈsɪ.kju.lə.buːˈləʊs/
týkající se puchýřků a velkých
puchýřů

viral /ˈvaɪə.rᵊl/ virový
vitamin /ˈvɪt.ə.mɪn/ vitamin,
vitaminový
waken /ˈweɪ.kən/ procitnout (probudit
se), budit se
xerostomia /ˈzɪə.rəˈstəʊ.mɪə/
xerostomie, suchost úst
zone /zəʊn/ zóna, oblast

Unit 10

Oral and Maxillofacial Surgery

Tissue Healing. Factors Influencing Healing. Exodontia. Apicectomy. Biopsy Technique. Suturing. Suture Removal. Laser Surgery and Cryosurgery. Infections. Spreading Infection. Patient Assessment in Infection. Swellings of Mouth, Face, and Neck. Tumours—Benign and Malignant. Oral Cancer. Cysts of the Jaws. Maxillofacial Trauma. Glasgow Coma Scale. Maxillofacial Emergency Action. Facial Skeleton Fractures.

Text 1

Tissue Healing

Surgery by definition results in **tissue damage**, thus, an understanding of factors influencing **wound healing** is important.

- **inflammatory phase** (0–4 days after injury—the vascular and cellular events in this phase produce a weak repair)
- **proliferative phase** (3–21 days after injury—at the end of this stage, the wound's strength has increased to 70% that of intact tissue)
- **remodelling phase** (21 days after injury onwards—contraction of newly formed scar tissue

eventually increases wound strength to 85%)

Factors Influencing Healing
Tissue factors
- **blood supply** (reduced in smoking, diabetes)
- **drainage** (e.g. venous, lymphatic—poor post radiography)
- **nutrition** (e.g. low protein level in debilitated patient)

Pre-existing infection

Acquired infection
- **general immune response** reduced (elderly, concurrent disease, steroids, immunosuppressives)
- **local** immune response reduced (radiotherapy, topical steroids)
- **adverse physical factors** (barriers cut, tissue planes opened, reduced salivary flow)
- **microbes** from patient (commensals or infective)
- microbes from other patient (via instruments/working surfaces)
- microbes from operator

Exodontia
Potential **complications of extraction** include:

- **failed local anaesthesia**
- **soft-tissue injuries**
- **nerve** injuries
- **fractured tooth**
- fractured **buccal plate** of bone
- fractured **maxillary tuberosity**
- **displaced roots**
- **lost tooth**
- **maxillary-antral perforation**
- postextraction **haemorrhage**
- **dry socket**
- **TMJ complications**—trismus, acute subluxation, dislocation
- **pain**—extraction of a painful tooth may not provide immediate relief
- **swelling**—particularly following surgical extraction

Apicectomy

Apicectomy is surgical **removal of the root apex** to allow the surgeon to visualise and gain access to the root canal. The main aim of the procedure is to establish an apical seat.

Biopsy Technique

Biopsy involves excision of tissue for histological examination.
Excisional biopsy – the lesion is excised in its entirety. This should include a small margin of healthy tissue surrounding the lesion.

Incisional biopsy – removal of a representative portion of the lesion should try to contain clinically healthy tissue at the margin. In potentially malignant lesions, the area most likely to show significant dysplasia should be included in the biopsy, e.g. the speckled part in a heterogeneous leukoplakia.

Punch biopsy – This has gained favour with clinicians and patients alike.

Suturing

Sutures are used to hold flaps and tissue in apposition to facilitate wound healing. There are a variety of suture **techniques** possible, e.g. **interrupted, vertical mattress, horizontal mattress, continuous**.

Suture Removal

Nonresorbable intraoral sutures are normally removed 7 days postoperatively. To remove, the **tied ends** of the suture are **grasped** in nontoothed forceps. **Fine point scissors** or a **stitch cutter** is inserted under the knot, and one side of the **suture is cut. By gently pulling** with the forceps, the suture is **removed**. Any adherent debris may be removed with chlorhexidine solution before the suture is removed.

Laser Surgery and Cryosurgery

Laser stands for amplification by the stimulated emission of radiation. Cryosurgery involves destruction of tissues by freezing.

Exercise 1
1. Which are the phases in tissue healing, and which are the factors influencing healing?
2. What can you say about pre-existing infection?
3. Describe potential complications of extraction.
4. What do you know about biopsy technique?
5. Talk about suture techniques and suture removal.

Translation 1
Faktory ovlivňující hojení ran, fáze zánětlivá, fáze bujení a nového modelování, tkáň netknutá, zjizvená, krevní zásobení, lymfatické a žilní odčerpání, výživa, oslabený, starší pacient, nepříznivé fyzické faktory, imunitní reakce snížená, možné komplikace extrakce, selhání místní anestézie, poranění měkkých tkání, nervu, zlomený zub, kost, ztracený zub, krvácení, suché lůžko, komplikace temporomandibulárního kloubu, otok, chirurgické odstranění hrotu kořene, biopsie, vyříznutí tkáně pro histologické vyšetření, malý okraj zdravé tkáně, obklopující ránu, u potenciálně maligní léze, výrazná dysplazie, šití, stehy, usnadnit hojení ran, odstranění stehů, nevstřebatelné stehy uvnitř úst, uchopit zavázané konce, pinzeta, nůžky, nůžky na stehy, vložit pod uzlík, ustřihnout, jemně zatáhnout.

Text 2
Infections
Infections that are dental in origin have a mixed bacterial aetiology, e.g. Streptococci (aerobic and anaerobic) and Bacteroides (anaerobic).

Spreading Infection
Whilst most infections remain localised, an infection may spread. **Pus from an infected tooth will spread** along the path of least resistance. This may be present as an extra- or intraoral sinus but can, on occasion, spread along tissue and fascial planes to produce severe, **life-threatening systemic infections**.

Patient Assessment in Infection
The following specific features should be recorded:
History
- **speed of onset**
- **malaise**
- **rigors**
- effect on **breathing and swallowing**
- **medical factors**—e.g. drugs, diabetes

Examination
- **temperature** (axillary)
- **heart rate**
- **trismus**
- **lymphadenopathy**
- **spread**—e.g. floor of mouth, tongue elevation, neck involvement, airway/voice

Bacteriology
- aspirate pus with a needle for an uncontaminated sample
- a pus specimen in a sterile pot is better than a swab in transport medium
- involve a bacteriologist early if there is a serious infection

Swellings of Mouth, Face, and Neck
A vast range of pathologies can present as a swelling.
History
In particular, note:
- **duration**
- variation in **size**
- **pain**—its nature and radiation
- any **neurological involvement**

Examination
Describe as follows:
- **look – site, size, shape, surface** (e.g. ulcerated), **colour**

- feel – consistency (e.g. **fluid filled, soft, firm, hard**)
- **relations** (e.g. attachment to or displacement of other **surrounding structures**)
- examine **lymph nodes**
- **special tests** – advanced imaging techniques such as **computer tomography (CT) scanning and magnetic resonance imaging (MRI)** may provide valuable information.

Exercise 2

1. Describe the ways in which infections spread.
2. Which specific features should be recorded?
3. How to take a sample for bacteriological tests?
4. History and examination in swellings of mouth, face, and neck.

Translation 2

Šíření infekce, hnis z infikovaného zubu, cestou nejmenšího odporu, závažné, život ohrožující systémové infekce, zaznamenat rychlost nástupu, malátnost, zimnici, účinek na dýchání a polykání, léky, teplotu, srdeční rytmus, křeč žvýkacího svalstva, onemocnění mízních uzlin, nasát jehlou, zkušební vzorek, sterilní kelímek, vata na špejli, otoky úst, obličeje a krku, trvání, povaha bolesti, postižení nervů, pohled, místo, velikost, tvar, povrch, barva otoku, pohmat, konsistence otoku, naplněný tekutinou, měkký, pevný, tvrdý, pokročilé zobrazovací metody, počítačová tomografie, skenování, zobrazování pomocí magnetické rezonance.

Text 3

Tumours—Benign and Malignant

Due to the large variation in presentation of growths in the head and neck region, categorisation is complex. The following is a basic classification:

Tumours

Tumours may be differentiated into **benign and malignant** varieties. A tumour is an **abnormal mass of tissue** whose growth exceeds and is uncoordinated with that of surrounding tissues. Abnormal growth continues after the stimulation which initiated it has ceased.

Benign tumours remain at their **site of origin**. Common examples include:
- **lipoma (fat)**
- **neuroma (nerve)**
- **papilloma (epithelium)**

Locally invasive tumours

As in benign tumours, growth is abnormal. Here is, in addition, **invasion into surrounding normal tissues**. Examples include:
- **ameloblastoma** (enamel-producing organ)
- **basal cell carcinoma** (skin), sometimes called rodent ulcer

Malignant tumours

In malignant tumours, there is **abnormal growth** with the potential for **local invasion** and **distant metastases**. The latter may be **via blood, lymphatic system, or body cavities. Carcinomas** are malignant tumours of **epithelial tissue**. The most common malignant tumour in the oral cavity is the **squamous cell carcinoma**. Sarcomas are malignant tumours of **connective tissue**, e.g. **liposarcoma** or **osteosarcoma**.

Oral Cancer
Assessment—particular note should be made of:
History
* **duration** of symptoms
* any **sensory nerve deficit**
* **pain**
* onset of difficulty **opening the mouth**, trismus
* **social habits and circumstances**
Examination
This should include an exhaustive description of the **primary lesion**, which is usually an **ulcer**: size, shape, colour, description of the ulcer edge, degree of hardness, whether bound down to other tissues, which tissues are involved clinically with the mass. The following special tests may be indicated:
* **blood tests** (full blood count and liver function tests, calcium and phosphate analysis)
* **imaging** (radiography of jaws and chest)
* **biopsy**
Treatment
This requires a team approach. **Surgeons** work together with **oncologists** as well as **specialist nurses, speech and dietetic specialists**. Considerable time needs to be spent with patients and their relatives to prepare them mentally and physically. They also need to feel part of the decision-making process.

There is very good evidence that **early small lesions treated properly have the best prognosis**.
If nodal metastases are present, the overall chance of cure decreases by 50%. There is evidence of increasing number of patients in whom, whilst the disease is controlled locally and regionally, distant metastatic disease results in death.
The need for early diagnosis cannot be overemphasized. **Careful screening of the oral mucosa** to detect potentially malignant and malignant lesions should be carried out routinely in any oral examination.

Cysts of the Jaws
A cyst may be defined as a **pathological cavity** having **fluid or semifluid contents** which has not been created by the accumulation of pus. It may or may not be lined by epithelium.

Exercise 3
1. What can you say about tumours?
2. Give some examples of benign tumours and locally invasive tumours.
3. Explain the term malignant tumours.
4. Think about important information concerning history and examination of oral cancer.
5. Think about possibilities of treatment of oral cancer.

Translation 3
Tumory nezhoubné, zhoubné, abnormální tkáňová hmota, nekoordinovaný růst, nezhoubné tumory, zůstávají na původním místě,

lipom, neurom, papilom, nezhoubné invazivní tumory, napadení okolních tkání, ameloblastom, hlodavý vřed, zhoubné tumory, abnormální růst, místní invaze, vzdálené metastázy, cestou krevní, lymfatickou, tělními dutinami, karcinomy, zhoubné nádory epitelové tkáně, karcinom dlaždicových buněk, sarkomy, zhoubné nádory pojivové tkáně, liposarkom, osteosarkom, rakovina úst, primární poranění, obvykle vřed, speciální testy, úplný krevní obraz, funkce jater, analýza kalcia a fosforečnanu, rentgen čelistí a hrudníku, biopsie, připravit pacienta duševně, fyzicky, příbuzní, součástí procesu rozhodování, potřeba včasné diagnózy, pečlivé prohlížení ústní sliznice, cysta na čelisti, patologická dutina s tekutým či polotekutým obsahem, která není vytvořena nahromaděním hnisu.

Text 4
Maxillofacial Trauma
Emergency receiving
Dealing with patients suffering facial trauma can be difficult. There are three main points which need to be **considered together**:
- **cervical spine**
- **airway**
- **bleeding**

The importance of these is closely followed by consideration of any other injury of significance to life, e.g. hidden haemorrhage from **intra-abdominal injury, fractured pelvis, femur**, etc. **Head injury** must be considered, particularly if there is deterioration in the **level of consciousness** determined by history

(from friend) or observation (Glasgow Coma Scale).

Glasgow Coma Scale
Best motor response
Obeys commands 6
Localises pain 5
Normal flexion to pain 4
Abnormal flexion to pain 3
Extension to pain 2
None 1
Best verbal response
Orientated 5
Confused conversation 4
Inappropriate words 3
Incomprehensible 2
None 1
Eyes open
Spontaneously 4
To speech 3
To pain 2
Do not open 1

Maxillofacial Emergency Action
If the patient arrives in obvious **respiratory distress** or with torrential **haemorrhage,** these will obviously **take precedence.** Never forget to **look for associated injuries.** A patient with a simple fractured zygoma may have fallen as a consequence of the blow and have sustained a significant head injury.

Cervical spine – any suspicion of neck injury makes temporary **immobilisation** with collar or sandbags essential.
Airway – the following objects may be causing upper airway **obstruction**: foreign bodies such as **teeth** or **denture** fragments, **vomit, or blood.**

It is essential to have good light and suction.

Lacerations – cleaning is very important. Any **cleaning solutions** should be used only on the intact skin (beware entry into the eyes). In the wound itself use normal saline. Take care to recognise **tattooing**, particularly with **road dirt**. A large scalpel blade to scrape skin margins or used tangentially on abrasions may be very helpful. Remember to check **tetanus prophylaxis**.

Facial Skeleton Fractures
Fractures may be classified **generally** as:
- simple
- compound
- comminuted
- greenstick
- pathological

Classified **according to site**:
- mandibular fractures
- maxillary (middle third of face) fractures
- zygomatic complex fractures
- nasal fractures

Treatment
As with any bone fracture, treatment involves:
- **reduction**
- **fixation and immobilisation**
- **prevention of infection**
- return to **function**

Exercise 4
1. Why is dealing with patients suffering facial trauma difficult?
2. Which life-threatening injuries should be considered?

3. Discuss the possibility of head injury and deterioration in the level of consciousness (Glasgow Coma Scale).
4. Talk about maxillofacial emergency action.
5. Describe possible associated injuries.
6. Classification and treatment of facial skeleton fractures.

Translation 4
Poranění horní čelisti a obličeje, naléhavý příjem, posuzovat společně krční páteř, dýchací cesty, krvácení, skryté krvácení ze zranění uvnitř břišní dutiny, zlomená pánev, stehenní kost, poranění hlavy, porucha úrovně vědomí, pozorování, Glasgow škála komatu, pohybová reakce, je poslušný pokynů, lokalizuje bolest, ohnutí, natažení na bolest, slovní reakce, orientovaná, zmatená konverzace, nepatřičná slova, nesrozumitelná, žádná, oči otevřené samovolně, na mluvení, na bolest, neotvírají se, pohotovostní akce, mít přednost, zjevná dechová tíseň, řinoucí se krvácení, podezření na poranění krční páteře, znehybnění pomocí límce, ucpání horních cest dýchacích, cizí tělíska, zuby, úlomky protéz, zvratky, krev, tržné rány, odřeniny, čistící roztoky, použít na neporušenou pokožku, v samotné ráně použít fyziologický roztok, zkontrolovat prevenci proti tetanu, zlomeniny v obličeji, uzavřené, otevřené, roztříštěné, částečné, patologické, zlomeniny dolní, horní čelisti, lícního komplexu, nosní, ošetření, redukce, fixace, znehybnění, prevence infekce, návrat k funkčnosti.

Vocabulary

abnormal /æbˈnɔː.məl/ abnormální

abrasion /əˈbreɪ.ʒən/ obrušování

according to /əˈkɔː.dɪŋ‚tuː/ podle

accumulation /ə‚kjuː.mjʊˈleɪ.ʃən/ nahromadění

acquire /əˈkwaɪəʳ/ získat

action /ˈæk.ʃən/ akce

adherent /ədˈhɪə.rənt/ přilepený

advanced /ədˈvɑːntst/ pokročilý

adverse /ˈæd.vɜːs/ nepříznivý

aerobic /eəˈrəʊ.bɪk/ aerobní

airway /ˈeə.weɪ/ dýchací cesty

alike /əˈlaɪk/ stejnou měrou

alloplastic /‚ælə'plæs.tɪk/ aloplastický

alloplasty /æl.ə‚plæs.tɪ/ aloplastika, plastika materiálem cizím lidskému tělu (stříbro, zlato, kovy)

ameloblastoma /æ‚me.lə.blæsˈtəʊ.mə/ ameloblastom, tumor dolní čelisti, vzniklý ze sklovinových buněk

amplification /‚æm.plɪ.fɪˈkeɪ.ʃən/ zesílení

anaerobic /‚æn.əˈrəʊ.bɪk/ anaerobní

analysis /əˈnæl.ə.sɪs/ analýza

antral /æn.trəl/ antrální, týkající se dutiny

apex /ˈeɪ.peks/ (pl. apices) vrchol, hrot

apposition /‚æ.pəˈzɪʃ.ᵊn/ přiložení, vzájemné dotýkání

approach /əˈprəʊtʃ/ přístup

aspirate /ˈæs.pɪ.rət/ nasátí

assessment /əˈses.mənt/ stanovení, určení

associated /əˈsəʊ.si.eɪ.tɪd/ spojený (přidružený)

attachment /əˈtætʃ.mənt/ připojení

axillary /æˈksɪl.ᵊr.i/ axilární, podpažní

bacteriologist /bæk‚tɪə.riˈɒl.ə.dʒɪst/ bakteriolog

Bacteroides /‚bæk.tɪəˈrɒɪ.diːz/ druh střevních bacilů

barrier /ˈbær.i.əʳ/ překážka

basal /ˈbeɪ.sl/ cell /sel/ bazální, základní buňka

benign /bɪˈnaɪn/ nezhoubný

beware /bɪˈweəʳ/ dát si pozor

bind /baɪnd/ down /daʊn/ svazovat

bleeding /ˈbliː.dɪŋ/ krvácení

blood /blʌd/ count /kaʊnt/ krevní obraz

blood /blʌd/ krev

blood /blʌd/ test /test/ krevní test

blow /bləʊ/ rána

body /ˈbɒd.i/ cavity /ˈkæv.ɪ.ti/ tělní dutina

bone /bəʊn/ kost

breathing /ˈbriː.ðɪŋ/ dýchání

buccal /bʌk.l/ bukální, tvářový, lícní

calcium hydroxide /‚kæl.si.əm. haɪˈdrɒk.saɪd/ hydroxid vápenatý

carcinoma /kɑː.sɪˈnəʊ.mə/ rakovinný nádor

carry /ˈkær.i/ out /aʊt/ provést (realizovat)

cause /kɔːz/ příčina, důvod, vyvolat, přinutit

cease /siːs/ ustat, zastavit se

cervical /səˈvaɪ.kəl/ collar /ˈkɒl.əʳ/ krční límec

cervical /səˈvaɪ.kəl/ krčkový

chance /tʃɑːnts/ šance, možnost

chest /tʃest/ hrudník, prsní

circumstance /ˈsɜː.kəm.stɑːnts/ okolnost, poměry

cleaning /ˈkliː.nɪŋ/ čištění, čistící

closely /ˈkləʊ.sli/ těsně

command /kəˈmɑːnd/ příkaz, nařídit, ovládat

commensal /ˈkɒm.əns.ᵊl/ symbiont

comminuted /ˈkɒ.mɪˈnjuː.tɪd/ fracture /ˈfræk.tʃəʳ/ roztříštěná zlomenina

complex /ˈkɒm.pleks/ komplex

compound /ˈkɒm.paʊnd/ **fracture** / ˈfræk.tʃəʳ/ otevřená zlomenina

computer /kəmˈpjuː.təʳ/ počítačový

concurrent /kənˈkʌr.ᵊnt/ souběžný

confused /kənˈfjuːzd/ zmatený

connective tissue /kəˌnek.tɪvˈtɪʃ.uː/ pojivová tkáň

consciousness /ˈkɒn.tʃə.snəs/ vědomí

consequence /ˈkɒnt.sɪ.kwənts/ následek

considerable /kənˈsɪd.ər.ə.bl̩/ značný

consideration /kənˌsɪd.əˈreɪ.ʃən/ úvaha

considered /kənˈsɪd.əd/ zvažován

consistency /kənˈsɪs.tᵊnt.si/ konzistence, tuhost

contain /kənˈteɪn/ obsahovat, pojmout, skládat se, zaujímat

content /ˈkɒn.tent/ obsah

continuous /kənˈtɪn.ju.əs/ souvislý, spojený

contraction /kənˈtræk.ʃən/ stah, smrštění

create /kriˈeɪt/ vytvořit

cryosurgery /kraɪ.əˈsɜːdʒər.i/ kryochirurgie, schlazení tkání pod minus 20 stupňů

cut /kʌt/ řezat, stříhat

cutting /ˈkʌt.ɪŋ/ řezací

cyst /sɪst/ cysta, váček

damage /ˈdæm.ɪdʒ/ poškození, zničení

death /deθ/ smrt

debilitate /dɪˈbɪl.ɪ.teɪt/ oslabit

debris /ˈdeb.riː/, /ˈdeɪ.briː/ úlomky

decision /dɪˈsɪʒ.ən/ **making** /ˈmeɪ. kɪŋ/ rozhodování

decision /dɪˈsɪʒ.ən/ rozhodnutí

decrease /dɪˈkriːs/ snížení, snížit se, být na ústupu

deficit /ˈdef.ɪ.sɪt/ deficit, nedostatek

denture/ˈden.tʃə/ zubní protéza

description /dɪˈskrɪp.ʃən/ popis

destruction /dɪˈstrʌk.ʃən/ ničení, zkáza, rozložení

detect /dɪˈtekt/ zjistit, objevit, určit

deterioration /dɪˌtɪə.ri.əˈreɪ.ʃən/ deteriorizace, zhoršení, chátrání, porucha

dietetic /ˌdaɪə.teˈtɪk/ dietetický, dietní

difficulty /ˈdɪf.ɪ.kəl.ti/ obtíž

dirt /dɜːt/ špína

dislocation /ˌdɪs.ləʊˈkeɪ.ʃən/ posunutí

displaced /dɪˈspleɪst/ **fracture** / ˈfræk.tʃəʳ/ dislokovaná zlomenina

displacement /dɪˈspleɪs.mənt/ posunutí

distant /ˈdɪs.tənt/ vzdálený

distress /dɪˈstres/ tíseň, stav ohrožení

drainage /ˈdreɪ.nɪdʒ/ odčerpání

dry /draɪ/ suchý

due /djuː/ **to** /tʊ/ kvůli, následkem, díky

duration /djʊəˈreɪ.ʃən/ trvání

dysplasia /disˈpleɪ.zɪə/ dysplazie, porucha vývoje nebo růstu

edge /edʒ/ okraj

effect /ɪˈfekt/ účinek, výsledek

elderly /ˈel.dəl.i/ postarší

elevation /ˌel.ɪˈveɪ.ʃᵊn/ vyvýšenina, pahrbek

emergency /ɪˈmɜː.dʒənt.si/ naléhavá nutnost, pohotovost

emission /ɪˈmɪʃ.ᵊn/ vysílání, vyzařování

emphasize /ˈemp.fə.saɪz/ zdůraznit

entirety /ɪnˈtaɪə.rɪ.ti/ celistvost

entry /ˈen.tri/ vstup

epithelium /e.pɪˈθiː.li.əm/ epitel, výstelka

essential /ɪˈsen.tʃəl/ základní, hlavní, nepostradatelný

establish /ɪˈstæb.lɪʃ/ zřídit, ustanovit, zabezpečit

event /ɪˈvent/ událost, případ, výsledek

eventually /ɪˈven.tju.əl.i/ nakonec

evidence /ˈev.ɪ.dᵊnts/ důkaz

exceed /ɪkˈsiːd/ převládat, přesahovat (míru)

excise /ekˈsaɪz/ odstranit, vyříznout

excision /ekˈsɪʒ.ᵊn/ excize, vyříznutí

exhaustive /ɪgˈzɔː.stɪv/ kompletní, důkladný

extension /ɪkˈsten.tʃən/ natažení, rozšíření

facial /ˈfeɪ.ʃᵊl/ obličejový

facilitate /fəˈsɪl.ɪ.teɪt/ usnadnit

fail /feɪl/ selhat, chybit

fascial /ˈfæ.ʃɪ.əl/ povázkový, týkající se povázky

fat /fæt/ tuk, tloušťka

favour /ˈfeɪ.vəʳ/ prospěch, pozornost

feature /ˈfiː.tʃəʳ/ charakteristická vlastnost

feel /fiːl/ cítit, procítit

femur /ˈfiː.məʳ/ femur, stehenní kost

fine /faɪn/ jemný, ryzí, ušlechtilý

firm /fɜːm/ pevný

fixation /fɪkˈseɪ.ʃᵊn/ fixace, upevnění

flap /flæp/ chlopeň, lalok

flexion /flek.ʃᵊn/ ohýbání

floor /flɔːʳ/ dno

fluid /ˈfluː.ɪd/ tekutina

following /ˈfɒl.əʊ.ɪŋ/ následující

forceps /ˈfɔː.seps/ lékařské kleště, pinzeta, nůžky, svorka

foreign /ˈfɒr.ən/ body /ˈbɒd.i/ cizí tělísko

fracture /ˈfræk.tʃəʳ/ fraktura, zlomenina

fragment /ˈfræg.mənt/ úlomek

freezing /ˈfriː.zɪŋ/ zmrazování

full /fʊl/ plný, úplný

function /ˈfʌŋk.ʃᵊn/ činnost, fungování

gain /geɪn/ získat

generally /ˈdʒen.ə r.əl.i/ zpravidla, obecně

gradual /ˈgræd.ju.əl/, /ˈgrædʒ.ʊ.əl/ postupný, pozvolný

grasp /grɑːsp/ pevně uchopit

greenstick /ˈgriːn.stɪk/ fracture / ˈfræk.tʃəʳ/ částečná zlomenina kosti

growth /grəʊθ/ růst

habit /ˈhæb.ɪt/ zvyk, návyk

haemorrhage /ˈhem.ᵊr.ɪdʒ/ vnitřní krvácení

hallucination /həˌluː.sɪˈneɪ.ʃᵊn/ halucinace, přelud

hard /hɑːd/ tvrdý, pevný, nesnadný

hardness /hɑːd.nəs/ odolnost, tvrdost

head /hed/ hlava, směřovat, hlavní

healing /ˈhiː.lɪŋ/ hojení

heart /hɑːt/ rate /reɪt/ srdeční frekvence

helpful /ˈhelp.fᵊl/ užitečný

heterogeneous /ˌhet.ər.əˈdʒiː.ni.əs/ heterogenní, různorodý

hide /haɪd/ skrýt

hold /həʊld/ držet

horizontal /ˌhɒr.ɪˈzɒn.tᵊl/ horizontální, vodorovný

imaging /ɪˈmɪdʒ.ɪŋ/ zobrazování

immediate /ɪˈmiː.di.ət/ bezprostřední

immobilization /ɪˌməʊ.bəl.aɪˈzeɪ.ʃən/ znehybnění

immune /ɪˈmjuːn/ imunní, odolný, bezpečný před něčím

immunosuppression /ˌɪm.jə.nəʊ. səˈpreʃ.ᵊn/ imunosuprese, snížení schopnosti organismu reagovat na cizí látky

importance /ɪmˈpɔː.tənts/ význam, závažnost

in /ɪn/ addition /əˈdɪʃ.ən/ kromě (čeho), navíc

inappropriate /ˌɪn.əˈprəʊ.pri.ət/ nepatřičný

incision /ɪnˈsɪʒ.ᵊn/ incise, naříznutí, vpich

incomprehensible /
ɪnˌkɒm.prɪˈhenʧ.sɪ.bl̩ /
nesrozumitelný

incorporated /ɪnˈkɔː.pər.eɪ.tɪd/
začleněný, vpravený

increase /ɪnˈkriːs/ zvýšit, zvětšování

inflammatory /ɪnˈflæm.ə.tər.i/ zánětlivý

initiate /ɪˈnɪʃ.i.eɪt/ zahájit, spustit

injury /ˈɪn.dʒ°r.i/ zranění, poškození

insert /ɪnˈsɜːt/ vložit

intact /ɪnˈtækt/ nedotčený, neporušený

interrupt /ˌɪn.tə°rʌpt/ přerušovat

intra-/ɪn.trə-/ abdominal /
æbˈdɒm.ɪ.nəl/ intraabdominální,
vnitrobřišní

intraoral /ɪn.trəˈɔː.rəl/ intraorální,
uvnitř úst

invasion /ɪnˈveɪ.ʒ°n/ invaze, napadení

invasive /ɪnˈveɪ.sɪv/ invazivní,
napadající

involvement /ɪnˈvɒlv.mənt/ postižení,
zapojení

jaw /dʒɔː/ čelist

knot /nɒt/ klička, uzel

laceration /ˌlæs.°rˈeɪ.ʃ°n/ lacerace,
tržná rána

least /liːst/ nejnižší

lesion /ˈliː.ʒ°n/ léze, zranění, poranění,
poškození, porucha

leukoplakia /ˌluːkə.ˈpleɪ.kɪə/
leukoplakie, bělavé skvrny na sliznici

level /ˈlev.°l/ stupeň, vrstva, stejná
rovina

life-threatening /ˈlaɪfˌθret.ən.ɪŋ/ život
ohrožující

light /laɪt/ světlo

line /laɪn/ lemovat

lipoma /lɪˈp.əʊ.mə/ lipom, nezhoubný
tukový nádor

liposarcoma /ˌlɪp.ə.sɑːˈkəʊ.mə/
liposarkom, zhoubný nádor z tukové
tkáně

liver /ˈlɪv.ə°r/ játra

local /ˈləʊ.k°l/ místní

localise /ˈləʊ.k°l.aɪz/ omezit na jedno
místo

locally /ˈləʊ.kəl.i/ lokálně, místně

look /lʊk/ podívat se, brát v úvahu

lost /lɒst/ ztracený

lymph /lɪmp f/ lymfa, míza

lymphadenopathy /
lɪmpˌfædɪˈnɒp.ə.θɪ/
lymfadenopatie, nepřesně určené
onemocnění mízních uzlin

lymphatic /lɪmp ˈfæt.ɪk/ lymfatický

magnetic /mægˈnet.ɪk/ magnetický

malaise /mælˈeɪz/ nevolnost, malátnost

malignant /məˈlɪg.nənt/ maligní,
zhoubný

mandibular /mæn.ˈdɪ.bjʊ.lə°r/
mandibulární

margin /ˈmɑː.dʒɪn/ okraj

mass /mæs/ hmota, masa

mattress /ˈmæt.rəs/ podložka

maxillary /mæˈksɪ.l°r.i/ čelistní

maxillofacial /ˌmæk.sɪ.ləˈfeɪ.ʃ°l/
maxilofaciální, týkající se horní
čelisti a tváře

medium /ˈmiː.di.əm/ medium,
přenašeč

mentally /ˈmen.t°l.i/ duševně,
psychicky

metastasis /metˈæs.tə.sɪs/ pl.
metastases metastáza

metastatic /ˌmet.əˈstæ.tɪk/
metastatický, týkající se metastázy

microbe /ˈmaɪ.krəʊb/ microb,
bakterie

motor /ˈməʊ.tər/ response /rɪˈspɒnt s/
pohybová reakce

mucosa /mjuːˈkəʊ.sə/ sliznice

nasal /ˈneɪ.zəl/ nosní

nature /ˈneɪ.tʃə°r/ povaha

neck /nek/ krk

needle /'niː.dl̩/ jehla

nerve /nɜːv/ nerv

neurological /ˌnjʊə.rə'lɒdʒ.ɪ.kᵊl/ neurologický

neuroma /ˌnjʊə'rəʊ.mə/ neurom, druh nádoru tvořený z nervových buněk

nodal /'nəʊ.dᵊl/ uzlový

node /nəʊd/ uzel, uzlina, otok

non- /nɒn-/ ne

none /nʌn/ žádný

nutrition /njuː'trɪʃ.ən/ výživa

obey /əʊ 'beɪ/ command /kə'mɑːnd/ být poslušný příkazu

object /'ɒb.dʒɪkt/ předmět

observation /ˌɒb.zə'veɪ.ʃᵊn/ pozorování, dodržování

obstruction /əb'strʌk.ʃᵊn/ překážka, ucpání

obviously /'ɒb.vi.ə.sli/ zjevně

on /ɒn/ occasion /ə'keɪ.ʒᵊn/ v případě nutnosti

oncologist /ɒŋ'kɒl.ə.dʒɪst/ onkolog

onset /'ɒn.set/ nástup, začátek

onwards /'ɒn.wədz/ dále

opening /'əʊ.pᵊn.ɪŋ/ otevření

orientated /ˌɔː.ri.ən'teɪ.tɪd/ orientovaný

origin /'ɒr.ɪ.dʒɪn/ původ, počátek

osteosarcoma /ˌɒs.tɪ.ə.sɑː'kəʊ.mə/ osteosarkom, maligní kostní nádor

overall /ˌəʊ.və'rɔːl/ celkový, všude, dohromady

painful /'peɪn.fᵊl/ bolestivý

papilloma /ˌpæp.ɪ.'ləʊ.mə/ papilom, nezhoubný epitelový nádor

part /pɑːt/ část, součást

particularly /pə'tɪk.jʊ.lə.li/ obzvláště

path /pɑːθ/ cesta

pathological /ˌpæθ.ə'lɒdʒ.ɪ.kᵊl/ patologický, chorobný

pelvis /'pel.vɪs/ pánev

perforation /ˌpɜː.fᵊr'eɪ.ʃᵊn/ proniknutí, propíchnutí

phase /feɪz/ fáze, etapa

phosphate /'fɒs.feɪt/ fosfát, fosforečnan

physically /'fɪz.ɪ.kli/ fyzicky

plane /pleɪn/ plocha (rovina)

plate /pleɪt/ deska

portion /'pɔː.ʃən/ část

post /pəʊst/ crown /kraʊn/ čepová korunka

pot /pɒt/ kelímek

potential /pəʊ 'ten.tʃᵊl/ potenciál, možný

presence /'prez.ᵊnts/ přítomnost (osoby, věci ap.), zevnějšek

present /'prez.ᵊnt/ přítomný

present /prɪ'z.ent/ představit se

primary /'praɪ.mə.ri/ primární, první, základní

proliferate /prə'lɪf.ᵊr.eɪt/ bujet

property /'prɒp.ə.ti/ kvalita, vlastnost

prophylaxis /ˌprɒf.ɪ'læk.sɪs/ profylaxe, prevence

protein /'prəʊ.tiːn/ protein, bílkovina

pull /pʊl/ táhnout, trhat (i s kořenem), zmítat

punch /pʌntʃ/ vytváření malých děr do tkáně

pus /pʌs/ hnis

radiation /ˌreɪ.di'eɪ.ʃᵊn/ radiace, záření

radiography /ˌreɪ.di'ɒg.rə.fi/ radiografie

receive /rɪ'siːv/ přijímat, získat

recognise /'rek.əg.naɪz/ rozpoznat

record /rɪ'kɔːd/ zaznamenat

reduction /rɪ'dʌk.ʃᵊn/ srovnání kosti, redukce

regionally /'riː.dʒᵊn.ᵊl.i/ regionálně

relation /rɪ'leɪ.ʃᵊn/ poměr (vztah)

relative /'rel.ə.tɪv/ příbuzný

relief /rɪ'liːf/ úleva

remain /rɪ'meɪn/ zbývat (zůstat)

remodel /ˌriːˈmɒd.əl/ přestavit, přemodelovat

removal /rɪˈmuː.vəl/ odstranění, vyjmutí

repair /rɪˈpeəʳ/ opravit, oprava

resistance /rɪˈzɪs.tənts/ odolnost, stálost, vzdor

resonance /ˈrez.ən.ənts/ rezonance

resorb /rɪˈzɔːb/ vstřebat se

respiratory /rɪˈspɪr.ə.tri/ **rate** /reɪt/ rytmus dýchání

respiratory /rɪˈspɪr.ə.tri/ respirační, dýchací

response /rɪˈspɒnts/ reakce

result /rɪˈzʌlt/ mít za následek

return /rɪˈtɜːn/ návrat

rodent /ˈrəʊ.dənt/ **ulcer** /ˈʌl.səʳ/ hlodavý vřed

root /ruːt/ kořen

routine /ruːˈtiːn/ rutina, běžná praxe

saline /ˈseɪ.laɪn/ fyziologický roztok

sample /ˈsɑːm.pl̩/ vzorek

sandbag /ˈsænd.bæg/ pytel písku na ochranu

sandblast /ˈsænd.blɑːst/ pískovat

sarcoma /sɑːˈkəʊ.mə/ sarkom, zhoubný nádor pojivových tkání

scalpel /ˈskæl.pəl/ **blade** /bleɪd/ čepelka skalpelu

scan /skæn/ skenovat, postupně snímat (po řádcích)

scar /skɑːʳ/ jizva

scrape /skreɪp/ oškrabat

screening /ˈskriː.nɪŋ/ podrobné prohlížení

seat /siːt/ dosedací plocha

semifluid /sem.i.ˈfluː.ɪd/ polotekutý

sensory /ˈsent.sər.i/ smyslový

shape /ʃeɪp/ tvar

side /saɪd/ strana

significance /sɪgˈnɪf.ɪ.kənts/ význam, hodnota

significant /sɪgˈnɪf.ɪ.kənt/ důležitý, význačný

simple /ˈsɪm.pl̩/ **fracture** /ˈfræk.tʃəʳ/ zavřená zlomenina

sinus /ˈsaɪ.nəs/ dutina

site /saɪt/ místo

size /saɪz/ velikost

skeleton /ˈskel.ɪ.tən/ kostra

skin /skɪn/ kůže

socket /ˈsɒk.ɪt/ dutina, ložisko

soft /sɒft/ **tissue** /ˈtɪʃ.uː/, /ˈtɪs.juː/ měkká tkáň

solution /səˈluː.ʃən/ roztok

specimen /ˈspes.ə.mɪn/ zkušební vzorek

speckled /ˈspek.l̩d/ skvrnitý (flíčky)

speech /spiːtʃ/ řeč

speed /spiːd/ rychlost

spine /spaɪn/ páteř

spontaneously /spɒnˈteɪ.ni.ə.sli/ spontánně

spread /spred/ šíření

squamous /skweɪ.məs/ **cell** /sel/ plochá (dlaždicová) buňka

stimulate /ˈstɪm.jʊ.leɪt/ stimulovat, podněcovat

stitch /stɪtʃ/ **cutter** /kʌt.əʳ/ nůžky na stehy

strength /streŋθ/ síla

Streptococcus /ˌstrep.təˈkɒk.əs/ (pl. **streptococci**) streptokok

subluxation /ˌsʌb.lʌkˈseɪ.ʃən/ subluxace, neúplné vykloubení

suction /ˈsʌk.ʃən/ odsávání

supply /səˈplaɪ/ dodávat, zásobovat, zásoba

support /səˈpɔːt/ podpora

surface /ˈsɜː.fɪs/ povrch, hladina, stěna

surgeon /ˈsɜː.dʒən/ chirurg

surrounding /səˈraʊn.dɪŋ/ okolní

suspicion /səˈspɪʃ.ən/ podezření

sustain /səˈsteɪn/ utrpět

suture /'suː.tʃəʳ/ sutura, šev, steh, sešití rány

swab /swɒb/ vata na špejli, vysušit tamponem

swallow /'swɒl.əʊ/ polykat

swelling /'swel.ɪŋ/ otok, nádor, boule

systemic /sɪ'stem.ɪk/ systemický, systémový

take /teɪk/ care /keəʳ/ dávat pozor, pečovat

take /teɪk/ precedence /'pres.ɪ.dᵊnts/ mít přednost

tangential /tæn'dʒen.tʃᵊl/ tangenciální, tečný

tattoo /tə'tuː/, /tæt'uːʳ/ tetovat

technique /tek'niːk/ pracovní postup, metoda

temperature /'tem.prə.tʃəʳ/ teplota

temporary /'tem.pᵊr.ᵊr.i/ dočasný

temporomandibular /ˌtem.pər.ə.mæn'dɪ.bjʊ.ləʳ/ joint /dʒɔɪnt/ kloub spánkový a dolní čelisti

tetanus /'tet.ᵊn.əs/ tetanus

thus /ðʌs/ tudíž

tie /taɪ/ zavázat

tomography /tə'mɒg.rə.fi/ tomografie

tongue /tʌŋ/ jazyk

toothed /tuːθt/ ozubený

torrential /tə'ren.tʃᵊl/ řinoucí se, proudící

transport /'træn.spɔːt/ transport, převoz

trauma /'trɔː.mə/, /'traʊ-/ trauma, úraz

trismus /trɪz.məs/ trizmus, křeč žvýkacího svalstva

tuberosity /'tjuː.bə'rɒs.ə.ti/ hrbol na kosti, drsnatina

tumour /'tjuː.məʳ/ tumor, nádor

ulcer /'ʌl.səʳ/ vřed

uncoordinated /ˌʌn.kəʊ'ɔː.dɪn.eɪ.tɪd/ nekoordinovaný, nesladěný

upper /'ʌp.əʳ/ horní, vrchní

valuable /'væl.jʊ.bl̩/ cenný, hodnotný

variation /ˌveə.ri'eɪ.ʃᵊn/ změna, různost

variety /və'raɪə.ti/ varianta, rozmanitost

vascular /'væs.kjʊ.ləʳ/ vaskulární, cévní

venous /'viː.nəs/ žilní

verbal /'vɜː.bəl/ slovní

vertical /'vɜː.tɪ.kᵊl/ vertikální, kolmý

visualise /'vɪʒ.u.ᵊl.aɪz/ vyšetřit zrakem

voice /vɔɪs/ hlas, hlasový, vyjádřit (názor, mínění)

vomit /'vɒm.ɪt/ zvracet, zvracení

weak /wiːk/ slabý, nedostatečný

whilst /waɪlst/ zatímco, kdežto, když

wound /wuːnd/ rána

zygomatic /zaɪ'gəʊ.mə.tɪk/ lícní

Unit 11

Periodontology

Structure of the Periodontal Tissues. Aetiology and Pathogenesis of Periodontal Disease. Stages in Periodontal Therapy. Hygiene Phase Therapy.

Text 1

Structure of the Periodontal Tissues

The periodontium consists of the tissues which **surround and support the teeth**. The periodontium can be divided into the **gingiva** and **periodontal ligament**.

Healthy gingivae have the following clinical features:

- **pale pink** in colour
- a **stippled** appearance
- a well-defined 'knife edge' **margin**
- scalloped **outline**
- **do not bleed** on gently probing with a periodontal probe

Aetiology and Pathogenesis of Periodontal Disease

Periodontal disease includes all pathological conditions of the periodontium but commonly refers to inflammatory diseases which are **plaque-induced**, i.e. **gingivitis** and **periodontitis**.

Gingivitis

In the absence of adequate oral hygiene, dental plaque accumulates and the gingival tissue will progress to an established or chronic gingivitis over a 3-week period.

They have the following **clinical features**:

- **red** in colour
- **swollen** appearance
- **stippling** is lost
- increased flow of gingival crevicular fluid
- **bleed readily** on probing

Periodontitis

Plaque accumulation always leads to gingivitis, but it does not invariably lead to periodontitis. **Breakdown of the periodontal ligament** and the development of a periodontal **pocket** is an unpredictable event. Cigarette smoking is a significant risk factor. Stopping smoking benefits periodontal health and improves the outcome of treatment.

Stages in Periodontal Therapy

Following **examination** and **diagnosis**, periodontal therapy is usually carried out in the following stages:

Hygiene phase

This stage of therapy comprises:
- dental health **education** and instruction in **plaque control**
- **elimination of obstacles** to effective oral hygiene, including defective restoration margins, grossly malpositioned teeth, and teeth of hopeless prognosis
- nonsurgical subgingival **scaling** and **root planing**

Reassessment
It is conducted 4–6 weeks after the completion of hygiene phase. This **indicates the success** of therapy and **highlights** specific **problems** or areas requiring further therapy.

Corrective phase
Disease is treated by further **root planing or surgery**.

Maintenance/recall phase
Patients should be **reviewed at regular intervals** to monitor oral hygiene and permit early detection of recurrent disease.

Exercise 1
1. Talk about the structure of the periodontal tissues.
2. Which are the clinical features of healthy gingivae?
3. Describe gingivitis and periodontitis.
4. Characterise individual stages in periodontal therapy.

Translation 1
Struktura tkání parodontu, dásně, periodontální vazivo, tkáně obklopují a podporují zuby, zdravé dásně, bledě růžová barva, vzhled s dolíčky, dobře patrný okraj, vroubkovaný obrys, při jemném použití sondy nekrvácí, zánětlivá onemocnění vyvolaná plakem, gingivitida, periodontitida, absence odpovídající ústní hygieny, dentální plak se hromadí, za tři týdny se objeví zánět dásní, klinické rysy zánětu dásní, rudá barva, oteklý vzhled, dolíčky se ztratí, při sondování ihned krvácí, akumulace plaku vede vždy k zánětu dásní, ale nevede nutně k zánětu parodontu, zničení vaziva parodontu a rozvoj chobotu, vyšetření a diagnóza, stádia léčby parodontu, fáze hygieny obsahuje, poučení o dentálním zdraví a kontrole, odstranění překážek efektivní orální hygieny, nechirurgické odstranění zubního kamene pod dásněmi a vyhlazení kořenů, nové posouzení provedené 4–6 týdnů po dokončení fáze hygieny, zdůraznit specifické problémy či oblasti vyžadující další léčbu, korektivní fáze, onemocnění je léčeno, udržovací fáze, pacienti jsou prohlíženi v pravidelných intervalech, monitorovat orální hygienu, včasné rozpoznání nového výskytu nemoci.

Text 2
Hygiene Phase Therapy
Oral hygiene instruction should be tailored to the circumstances and needs of the individual patient. Begin by **explaining** the **nature of periodontal disease**, the role of dental plaque, and the **need to improve cleaning** in areas particularly difficult to reach.
- **models** and information **leaflets** may help understanding

- **visualisation of plaque** can be enhanced by the use of **disclosing agents** and a handheld **mirror**
- it is important to establish deficiencies in current practice and **offer advice**

Tooth-brushing technique

Numerous tooth brushing techniques have been described, of which the modified Bass technique is probably the simplest and most effective.

The **head of the toothbrush** should be angled so that the **filaments are at 45 degrees** to the long axis of the tooth and should be placed **at the gingival margin** to allow the tips of the filaments just to enter the gingival crevice. A **back-and-forth movement** should be used to facilitate plaque removal.

It should be stressed that accessing the awkward areas is more important than continually cleaning the more easily accessible surfaces. Scrub techniques and toothbrushes with hard filaments should be avoided as these can cause gingival recession.

Patients must also be instructed in **interproximal plaque control** techniques. A variety of aids for between-tooth cleaning are available.

Oral hygiene aids
Toothbrushes

The most important features are the **size of the head**, **medium** texture filaments, and **rounded ends** to the bristles.

Electric toothbrushes are of benefit in patients with reduced manual dexterity.

Single-tufted brushes help cleaning around alone-standing teeth, partially erupted third molars, proximal spaces adjacent to saddle areas in partially dentate patients.

Floss can be waxed or unwaxed. Waxed may be easier for first-time users.

Tape is broader than floss and passes between teeth more easily. May be beneficial where interproximal restorations are present.

Superfloss is used for cleaning under bridge pontics.

Floss threader is used to pass floss beneath pontics.

Interproximal (bottle) brushes are available in a range of sizes. Choose the largest size which passes between the teeth without causing discomfort.

Wooden sticks are not as effective as interproximal brushes.

Scaling and root planing

Scaling and root planing can be achieved using either hand instruments or ultrasonic scalers.

Hand instruments

Scaling instruments can be classified as **chisels, sickles, hoes, and curettes**. To be effective, instruments should be **sharpened** regularly.

Ultrasonic scalers

Ultrasonic scalers are composed of an electric power generator, a **handpiece**, and an **insert** with a **working tip**.

A fine **water jet** is directed onto the vibrating tip, acting as a coolant.

Exercise 2

1. How would you give effective oral hygiene instructions?
2. Describe tooth-brushing techniques.
3. Give information about oral hygiene aids.
4. Which instruments for scaling and root planing do you know?

Translation 2

Vysvětlit povahu nemoci parodontu, úlohu dentálního plaku, zlepšit čistění, modely, informační letáky, zviditelnění plaku, odhalující prostředek, rukou držené zrcadlo, technika čistění zubů, modifikovaná Bassova technika je nejjednodušší a nejúčinnější, naklonit hlavu kartáčku, vlákna jsou ve 45 stupních k dlouhé ose zubu, umístit k dásňovému okraji, umožnit špičkám vláken vstoupit do dásňové skuliny, pohyb dozadu a dopředu, vyhnout se technikám drhnutí a kartáčkům s tvrdými vlákny, které způsobují ústup dásní, pomůcky pro mezizubní čistění, kartáčky, velikost hlavy, střední struktura vlákna, kulaté konce štětin, elektrické kartáčky, prospěšné pro pacienty s omezenou manuální zručností, kartáčky s jedním chomáčkem pro čistění kolem osamocených nebo částečně prořezaných zubů, nit voskovaná, nevoskovaná, páska, širší než nit, snadněji prochází mezi zuby, mezizubní kartáčky dostupné v řadě velikostí, odstraňování zubního kamene a leštění kořenů, ruční nástroje, dlátka, srpky, motyčky a kyrety, ultrazvukové odstraňovače zubního kamene, násadec a vložka s pracovním hrotem, chladicí prostředek, jemný trysk vody směrovaný na vibrující hrot.

Vocabulary

access /ˈæk.ses/ přístup, vstup

accessible /əkˈses.ə.bļ/ dostupný

accumulate /əˈkjuː.mjʊ.leɪt/ hromadit se

angled /ˈæŋ.gļd/ šikmý

awkward/ˈɔː.kwəd/ špatně přístupný, nešikovný

axis /ˈæk.sɪs/ osa

beneficial /ˌben.ɪˈfɪʃ.əl/ prospěšný

bottle /ˈbɒt.l/ brush /brʌʃ/ malý mezizubní kartáček

bridge /brɪdʒ/ zubní můstek

bristle /brɪs.l/ štětina

chisel /ˈtʃɪz.əl/ dláto, sekáč

completion /kəmˈpliː.ʃən/ ukončení

comprise /kəmˈpraɪz/ zahrnovat, obsahovat

conduct /kənˈdʌkt/ vést, řídit

continually /kənˈtɪn.ju.ə.li/ nepřetržitě

coolant /ˈkuː.lənt/ chladivo, ochlazovací prostředek

corrective /kəˈrek.tɪv/ nápravný, opravný

crevice /ˈkrev.ɪs/ prasklina, škvíra

crevicular /ˈkre'v.ɪ.kjʊ.ləʳ/ štěrbinový

curette /kjʊəˈret/ kyreta

current /ˈkʌr.ənt/ aktuální, současný

defective /dɪˈfek.tɪv/ vadný, porušený

degree /dɪˈgriː/ stupeň

dentate /den.teɪt/ ozubený, zubatý, vroubkovaný

detection /dɪˈtek.ʃən/ odhalení, vypátrání

direct /daɪˈrekt/ nasměrovat, zamířit

disclose /dɪˈskləʊz/ odhalit, prozradit

edge /edʒ/ okraj, hrana

education /ˌed.jʊˈkeɪ.ʃ°n/ školení, instruktáž

elimination /ɪˌlɪm.ɪˈneɪ.ʃᵊn/ vyloučení, vyřazení
enhance /ɪnˈhɑːnts/ zlepšit kvalitu, zvětšit
event /ɪˈvent/ událost, případ, výsledek
filament /ˈfɪl.ə.mənt/ vlákno
fine /faɪn/ jemný
floss /flɒs/ hedvábí, hedvábná voskovaná nit
flow /fləʊ/ tok, výtok
forth /fɔːθ/ dopředu, dále
generator /ˈdʒen.ə.reɪ.təʳ/ zdroj, původce
gingival /ˌdʒɪn.dʒɪ.val/ gingivální, dásňový
grossly /ˈgrəʊ.sli/ hrubě
handheld /ˌhændˈheld/ ruční (držený v ruce), přenosný
handpiece /hænd.piːs/ násadec, rukojeť
hard /hɑːd/ tvrdý, nesnadný
highlight /ˈhaɪ.laɪt/ zdůraznit
hoe /həʊ/ motyčka
hopeless /ˈhəʊ.pləs/ beznadějný, bezvýhledný
insert /ɪnˈsɜːt/ vložka
interproximal /ɪn.təʳ.prɒkˈsɪ.məl/ interproximální
invariably /ɪnˈveə.ri.ə.bli/ trvale, pravidelně
jet /dʒet/ proud vody, stříkat
ligament /ˈlɪg.ə.mənt/ ligament, vaz
malposition /mæl.pəˈzɪʃ.ᵊn/ chybná poloha, špatné úmístění
medium /ˈmiː.di.əm/ střed, prostřední
mirror /ˈmɪr.əʳ/ zrcadlo
model /ˈmɒd.ᵊl/ model, vzor
modify /ˈmɒd.ɪ.faɪ/ upravit, uzpůsobit
need /niːd/ potřeba
nonsurgical /nɒnˈsɜː.dʒɪ.kᵊl/ nechirurgický
obstacle /ˈɒb.stɪ.kl̩/ překážka
outcome /ˈaʊt.kʌm/ výsledek, závěr
outline /ˈaʊt.laɪn/ obrys, náčrt, přehled
pale /peɪl/ bledý
pathogenesis /ˌpæθəˈdʒen.ɪ.sɪs/ patogeneze, vznik a vývoj onemocnění
periodontitis /ˌper.ɪ.əˈdɒn.ˈtaɪ.tɪs/ periodontitida, zánět závěsného aparátu
periodontium /ˌper.ɪ.əˈdɒn.ʃiəm/ periodoncium, parodont
permit /pəˈmɪt/ dovolit, tolerovat, připustit
pink /pɪŋk/ růžová barva
place /pleɪs/ umístit, prostor
pontic /ˌpɒnt.ɪk/ umělý zub umístěný na můstku
probe /prəʊb/ zubařská sonda
prognosis /prɒgˈnəʊ.sɪs/ (pl. prognoses) prognóza, předpověď
progress /prəˈgres/ postupovat, vyvíjet se
proximal /prɒˈk.sɪ.məl/ proximální
readily /ˈred.ɪ.li/ pohotově, ihned
reassess /ˌriː.əˈses/ přehodnotit
recession /rɪˈseʃ.ᵊn/ odstoupení, ústup
removal /rɪˈmuː.vᵊl/ odstranění, vyjmutí
review /rɪˈvjuː/ zhodnotit, prohlédnout opět
root /ruːt/ planing /pleɪn.ɪŋ/ vyhlazení stěn kořene
rounded /ˈraʊn.dɪd/ zakulacený
saddle /ˈsæd.l̩/ sedlo
scaler /skeɪl.əʳ/ škrabka
scalloped /ˈskɒl.əpd/ vroubkovaný, zoubkovaný
scrub /skrʌb/ drhnout (kartáčem)
sickle /ˈsɪk.l̩/ srpek
simple /ˈsɪm.pl̩/ jednoduchý

single /ˈsɪŋ.gl̩/ jednotlivý, samostatný

stick /stɪk/ tyčinka, přilepit

stippled /ˈstɪp.l̩d/ dolíčkovaný, tečkovaný

stippling /ˈstɪp.lɪŋ/ tečkování, dolíčkování

support /səˈpɔːt/ podpora, podpírat

surround /səˈraʊnd/ obklopit, okraj

tailored /ˈteɪ.ləd/ upravený na míru

tape /teɪp/ proužek, stužka

texture /ˈteks.tʃəʳ/ struktura, tkáň, vazba

threader /ˈθred.əʳ/ závitnice

tip /tɪp/ hrot, špička, naklonit

tufted /ˈtʌf.tɪd/ chomáčkovitý

ultrasonic /ˌʌl.trəˈsɒn.ɪk/ ultrazvukový

user /ˈjuː.zəʳ/ uživatel

vibrate /vaɪˈbreɪt/ vibrovat (kmitat), chvět se

visualisation /ˌvɪʒ.u.əl.aɪˈzeɪ.ʃ°n/ znázornění (vizuální)

waxed /wækst/ voskovaný

wooden /ˈwʊd.°n/ dřevěný

Unit 12

Restorative Dentistry

Importance of Moisture Control.
Methods Available to Achieve Moisture
Control. Restorative Techniques.
Acrylic Denture Provision. Reasons
for Root Treatments. Reasons for
Immediate Replacement.

Text 1

Importance of Moisture Control

The dentist will have **poor visibility**
without it and **may injure** the patient
or perform dental treatment to a low
standard without realising it.

It will be **uncomfortable for the patient**
to have a mouthful of water and saliva,
especially if being treated in the supine
position. The patient may keep trying
to swallow or want to spit out, both of
which tend to interrupt the treatment.
The tooth being treated will become
contaminated with water or saliva and
allow bacteria to wash into the cavities
or onto the tooth preparations. This is
especially important during endodontic
treatment.

All dental **filling materials are**
adversely affected by moisture
contamination as follows:

- **composites** do not lock into the
  etched enamel surface

- **amalgam** expands as the zinc
  content reacts and produces gas
  bubbles
- **glass ionomers** do not set
  correctly and the resulting filling is
  weak
- **lining cements** do not adhere to
  the cavity floor
- **luting cements** do not adhere
  to the preparation walls and the
  restoration may become loose
- **Impression materials**, other than
  alginate, will have their surface set
  contaminated by moisture bubbles,
  which will result in inaccurate
  impressions and casts.

Methods Available to Achieve
Moisture Control

- **Slow-speed aspiration** using a
  saliva ejector, which the **patient**
  can hold beneath the tongue
  to prevent saliva pooling in the
  floor of the mouth. Some ejectors
  also have flanges to help keep the
  tongue to one side.

- **High-speed aspiration** with
  a wide-bore suction tip, for
  immediate and fast moisture
  removal. This is **essential**
  whenever the air turbine is

being used because of the copious amounts of water produced.

- **Isolation** of the tooth undergoing treatment from the rest of the mouth by the use of **rubber dam**—a special sheet of rubber that is pierced and through which the tooth is poked. It is held in place with special **tooth clamps** and supported on the patient's face with a **frame**. Isolation of the tooth by **cotton wool rolls** placed in the sulci. Being absorbed they tend to soak up pooling moisture and prevent contamination. **Cavities and tooth preparations** themselves can be wiped dry using **cotton wool pledgets held in forceps**. They can also **be blown dry using the triple syringe**, although it is possible that the air is minutely contaminated with water already within the nozzle of the syringe. **Gingival retraction cord** placed in the gingival crevice of the tooth being treated. The cord is soaked in either alum or adrenaline to prevent bleeding at the site, but it also absorbs traces of crevicular fluid from the area. **Specially made discs of absorbent material** placed in the buccal sulcus, especially those that fit over the Wharton's duct from the parotid gland and directly absorb salivary secretions—dry guards. They contain an absorbent material similar to that used in babies' nappies. Patients undergoing intravenous sedation can also be given **an intravenous injection of atropine**, which acts on the salivary glands to reduce their saliva production and secretion, but this is reserved for extreme cases.

Exercise 1
1. Why is moisture control important during restorative dentistry?
2. Discuss the methods available to achieve it.

Translation 1
Kontrola vlhkosti, špatná viditelnost, provést zubní ošetření, nepříjemné pro pacienta, poloha vleže, polknout, vyplivnout, přerušit ošetření, amalgam zvětšuje objem, plynové bubliny, tuhnout správně, výplň je slabá, cementy nedrží, náhrady se uvolňují, nepřesné otisky a odlitky, pomalé odsávání, vysokorychlostní odsávání, odsavač slin, držet pod jazykem, špička savky, okamžité a rychlé odstranění vlhkosti, použít vzduchovou turbínu, izolace ošetřovaného zubu, použití gumové blány, držet na místě, svitky vaty, nasáknout hromadící se vlhkost, vysušit vatovými tamponky, uchopený v kleštích, vyfoukat trojitou stříkačkou, šňůrka na odtažení dásně, fyziologický dásňový chobot, zabránit krvácení v místě, umístěný do tvářové rýhy, nitrožilní injekce, v extrémních případech.

Text 2
Restorative Techniques
A mesial-occlusal-distal (MOD) cavity with a buccal extension is a large cavity, requiring adequate restoration if the tooth is to be returned to its

full function. Lower molar teeth are used for heavy mastication, so the restoration chosen will be expected to be able to withstand heavy occlusal loads. The buccal involvement may be just the buccal groove, or it may be the whole buccal wall, so restorative techniques will be described for both scenarios.

For an MOD with buccal groove involvement
A class 2 amalgam restoration with buccal extension is probably the restoration most commonly used in this situation.

- A composite material designed with a higher filler content than usual, for use specifically as a posterior, aesthetic filling material, is employed using a direct technique (formed and placed at the chairside).
- An indirect technique is using a composite inlay, which is formed at the laboratory using impression taken of the cavity after tooth preparation.
- A gold inlay, formed as above.
- A porcelain inlay, formed as above.

All the indirect inlay techniques involve a two-visit procedure for the patient and necessitate the placement of a temporary filling while the inlay is being made at the laboratory.

For an MOD with whole buccal wall involvement
There will be no retention on any restoration buccally, unless provided artificially.

- A pinned amalgam restoration, with two dentinal pins placed at the corners of the buccal side of the cavity to prevent the restoration slipping sideways out of the cavity during mastication, as amalgam is nonadhesive to tooth.
- A pinned posterior composite, with dentinal pins placed as above, to give added retention besides that provided by the mechanical locking of the composite to all etched enamel.
- A full coverage restoration using the remaining tooth tissue to prevent sideways slipping during mastication.

They can either be a full gold crown or a bonded porcelain crown. Whichever is used, a strong core must be produced beneath it to provide adequate strength to resist occlusal forces. This can be provided by a pinned restoration of amalgam, posterior composite, or reinforced glass ionomer cement. If the tooth is root-filled, more retention could be provided by the use of posts placed in the root canals.

Role of the dental nurse
To:

- have all necessary **instruments sterilised and to hand** ready for use, whichever procedure is adopted
- ensure that all necessary **materials are available** for use
- **pass and receive** the necessary **local anaesthesia**, if it is required
- provide good **aspiration, soft-tissue retraction, and moisture control** during tooth preparation

- **mix any restorative** material **or impression material** correctly and efficiently, and pass it to the dentist with adequate working time available for its use
- provide **good moisture control during placement** of the restoration, and be **available to aspirate** as necessary during any adjustment to the restoration
- **disinfect all impressions**, if laboratory work is involved, and **pack them correctly** ready for transportation to the laboratory, together with the **completed dockets**
- **mix and help place any temporary filling or covering** that may be necessary in the meantime
- see that the used **instruments are cleaned and sterilised after use**, that all unused **materials are disposed of,** and that the **surgery is tidied and made ready** for the next patient

Exercise 2
1. Discuss the methods available for restoring a lower molar tooth with a mesial-occlusal-distal cavity with a buccal extension.
2. How would the dental nurse assist the dentist during the restoration?

Translation 2
Konzervační techniky, vrátit zubu úplnou funkčnost, dolní stoličky, silné žvýkání, vydržet velkou zátěž skusu, postižení tváře, použitý výplňový materiál, vytvořit a umístit u křesla, vytvořený v laboratoři, vzít otisk

dutiny, zahrnovat postup dvou návštěv, umístění dočasné výplně, úloha zubní sestry, předat připravené k použití, zajistit správně odsávání, odtažení měkké tkáně, kontrola vlhkosti, preparace zubu, podávat nástroje lékaři, být k dispozici, během úpravy a umístění náhrady, dezinfikovat otisky, zabalit a připravit pro převoz do laboratoře, vyplněné stvrzenky, míchat a pomáhat umístit dočasné výplně a pokrytí, dohlédnout, aby nástroje byly vyčištěny a sterilizovány po použití, všechny nepoužité materiály jsou odklizeny, ordinace je uklizena a připravena pro dalšího pacienta.

Text 3
Acrylic Denture Provision
Acrylic denture provision **for an edentulous patient can take at least four visits**, possibly five if the prostheses have to be retried for any reason.
It is assumed that, on each visit, the **dental nurse will receive the patient** into the clinical area, **seat them** comfortably and put a **protective bib** in place. **After each appointment**, the dental nurse will **provide tissues and mouthwash** as required.

Stages of provision: role of the nurse
Impressions
To:
- choose the correct edentulous **impression trays** and place the necessary **adhesive** on them
- **mix** the chosen **impression material** (usually alginate) to a smooth, air-free consistency and either load each tray at a time or

155

present the mix to the dentist for loading

- **clean mixing bowls and spatulas** thoroughly after each mix
- **fill in the laboratory sheet** correctly with the patient's details and the necessary instructions
- **sterilise impressions** once they are out of the patient's mouth, by running them **under the cold tap** and then immersing them in **a fresh solution of 10% sodium hypochlorite** for 10 minutes
- cover them with a **wet piece of gauze and seal them in an airtight bag** ready for transport to the laboratory
- hand the shade guide to the dentist and **record the chosen shade correctly on the laboratory sheet**
- place the **package of impressions and laboratory sheets ready for collection**

Bite record and second impressions
To:

- **set out the correct laboratory work ready** for use
- place the **flame heater, wax knife,** and possibly, a Le Cron **carver** ready for use should the dentist require them

Some dentists also use a Willis gauge to determine the correct occlusal face height of the patient, in which case this should also be placed ready for use. If **occlusal registration paste** is used to record the patient's bite, the dental nurse must have the **correct proportions laid out on a clean paper pad** and should mix the constituents correctly and thoroughly. The mixture should be presented to the dentist for use with the spatula wiped clean. Once completed, the **occlusal rims should be rinsed in cold disinfectant solution** before being packed and placed for collection.

Try-in
To:

- **set out the correct laboratory work**
- set out **pink wax, a flame, wax knife,** and possibly, a Le Cron **carver and articulating paper** ready for use by the dentist
- **hold a mirror for the patient** to view the trial dentures and **discuss their fit and appearance** with the dentist
- **disinfect the trial dentures** again, once the patient and dentist are satisfied with them, with cold solution before **packing and placing them ready for collection** by the laboratory

Retry of trial dentures
This stage is not always necessary. If it is, however, then the surgery procedure is repeated as for the original trial insertions to ensure that any previous problems or areas of dissatisfaction have been corrected.

Fitting of completed dentures
To:

- set out correct **laboratory work** ready for use
- lay out a **straight handpiece** and selection of **stainless steel acrylic trimming burs** ready for use
- place **articulating paper** ready for use, some dentists prefer to

use occlusal indicator wax to determine the presence of any premature occlusal contacts
- have **pressure indicating cream** at hand; this may also be used to determine the presence of high spots on the fitting surface of the dentures so they can be removed using the acrylic trimming burs
- hold the **mirror** for the patient to view the completed dentures
- **hand and explain written denture-care instructions**, if used, to the patient before they leave the surgery
- ensure the **patient is told to contact the surgery** at their earliest convenience to report any problems with the new dentures

Exercise 3

1. Describe the role of the dental nurse at each stage of the provision of an acrylic denture to an edentulous patient.

Translation 3

Akrylátová náhrada, bezzubý pacient, protézy musí být znovu vyzkoušeny, přijmout pacienty, usadit je pohodlně, umístit ochranou náprsenku, po každém setkání, poskytnout kapesníčky a výplach úst, vybrat správné otiskovací lžíce, naplnit každou lžíci, vyčistit důkladně míchací misky a lopatky, vyplnit záznam pro laboratoř, podrobnosti o pacientech a nezbytné pokyny, sterilizovat otisky, omytí náhrady pod studenou vodou z kohoutku, ponoření do roztoku chlornanu sodného na 10 minut, přikrýt vlhkým kouskem gázy, uzavřít

do neprodyšného vaku, připraven na převoz do laboratoře, odevzdat vzorník odstínů zubaři, zaznamenat vybraný odstín, připravit k vyzvednutí balíček otisků a dokumentů, záznam skusu, připravit k použití, registrační pasta, čistý papírový čtverec, míchat důkladně, podat lékaři, propláchnout v desinfekčním roztoku, držet pacientovi zrcátko, vzhled a upevnění, pacient je spokojen, upevnění dokončených protéz, rovný násadec, nerez ocel, fréza na pryskyřici, artikulační papír, písemné instrukce o dentální péči, než pacient odejde z ordinace, kontaktovat ordinaci, hlásit jakékoli problémy s novou protézou.

Text 4

Instruments and materials that may be required to extirpate the pulp of a tooth and to dress the tooth for a period before root filling
- **Local anaesthetic**: suitable loaded syringe, topical anaesthetic if required
- **Rubber dam**: rubber dam sheet, rubber dam punch and forceps, suitable clamp, disinfectant wash
- **Full conservation tray**: mirror, probe, forceps, small and large spoon excavators, amalgam plugger and burnisher, flat plastic instrument
- **Handpieces and attachments**: air turbine and suitable diamond bur for access cavity, slow-speed handpiece and rosehead bur for final access, engine reamers if necessary to locate canal entrance
- **Endodontic instruments and materials**: barbed broach, set of

endodontic hand files or reamers
for debridement, selection of paper
points for drying and dressing,
irrigation syringes, suitable
irrigation solution, proprietary
antiseptic mouthwash or sodium
hypochlorite, antiseptic dressing,
creosote, parachlorphenol,
temporary filling material to seal
access cavity

Reasons for Root Treatments
- **To save a tooth when extraction is the only other course of treatment** possibly due to:
- **pulpitis** being present as a result of, for example, caries, irritant deep filling, irritant unlined filling, iatrogenic (caused by dentist), trauma
- **problems during attempted restoration**, such as traumatic exposure, non-use of water spray on air turbine handpiece
- **traumatic injury** resulting in direct pulp exposure because of crown fracture or death of the tooth with time
- presence of an **apical abscess in a nonvital tooth**
- To save a tooth **when it is required** as a bridge retainer or as a denture abutment
- To save a tooth when the **patient's medical history contraindicates extraction,** e.g. any bleeding disorder

Exercise 4
1. List the instruments and materials that may be required to extirpate the pulp of a tooth and to dress the tooth for a period before root filling.

2. Why may a tooth require root treatment?

Translation 4
Nástroje a materiály, naplněná stříkačka, gumová blána, dírkovač kofferdamu, pinzeta, svorka, dezinfekční roztok, miska na nástroje, zrcátko, sonda, kleště, malý a velký lžícový exkavátor, cpátko na amalgam, hladítko, plochý plastový nástroj, násadce a doplňky, vzduchová turbinka, diamantový brousek, rozšiřovač, pulpextraktor, pilníky, papírové čípky, zavlažovací stříkačky, zavlažovací roztok, registrovaný antiseptický výplach, antiseptický obvaz, dočasný výplňový materiál, léčba kořene, zachránit zub, zánět dřeně, kaz, dráždivá hluboká výplň, traumatické obnažení, poranění, fraktura korunky, odumření zubu, apikální absces, devitalizovaný zub, držák můstku, pilíř náhrady, kontraindikace vytržení, porucha krvácení.

Text 5
Reasons for Immediate Replacement
An anterior tooth requires extraction and the patient requests an artificial replacement.
The patient is to have their remaining teeth extracted but is not prepared to wait several months before a denture is constructed while bone resorption occurs.

Further treatment
Once a tooth has been extracted the surrounding **alveolar bone gradually resorbs and remodels**

itself. This occurs most rapidly in the first 6 months after extraction but usually continues until 12 months postextraction.

Thus, within a short time after fitting the **immediate replacement denture**, the prosthesis will become **loose-fitting and unstable** in the mouth. The patient may then have to rely on **denture adhesives** in order to continue wearing the denture fully and especially for eating food. If anterior teeth are replaced, the laboratory quite often sets them as fitting against the gingivae, with no acrylic flange present.

Once bone resorption occurs, this area will **allow food to collect beneath the denture** because a space develops between the shrinking gingivae and the denture. This is **uncomfortable** for the patient and most annoying for them to have to keep removing the prosthesis and rinsing it clean.

For all these reasons, it is quite normal for the patient to **attend on a regular basis for chairside relining of the denture.**

The dentist can **add cold-cured acrylic to the fitting surface** of the denture and so replace the lost bone, without the patient having to leave the denture at the surgery.

If a great deal of resorption has occurred, it may be necessary for a wash impression of the fitting surface to be taken and then **the denture returned to the laboratory** for a heat-cured acrylic reline. However, the patient will not be keen to have to leave the denture out for any length of time. This relining process may need to be carried out for **up to 12 months**

after the teeth were extracted and the prosthesis fitted. If a 'gum fitted' appliance was originally made, softened gutta-percha may be used to border-mould the area and allow the technician to construct an acrylic flange while also carrying out a reline. After 12 months, when it can be assumed that the majority of the bone resorption has occurred, a decision has to be made as to **whether a completely new prosthetic appliance** needs to be constructed or whether **the relined appliance is satisfactory** in both its **fit and appearance.**

Oral hygiene instructions

Patients with an immediate replacement have undergone **both a surgical procedure** in having a tooth extracted **and** have had **a new prosthetic appliance** fitted. They must, therefore, be given instructions covering both procedures, as follows:

- **keep the denture in the mouth 24 hours after the extractions** have been performed in order to protect the blood clots and hopefully avoid a postoperative infection
- **brush all the mouth as normal** on the night of the procedure
- on removing the **denture** (over a sink of water to prevent any breakages), **rinse it under the cold tap to remove debris**
- **brush the denture and your own teeth** at the same time with a toothbrush and toothpaste, taking care not to knock the extraction socket(s)
- **rinse the surgical area with hot, saltwater mouthwashes** several

times each day for one week to promote healing and prevent postoperative infection

- **report any severe pain or bleeding** to the dental surgery as soon as possible
- during the first few weeks of wear, **you can sleep with the prosthesis** in place if you wish, to **enable bedding of the appliance into the soft tissues**

However, unless the patient's standard of oral hygiene is excellent, this should not be recommended as routine. This is because the soft tissues need to recover from having the appliance in situ all day. In addition, the patient should be advised that:

- **Candidal infections** are quite common beneath upper acrylic dentures **due to poor oral and denture hygiene** and are especially common under dentures that are rarely removed.
- **while out of the mouth overnight, keep the denture moist**; otherwise, the acrylic tends to dry out.
- **immerse it in cold water, or a nonstaining proprietary mouthwash solution**, after being brushed clean.
- dentures can be **soaked in a sodium hypochlorite** solution overnight, but take care **not to use too strong a concentration** as the denture teeth may well be bleached to a lighter shade.
- the dentures can be soaked overnight in a **proprietary denture cleanser.**

Exercise 5

1. Why might an immediate replacement denture be provided?
2. What further prosthetic treatment may be required to the denture after fitting, and why?
3. What oral hygiene instructions would the dental nurse give to the patient after the immediate denture has been fitted?

Translation 5

Okamžitá náhrada, přední zub potřebuje vytrhnout, požadovat umělou náhradu, vytrhnout zbývající zuby, čekat, než se vyrobí protéza, další léčba, resorpce okolní dásňové kosti, pokračovat po 12 měsíců po extrakci, protéza se uvolní, nestabilní v ústech, spoléhat na lepidla na protézy, potrava se hromadí pod protézou, navštěvovat pravidelně, obnova vnitřní strany protézy, nechat protézu v ordinaci, vrátit do laboratoře, upevnit protézu, je třeba učinit rozhodnutí, vytvořit úplně novou náhradu, padnutí a vzhled, pokyny pro ústní hygienu, podstoupit chirurgickou proceduru, nechat náhradu v ústech 24 hodin, ochránit krevní sraženinu a zabránit infekci, čistit ústa jako obvykle, vyjmout protézu a propláchnout pod studenou vodou, odstranit zbytky, čistit protézu i vaše vlastní zuby kartáčkem a pastou, neuhodit se do jamky po vytržení, vypláchnout teplou slanou vodou, podporovat hojení, ohlásit co nejdříve silnou bolest či krvácení, poradit pacientovi, infekce kandidózy pod protézou, mimo ústa, udržovat protézu vlhkou, ponořit do studené vody, ústní vody, čističe na protézy, být namočen do roztoku chlornanu sodného přes noc, příliš silná koncentrace, vybělit do světlejšího odstínu.

Text 6

Dental nurse assistance during **the provision of an anterior composite restoration to an adult patient, under local anaesthesia**

- The nurse would **seat the patient** in the dental chair and cover them with a **protective bib and safety glasses**.
- The **correct notes and charting** would be available for the dentist to read.
- A local anaesthetic **syringe would be loaded with the cartridge** of choice, **fitted with a short needle,** and held correctly to be passed to the dentist for use.
- A **full sterile conservation tray** would have been set out ready for use with cotton wool rolls available, as well as a celluloid matrix strip if the cavity requires one.
- **Handpieces would be connected ready** for use by the dentist, with the bur selection to hand.
- **Mouthwash and tissues** would be available for patient use throughout the procedure.
- If **rubber dam** is to be used, all the necessary equipment would be sterile and laid out ready for use by the dentist.
- Once **anaesthesia has been achieved**, the dental nurse would assist by providing **adequate aspiration** so the patient would not be choking but **without obscuring the dentist's vision**.

- **Once cavity preparation is completed**, the dental nurse would assist by **having the filling materials ready**, which would be handed to the dentist as required and in the appropriate order.
- **A lining** would be placed first, followed by **enamel etching**.
- The dental nurse would provide adequate aspiration as the **etchant is washed off**, and the **tooth would then be dried**.
- **Bonding resin** would then be passed to the dentist, with its appropriate **applicator**.
- **The composite shade guide** would be required at some point of the procedure (the dentist would decide when), and then the dental nurse would **load the correct choice** into the applicator if compoules are used or have the correct choice ready to be dispensed onto a paper pad.
- If the dentist wanted to **use light-cured material**, the dental nurse would have to **operate the curing lamp** while the dentist adapted the matrix strip to the tooth.
- **The protective shield** would also need holding correctly to avoid viewing the blue light.
- The dental nurse would then **aspirate as the restoration is polished and completed**.
- Once the patient had left the surgery, **all disposables would be correctly discarded** in either the sharps bin or the clinical waste bag.
- **All instruments** would be **scrubbed clean and autoclaved** ready for reuse.

- All **work surfaces** would be **wiped over with disinfectant** before the next patient was admitted.

Exercise 6

1. Describe how the dental nurse would assist during the provision of an anterior composite restoration to an adult patient under local anaesthesia.

Translation 6

Asistence zubní sestry, usadit pacienta do křesla, ochranná náprsenka a bezpečnostní brýle, poznámky a diagramy, naplněná stříkačka, vybraná náplň, upevnit jehlu, správně držet a podat, připravit k použití vatové tampóny, celuloidová páska, spojit násadce s vrtáčky, vypláchnutí úst a ubrousky, dostupné pacientovi k použití, po celou dobu procedury, připravit pro lékaře k použití, sterilní vybavení, poskytnout vhodné odsávání, nezakrývat lékaři výhled, mít připravené výplňové materiály, podávat lékaři podle potřeby, vyložení, leptání skloviny, vypláchnout leptadlo, vysušit zub, pojivová pryskyřice s vhodným aplikátorem, vzorník odstínů kompozitních výplňových materiálů, naplnit do aplikátoru, rozdělit na papírový čtverec, světlem tvrzený materiál, obsluhovat polymerační lampu na tuhnutí kompozit, upravovat pojivo do zubu, držet ochranný štít, leštit a dokončit, jakmile pacient opustil ordinaci, pomůcky na jedno použití, vyhodit do nádoby na ostré předměty, pytel na klinický odpad, vydrhnout všechny nástroje, být dán

do autoklávu, přetřít všechny pracovní povrchy dezinfekcí, přijmout dalšího pacienta.

Text 7

Dental nurse assistance during the fitting of a crown

- **A full, sterile conservation tray of instruments** would be set out ready for use.
- The **correct item of laboratory work** would be set ready for use.
- **Articulating paper and holders** would be laid out and **dental floss** ready to enable the interproximal removal of cement.
- Suitable **local anaesthesia** would be prepared if necessary.
- Once the **temporary crown has been removed** and the **permanent replacement tried for fit and occlusion**, the dental nurse would **mix the luting cement** chosen by the dentist. The cement would be mixed thoroughly and efficiently to the correct **creamy consistency**. It would then **be placed** into the crown and then placed firmly over the prepared tooth. **During setting**, the dental nurse would either **provide good moisture control or hold the crown** in place.
- Once setting has occurred, adequate **aspiration** would be provided while **excess cement** was **removed**. Aspiration would also be provided during any necessary **occlusal adjustments.**
- Once the treatment is complete, the dental nurse would **escort the patient from the surgery,**

then clean and sterilise the used instruments.

Luting cements available
Luting cements are those mixed to a creamy consistency to **allow the accurate placement of crowns, bridges, and inlays**.

Zinc phosphate cement
Zinc oxide powder and phosphoric acid, mixed on a cooled glass slab with a metal spatula. Powder is spatulated by portions into the liquid to produce a creamy consistency.

Zinc polycarboxylate cement
Zinc oxide powder and polyacrylic acid, mixed on a glass slab with a metal spatula. Powder is spatulated by portions into the liquid to produce a creamy consistency.

Luting glass ionomer cement
Fine-particle glass ionomer powder containing polyacrylate and aluminosilicates, with pure water, mixed on a glass slab or a waxed paper pad with a metal spatula. Powder is spatulated by portions into the liquid to produce a creamy consistency. Nowadays, machines are available that self-mix some of the materials, especially dual-cure composites and glass ionomer cements.

Exercise 7
1. How might the dental nurse assist during the fitting of a crown?
2. What materials are available for the cementation of the crown, and how is each mixed?

Translation 7
Upevnění korunky, artikulační papír, držáky, zubní nit, vhodná místní anestézie, dočasná korunka, stálá korunka, vyzkoušet zapadnutí a skus, smíchat důkladně tmelící cement, krémová konsistence, během tuhnutí, odstranit nadbytečný cement, nezbytné úpravy skusu, doprovodit pacienta z ordinace, vyčistit a sterilizovat použité nástroje, umožnit přesné umístění, prášek zinkové běloby a kyselina fosforečná, zchlazená skleněná destička, kovová třecí lopatka, roztírat po částech, kyselina polyakrylová, sklo-ionomerní cement, jemné částice, polyakrylát, aluminosilikát (hlinito-křemičitan), čistá voda, čtverec voskového papíru, stroje na samočinné míchání, dvojitě vytvrzované kompozity.

Text 8
Methods available for restoring a **root-filled central incisor which has fractured at the gingival margin**
Fracture at the gingival level indicates that no clinical crown remains. Therefore, a post needs placing into the root canal to provide a core on which the clinical crown can be made. Root-filling material is drilled out of the canal using Gates-Glidden drills and a slow handpiece. A post hole is then prepared to know width and depth using the Parapost system. The root face is prepared for the crown. Impressions are taken of post hole and prepared tooth, then a post crown restoration is made in the laboratory. Alternatively, a prefabricated post can be cemented immediately and an impression taken for just a crown to

be constructed over the core. No other technique can be used in this situation, as only a post cemented into the root canal will provide adequate support for a functional restoration.

Methods available for restoring a class 2 cavity which involves two surfaces of posterior teeth

Premolars may or may not be visible when the patient talks and smiles. The majority of these cavities are restored with an amalgam filling. Some patients may choose to have a posterior composite filling placed (privately). This is acceptable in a small cavity and where the patient has no grinding habits. The cavity is cleared of all caries by first using the air turbine and diamond burs, then by round burs in the slow handpiece. The cavity is then lined with calcium hydroxide. Following application of a matrix band, an amalgam filling can be placed and anatomically carved to restore the tooth to full function. Alternatively, the enamel margins can be acid-etched, washed, and dried, then resin and a posterior composite filling material can be placed. Light-cured varieties tend to be used today, so a celluloid matrix strip is required around the tooth to prevent overspill interproximally. A small class 2 cavity could also be restored with a gold inlay, but this restoration is very costly, and in a small cavity, would have no benefit over the other two techniques.

Methods available for restoring a class 4 cavity in an upper central incisor

A class 4 cavity involves an interproximal surface and incisal edge of an anterior tooth. Restoration in this situation has to be strong enough to withstand biting forces but must also be of acceptable appearance to the patient. The ideal restoration is an acid-etched composite matched to the colour of the tooth. Depending on the size of the fracture, a dentinal pin may also be used for added strength and retention. Rubber dam may also be used to isolate the tooth, if possible. The tooth is prepared by exposing as much enamel as possible to provide retention. Any dentine is covered with calcium hydroxide. The enamel is acid-etched, washed, and dried. The adjacent teeth can be separated by celluloid matrix strips, or a crown former can be used. This prevents the composite from being inadvertently sealed to the contact points of the adjacent teeth. Resin is coated over the etched enamel then the composite is applied. The majority of materials available are light-cured. The restoration can be trimmed and polished as necessary. The alternative restoration would be either a porcelain veneer or a crown. A porcelain veneer would provide no extra retention, and the cavity would still require restoration behind the veneer. A crown would only be indicated if the tooth is likely to suffer further trauma and continue to fracture.

Methods available for restoring a deep class 5 cavity in a molar

A class 5 cavity involves the gingival one-third of the tooth. The enamel is thin in this position, and the pulp chambers are not too deep beneath the dentine. If adequate retention can be gained by undercutting the cavity, a well-lined amalgam restoration can be placed. If access is difficult, or if there is a danger of pulp exposure during undercutting, then a glass ionomer cement is the restoration of choice. Glass ionomers are irritant to the pulp, so a calcium hydroxide lining is also required. Glass ionomers are adhesive to dentine and enamel, so no cavity undercutting is necessary. Moisture control must be thorough during filling, as glass ionomers are very sensitive to moisture contamination. A surface varnish is required as soon as surface setting has occurred.

Exercise 8
1. Describe the methods available for restoring the following:
a. a root-filled central incisor which has fractured at the gingival margin
b. a small class 2 cavity in a premolar
c. a class 4 cavity in an upper central incisor
d. a deep class 5 cavity in a molar

Translation 8
Řezák s vyplněným kořenem, fraktura v dásňovém okraji, nezůstává korunka, podpěra v kořenovém kanálku, střed pro korunku, materiál pro výplň kořene, vrtačka, vyvrtat, připravit otvor pro čep, znát šířku a hloubku, připravit kořenovou frézu, vzít otisky, čepová korunka, zatmelit čep do kořenového kanálku, poskytnout adekvátní podporu, funkční obnova, premoláry

mohou být vidět, když pacient mluví a usmívá se, opravit amalgámovou výplní, návyk skřípat zuby, dutina je vyčištěna od kazů, vzduchová turbinka, diamantový brousek, kulatý vrtáček, dutina je obložena, aplikace matriční pásky, umístit výplň, okraje skloviny mohou být leptány, vypláchnuty a vysušeny, světlem tvrzené varianty, celuloidová páska kolem zubu, zabránit styčnému předávkování, zlatá výplň je velmi nákladná, nemá žádnou výhodu proti ostatním technikám, horní střední řezák, hrana řezáku, přední zub, zadní zub, vydržet sílu při kousání, přijatelný vzhled, hodit se k barvě zubu, izolovat zub, odhalit sklovinu co nejvíce, sousední zuby, šablona na korunku, potáhnout leptanou sklovinu, aplikovat kompozit, vyčistit (oříznout) a vyleštit, porcelánová fazeta, indikovat korunku, zub se pravděpodobně bude dále lámat, utrpět další úraz, přístup je obtížný, nebezpečí odhalení dřeně, sklo-ionomerní cement, dráždivý pro dřeň, sklo-ionomery jsou přilnavé k zubovině i sklovině, kontrola vlhkosti musí být důkladná během plnění, tuhnutí povrchu, lak na povrch.

Exercise 9/ Homework
The sentences have been divided into separate halves. Match the half-sentences in column A with the half-sentences in column B to make sentences which are complete and correct.

A
1. Celluloid matrix strips are used by the dentists to . . .
2. A Black's class 3 cavity is one which involves . . .

3. Linings should be placed beneath amalgam fillings to prevent . . .
4. Wooden wedges may be required during tooth restoration to . . .
5. A Moore's mandrel holds . . .
6. The speed of an air turbine handpiece is approximately . . .
7. Waste amalgam should be handled with care due to . . .
8. A reinforced glass ionomer cement is one that contains . . .
9. Zinc phosphate cement should be mixed on . . .
10. Cavity margins can be trimmed by hand, using . . .
11. A ball-ended burnisher is used by the dentist to . . .
12. The instrument required to pack amalgam into a cavity is . . .
13. In restorative dentistry, articulating paper is used to show . . .
14. Friction-grip white stones are used to . . .

B

a. *show premature contacts on fillings, crowns, bridges, and dentures.*
b. *cervical margin trimmer.*
c. *burnish the margins of amalgam fillings and the thin edges of gold crowns to the tooth surface.*
d. *mercury content.*
e. *the mesial or distal surface of an incisor or canine tooth.*
f. *an amalgam plugger.*
g. *thermal conduction and irritation of the pulp.*
h. *hold composite fillings in place and separate them from adjacent teeth during setting.*
i. *adapt metal matrices to the tooth at the gingival margin.*

j. *polishing discs during the finishing of composite restorations.*
k. *polish composite restorations.*
l. *500,000 revolutions per minute.*
m. *silver particles to give more strength.*
n. *glass slab with a metal spatula.*

Exercise 10 / Homework

The sentences have been divided into separate halves. Match the half-sentences in column A with the half-sentences in column B to make sentences which are complete and correct.

A

1. Gingival retraction cord is soaked in . . .
2. Impressions should be soaked in . . .
3. Full tooth coverage to deciduous molar teeth is achieved using . . .
4. A bridge with retainers on just one side of the pontic is called a . . .
5. A full gold pontic providing an occlusal surface but no gingival contact is called . . .
6. Crowns made with a metallic inner surface and porcelain overlaid are . . .
7. Laboratory-made permanent posts for use in root-filled teeth when fitting a post crown are made of . . .
8. Bridges made as immediate tooth replacement following extraction are made . . .
9. Bridges cemented with composite material are called . . .
10. Finger pluggers are used in endodontics to . . .
11. A rubber dam clamp is used to . . .

12. The three types of preformed points used to fill root canals are . . .
13. Medicinal creosote is used in endodontics to . . .
14. A periapical area of bone loss appearing on a radiograph is likely to be . . .

B

a. *bonded crowns.*
b. *hold the sheet of rubber dam tightly down at the gingival margin around the tooth on which it is placed.*
c. *a periapical abscess.*
d. *disinfect the root canal for some time before root-filling.*
e. *cast precious or nonprecious metal alloys.*
f. *gutta-percha points, acrylic points, and silver points.*
g. *acid-etch bridges.*
h. *squeeze gutta-percha against the sides of the canal and ensure its width is fully obturated by creating space for accessory points.*
i. *10% sodium hypochlorite for 10 minutes to disinfect them before sending to the laboratory.*
j. *adrenaline or alum and is used to retract gingivae at cavity edges and crown/bridge preparation margins.*
k. *preformed stainless steel crowns.*
l. *a simple cantilever bridge.*
m. *a hygienic pontic.*
n. *heat-cured acrylic.*

Exercise 11/ Homework

The sentences have been divided into separate halves. Match the half-sentences in column A with the half-sentences in column B to make sentences which are complete and correct.

A

1. A root canal must be filled to its full length and width . . .
2. A tooth which is correctly root-filled but has residual periapical pathology may require . . .
3. Gutta-percha may be used during endodontic treatment to . . .
4. An anterior tooth which may require a post crown eventually must not be root-filled with . . .
5. Denture stomatitis is . . .
6. Partial dentures can be constructed of both acrylic and . . .
7. Impression paste consists of . . .
8. Titanium implants can be used in edentulous patients to . . .
9. A Willis gauge is used to . . .
10. A latch-grip pink stone is used in prosthetics to . . .
11. Candidal infection is best treated with . . .
12. An overdenture is used to . . .
13. Dentures with metal components should not be cleaned with . . .
14. Xerostomia is . . .

B

a. *acrylic and chrome-cobalt.*
b. *prevent bacterial entry and reinfection.*
c. *increase the patient's occlusal face height and relieve strain on the temporomandibular joint and masticatory muscles.*
d. *dry mouth.*

167

e. *a fungal infection beneath dentures, caused by Candida albicans.*

f. *provide support for a more retentive prosthesis to be placed, which can clip onto the implants.*

g. *record the occlusal face height of a patient.*

h. *an antifungal agent, such as nystatin or micozanole.*

i. *sodium hypochlorite.*

j. *an apicectomy.*

k. *fill the root canal, and if warmed, to test for vitality before extirpation commences.*

l. *a full–length silver point.*

m. *trim and polish chrome-cobalt dentures.*

n. *zinc oxide and eugenol modified into paste form.*

Exercise 12 / Homework

Fill in the missing words. Choose the correct ones.

| 1. Acid etchant used for composite fillings contains 33% phosphoric acid. Polyacrylic acid is used as a tooth _____ before the placement of glass ionomer _____. Both hydrogen peroxide and hydrochloric acid were used in the past for _____ procedures, but neither have a _____ in the UK now. | Licence, fillings, conditioner, tooth-bleaching, etchant | |
| 2. The dental nurse's most vital role during the _____ of a filling is adequate moisture control. | Correct, batch, placement, failure, procedure, before | |

Radiographs would be viewed _____ the procedure begins, not after the cavity has been cut. The procedure cannot be stopped before completion whether it runs over or not, as sometimes this is unavoidable. Ideally, the _____ amount of material is mixed first time to avoid waste and unnecessary expense, but another _____ can soon be mixed. However, poor moisture control will inevitably result in _____ of the restoration at some point, and then the whole _____ has to be repeated.

| 3. The following is not suitable as a lining beneath a composite filling: zinc phosphate cement. Zinc phosphate cement _____ chemically with composite materials, and this affects the _____. They should, therefore, not be placed beneath these _____. Both glass ionomer cements and calcium hydroxide cements are _____ alternatives. | suitable, reacts, restorations, setting |
| 4. A Siqveland matrix band and a holder are required for a class 2 amalgam restoration. This metal matrix band is placed _____ molar and premolar teeth with a two-surface cavity present and tightened before _____ with amalgam, which sets chemically. It cannot be used for any procedure involving _____-_____ materials as the light cannot shine through _____, and class 1 cavities do not require any | metal, light-cured, gingivally, around, filling, used |

type of matrix band to be ____. The Siqveland band could not be accurately adapted around the tooth _____ to allow a class 5 restoration to be placed.		8. Opposing arch impressions during crown preparation are usually taken in alginate. The full _____ arch has to be recorded to allow the _____ produced to be articulated into the correct biting _____. The crown can then be constructed to fit accurately into that ____. Alginate will record the arch accurately enough, without being overly _____.	bite, models, expensive, position, opposing
5. Beebee shears (_____) are required when the following procedure is being carried out: shaping temporary crowns. These shears have been specifically _____ to allow shaping of the softer types of temporary _____. Harder varieties require trimming with acrylic ____, as to denture teeth. _____ veneers are likely to be shattered by any attempt to adjust them, because they are so _____. Celluloid matrix strips can be cut with ordinary scissors, if necessary.	Porcelain, crowns, fragile, scissors, burs, designed		
		9. Bonded crowns can be cemented with all of the following: zinc phosphate cement, glass ionomer cement, polycarboxylate cement, except light-cured composite cement. The other three examples can all be mixed as luting cements as required for crown _____, whereas light-cured _____ has its own, fairly stiff, predeterminated _____. Obviously, its setting would be _____ beneath all-metallic and bonded crowns.	Impossible, composite, consistency, cementation
6. Glass ionomers should be mixed on a _____ slab with a metal spatula or waxed paper pad with a metal spatula. They should not, however, be mixed on _____ (unwaxed) paper pads as the water _____ __ during mixing and incorrect _____ result.	soaks in, quantities, ordinary, glass		
		10. A bridge which has retainers several teeth away from the pontic is called a spring cantilever bridge. Both _____-_____ and fixed-movable bridges are retained at either end of the span, whereas a _____ cantilever bridge is retained on one side of the pontic only. The _____ spring cantilever bridge is one replacing an upper anterior tooth with the retainers being _____ via a palatal bar.	connected, fixed-fixed, commonest, simple
7. The bur usually used to cut a tooth for a crown preparation is a high-speed tapered _____ bur. Slow-speed stainless steel burs will not cut _____ enamel, and crown preparations need to be parallel-sided at the most to allow their placement. Under no _____ should undercuts be produced in the preparation, or the crown will not seat ____.	circumstances, fully, through, diamond		

11. Maryland and Rochette bridges are examples of those retained by light-cured composites. These are common _____ of acid-etch retained bridges, where _____ tooth preparation is carried out and the bridge is _____ by the bond between composite and tooth. Theoretically, orthodontic adhesives work on the same _____, but they are not intended to cement _____ in place permanently.	principle, minimal, retained, brackets, examples
12. Patient should be advised to clean beneath fixed-fixed-type bridges with superfloss. Superfloss is special floss with a _____ end which can be threaded _____ the pontic so that the area can be _____ thoroughly. Food does collect beneath the pontic, even in the best-cared-for mouths. _____ develops and can cause problems _____ removed regularly.	Plaque, unless, cleaned, stiff, beneath
13. A fixed-movable-type bridge is necessary in some circumstances to allow slight _____ at the bridge joint. Bridges, by definition, are designed to be _____ in place and should not be removed by the patient for _____ or for any other reason. Under no circumstances should a bridge be _____ onto loose teeth, as the problem will only be exacerbated and other teeth may well be _____ as excess movement occurs.	cleaning, loosened, permanently, fitted, movement

14. Which of the following should be recorded on a laboratory sheet after a bridge preparation: the chosen _____ of the bridge, the patient's name, the _____ of retainers and pontics? All of this information is required by the _____ before the bridge can be constructed. Teeth acting as _____ and those missing and to be replaced by pontics may be obvious in the patient's mouth but are not necessarily so on a laboratory _____.	model, technician, notation, shade, retainers
15. A barbed broach is used in endodontics to remove the canal contents. This hand _____ is specifically designed with tiny hooks on its apical portion. These dig into the canal contents so that they are _____ ___ as the instrument is withdrawn from the canal. Files and reamers are used to smooth the canal walls and for determining the _____ length of the root, and plain _____ are used to help _____ the canal entrance, where this is not obvious.	pulled out, locate, diagnostic, broaches, instrument
16. The inhalation or _____ of endodontic instruments can be prevented by the use of parachute chains, rubber dam, floss tied around the instruments. Although the use of rubber dam is the best _____ method, because its use physically prevents any instruments _____ ____ to the pharynx, the other two examples are _____ if used correctly.	falling back, effective, preventive, swallowing

17. The successful obturation of the root canal is aided by the use of lateral condensers. Engine reamers are used in the canal _____ before root filling, and an apex locator is an electric device used to _____ determine the diagnostic length of the root without using _____. Rubber dam is a sheet of rubber material used to _____ the tooth undergoing treatment and to prevent instruments falling into the pharyngeal region and being swallowed or _____.	isolate, painlessly, inhaled, preparation, radiographs
18. The vitality of a tooth can be tested by the use of all of the following: ethyl chloride, warmed _____-_____, an electric pulp tester, except radiographs. Even teeth with obvious periapical abscesses showing on radiographs can retain their vitality and require _____ before endodontic therapy can commence. A ___-_____ tooth appears no different than a vital one on a radiograph. The other three choices all rely on nerve stimulation of the tooth which the patient can _____ to the dentist. Loss of sensation indicates _____ of vitality.	loss, report, analgesia, nonvital, gutta-percha
19. All root-filling materials must have the following properties: be radio-opaque, be biocompatible, be nondegradable, except be bactericidal. Not all teeth become nonvital and require _____ therapy because of _____ attack, so the need for	visible, endodontic, nonreactive, bacterial

antibiotic-containing materials is not always called for. However, they must all be ___-_____ to body tissues, be clearly _____ on radiographs, and be permanent.	
20. The impression material often used for denture construction is alginate. Impressions of the whole tooth-bearing areas are required for _____ construction, so the material commonly used has to be cost-effective, _____ enough to pull out of _____, and accurate enough to record the tissues with the _____ of distortion. Alginate meets all these _____.	Pliable, minimum, criteria, denture, undercuts
21. Clasps fitted to an acrylic denture are usually constructed from stainless steel. Although clasps can be constructed from _____ alloy and gold, they would be far too costly for _____ use. Chrome-cobalt clasps are an integral _____ of metal dentures and have to be cast _____ as part of the _____ plate itself.	Individually, routine, part, precious, base
22. When a denture requires relining, an impression is taken using impression paste. Relining is necessary when the ___ of the denture deteriorates, usually due to ridge _____. The inaccuracy present is usually small and can be recorded by taking an _____ of the denture-bearing area with the _____ as the tray. Only a smear of impression material is required, so one is used which does not _____ in thin section like alginate	tear, fit, denture, impression, paste, resorption

171

does. Registration _____ is used to record the patient's bite.	
23. An upper full denture is retentive due to surface tension. The surface _____ of the film of saliva lying between the denture and the hard palate is the main _____ that holds an _____ denture in place. Muscle contractions are more important for the _____ of lower dentures, and _____ should only be necessary in accurate dentures present in poor-shaped mouths. Suction pads used to be available many years ago but have since been linked with malignant _____ tumours.	Upper, palatal, adhesives, retention, tension, force
24. Common oral pathologies seen in denture wearers include all the following: hyperplasia, oral candida, mouth ulcers, except oral cancer. Oral cancer is no more _____ in denture wearers than it is in nonwearers and is fortunately rare. It can be linked to smoking and _____. Hyperplasia and ulceration are common _____ when dentures are _____ rubbing the soft tissues. Oral candida (thrush) is a commonly seen _____ infection beneath unclean dentures.	Prevalent, fungal, continually, occurrences, drinking
25. Marginal leakage occurs around restorations. This is a _____ that can occur around restorations due to _____ or poor placement _____, whereby oral _____ seep down the microscopic gaps	Phenomenon caries, fluids, technique, shrinkage

present and allow _____ to develop or allow luting cements to gradually dissolve so that crowns etc. are lost.	
26. A root filling placed from the crown end of a tooth is called orthograde. This is the conventional type of root _____ procedure, whereas a _____ root filling is carried out _____ an apicectomy procedure. Lateral condensation is the technique of fully sealing the root canal with gutta-percha and _____ during the root-filling process, and _____ is the removal of the pulp from the root canal as root canal therapy commences.	Filling, sealant, extirpation, following, retrograde
27. Irreversible pulpitis can be treated by extraction. A tooth _____ with irreversible pulpitis can only be treated by root canal _____ or extraction, as the pulp is dying or _____. A crown or an amalgam filling may be required to restore the tooth once a root filling has been placed, but neither will actually treat the initial _____. Subgingival scaling will have no effect on _____ pulpitis whatsoever.	suffering, irreversible, problem, dead, therapy

Solution to Exercise 9

1h, 2e, 3g, 4i, 5j, 6l, 7d, 8m, 9n, 10b, 11c, 12f, 13a, 14k

Solution to Exercise 10

1j, 2i, 3k, 4l, 5m, 6a, 7e, 8n, 9g, 10h, 11b, 12f, 13d, 14c

Solution to Exercise 11
1b, 2j, 3k, 4l, 5e, 6a, 7n, 8f, 9g, 10m,
11h, 12c, 13i, 14d

Vocabulary

abutment /ə'bʌt.mənt/ vyztužení, podpěra

acceptable /ək'sept.ə.bḷ/ přijatelný, vhodný

access /'æk.ses/ přístup

accurate /'æk.jʊ.rət/ pečlivý, přesný

acid /'æs.ɪd/ kyselina

acid-/'æs.ɪd/ **etch** /'etʃ/ leptat kyselinou

act /ækt/ působit

adapted /ə'dæp.tɪd/ přizpůsobený, upravený

add /æd/ přidat, přimísit

adequate /'æd.ə.kwət/ přiměřený, dostačující

adhere /əd'hɪəʳ/ držet na, lepit se na

adhesive /əd'hiː.sɪv/ lepidlo, přilnavý

adjacent /ə'dʒeɪ.sənt/ přiléhající, sousední

adjust /ə'dʒʌst/ přizpůsobit, nastavit přístroj

adjustment /ə'dʒʌst.mənt/ nastavení, přizpůsobování

admit /əd'mɪt/ přijmout, připustit

adopted /ə'dɒp.tɪd/ přijatý

adrenaline /ə'dren.əl.ɪn/ adrenalin, epinefrin

adult /'æd.ʌlt/ dospělý člověk

adversely /'æd.vɜː.sli/ příčně, nepříznivě

advised /əd'vaɪzd/ doporučený

affect /ə'fekt/ postihnout, působit

affected /ə'fek.tɪd/ ovlivněný, zasažený

agent /'eɪ.dʒᵊnt/ činitel, faktor, přísada

airtight /'eə.taɪt/ vzduchotěsný

allow /ə'laʊ/ dovolovat, poskytnout

alloy /'æl.ɔɪ/ slitina, příměs, směs

alternatively /ɒl'tɜː.nə.tɪv.li/ eventuálně, střídavě

alum /'æl.əm/ kamenec, ledek

aluminosilicate /ˌæl.jʊ'mɪn.ə'sɪl.ɪ.kət/ aluminosilikát, hlinito-křemičitan

amount /ə'maʊnt/ množství

anaesthetic /ˌæn.əs'θet.ɪk/ působící znecitlivění, anestetikum

annoying /ə'nɔɪ.ɪŋ/ nepříjemný, otravný

antifungal /ˌæn.ti'fʌŋ.gəl/ proti houbám, fungicidní

apex /'eɪ.peks/ (pl. apices) vrcholový bod, špička

apical /'eɪ.pɪ.kəl/ apikální, v okolí hrotu

apicectomy /æ.pɪ'sek.tə.mɪ/ resekce kořenového hrotu

appearance /ə'pɪə.rənts/ zevnějšek, vzhled

appliance /ə'plaɪ.ənts/ zařízení, přístroj, obklad

application /ˌæp.lɪ'keɪ.ʃən/ použití, léčebný prostředek, přiložení (obkladu)

applicator /'æp.lɪ.keɪ.təʳ/ aplikátor, štětec

applied /ə'plaɪd/ použitý, přiložený

appointment /ə'pɔɪnt.mənt/ schůzka, úmluva, jmenování

appropriate /ə'prəʊ.pri.ət/ náležitý, vhodný

approximately /ə'prɒk.sɪ.mət.li/ přibližně

arch /ɑːtʃ/ oblouk

articulated /ɑː'tɪk.jʊ.leɪ.tɪd/ kloubový, spojený

articulating /ɑː'tɪk.jʊ.leɪ.tɪŋ/ **paper** / 'peɪ.pəʳ/ artikulační papír

artificially /ˌɑː.tɪ'fɪʃ.ᵊl.i/ uměle

aspiration /ˌæs.pɪˈreɪ.ʃən/ vdech, odsávání (nečistot)

assistance /əˈsɪs.tənts/ podpora, pomoc

assume /əˈsjuːm/ předpokládat, přijmout

at /ət/ hand /hænd/ k dispozici, po ruce

atropine /æt.rəp.ɪn/ atropin

attachment /əˈtætʃ.mənt/ připojení, připevnění

attack /əˈtæk/ útok, záchvat postihnout (nemocí apod.)

attempt /əˈtempt/ pokusit se, snažit

attend /əˈtend/ navštěvovat, ošetřovat

autoclave /ˈɔː.təʊ.kleɪv/ autoklávovaný

available /əˈveɪ.lə.bļ/ dostupný, vhodný

avoid /əˈvɔɪd/ uchránit se, vyhýbat se

bag /bæg/ taška, pytel, sáček

ball-ended /bɔːl.ˈen.dɪd/ zakončený kuličkou

band /bænd/ páska, proužek

barbed /bɑːbd/ opatřený ozubcem, ostnatý

batch /bætʃ/ dávka

bearing /ˈbeə.rɪŋ/ opěrný, nosný

bedding /ˈbed.ɪŋ/ podklad, navrstvení

bee /biː/ včela, včelí

benefit /ˈben.ɪ.fɪt/ prospěch, užitek

bib /bɪb/ náprsenka, bryndáček

bin /bɪn/ koš (na odpadky), popelnice

biocompatible /ˌbaɪ.əʊ.kəmˈpæt.ɪ.bᵊl/ biokompatibilní, biologicky slučitelný

bite /baɪt/ kousat, stisková linie

biting /ˈbaɪ.tɪŋ/ kousání, kousající

bleach /bliːtʃ/ bělit, vybělit

bleaching /bliːtʃ.ɪŋ/ bělení, bělicí

bleeding /ˈbliː.dɪŋ/ krvácení

blown /bləʊn/ dry /draɪ/ vyfoukat, vysušit

bond /bɒnd/ spojovat, vazba (chemická ap.)

bond /bɒnd/ tmelit, lepit

bonding /ˈbɒnd.ɪŋ/ spojení lepidlem, vázání, slučování

border /bɔː.dəʳ/ okraj

bore /bɔːr/ vrtání, vývrt

bowl /bəʊl/ miska, kalíšek

bracket /ˈbræk.ɪt/ podpěra, spojit svorkou

breakage /ˈbreɪ.kɪdʒ/ rozbití, zlom

bridge /brɪdʒ/ můstek

broach /brəʊtʃ/ bodec, kořenová jehla, sonda, čep

brush /brʌʃ/ kartáček, vyčistit si kartáčkem

buccal /bʌk.l/ tvářový, lícní

bur /bɜːr/ vrtáček

burnisher /ˈbɜː.nɪʃ.əʳ/ leštítko, hladítko, cpátko

by /baɪ/ hand /hænd/ ručně, za ruku

calcium hydroxide /ˌkæl.si.əm. haɪˈdrɒk.saɪd/ hydroxid vápenatý

call /kɔːl/ for /fɔːr/ vyžadovat, požadovat

cantilever /ˈkæn.ti.liː.vəʳ/ bridge / brɪdʒ/ samonosný můstek

care /keəʳ/ péče, pozornost

caries /ˈkeə.riːz/ zubní kaz

cartridge /ˈkɑː.trɪdʒ/ kazeta, náplň, zásobník

carve /kɑːv/ vyřezat

carver /ˈkɑː.vəʳ/ modelovací nůž, kráječ, rydlo

case /keɪs/ případ

cast /kɑːst/ odlít, odlitek

celluloid /ˈsel.jʊ.lɔɪd/ strip /strɪp/ celuloidová páska

cervical /səˈvaɪ.kəl/ cervikální, krčkový

chain /tʃeɪn/ řetízek

chairside /tʃeəʳ.saɪd/ vedle křesla

chamber /ˈtʃeɪm.bəʳ/ vyhloubit

chart /tʃɑːt/ sestavovat diagramy

choice /tʃɔɪs/ volba, výběr, sortiment

choke /tʃəʊk/ dusit se

choose /tʃuːz/ vybrat si

circumstance /ˈsɜːʔ.kəm.stɑːnts/ okolnost

clamp /klæmp/ upnout, výztuha, svorka

clasp /klɑːsp/ háček, opatřit sponou

cleanser /ˈklen.zəʳ/ čisticí prostředek

clear /klɪəʳ/ **off** /ɒf/ očistit, vyprázdnit

clip /klɪp/ sepnout (spínátkem), štípat

clot /klɒt/ sraženina

coated /ˈkəʊ.tɪd/ pokrytý, potažený

cold-cure /ˈkəʊld.kjʊəʳ/ tuhnout za studena

collect /kəˈlekt/ hromadit se

common /ˈkɒm.ən/ běžný, obvyklý, společný

complete /kəmˈpliːt/ doplnit, dokončit

completion /kəmˈpliː.ʃən/ dokončení, dohotovení

concentration /ˌkɒnt.sənˈtreɪ.ʃʰn/ hustota, koncentrace

condenser /kənˈden.səʳ/ chladič

conditioner /kənˈdɪʃ.ʰn.ʰr/ kondicionér

conduction /kənˈdʌk.ʃən/ vodivost, přenos

connected /kəˈnek.tɪd/ připojený, spojený

conservation /ˌkɒnt.səˈveɪ.ʃʰn/ ochrana, zachování

consistency /kənˈsɪs.tʰnt.si/ soudržnost, tuhost

constituent /kənˈstɪt.ju.ənt/ prvek (složka, člen, součást)

construct /kənˈstrʌkt/ vybudovat

content /ˈkɒn.tent/ obsah, objem

continually /kənˈtɪn.ju.ə.li/ nepřetržitě, ustavičně

contraction /kənˈtræk.ʃən/ stažení, kontrakce

convenience /kənˈviː.ni.ənts/ výhoda, vhodnost, příležitost (vhodná)

conventional /kənˈvent.ʃən.əl/ konvenční, tradiční

cooled /kuːld/ chlazený, zchlazený

copious /ˈkəʊ.pi.əs/ hojný, bohatý

cord /kɔːd/ šňůra, lanko

core /kɔːʳ/ nitro, střed

corner /ˈkɔː.nəʳ/ roh, kout, úhel

correctly /kəˈrekt.li/ správně, přesně

cost /kɒst/ **-effective** /ɪˈfek.tɪv/ cenově přístupný

costly /ˈkɒst.li/ nákladný, drahý

cotton /ˈkɒt.ʰn/ **wool** /wʊl/ vata

course /kɔːs/ průběh, postup

cover /ˈkʌv.əʳ/ pokrýt, kryt

coverage /ˈkʌv.ʰr.ɪdʒ/ pokrytí, rozsah, šíře záběru

covering /ˈkʌv.ʰr.ɪŋ/ překrytí, obložení

cream /kriːm/ pasta

creosote /ˈkriː.ə.səʊt/ kreozot (chem.)

crevice /ˈkrev.ɪs/ štěrbina, trhlina (úzká)

crevicular /ˈkreˈv.ɪ.kjʊ.ləʳ/ štěrbinový

criterion /kraɪˈtɪə.ri.ən/ **(pl. criteria)** měřítka

crown /kraʊn/ korunka (zubu)

cure /kjʊəʳ/ vyléčit se, léčba, kúra (léčebná)

cure /kjʊəʳ/ vytvrdit

curing /kjʊəʳ.ɪŋ/ **lamp** /læmp/ polymerační lampa

dead /ded/ odumřelý

deal /dɪəl/ část, hodně

death /deθ/ zánik

debridement /dɪˈbriːd.mənt/ excise kavity, odstranění nekrotické tkáně

debris /ˈdeb.riː/, /ˈdeɪ.briː/ zbytky, nečistota

deciduous /dɪˈsɪd.ju.əs/ **teeth** /tiːθ/ dočasný, mléčný chrup

decision /dɪˈsɪʒ.ən/ rozhodnutí, nález

deep /diːp/ hluboký

degradable /dɪˈgreɪ.də.bl̩/ rozložitelný, odbouratelný

dentures /ˈden.tʃəz/ zubní protéza

depend /dɪˈpend/ záviset, záležet na

depth /depθ/ hloubka

deteriorate /dɪˈtɪə.ri.ə.reɪt/ kazit se, chátrat, zhoršit

determine /dɪˈtɜː.mɪn/ určit, stanovit

develop /dɪˈvel.əp/ vyvinout se, projevit

device /dɪˈvaɪs/ zařízení, záměr

diamond /ˈdaɪə.mənd/ bur /bɜːˀr/ diamantový brousek

diamond /ˈdaɪə.mənd/ diamant

dig /dɪg/ vrtat, dloubat

disc /dɪsk/ kotouč

discard /dɪˈskɑːd/ vyřadit

disinfect /ˌdɪs.ɪnˈfekt/ dezinfikovat

disorder /dɪˈsɔː.dəʳ/ porucha (zdraví)

dispense /dɪˈspents/ rozdělit, připravovat léky

disposable /dɪˈspəʊ.zə.bl̩/ k jednou použití (pouze)

dispose /dɪˈspəʊz/ of /əv/ naložit s, zbavit se

dissatisfaction /dɪsˌsæt.ɪsˈfæk.ʃən/ nespokojenost

dissolve /dɪˈzɒlv/ rozpustit, odstranit

distortion /dɪˈstɔː.ʃən/ zkřivení, zkroucení

docket /ˈdɒk.ɪt/ stvrzenka, nálepka

dressing /ˈdres.ɪŋ/ obvaz

dried /draɪd/ vysušený, zaschlý

drill /drɪl/ vrták, vrtačka

dry /draɪ/ out /aʊt/ vysušit

dual /ˈdjuː.əl/ dvojitý, obousměrný

duct /dʌkt/ kanálek, trubice

dying /ˈdaɪ.ɪŋ/ hynoucí

edentulous /əˈden.tju.ləs/ bezzubý

edge /edʒ/ okraj, hrot

effective /ɪˈfek.tɪv/ účinný (vysoce)

efficiently /ɪˈfɪʃ.ənt.li/ efektivně

either /ˈaɪ.ðəʳ/ or /ɔːʳ/ buď, jeden nebo druhý

ejector /ɪˈdʒek.təʳ/ ejektor, sací pumpa

employed /ɪmˈplɔɪd/ použitý

enable /ɪˈneɪ.bl̩/ umožňovat, uzpůsobit

engine /ˈen.dʒɪn/ stroj

enough /ɪˈnʌf/ dostatečně

ensure /ɪnˈʃɔːʳ/ zabezpečit, zajistit

entrance /ˈen.trənts/ přístup

entry /ˈen.tri/ vstup, záznam, údaj

equipment /ɪˈkwɪp.mənt/ vybavení, zařízení

escort /ɪˈskɔːt/ doprovodit

essential /ɪˈsen.tʃəl/ nezbytný, podstatný

etch /etʃ/ leptat

etchant /etʃ.ənt/ leptadlo

exacerbate /ɪgˈzæs.ə.beɪt/ zhoršit, přitížit

except /ɪkˈsept/ kromě, vyjmout

excess /ekˈses/ nadbytek, nadměrný

expand /ɪkˈspænd/ rozšířit se, zvětšit

expense /ɪkˈspents/ výdaje, náklady

expose /ɪkˈspəʊz/ odkrýt, uvolnit

extirpation /ˌek.stɜːˈpeɪ.ʃən/ extirpace, totální vynětí nervového cévního svazku

extreme /ɪkˈstriːm/ mimořádný

fall /fɔːl/ back /bæk/ ustoupit, stáhnout se (zpět)

fast /fɑːst/ rychlý

file /faɪl/ pilníček

filler /ˈfɪl.əʳ/ náplň, vložka, plnič

filling /ˈfɪl.ɪŋ/ výplň, plnění

final /ˈfaɪ.nəl/ konečný, finální

fine /faɪn/ jemný

firmly /ˈfɜːm.li/ pevně

fit /fɪt/ vhodný, upravit

fitting /ˈfɪt.ɪŋ/ úprava, instalace, příhodný

flame /fleɪm/ plamen

flange /flændʒ/ výčnělek, křídlo

floor /flɔːʳ/ dno

floss /flɒs/ hedvábná voskovaná nit

follow /ˈfɒl.əʊ/ následovat

force /fɔːs/ síla

forceps /ˈfɔː.seps/ lékařské kleště, pinzeta

former /ˈfɔː.məʳ/ tvarovač

fortunately /ˈfɔː.tʃ°n.ət.li/ naštěstí

fragile /ˈfrædʒ.aɪl/ křehký

frame /freɪm/ rámeček

free /friː/ zbavený, volný

fresh /freʃ/ čerstvý

friction /ˈfrɪk.ʃ°n/ tření

full /fʊl/ plný

functional /ˈfʌŋk.ʃ°n.°l/ funkční, fungující

fungal /ˈfʌŋ.gəl/ houbový, plísňový

further /ˈfɜː.ðəʳ/ další, vzdálenější

gain /geɪn/ získat

gap /gæp/ trhlina

gauge /geɪdʒ/ standardní míra, zkušební přístroj

gauze /gɔːz/ gáza, mul

glass /glɑːs/ sklo, sklenice

glasses /glɑːs.ɪz/ brýle

grind /graɪnd/ skřípat

grip /grɪp/ uchopit, upínadlo

groove /gruːv/ rýha

guard /gɑːd/ ochrana

guide /gaɪd/ šablona, příručka

habit /ˈhæb.ɪt/ zvyk

hand /hænd/ předat, podat

handle /ˈhæn.dl̩/ ovládat

handpiece /ˈhænd.piːs/ držadlo, násadec

hard /hɑːd/ palate /ˈpæl.ət/ tvrdé patro

healing /ˈhiː.lɪŋ/ hojení, léčivý

heat /hiːt/ způsobený teplem

heater /ˈhiː.təʳ/ zahřívač (přístroj)

height /haɪt/ výška, úroveň

held /held/ držený

high-speed /ˌhaɪˈspiːd/ vysokorychlostní

holder /ˈhəʊl.dəʳ/ držadlo

holding /ˈhəʊl.dɪŋ/ držení

hole /həʊl/ dírka

hook /hʊk/ háček

however /ˌhaʊˈev.əʳ/ avšak

hydrochloric acid /ˌhaɪd.rə.klɒr.ɪkˈæs.ɪd/ kyselina chlorovodíková

hydrogen /ˈhaɪ.drɪ.dʒən/ peroxide /pəˈrɒk.saɪd/ peroxid vodíku

hygienic /haɪˈdʒiː.nɪk/ hygienický

hyperplasia /ˌhaɪ.pəˈpleɪ.zɪ.ə/ hyperplazie, zbytnění

iatrogenic /aɪˌætrəˈdʒen.ɪk/ iatrogenní

immediate /ɪˈmiː.di.ət/ okamžitý

immerse /ɪˈmɜːs/ ponořit

implant /ɪmˈplɑːnt/ implantát

impression /ɪmˈpreʃ.°n/ otisk

in /ɪn/ addition /əˈdɪʃ.°n/ vedle (navíc)

in situ /ˌɪnˈsɪt.juː/ na původním místě

inaccuracy /ɪnˈæk.jʊ.rə.si/ nepřesnost, chyba

inaccurate /ɪˈnæk.jʊ.rət/ nesprávný, nepřesný

inadvertently /ˌɪn.ədˈvɜː.t°nt.li/ nedopatřením

incisal /ɪnˈsɪ.z°l/ edge /edʒ/ řezáková hrana

incisor /ɪnˈsaɪ.zəʳ/ řezák

incorrect /ˌɪn.kərˈ°kt/ nesprávný, nevhodný

indicate /ˈɪn.dɪ.keɪt/ indikovat, označit, ukazovat, signalizovat

indicator /ˈɪn.dɪ.keɪ.təʳ/ ukazatel

inevitably /ɪˈnev.ɪ.tə.bli/ nevyhnutelně

inhalation /ˌɪn.həˈleɪ.ʃ°n/ vdechování

initial /ɪˈnɪʃ.°l/ původní, výchozí

inner /ˈɪn.əʳ/ vnitřní

insertion /ɪnˈsɜː.ʃ°n/ zasazení, aplikace (vložka)

instrument /ˈɪn.strə.mənt/ nástroj

integral /ˈɪn.tɪ.grəl/ nedílný

intended /ɪnˈten.dɪd/ zamýšlený, plánovaný

interproximal /ˌɪn.təˈprɒk.sɪ.m°l/ aproximální, styčný

interrupt /ˌɪn.təˈrʌpt/ přerušit

involve /ɪnˈvɒlv/ obsahovat

involvement /ɪnˈvɒlv.mənt/ zapojení, postižení, komplikace

irreversible /ˌɪr.ɪˈvɜː.sɪ.bļ/ nezvratný

irrigation /ˌɪr.ɪˈgeɪ.ʃ°n/ zavlažování, výplach

irritant /ˈɪr.ɪ.tənt/ dráždivý

isolate /ˈaɪ.sə.leɪt/ odloučit, izilovat

item /ˈaɪ.təm/ položka, jednotlivost

joint /dʒɔɪnt/ kloub, spojení

keen /kiːn/ nadšený

keep /kiːp/ ponechat, udržovat

knock /nɒk/ uhodit

latch /lætʃ/ západka, zaklapnout

lateral /ˈlæt.r°l/ postranní, příčný

lay /leɪ/ out /aʊt/ vyložit, dimenzovat

leakage /ˈliː.kɪdʒ/ unikání, propouštění

length /leŋk θ/ délka, trvání

licence /ˈlaɪ.s°nts/ oprávnění, povolení

light /laɪt/ světlo - cured /kjʊəʳ.d/ světlem tuhnoucí

light /laɪt/ světlý

likely /ˈlaɪ.kli/ pravděpodobně

lined /laɪnd/ vyztužený, obložený

lined /laɪnd/ with /wɪð/ lemovaný

lining /ˈlaɪ.nɪŋ/ vložka, výplněk

linked /lɪŋkt/ to /tʊ/ spojený s

liquid /ˈlɪk.wɪd/ tekutina, kapalný

load /ləʊd/ náplň, zatížit, plnit

local /ˈləʊ.kəl/ místní

locate /ləʊ ˈkeɪt/ zjistit polohu (místo), vyhledat

locator /ləʊ ˈkeɪ.təʳ/ vyhledávač, lokátor

lock /lɒk/ zámek, zavřít

locking /lɒk.ɪŋ/ uzavírání, blokování

loose /luːs/ uvolněný

loose-fitting /ˌluːsˈfɪt.ɪŋ/ volný

loosen /ˈluː.s°n/ rozviklat, povolit

loss /lɒs/ ztráta, úbytek

luting /luːt.ɪŋ/ utěsňování

main /meɪn/ hlavní, silný

majority /məˈdʒɒr.ə.ti/ většina

malignant /məˈlɪg.nənt/ zhoubný, škodlivý

mandrel /ˈmæn.drəl/ vřeteno, trn, jádro

margin /ˈmɑː.dʒɪn/ pokraj, lem

marginal /ˈmɑː.dʒɪ.nəl/ okrajový

mastication /ˌmæs.tɪˈkeɪ.ʃ°n/ žvýkání, mastikace

matched /mætʃt/ vyrovnaný, sesazený

matrix /ˈmeɪ.trɪks/ matrice, forma

matrix /ˈmeɪ.trɪks/ band /bænd/ matriční páska

meantime /ˈmiːn.taɪm/ mezitím

metal /ˈmet.°l/ kov, kovový, vylít kovem

minutely /maɪˈnjuːt.li/ nepatrně

mirror /ˈmɪr.əʳ/ zrcátko, odrážet se

mixture /ˈmɪks.tʃəʳ/ směs, příměs

modify /ˈmɒd.ɪ.faɪ/ upravit, přizpůsobit

moist /mɔɪst/ vlhký, mokrý

moisture /ˈmɔɪs.tʃ°r/ vlhkost

mould /məʊld/ tvar, modelovat, formovat

mouthful /ˈmaʊθ.fʊl/ plná ústa

mouthwash /ˈmaʊθ.wɒʃ/ ústní voda, kloktadlo

nappy /ˈnæp.i/ plenka

necessitate /nəˈses.ɪ.teɪt/ nutně vyžadovat

178

needle /ˈniː.dl̩/ jehla, vpichovat, očkovat

neither /ˈnaɪ.ðəʳ/ aniž (a také ne), žádný (z obou)

nonstaining /nɒn.ˈsteɪn.ɪŋ/ nešpinící

nonvital /nɒn.ˈvaɪ.tᵊl/ devitalizovaný

non-/nɒn-/ ne (záporná předpona)

notation /nəʊ ˈteɪ.ʃᵊn/ záznam, označovací soustava

note /nəʊt/ poznámka

nozzle /ˈnɒz.l̩/ tryska, hubička, licí koncovka

obdurate /ˈɒb.djʊ.rət/ zacpat, utěsnit

obscure /əbˈskjʊər/ zakrýt, zastírat

obturation /ˌɒb.tjʊ.əˈreɪ.ʃᵊn/ utěsnění, uzavření

obviously /ˈɒb.vi.ə.sli/ zřejmě, evidentně

occlusion /əˈkluː.ʒᵊn/ skus, okluze, zátvor

occur /əˈkɜːʳ/ vyskytovat se, nastat, napadnout (přijít na mysl)

occurrence /əˈkʌr.ᵊnts/ výskyt, případ, událost

once /wʌnts/ jednou, jakmile jednou, svého času

operate /ˈɒp.ᵊr.eɪt/ řídit, fungovat, obsluhovat (stroj ap.), působit (o léku ap.)

opposing /əˈpəʊ.zɪŋ/ protichůdný, čelící

order /ˈɔː.dəʳ/ pořadí, postup, objednávka

ordinary /ˈɔː.dɪ.nə.ri/ obyčejný, obvyklý, běžný

orthograde /ɔːˈθəʊ.greɪd/ ortográdní

otherwise /ˈʌð.ə.waɪz/ jinak, nebo, z jiného hlediska

over /ˈəʊ.vəʳ/ přes, nad, u konce, pokrytí celku

overlay /ˌəʊ.vəˈleɪ/ překrýt (vrstvou)

overly /ˈəʊ.vᵊl.i/ moc, příliš

overnight /ˌəʊ.vəˈnaɪt/ přes noc (též přen.)

overspill /ˈəʊ.və.spɪl/ přelití, přebytek

pack /pæk/ balíček, balit

package /ˈpæk.ɪdʒ/ balení, zabalit

pad /pæd/ podložit (vatou), těsnit, blok (na psaní), polštář

pain /peɪn/ bolest, trápit

painlessly /ˈpeɪn.lə.sli/ bezbolestně

palatal /ˈpæ.lə.tl̩/ bar /bɑːʳ/ patrový třmen

paper /ˈpeɪ.pəʳ/ point /pɔɪnt/ papírový čípek

parachlorphenol /pær.əˌklɒrˈfiː.nɒl/ parachlorfenol

parachute /ˈpær.ə.ʃuːt/ padákový

parotid /pəˈrɒt.ɪd/ gland /glænd/ příušní žláza

particle /ˈpɑː.tɪ.kl̩/ částečka

pass /pɑːs/ podat, projít

past /pɑːst/ poslední, minulý, za, přes

paste /peɪst/ pasta, lepidlo, přilepit

pathology /pəˈθɒl.ə.dʒi/ patologie

perform /pəˈfɔːm/ provést

perform /pəˈfɔːm/ vykonat, fungovat, předvést

permanent /ˈpɜː.mə.nənt/ stálý, trvalý, nepřetržitý

pharynx /ˈfær.ɪŋks/ hltan

phenomenon /fəˈnɒm.ɪ.nən/ fenomén (úkaz, jev, div), vlastnost

phosphoric /fɒsˈfɒr.ɪk/ acid /ˈæs.ɪd/ kyselina fosforečná

piece /piːs/ kus

pierce /pɪəs/ probodnout, prorazit

pin /pɪn/ kolík, čípek, špendlík, svorka, připevnit, přišpendlit

pink /pɪŋk/ růžový

placement /ˈpleɪs.mənt/ umístění, uspořádání

plain /pleɪn/ rovina, jednoduchý, jasný (zřetelný)

plate /pleɪt/ plát (deska), patro (umělého chrupu)

pledget /pledʒ.ɪt/ tampon z vaty

pliable /ˈplaɪ.ə.bl̩/ ohebný, pružný, plastický

plugger /plʌg.əʳ/ cpátko

point /pɔɪnt/ bod, hrot

poke /pəʊk/ strkat, dloubnout, rýpat

polish /ˈpɒl.ɪʃ/ leštit

polyacrylic /ˈpɒl.i.əˈkrɪl.ɪk/ acid /ˈæs.ɪd/ kyselina polyakrylová

polycarboxylate /pɒl.i.kɑːˈbɒk.sɪl.eɪt/ polykarboxylát

pontic /ˌpɒnt.ɪk/ umělý zub umístěný na můstku

pooling /puː.lɪŋ/ sdílení, shromažďující

poor /pɔːʳ/ špatný, slabý

porcelain /ˈpɔː.səl.ɪn/ porcelán (jemný)

portion /ˈpɔː.ʃən/ část, podíl

position /pəˈzɪʃ.ən/ postavení (poloha)

post /pəʊst/ stojan, sloupek, podpěra

post /pəʊst/ crown /kraʊn/ čepová korunka

powder /ˈpaʊ.dər/ prášek, rozemlít

precious /ˈpreʃ.əs/ drahý, vzácný

prefabricated /ˌpriːˈfæb.rɪ.keɪ.tɪd/ stavebnicový, předmontovaný

premature /ˈprem.ə.tʃəʳ/ předčasný, raný

preparation /ˌprep.ərˈeɪ.ʃən/ příprava, preparace

present /ˈprez.ənt/ přítomný, nabídnout

prevalent /ˈprev.əl.ənt/ obvyklý, převládající

prevent /prɪˈvent/ předejít, zabránit

principle /ˈprɪnt.sɪ.pl̩/ základní pravidlo

probe /prəʊb/ zubařská sonda, zkoumat sondou

procedure /prəˈsiː.dʒəʳ/ procedura (postup)

promote /prəˈməʊt/ napomáhat, podporovat

proprietary /prəˈpraɪə.tri/ patentovaný

prosthesis /ˈprɒs.θiː.sɪs/ (pl. prostheses) protetika, protéza

protective /prəˈtek.tɪv/ ochranný, bezpečnostní

provision /prəˈvɪʒ.ən/ zajištění (zabezpečení)

pull /pʊl/ out /aʊt/ vytáhnout

pulpitis /pʌlˈaɪ.tɪs/ zánět dřeně

punch /pʌntʃ/ úder, propíchnout

quantity /ˈkwɒn.tɪ.ti/ množství

radio-opaque /ˈreɪ.di.əʊ.əʊˈpeɪk/ nepropustný pro záření

rapidly /ˈræp.ɪd.li/ rychle

rare /reəʳ/ vzácný

rarely /ˈreə.li/ zřídka

realise /ˈrɪə.laɪz/ uvědomit si, chápat

reamer /ˈriː.məʳ/ výstružník, rozšiřovač

reason /ˈriː.zən/ důvod

receive /rɪˈsiːv/ dostat

record /rɪˈkɔːd/ zaznamenat

recover /rɪˈkʌv.ər/ objevit

registration /ˌredʒ.ɪˈstreɪ.ʃən/ zápis, zaznamenávání

regularly /ˈreg.jʊ.lə.li/ pravidelně

reinforce /ˌriː.ɪnˈfɔːs/ zesílit, vyztužit

relieve /rɪˈliːv/ ulevit, zmírnit

reline /riːˈlaɪn/ obložit, vyměnit obložení

rely /rɪˈlaɪ/ on /ɒn/ spoléhat

remain /rɪˈmeɪn/ zbývat, zůstat, vytrvat

remaining /rɪˈmeɪ.nɪŋ/ zbývající, zůstávající

removal /rɪˈmuː.vəl/ vyjmutí, odstranění, přesun

repeated /rɪˈpiː.tɪd/ opakovaný, častý

replacement /rɪˈpleɪs.mənt/
nahrazování, náhrada (vadné
součásti)

report /rɪˈpɔːt/ hlásit, podat zprávu,
udělat zápis

require /rɪˈkwaɪəʳ/ nutně potřebovat,
požádat

residual /rɪˈzɪd.ju.əl/ zbývající, zbytek

resin /ˈrez.ɪn/ pryskyřice

resist /rɪˈzɪst/ odolávat, vydržet

resorption /rɪˈsɔːp.ʃən/ rozpuštění

restorative /rɪˈstɒr.ə.tɪv/ obnovující

restore /rɪˈstɔːʳ/ obnovit,
rekonstruovat

retainer /rɪˈteɪ.nəʳ/ úchytka

retention /rɪˈten.tʃən/ zadržení,
nahromadění

retentive /rɪˈten.tɪv/ zadržující,
retenční

retract /rɪˈtrækt/ odtáhnout

retraction /rɪˈtræk.ʃən/ stahování,
smršťování

retrograde /ˈret.rəʊ.greɪd/
odvrácený, zpětný

retry /ˌriːˈtraɪ/ nový pokus, zkoušet
znova

reuse /ˌriːˈjuːz/ znovu použít,
opakované použití

revolution /ˌrev.əˈluː.ʃən/ otáčka

ridge /rɪdʒ/ vyvýšenina, okraj

rim /rɪm/ lem, hrana, okraj, obroučka

rinse /rɪnts/ vypláchnout, proprat

roll /rəʊl/ svitek

root /ruːt/ **face** /feɪs/ kořenová fréza

rose /rəʊz/ -**head** /hed/ **bur** /bɜːr/
vrtáček ve tvaru špičatého poupěte

rose /rəʊz/ růže

round /raʊnd/ **bur** /bɜːr/ kulatý
vrtáček

rub /rʌb/ dřít, drhnout

rubber /ˈrʌb.əʳ/ **dam** /dæm/ gumová
blána

safety /ˈseɪf.ti/ bezpečnostní

salt /sɒlt/ - **water** /ˈwɔː.təʳ/ slaná voda

satisfied /ˈsæt.ɪs.faɪd/ spokojený

save /seɪv/ zachránit

scale /skeɪl/ odstranit zubní kámen

scenario /sɪˈnɑː.ri.əʊ/ scénář, postup

scissors /ˈsɪz.əz/ nůžky, kleštičky

scrub /skrʌb/ vydrhnout

seal /siːl/ uzavřít těsně, zaplombovat,
utěsnění

sealed /siːld/ utěsněný, hermeticky
uzavřený, zaplombovaný

seat /siːt/ usadit, sedadlo

seep /siːp/ prosakovat

selection /sɪˈlek.ʃən/ výběr, volba

self-/self/ sebe-, sobě

self-/self/ **limiting**/ˈlɪm.ɪ.tɪŋ/
spontánně mizející

sensation /senˈseɪ.ʃən/ smyslové
vnímání

sensitive /ˈsent.sɪ.tɪv/ citlivý (na něco)

separate /ˈsep.ər.ət/ oddělit, odtrhnout

set /set/ **out** /aʊt/ stanovit, vytyčovat

set /set/ vsadit, zasadit, sestavit, upravit

setting /ˈset.ɪŋ/ tuhnutí, nasazení,
seřízení

severe /sɪˈvɪəʳ/ těžký, vážný, prudký
(bolest ap.)

shade /ʃeɪd/ odstín

shape /ʃeɪp/ formovat, tvarovat

shaped /ʃeɪpt/ tvarovaný, zformovaný

sharp /ʃɑːp/ ostrý předmět

shattered /ˈʃæt.əd/ zničený, rozpadlý,
rozdrcený

shears /ʃɪəz/ kleště, nůžky (velké)

sheet /ʃiːt/ arch, tenká deska, výkaz

shield /ʃiːld/ ochrana (přen.), ochranný
štít

shine /ʃaɪn/ zářit, lesknout se

shrink /ʃrɪŋk/ srážet se, smršťovat

shrinkage /ˈʃrɪŋ.kɪdʒ/ ztráta na
objemu

side /saɪd/ strana, vedlejší

sideways /'saɪd.weɪz/ stranou

simple /'sɪm.pl̩/ prostý, jednoduchý

sink /sɪŋk/ dřez

site /saɪt/ místo, být umístěn

size /saɪz/ velikost

slab /slæb/ destička

slight /slaɪt/ tenký, lehký

slip /slɪp/ prokluzovat

slow-speed /sləʊ.spiːd/ pomalý

smear /smɪəʳ/ skvrna, šmouha, namazet

smile /smaɪl/ usmívat se

smooth /smuːð/ hladký

soak /səʊk/ up /ʌp/ nasakovat, vstřebat

soaked /səʊkt/ prosáknutý

socket /'sɒk.ɪt/ zubní lůžko

sodium /'səʊ.di.əm/ hypochlorite / haɪ.pəʊ'klɔː.raɪt/ chlornan sodný

soften /'sɒf.ᵊn/ změkčit, sejmout

solution /sə'luː.ʃən/ roztok, řešení

space /speɪs/ volný prostor, mezera

span /spæn/ šíře, rozpětí, oblouk

spatula /'spæt.jʊ.lə/ lopatička

spit /spɪt/ out /aʊt/ vyplivnout

spoon /spuːn/ lžíce, lopatka

spot /spɒt/ tečka, skvrna, kapka

spray /spreɪ/ rozprašovat

spring /sprɪŋ/ tryskat, pramen

squeeze /skwiːz/ protlačit, mačkat

stage /steɪdʒ/ etapa (období)

stainless steel /ˌsteɪn.ləs'stiːl/ nerezavějící ocel

standard /'stæn.dəd/ norma, pravidlo (určitý poměr)

stiff /stɪf/ tuhý

stimulation /ˌstɪm.jʊ'leɪ.ʃᵊn/ podráždění (svalů, nervů)

stone /stəʊn/ kámen

straight /streɪt/ přímo, přímý, rovný

strain /streɪn/ napětí, napnout

strip /strɪp/ proužek, plátek

suction /'sʌk.ʃᵊn/ odsávání, nasávání (vzduchu)

suffer /'sʌf.əʳ/ trpět, utrpět, být poškozen

suitable /'sjuː.tə.bl̩/ vhodný, přiměřený

sulcus /sʌl.kəs/ (pl: sulci) rýha, sulkus

super /'suː.pəʳ/ extra, výborný

supine /'suː.paɪn/ ležící tváří vzhůru

support /sə'pɔːt/ podpora, podpírat

surface /'sɜː.fɪs/ povrch (též přen.), opracovat povrch

surgery /'sɜː.dʒər.i/ ordinace, operace

surgical /'sɜː.dʒɪ.kᵊl/ chirurgický, pooperační

surrounding /sə'raʊn.dɪŋ/ obklopující, sousední (tkáň)

swallow /'swɒl.əʊ/ polykat

syringe /sɪ'rɪndʒ/ stříkačka

talk /tɔːk/ hovor, mluvit

tapered /'teɪ.pəʳ/ zužující se, zahrocený, kuželový

tear /teəʳ/ roztrhnout se, trhlina

temporary /'tem.pᵊr.ᵊr.i/ dočasný, prozatímní

tend /tend/ to /tʊ/ mít sklon, inklinovat

tension /'tenʃ.ʃᵊn/ napínání (tahem)

theoretically /θɪə'ret.ɪ.kli/ teoreticky

therefore /'ðeə.fɔːʳ/ z toho důvodu

thin /θɪn/ tenký, řídký

thorough /'θʌr.ə/ dokonalý, úplný

thoroughly /'θʌr.ə.li/ řádně, důkladně

threaded /θred.ɪd/ navlečený, niťový, se závitem

throughout /θruː'aʊt/ úplně (veskrze), všude v

tidy /'taɪ.di/ uklidit

tie /taɪ/ svázat

tighten /'taɪ.tᵊn/ utažený, napjatý

tiny /'taɪ.ni/ tenounký (nepatrný)

tip /tɪp/ špička

tissue /ˈtɪʃ.uː/ papírový kapesník, tkáň

topical /ˈtɒp.ɪ.kᵊl/ místní

trace /treɪs/ stopa

trauma /ˈtrɔː.mə/ trauma, úraz

tray /treɪ/ tác, miska, otiskovací lžíce

trial /ˈtraɪəl/ zkouška, pokus

trim /trɪm/ úprava, oříznout

trimming /ˈtrɪm.ɪŋ/ upravování

triple /ˈtrɪp.l̩/ trojitý

try /traɪ/ zkouška

tumour /ˈtjuː.məʳ/ otok, tumor

turbine /ˈtɜː.baɪn/ turbína

ulcer /ˈʌl.səʳ/ vřed, nádor

unavoidable /ˌʌn.əˈvɔɪ.də.bl̩/ nevyhnutelný

uncomfortable /ʌnˈkʌmp f.tə.bl̩/ nepříjemný, nepohodlný

undercut /ˌʌn.dəˈkʌt̩/ podříznout, zářez

undergo /ˌʌn.dəˈgəʊ/ podstoupit

unless /ənˈles/ pokud ne

unnecessary /ʌnˈnes.ə.ser.i/ zbytečný (nepodstatný)

unstable /ʌnˈsteɪ.bl̩/ nepevný, pohyblivý

unused /ʌnˈjuːzd/ nepoužitý

varnish /ˈvɑː.nɪʃ/ lak, nalakovat

veneer /vəˈnɪəʳ/ tenká vrstva, nátěr, obložení

view /vjuː/ pohled, dívat se

wash /wɒʃ/ mýt, promýt, prát

waste /weɪst/ odpad

wax /wæks/ vosk

waxed /wækst/ voskovaný

weak /wiːk/ slabý, křehký

wearer /ˈweə.rəʳ/ nositel

wedge /wedʒ/ klín, vtlačit, zaklínit

well /wel/ správně (dobře)

wet /wet/ namočit (navlhčit)

whatsoever /ˌwɒt.səʊˈev.əʳ/ vůbec

whereas /weəˈræz/ kdežto (zatímco naopak)

whereby /weəˈbaɪ/ čímž (pomocí něhož)

whether /ˈweð.əʳ/ jestli

whichever /wɪˈtʃev.əʳ/ kterýkoli (z určitého počtu)

whole /həʊl/ celý, celistvý

wide /waɪd/ široký

width /wɪtθ/ šíře, vůle

wipe /waɪp/ utřít

withdrawn /wɪðˈdrɔːn/ stáhnutý

withstand /wɪðˈstænd/ odolávat, snést

wooden /ˈwʊd.ᵊn/ dřevěný

xerostomia /ˈzɪə.rəˈstəʊ.mɪə/ xerostomie, suchost úst

zinc /zɪŋk/ oxide/ oxide /ˈɒk.saɪd/ zinková běloba

zinc /zɪŋk/ phosphate /ˈfɒs.feɪt/ fosforečnan zinečnatý

Unit 13

Operative Dentistry

Diagnosis of Pulpal Pain. Treatment Planning. Management of the Deep Carious Lesion. Principles of Cavity Preparation. Plastic Restorations. Crowns. Veneers. Inlays and Onlays. Fixed Bridges. Fixed-Movable Bridges. Adhesive Bridges. Tooth Wear. Bleaching and Microabrasion. Endodontics. Surgical Endodontics. Relationship within Restorative Dentistry.

Text 1

Diagnosis of Pulpal Pain

Pain history is important—**sharpness, dullness, throbbing, duration** (short, constant), **reaction to heat**, reaction to **cold**, reaction to **pressure**, reaction to **sweet** stimuli, **site**, and **radiation**; pulpal pain is often worse at night.

Clinical examination:

visual
probing
percussion
sensibility testing
laser doppler
radiographs
transillumination
tooth 'sloth'

Treatment Planning

History taking:

patient complaints
history of treatment to teeth
general dental history
medical history
social history

Examination—extraoral, intraoral, radiographic

Diagnosis—potential categories of dentate patient:

- dental pain
- nondental pain
- caries
- tooth wear
- periodontal disease
- previous misdiagnosis
- iatrogenic problems
- routine, e.g. symptom-free patient attending for check-up
- aesthetic problem, e.g. discoloration
- occlusal problem
- functional problem, e.g. insufficient teeth to chew adequately
- traumatic problem, e.g. broken teeth following acute trauma
- management problem, e.g. dental phobic

Definite treatment includes:

- premolar and molar endodontics

- endodontic retreatment
- provision of post cores
- crown and bridgework
- removable prosthesis construction
- implants

When planning treatment in operative dentistry the dentist takes into account not just the teeth but the individual patient's total oral health and general health needs.

Occlusion

Occlusion is the relationship of cusps or masticating surfaces of maxillary and mandibular teeth.

Retruded contact position – position of the mandible when the condyles are in their most retruded position in the glenoid fossa, and there is occlusal contact of the teeth.

Intercuspal position – the position of maximum intercuspation of the teeth.

Stable occlusion – an occlusion in which overeruption, tilting, and drifting of teeth cannot cause new occlusal interferences.

Occlusal harmony – the absence of occlusal interferences which allows mandibular movement in all excursions (with the teeth together) and does not result in discomfort, strain, or harm to the teeth or masticatory apparatus.

Exercise 1
1. What can you tell about the pulpal pain?
2. Talk about the diagnosis.

3. Talk about the treatment plan and definite treatment in operative dentistry.
4. What is occlusal harmony, and which deviations do you know?

Translation 1
Diagnóza dřeňové bolesti, ostrá, tupá, tepající, stálá, místo a vyzařování reakce na teplo, chlad, tlak, na sladké, klinické vyšetření, zrakem, sondou, poklepem, testováním citlivosti, pomocí laseru, rentgenových snímků, prosvícení, anamnéza lékařská, sociální, obtíže pacienta, bolest zubů, kazy, opotřebení zubů, onemocnění parodontu, kontrola, problém estetický, okluze, funkční, traumatický, endotontická léčba, zhotovení korunek a můstků, vyjímatelných náhrad, implantátů, okluze, hroty, žvýkací povrchy, zuby horní a dolní čelisti, okluzní harmonie, pohyb dolní čelisti ve všech směrech, žádné nepohodlí, napětí, či poškození zubů ani žvýkacího aparátu.

Text 2
Management of the Deep Carious Lesion
A deep carious lesion occurs when the caries lies in close proximity to the dental pulp.

Principles of Cavity Preparation
Objectives of cavity preparation:
- removal of carious or fractured tooth tissue
- secondary prevention of caries
- minimise pulpal or periodontal damage

- cavity should be prepared such that the filling material to be used can restore function and appearance of the tooth and is retained in the tooth

Stages in cavity preparation
- outline form
- resistance form
- retention form
- management of remaining caries
- enamel margin finishing
- cavity toilet

Resistance form refers to the features of the cavity design which resist occlusal forces. **Retention form** refers to the features of the cavity design which resist displacement of the final restoration.

Black's classification of cavities

I. cavity originating in anatomical pit or fissure
II. cavity originating on mesial or distal aspect of molar/premolar teeth
III. cavity originating on mesial or distal aspect of incisors/canines not involving incisal edge
IV. cavity originating on mesial or distal aspect of incisors/canines involving incisal edge
V. cavity originating in cervical third of buccal/lingual/palatal aspects of teeth (excluding anatomical pits)

Plastic Restorations

Plastic restorations are used intracoronally. Materials include amalgam, resin composite, glass ionomer.

Crowns

A crown is a restoration which encompasses coronal tooth tissue, covering remaining tooth substance and restorations. When insufficient tooth tissue remains, the root canal can be used to aid retention—a post crown.

Assessment of teeth for crowns:
- tooth vitality
- periodontal support and gingival condition
- oral hygiene
- caries control
- occlusion
- radiographic appearance
- aesthetics
- adjacent teeth

Veneers

A veneer is essentially a facing placed on a tooth. Types of veneers:
- labial veneers
- palatal veneers
- reverse three-quarter
- dentine-bonded crowns

Clinical stages: preparation, impressions, temporisation, cementation

Inlays and Onlays

Inlays are intracoronal restorations which are manufactured in the laboratory and cemented into place. Types: gold inlays, composite inlays, porcelain inlays.

Onlays are extracoronal restorations on the occlusal surface of a tooth. Types: gold onlays, composite onlays, porcelain onlays.

Fixed Bridges

A bridge is a dental prosthesis which replaces a missing tooth or teeth and is attached permanently to one or more natural teeth (or implants). It is not removable by the patient.

Definitions:

Abutment tooth – a tooth which supports a bridge
Retainer – part of a bridge which is cemented to an abutment tooth
Pontic – each replacement tooth in a bridge
Unit – each part of a bridge, i.e. abutment or pontic, is referred to as a unit. Thus two abutments and one pontic constitutes a three-unit bridge
Pier – nonterminal abutment
Cantilever bridge – this type has a pontic connected to a retainer at one end only

Fixed-Movable Bridges

A fixed-movable bridge has a joint allowing limited movement between pontic and retainer.
Spring cantilever bridges support a pontic at some distance from the retainer. A gold bar which is in contact with palatal mucosa connects pontic to retainer.

Adhesive Bridges

Modern adhesive bridgework relies on the micromechanical bonding of composite resin or chemically active resin to etched enamel or sandblasted metal.

Exercise 2

1. Give principles of cavity preparation and name the stages in cavity preparation.
2. What does Black's classification of cavities mean?
3. What do you know about crowns and assessment of teeth for crowns?
4. Which types of veneers do you know?
5. What is meant by clinical stages in connection with veneers?
6. What are inlays and onlays?
7. Talk about fixed bridges, fixed-movable bridges, and adhesive bridges.

Translation 2

Hluboké poškození kazem, cíle preparace kavity, odstranění zubní tkáně, sekundární prevence, minimalizovat poškození, obrys, tvar zajišťující odolnost výplně, retenční tvar, ošetření zbylých kazů, dokončení okraje skloviny, toaleta kavity, klasifikace kavit, jamka, fisura, stoličky, třenové zuby, řezáky, strana lícní, jazyková, patrová, výplně, amalgám, pryskyřičný kompozit, fazetovaná korunka, zhodnocení zubu pro korunky, vitalita zubu, stav dásní, ústní hygiena, kontrola kazu, okluze, vzhled na rentgenu, estetika, sousední zuby, klinická stádia, příprava, otisky, vyčkání, přitmelení, inleje, vyrobené v laboratoři, zlaté, kompozitní, porcelánové, onleje, na okluzním povrchu zubu, pevné můstky, nahrazují chybějící zub, připojeny nastálo, pilíř, držák, umělý zub na můstku, pilířový zub, krakorcový můstek, fixní pohyblivé můstky, spojení umožňující omezený pohyb, moderní adhesivní můstky, mikro-mechanické připojení k leptané sklovině.

Text 3

Tooth Wear

Tooth wear is also known as tooth surface loss, noncarious tooth surface loss, and nonbacterial tooth surface loss.

Attrition is the loss of tooth substance by wear **due to mastication** or contact between occluding surfaces.
Aetiology of attrition:
- **bruxism** (grinding, clenching)
- lack of posterior support and **occlusal collapse**
- **salivary flow** and composition
- **tooth structure**

Abrasion is the loss of tooth substance by wear due to factors other than tooth contact.
Aetiology of abrasion:
- **aggressive oral hygiene** techniques (toothbrush, toothpaste, interdental cleaning)
- **habitual chewing** (pens/pencils, fingernails, nut shells)
- occupational chewing (electrical wire, fishing line, ironmongery, etc.)

Erosion is the progressive loss of hard dental tissues by a **chemical process not involving bacterial action.**
Aetiology of erosion:
- **acidic** diet (carbonated drinks, fruit juices, citrus fruits, pickled foods, mouthwashes)
- acid **regurgitation** (bulimia nervosa, gastrointestinal problems, chronic alcoholism, morning sickness)
- **industrial** processes (armament production, battery workers)
- **medical** problems (compulsive achievers, 'chewing the cud')
- **leisure** activities (swimming)
- **tooth structure**
- **salivary flow** and salivary composition

Management of tooth wear

In general the following basic principles apply:
- control of aetiological factors
- pain and caries control
- period of observation to determine if wear is progressing
- provisional intervention
- definitive restorations (crown restoration, definitive dentures/overdentures)
- review

Bleaching and Microabrasion

Bleaching techniques aim to whiten discoloured teeth.

Endodontics

Endodontics involves treatment of the dental pulp.
Causes of pulpal damage:
- dental caries
- trauma
- periodontal disease
- damage during operative procedures

Instrumentation

There are many instruments in use in root canal treatment.

Commonly used instruments include:

- **files** – used to widen the root canal. Files may be handheld or operated in a handpiece or ultrasonic handpiece.
- **rotary files** – used to widen the root canal, especially the coronal part.
- **broaches** – these instruments, e.g. barbed broach, are used for vital tissue removal.
- **side-cutting burs** – used for preparation of the coronal two-thirds of the root canal.
- **spiral paste fillers** – used for placing sealer or intracanal dressings into the pulp cavity.
- **spreaders and compactors** – used in root canal obturation.

Surgical Endodontics

Apicectomy is the surgical removal of the root apex and surrounding tissue and is often combined with retrograde filling.

Other types of procedures in surgical endodontics:

- root amputation
- hemisection
- periapical curettage
- 'Through and through' root filling
- reimplantation of teeth
- transplantation of teeth
- incision and drainage of endodontically associated swellings
- perforation repair

Relationship within Restorative Dentistry

Total patient care often requires a combined approach between the disciplines of fixed prosthodontics, periodontology, and endodontics.

Exercise 3
1. What do you understand by tooth wear?
2. Talk about attrition, abrasion, and erosion.
3. Which are the basic principles in the management of tooth wear?
4. Describe procedures in surgical endodontics.
5. Give the names and characteristics of commonly used instruments.

Translation 3

Opotřebování zubů, otírání, bruxismus, skřípání, svírání, nedostatek podpory, kolaps okluze, tok slin, složení, struktura zubu, obrušování, agresivní čistění, kartáček, pasta, mezizubní čistění, zlozvyk okusování, nehty, skořápky ořechů, odírání, ztráta tvrdých tkání, sycené nápoje, ovocné džusy, citrusové ovoce, potraviny v kyselém nálevu, ústní vody, opakované zvracení, bulimie, gastrointestinální problémy, alkoholismus, ranní nevolnost, opětovná kontrola, určit, zda opotřebování pokračuje, provizorní zásah, definitivní výplně, náhrady, ošetření kořenových kanálků, nástroje, pilník, násadec, kořenová jehla, pulpextraktor, vrtáček, plnič, pečetidlo, cpátko pro kořenové kanálky, ucpání kořenových kanálků, chirurgická endodoncie, resekce kořenového hrotu, amputace kořene, hemisekce, reimplantace zubů, rozříznutí a drenáž.

189

Vocabulary

abrasion /ə'breɪ.ʒən/ obrušování

abutment /ə'bʌt.mənt/ pilíř zubního můstku, nástavec, sekundární díl

achieve /ə'tʃiːv/ dosáhnout

achiever /ə'tʃiː.vər/ úspěšný člověk

acid /'æs.ɪd/ kyselina

acidic /'æs.ɪ.dɪk/ acidický, kyselinotvorný

acute /ə'kjuːt/ akutní

adequately /'æd.ə.kwət.li/ přiměřeně, dostatečně

adhesive /əd'hiː.sɪv/ přilnavý, lepicí páska, přilnavý, ulpívající

adjacent /ə'dʒeɪ.sənt/ přiléhající, sousední

aetiology /ˌiː.ti'ɒl.ə.dʒi/ etiologie, nauka o původu a příčinách

aggressive /ə'gres.ɪv/ agresivní

aim /eɪm/ záměr, cíl

alcoholism /'æl.kə.hɒl.ɪ.zəm/ alkoholismus

allow /ə'laʊ/ umožnit

amalgam /ə'mæl.gəm/ amalgám

amputation /ˌæm.pjʊ'teɪ.ʃən/ amputace, odstranění

apex /'eɪ.peks/ **(pl. apices)** vrchol, hrot

apicectomy /æ.pɪ'sek.tə.mɪ/ apikektomie, resekce kořenového hrotu

apparatus /ˌæp.ə'reɪ.təs/ ústrojí

armament /'ɑː.mə.mənt/ armáda, zbrojní

aspect /'æs.pekt/ pohled

attached /ə'tætʃt/ spojený, připojený

attrition /ə'trɪʃ.ən/ otírání

barbed /bɑːbd/ **broach** /brəʊtʃ/ pulpextraktor

barbed /bɑːbd/ opatřený ostny

battery /'bæt.ər.i/ baterie

bleach /bliːtʃ/ bělit

bond /bɒnd/ tmelit, spojit

bonding /'bɒnd.ɪŋ/ vazba, tmelení, spojení, lepit, materiál umožňující spojení

bridge /brɪdʒ/ můstek

bridgework /brɪdʒ.wəːk/ zhotovení můstku

broach /brəʊtʃ/ kořenová sonda, jehla

broken /brəʊ.kᵊn/ zlomený, rozbitý

bruxism /bruːk.sɪ.zəm/ bruxismus, skřípání zuby

bulimia /bʊˌlɪm.i.ə/ chorobná chuť k jídlu

bur /bɜːr/ vrtáček

canal /kə'næl/ kanálek

canine /'keɪ.naɪn/ zub špičák

cantilever /'kæn.ti.liː.vəʳ/ samonosný

carbonated /'kɑː.bən.eɪ.tɪd/ perlivý

caries /'keə.riːz/ kaz

carious /'keər.ɪ.əs/ zkažený

cavity /'kæv.ɪ.ti/ dutina, prohloubení, zubní kaz

cementation /ˌsiː.men'teɪ.ʃᵊn/ nacementování, přitmelení

cervical /sə'vaɪ.kəl/ krčkový

check-up /tʃek. ʌp/ kontrola

chew /tʃuː/ **the cud** /kʌd/ přežvykovat

citrus /'sɪt.rəs/ citrus

classification /ˌklæs.ɪ.fɪ'keɪ.ʃᵊn/ klasifikace, třídění

clench /klentʃ/ sevřít, zatnout

collapse /kə'læps/ kolaps, zhroucení

combine /kəm'baɪn/ kombinovat, spojit

compactor /kəm'pæk.təʳ/ lis, zhutňovač

complaint /kəm'pleɪnt/ stížnost, potíž

composite /'kɒm.pə.zɪt/ kompozitní výplňový materiál

composition /ˌkɒm.pə'zɪʃ.ən/ složení

compulsive /kəm'pʌl.sɪv/ nutkavý (psych.)

condition /kən'dɪʃ.ən/ stav, kondice, podmínka, podmiňovat, poměry, okolnost

condyle /ˌkɒn.daɪl/ kondyl, kloubní hrbol

constant /ˈkɒnt.stᵊnt/ stálý

constitute /ˈkɒn.stɪ.tjuːt/ vytvářet

copy /ˈkɒp.i/ kopie

crown /kraʊn/ korunka

curettage /ˌkjʊəˈret.ɪdʒ/ kyretáž, výškrab

cusp /kʌsp/ vrcholek, hrbolek

cutting /ˈkʌt.ɪŋ/ řezací

damage /ˈdæm.ɪdʒ/ poškození, zničení

deep /diːp/ hluboký

definitive /dɪˈfɪn.ɪ.tɪv/ definitivní

dentine /ˈden.tiːn/ dentin, zubovina

design /dɪˈzaɪn/ návrh

diagnosis /ˌdaɪ.əgˈnəʊ.sɪs/ diagnóza, rozpoznání (choroby), určení, popsání

discoloration /dɪˌskʌl.əˈreɪ.ʃən/ změna barvy zubů

discomfort /dɪˈskʌmp.fət/ nepohoda

distal /dɪ.stəl/ vzdálený, zadní (zuby)

distance /ˈdɪs.tənts/ vzdálenost

doppler /ˈdɒp.ləʳ/ dopler

dressing /ˈdres.ɪŋ/ obvaz, úprava

drift /drɪft/ rozšiřovat, vybočit

dullness /ˈdʌl.nəs/ tupost (přen.)

duration /djʊəˈreɪ.ʃən/ trvání

edge /edʒ/ okraj, hrana

enamel /ɪˈnæm.ᵊl/ sklovina

essentially /ɪˈsen.tʃᵊl.i/ v podstatě, nezbytně

etching /ˈetʃ.ɪŋ/ leptání

excursion /ɪkˈskɜː.ʃᵊn/ odchýlení, odbočení

facing /ˈfeɪ.sɪŋ/ fazeta

file /faɪl/ pilník

filler /ˈfɪl.əʳ/ plnivo, plnič

filling /ˈfɪl.ɪŋ/ material /məˈtɪə.ri.əl/ materiál na výplně

final /ˈfaɪ.nᵊl/ konečný

finish /ˈfɪn.ɪʃ/ dokončení

fishing /ˈfɪʃ.ɪŋ/ line /laɪn/ vlasec

fissure /ˈfɪʃ.əʳ/ fisura, prasklina

fixed /fɪkst/ pevný

flow /fləʊ/ tok

fossa /fɒs.ə/ jamka

fracture /ˈfræk.tʃəʳ/ fraktura, zlomenina

function /ˈfʌŋk.ʃᵊn/ činnost, fungování

functional /ˈfʌŋk.ʃᵊn.ᵊl/ funkční

gastrointestinal /ˌgæs.trəʊˌɪn.tesˈtaɪ.nᵊl/ gastrointestinální, týkající se žaludku a střeva

general /ˈdʒen.ᵊr.ᵊl/ hlavní, všeobecný, celkový

glass /glɑːs/ ionomer /ˈaɪ.əˌnɒ.məʳ/ sklo-ionomer

glenoid /glɪː.nɒɪd/ fossa /fɒs.ə/ jamka lopatky pro skloubení v ramenním kloubu

glenoid /glɪː.nɒɪd/ glenoidální, vyhloubený

glucose /ˈgluː.kəʊs/ glukóza, hroznový cukr

gold /gəʊld/ zlato, zlatý

grinding /ˈgraɪn.dɪŋ/ skřípání

habitual /həˈbɪtʃ.u.əl/ habituální, navyklý, častý, notorický

handheld /ˌhændˈheld/ ruční (držený v ruce), přenosný

handpiece /hænd.piːs/ násadec, rukojeť

harm /hɑːm/ poškození, zranění

hemisection /ˈhem.ɪ.ˈsek.ʃᵊn/ hemisekce, řez v polovině orgánu

iatrogenic /aɪˌætrəˈdʒen.ɪk/ iatrogenní, lékařem vyvolaný

incision /ɪnˈsɪʒ.ᵊn/ incise, naříznutí, vpich, incise, vyříznutí, chirurgické otevření

incisor /ɪnˈsaɪ.zəʳ/ řezák

instrumentation /ˌɪn.strə.menˈteɪ.ʃᵊn/ vybavení nástroji

insufficient /ˌɪn.səˈfɪʃ.ənt/
nedostatečný

intercuspal /ˌɪn.təˈkʌsp.ᵊl/ mezi
hrboly, hroty

interference /ˌɪn.təˈfɪə.rᵊnts/ rušivé
ovlivňování

intervention /ˌɪn.təˈven.ʃᵊn/
intervence, zásah

intracanal /ɪn.trə.kəˈnæl/ uvnitř kanálku

intracoronally /ɪn.trəˈkɒr.ᵊn.ᵊl.i/ mezi
korunkami

involve /ɪnˈvɒlv/ zahrnovat, znamenat,
postihnout

iron /aɪən/ železo

ironmongery /ˈaɪənˌmʌŋ.gər.i/ práce
se železem

joint /dʒɔɪnt/ místo připojení, kloub

labial /ˈleɪ.bi.əl/ retný

lack /læk/ nedostatek

large /lɑːdʒ/ intestine /ɪnˈtes.tɪn/
tlusté střevo

laser /ˈleɪ.zəʳ/ laserový

leisure /ˈleʒ.əʳ/ volný čas

lesion /ˈliː.ʒᵊn/ léze, zranění

limit /ˈlɪm.ɪt/ omezit

lingual /ˈlɪŋ.gwəl/ jazykový

loss /lɒs/ ztráta

management /ˈmæn.ɪdʒ.mənt/
ošetření, léčba, zvládnutí

manufacture /ˌmæn.jʊˈfæk.tʃəʳ/
tvořit, zpracovat

margin /ˈmɑː.dʒɪn/ okraj

masticate /ˈmæs.tɪ.keɪt/ žvýkat

mastication /ˌmæs.tɪˈkeɪ.ʃᵊn/
mastikace, žvýkání

material /məˈtɪə.ri.əl/ materiál

mesial /miː.zjəl/ střední

metal /ˈmet.əl/ kov

minimise /ˈmɪn.ɪ.maɪz/
minimalizovat, zmenšit

misdiagnosis /mɪsˌdaɪ.əgˈnəʊ.sɪs/
chybná diagnóza

molar /ˈməʊ.lᵊr/ stolička

mouthwash /ˈmaʊθ.wɒʃ/ výplach úst,
ústní voda

movable /ˈmuː.və.bl̩/ pohyblivý

mucosa /mjuːˈkəʊ.sə/ sliznice

nail /neɪl/ nehet

natural /ˈnætʃ.ᵊr.ᵊl/ přirozený, přírodní

non-/nɒn-/ ne

nut /nʌt/ oříšek

objective /əbˈdʒek.tɪv/ cíl

observation /ˌɒb.zəˈveɪ.ʃᵊn/
pozorování, dodržování

obturation /ˌɒb.tjʊ.əˈreɪ.ʃᵊn/ utěsnění,
uzavření, ucpání

occlude /əˈkluːd/, /ɒkˈluːd/ uzavřít

occupational /ˌɒk.jʊˈpeɪ.ʃᵊn.ᵊl/
pracovní

onlay /ˈɒn.leɪ/ onlej, štěp aplikovaný
na povrch tkáně

operative /ˈɒp.ᵊr.ə.tɪv/ operační,
operativní

originate /əˈrɪdʒ.ɪ.neɪt/ začínat

outline /ˈaʊt.laɪn/ obrys, nárys,
náčrtek, kontura, vytyčit, zakreslit

overdentures /ˈəʊ.və.ˈden.tʃəz/
hybridní protézy

overeruption /ˈəʊ.və.ɪˈrʌp.ʃᵊn/
supraokluze

palatal /ˈpæ.lə.tl/ patrový

paste /peɪst/ pasta

percussion /pəˈkʌʃ.ᵊn/ poklep

perforation /ˌpɜː.fᵊrˈeɪ.ʃᵊn/ proniknutí,
propíchnutí

periapical /per.ɪˈeɪ.pɪk.l/ periapikální,
v okolí hrotu kořene

period /ˈpɪə.ri.əd/ doba, období

periodontology /ˌper.ɪ.ədɒnˈtɒl.ə.dʒɪ/
periodontologie, odvětví
specializující se na léčení tkáně
kolem zubů

permanently /ˈpɜː.mə.nənt.li/ stále

phobic /ˈfəʊ.bɪk/ týkající se fobie, ustrašený

pickled /ˈpɪk.l̩d/ **food** /fuːd/ potraviny nakládané do kyselého nálevu

pier /pɪəʳ/ pilíř, pilířový zub

pit /pɪt/ jamka

plastic /ˈplæs.tɪk/ pružná hmota, plast

pontic /ˌpɒnt.ɪk/ umělý zub umístěný na můstku

porcelain /ˈpɔː.səl.ɪn/ porcelán

post /pəʊst/ čep, sloupek, podpěra

posterior /pɒsˈtɪə.ri.əʳ/ zadní

premolar /ˌpriːˈməʊ.ləʳ/ třenový zub

preparation /ˌprep.əˈreɪ.ʃən/ úprava, příprava, přípravek, preparace

probing /ˈprəʊ.bɪŋ/ sondáž

progressive /prəˈgres.ɪv/ progresivní, postupující

prosthesis /ˈprɒs.θiː.sɪs/ protéza, náhrada

prosthodontics /ˌprɒs.θəˈdɒnt.ɪks/ protetická stomatologie

provision /prəˈvɪʒ.ən/ poskytnutí

provisional /prəˈvɪʒ.ən.əl/ provizorní, dočasný

proximity /prɒkˈsɪm.ɪ.ti/ blízkost

pulpal /pʌlp.əl/ dřeňový

radiograph /reɪ.di.ə.grɑːf/ rentgenový snímek

radiographic /ˌreɪ.diˈɒg.rə.fik/ rentgenový

regurgitation /rɪˌgɜː.dʒɪˈteɪ.ʃən/ opakované zvracení

reimplantation /ˌriː.ɪm.plɑːnˈteɪ.ʃən/ reimplantace, nahrazení odejmuté časti

relationship /rɪˈleɪ.ʃən.ʃɪp/ vztah

rely /rɪˈlaɪ/ **on** /ɒn/ spoléhat se na

remaining /rɪˈmeɪ.nɪŋ/ zbývající

removable /rɪˈmuː.və.bl̩/ pohyblivý

repair /rɪˈpeəʳ/ opravit, oprava

replace /rɪˈpleɪs/ nahradit

replacement /rɪˈpleɪs.mənt/ nové umístění, náhrada

resin /ˈrez.ɪn/ **composite** /ˈkɒm.pə.zɪt/ kompozitní pryskyřice

resistance /rɪˈzɪs.tənts/ odolnost, stálost, vzdor

restoration /ˌres.təˈreɪ.ʃən/ výplň, vyplnění, obnova, náhrada

restorative /rɪˈstɒr.ə.tɪv/ opravený, obovený, konzervační

restore /rɪˈstɔːʳ/ opravit, obnovit, navrátit do původního stavu

retained /rɪˈteɪnd/ ponechaný, zadržený

retainer /rɪˈteɪ.nəʳ/ napínač, držák, retenční přístroj

retention /rɪˈten.tʃən/ zadržení, retence

retrograde /ˈret.rəʊ.greɪd/ retrográdní, obrácený

retruded /rɪˈtruː.dɪd/ ustouplý zpět

root /ruːt/ **canal** /kəˈnæl/ kořenový kanálek

rotary /ˈrəʊ.tər.i/ otočný, otáčivý, rotační

salivary /səˈlaɪ.vər.i/ slinný

sandblast /ˈsænd.blɑːst/ pískovat

sealer /ˈsiː.ləʳ/ pečetidlo, prostředek pro utěsnění

secondary /ˈsek.ən.dri/ sekundární (druhotný), závislý-porucha

sensibility /ˌsent.sɪˈbɪl.ɪ.ti/ citlivost

sharpness /ˈʃɑːp.nəs/ ostrost

shell /ʃel/ skořápka

sickness /ˈsɪk.nəs/ nevolnost

side /saɪd/ strana

site /saɪt/ místo

sloth /sləʊθ/ loudavost, nemotornost

spiral /ˈspaɪə.rəl/ spirálovitý

spreader /spred.əʳ/ cpátko pro kořenové kanálky

spring /sprɪŋ/ pero, pružina

stable /ˈsteɪ.bl̩/ stabilní, stálý

stage /steɪdʒ/ stupeň, stádium (období)

stimulus /ˈstɪm.jʊ.ləs/ (pl. **stimuli**) podnět

strain /streɪn/ napětí, napnout, usilovat, námaha

surface /ˈsɜː.fɪs/ povrch, hladina, stěna

surgical /ˈsɜː.dʒɪ.kəl/ chirurgický

surrounding /səˈraʊn.dɪŋ/ okolní

swelling /ˈswel.ɪŋ/ otok, nádor, boule

take /teɪk/ **into** /ˈɪn.tuː/ **account** / əˈkaʊnt/ vzít v úvahu

technique /tekˈniːk/ pracovní postup, metoda

temporisation /tem.pə.raɪˈzeɪ.ʃən/ vyčkávání

terminal /ˈtɜː.mɪ.nəl/ koncový

throb /θrɒb/ tepat, tep

through and through /θruː/ skrz naskrz

tilt /tɪlt/ nachýlit, naklonit, vyklonit, sklon

tissue /ˈtɪʃ.uː/, /ˈtɪs.juː/ tkáň, papírový kapesník

toilet /ˈtɔɪ.lət/ toaleta, čistění

tooth /tuːθ/ **wear** /weəʳ/ opotřebení zubů

transillumination /ˌtræn.zɪˈluː. mɪˈneɪ.ʃən/ prosvícení

transplantation /ˌtræn.splɑːnˈteɪ.ʃən/ transplantace

trauma /ˈtrɔː.mə/, /ˈtraʊ-/ trauma, úraz

traumatic /trɔːˈmæt.ɪk/, /traʊ-/ traumatický, úrazový

ultrasonic /ˌʌl.trəˈsɒn.ɪk/ ultrazvukový

unit /ˈjuː.nɪt/ jednotka, celek

veneer /vəˈnɪəʳ/ dýha, fazeta, obložení

visual /ˈvɪʒ.u.əl/ zrakový

vitality /vaɪˈtæl.ɪ.ti/ životnost

wear /weəʳ/ opotřebování

whiten /ˈwaɪ.tən/ bělit

widen /ˈwaɪ.dən/ rozšířit

wire /waɪəʳ/ drát

worker /ˈwɜː.kəʳ/ dělník, pracovník

Unit 14

Minor Oral Surgery

List of Instruments. Dental Nurse Assistance. Complications Following Extraction. Localised Osteitis. Avoiding Postoperative Complications.

Text 1

List of Instruments

- **Full conservation tray**: mirror, probe, tweezers, small and large excavators, amalgam plugger, burnisher, flat plastic instrument
- **Surgical instruments**: scalpel blade and handle, Mitchell's trimmer, periosteal elevator, retractors, needle holders, suture, dissecting forceps, surgical handpiece and burs, Hunt's water syringe, set of elevators, suction tips, scissors
- **Special instruments**: microhead for air turbine for retrograde cavity, surgical amalgam carrier, bone wax
- **Local anaesthetic**: loaded syringe ready for use

Dental Nurse Assistance

Have all instruments and equipment sterile, laid out, and ready for use before the procedure begins. **Seat the** patient comfortably in the chair with bib and safety glasses on. **Pass and retrieve local anaesthetic syringe;** help the patient to swill out. Supply full **chairside nursing** during the procedure, as follows:

- ensure adequate **aspiration of surgical area** to allow good vision
- **retract soft tissues**, as necessary
- anticipate the order of instrumentation and **have the instruments to hand,** as required
- **reassure the patient** throughout the procedure without disturbing the dentist or slowing the procedure down
- **remove pathological debris** from the area, as necessary
- **mix materials** as required, correctly and efficiently
- **develop intraoperative radiographs**, as necessary

Help patient from surgery after the procedure, then **clean and sterilise instruments**, dispose of disposables, and **prepare surgery** for next patient.

Postoperative instructions to patient
Warn that the **area** may be **sore, bruised, and swollen for next few days**. Talk about adequate **analgesia**, as advised by the dentist. Explain that

the **area will be numb** for several hours, so no attempt should be made at chewing or drinking until the anaesthesia has worn off. Tell the patient **not to drink alcohol and hot drinks or exercise** for the remainder of the day.

Give advice about **hot, saltwater mouthwash** to begin on the day after the operation and to continue until suture removal appointment.

Provide **advice in case of emergency**, according to practice protocol. Make an **appointment for suture removal**, as requested by the dentist.

Exercise 1

1. List the instruments the dental nurse would set out for an apicectomy procedure of an upper incisor tooth.

2. How would the dental nurse assist during this procedure, and what postoperative instructions should be given to the patient?

Translation 1

Nástroje konzervační, miska, zrcadélko, sonda, pinzeta, exkavátory, cpátko na amalgam, hladítko, plochý tvárlivý nástroj, nástroje chirurgické, čepel skalpelu, rukojeť, Mitchellův ořezávací nůž, raspatorium, držáky, držátka na jehly, šití, kleště na oddělování tkání, chirurgický násadec a vrtáčky, vodní stříkačka, sada pák, sací špičky, nůžky, mít všechny nástroje a vybavení připravené k použití, usadit pacienta do křesla, náprsenka, ochranné brýle, ošetřování u křesla, podávat a brát zpět nástroje, pomoci vypláchnout, zajistit dostatečné odsávání, odtahovat měkké tkáně, mít nástroje po ruce, nerušit lékaře, odstraňovat patologické úlomky, vyvolat rentgenové snímky, pomoci pacientovi z ordinace, vyčistit a sterilizovat nástroje, vyhodit pomůcky a jedno použití, připravit ordinaci pro dalšího pacienta, pooperační pokyny, oblast může být bolestivá, zhmožděná, oteklá, analgesie, oblast necitlivá několik hodin, nežvýkat, nepít alkohol, horké nápoje, necvičit po zbytek dne, výplach teplou slanou vodou, do vyjmutí stehů.

Text 2
Complications Following Extraction Bleeding

- **Reactionary haemorrhage**: occurs **within 24 hours** after the procedure, either due to patient not following postoperative instructions given—for example, **drinking alcohol, having hot drinks, exercising, lying down in hot room**—or very rarely, it may be due to the patient having an undiagnosed blood disorder which affects blood clotting.

- **Secondary haemorrhage**: occurs **within 7 days** of the procedure and usually results **from an infection** occurring at the site of the extraction. This may be **due to poor oral hygiene** by the patient or by the patient continually touching the site with dirty fingers or by the dentist failing to prescribe **antibiotics** for patients likely to acquire an infection, such as **diabetics**.

Localised Osteitis

Dry socket, which is the **loss of the blood clot from the socket**, leaving the **bare alveolar bone** open to the oral cavity and its bacterial flora, with **acute inflammation** ensuing.

It occurs a few days after the procedure, is **very painful,** and requires further dental treatment. **The blood clot can be lost physically,** either by the patient not following the postoperative instructions given, as above, or **through destruction by bacterial invasion** of the clot from the oral bacteria.

Poor blood clot development can also occur, especially **after difficult extractions where considerable pressure** has been put **on the socket walls,** so that the end blood vessels are crushed and inadequate bleeding and clot formation occurs.

Avoiding Postoperative Complications

Ensure correct postoperative instructions are given and understood, and stress the importance of those instructions being followed.

Preoperative tooth scaling of patients with neglected oral hygiene should reduce the incidence of dry socket. Ask the patient to use an **antiseptic mouthwash just prior to extraction,** which should help.

Consider the necessity of **preventive measures** following difficult extractions, such as immediately **placing antiseptic dressings** to help ward off infection. Consider **antibiotic therapy** for patients with a known likelihood of postoperative infection.

Postoperative instructions to patient

Do not drink alcohol and hot drinks or take exercise for the rest of the day. **Stay sitting upright** for several hours. **Avoid being in a warm room** if possible. **Do not touch,** poke, or fiddle with **the extraction site.** Take **adequate analgesics,** as required, but avoid aspirin-based ones for at least the first day. Begin frequent hot, **saltwater mouthwashes the day after extraction,** and continue for up to a week after the procedure. **Do not eat any spicy or acidic foods** for a few days, as these may irritate the socket. Contact the surgery as soon as possible if prolonged bleeding or severe pain occurs.

Exercise 2

1. Discuss the complications that may arise following an extraction procedure and how they can be avoided.
2. What postoperative instructions would the dental nurse give to the patient?

Translation 2

Komplikace po extrakci, reakční krvácení, do 24 hodin po proceduře, nediagnostikovaná porucha srážlivosti krve, druhotné krvácení do 7 dnů od procedury, infekce v místě vytržení, osteitida, obnažené lůžko, ztráta krevní sraženiny z jamky, odhalená dásňová kost, napadení bakteriemi, akutní zánět, extrakce obtížné, značný tlak na stěny lůžka, konce krevních cév jsou rozdrcené, vyhnutí se pooperativním komplikacím, důležitost dodržení pokynů, zanedbaná ústní hygiena, odstranění zubního kamene, preventivní opatření, umístění antiseptických obvazů, uvážit léčbu antibiotiky, zůstat sedět zpříma, vyhýbat se dotýkání, šťourání či nervózního pohrávání v místě po vytržení, nejíst kořeněné a kyselé potraviny, které mohou dráždit jamku.

Text 3

List of Instruments and Their Uses

- **Mouth mirror**: for viewing the surgical area fully
- **Probe and tweezers**: for testing for anaesthesia, if necessary, and for removing tooth and filling spicules, if necessary
- **Upper molar forceps**: to attempt whole removal of tooth once surgery has been performed and bone removed
- **Elevators**: to loosen and elevate roots if they are separated; a range of elevators should be laid out, unless the dentist has a special preference
- **Air turbine and burs**: for separating the roots to be elevated singly, if necessary
- **Coupland's chisel**: to split the roots following drilling
- **Slow-speed handpiece and burs**: for bone removal, if necessary
- **Scalpel blade and handle**: for cutting the periosteal flap
- **Mitchell's trimmer**: to raise the corner of the flap initially
- **Periosteal elevator**: to raise the flap completely off the bone and allow access for bone removal
- **Hunt's water syringe**: for irrigation while using the slow handpiece

- **Retractors**: range of cheek and tissue retractors as necessary, to be held by dental nurse
- **High-speed suction tip**: necessary if tooth sectioning is carried out with air turbine
- **Surgical fine suction tip**: for blood and irrigation solution removal at the surgical site
- **Needle holder**: for holding the needle during suturing following the complete tooth removal
- **Suture**: usually black braided silk on a curved 3.0 needle, for repositioning and holding the flap after surgery
- **Dissecting forceps**: to hold the corners of the flap while passing the needle through during suturing
- **Scissors**: to cut the suture ends

Exercise 3

1. A grossly carious upper first permanent molar tooth is to be surgically extracted. What instruments should be set out, and how are they used during the procedure?

Translation 3

Seznam nástrojů a jejich užití, ústní zrcadélko, prohlédnutí operačního místa, sonda, pinzety, testování anestézie, odstraňování úlomků zubu a výplní, kleště na horní moláry, odstranění zubu, jakmile je proveden chirurgický zákrok a odstraněna kost, zvedače, uvolnit a zvednout kořeny, jestliže jsou odděleny, vzduchová turbinka a vrtáčky, oddělení kořenů jednotlivě, Couplandovo dlátko, oddělit kořeny po vrtání, násadec s pomalou rychlosti a vrtáčky, odstranění kosti, čepel skalpelu a rukojeť, odříznutí útržku, Mitchellův ořezávací nůž, nejprve zvednout koutek, raspatorium, úplně zvednout útržek, umožnit přístup pro odstranění kosti, Huntova vodní stříkačka, pro zavlažení při užití pomalé vrtačky, tvářové a tkáňové držáky, vysoko-rychlostní sací hrot, nezbytný při provádění průřezu zubu, chirurgický jemný sací hrot, odstraňování krve a zavlažovacího roztoku v operačním místě, držátko jehel, držení jehly během šití po úplném odstranění zubů, šití, černé opředené hedvábí na zahnuté 3.0 jehle, opětné přiložení a držení chlopně po chirurgickém zákroku, disekční kleště, držet koutky chlopně při procházení jehly během šití, nůžky, ustřihnout konce.

Exercise 4 / Homework

The sentences have been divided into separate halves. Match the half-sentences in column A with the half-sentences in column B to make sentences which are complete and correct.

A

1. The instruments used to extract teeth are . . .
2. Straight-bladed forceps with the handles in line with the blades are used to extract . . .
3. Double-beaked forceps are used to extract . . .
4. Three types of elevators routinely used in the extraction of teeth are . . .
5. Upper molar forceps have one beaked blade to engage . . .

6. Bite packs are used postoperatively to . . .
7. Bleeding during extraction or immediately afterwards is called a . . .
8. Warwick James' elevators are made in sets of three called . . .
9. Aspirin should not be recommended as a postoperative analgesic because . . .
10. Localised osteitis is . . .
11. The most likely place for an upper molar root apex to be displaced to is . . .
12. An inhaled root fragment will probably become lodged in the . . .
13. The surgical procedure used to alter the shape of the alveolar ridge is called . . .

B

a) *act as pressure pads and prevent haemorrhage.*
b) *an infection of the bony extraction socket, which is caused by loss of the postoperative blood clot and subsequent infection by the oral bacteria.*
c) *right bronchus or right lung.*
d) *upper incisors and canine teeth.*
e) *lower molar teeth.*
f) *the buccal furcation of the mesial and distal roots.*
g) *Cryer's, Winter's, and Warwick James' elevators.*
h) *alveolectomy and is carried out to remove ridge undercuts and unevenness before prostheses are provided.*
i) *primary haemorrhage.*
j) *straight, left-curved, and right-curved.*

k) *forceps and elevators.*

l) *the maxillary antrum.*

m) *it may allow haemorrhage to continue due to its antiplatelet property.*

Exercise 5 / Homework

The sentences have been divided into separate halves. Match the half-sentences in column A with the half-sentences in column B to make sentences which are complete and correct.

A

1. The most likely tooth to be impacted is the . . .
2. Forceps with straight blades at right angles to the handle are used to . . .
3. Gingivectomy is the surgical procedure carried out to . . .
4. Reactionary haemorrhage occurs when . . .
5. A tissue rake is used to . . .
6. When a cyst is enucleated it is . . .
7. Apicectomy is . . .
8. Periosteal elevators are used surgically to . . .
9. An Austin retractor is used to . . .
10. Absorbable packs used to control postoperative haemorrhage contain . . .
11. Secondary haemorrhage occurs . . .
12. Frenectomy is . . .
13. Patients should be advised not to drink hot liquids or . . .
14. An oroantral fistula occurs when . . .
15. Radiographs are required before the surgical removal of lower third molars to show . . .

B

a) *extract lower premolars, lower canines, lower incisors, and all lower roots.*

b) *oxidised cellulose, fibrin, or gelatine and act by encouraging blood to clot, hence controlling haemorrhage.*

c) *is the angle of impaction, the number of roots and any curvature, the proximity of the inferior dental nerve, and the amount of overlying bone, if any.*

d) *the surgical dissection of the lingual or labial frenum to allow greater mobility of the tongue or lip.*

e) *peel the periosteum from the underlying bone and raise the periosteal flap.*

f) *remove gingivae at the site of periodontal pockets.*

g) *removed completely from the cystic cavity with its capsule intact.*

h) *the patient has not followed the postoperative instructions given, and bleeding occurs within 24 hours of the surgery.*

i) *retract the patient's cheek to allow better access and vision to the surgical area.*

j) *lower third molar, and when partially erupted is often troubled by pericoronitis.*

k) *the amputation and removal of a root apex, with any associated pathological lesion attached.*

l) *within 7 days after operation and is due to an infection at the surgical site.*

m) *retract the periosteal flap raised during a surgical procedure.*

n) *alcohol after an extraction.*
o) *an unnatural connection is made*
    between the oral cavity and the
    maxillary antrum, usually through
    an extraction socket.

Exercise 6 / Homework

The sentences have been divided
into separate halves. Match the
half-sentences in column A with the
half-sentences in column B to make
sentences which are complete and
correct.

A

1. High-speed aspiration may be
    required during extraction to . . .
2. Bite packs are made up in the
    surgery by . . .
3. Patients who have undergone
    minor oral surgery must not be
    allowed to leave the practice
    until . . .
4. A local anaesthetic containing
    adrenaline is useful for extractions
    because . . .
5. Irrigation is provided during minor
    oral surgery using . . .
6. Bone rongeurs are used to . . .
7. Another instrument with the same
    use as bone rongeurs is . . .
8. Air turbine handpieces should
    not be used during bone surgery
    because of the risk of . . .
9. Periosteal flaps are held for
    suturing using . . .
10. A Mitchell's trimmer is mainly
    used to . . .
11. A vertically impacted lower third
    molar is positioned . . .
12. A cyst which develops around the
    crown of an unerupted tooth is
    called . . .

13. Normal consequences of minor
    oral surgery are . . .
14. A surgical blade should be
    removed from the handle by . . .

B

a) *its vasoconstrictor action helps*
    reduce bleeding at the site, as well
    as helping to maintain anaesthesia
    for the duration of prolonged
    surgical procedures.
b) *a bone file.*
c) *bruising of the area, and possibly*
    the lips, and swelling of the area.
d) *postoperative haemorrhage has*
    ceased.
e) *remove sudden spurts of blood or*
    pus, to catch any loose pieces of
    tooth, or to catch the extracted
    tooth if it falls from the grip of the
    forceps.
f) *sterile saline or sterile water,*
    which is administered from a
    Hunt's irrigation syringe.
g) *surgical emphysema, which occurs*
    when air is forced at high pressure
    under the soft tissues during
    surgery.
h) *holding it firmly in a locked pair*
    of Spencer-Wells forceps while the
    blade handle is eased free.
i) *wrapping gauze squares around*
    cotton wool rolls and can be
    sterilised by autoclaving, with a
    drying cycle being chosen.
j) *dissecting forceps or rat-toothed*
    forceps.
k) *help enucleate cysts and to scrape*
    pathological debris from surgical
    sites.
l) *a dentigerous cyst.*

m) *upright and partially impacted into the ascending ramus of the mandible.*

n) *remodel prominent bony projections remaining after the extraction (surgical or routine) of teeth.*

Exercise 7 / Homework

Fill in the missing words. Choose the correct ones.

1. The roots of which teeth may be close to or penetrate the maxillary antrum: upper molars or upper premolars? The maxillary _____ is the air space lying above the hard palate and around the _____ _____. It extends anteriorly as far forwards as the first _____ _____ and can be seen clearly on radiographs of the area, dipping down between the roots of the _____ molars and premolars.	Nasal cavity, premolar teeth, upper, antrum
2. The commonest postoperative extraction complication is a localised osteitis. _____ _____ _____ is an expected event following tooth extraction; it is not a complication of the procedure. Oroantral fistula is a rare complication of upper tooth extraction, where an abnormal _____ is formed between the oral cavity and the maxillary antrum. Very rarely, a premolar can be _____ avulsed during the extraction of its overlying deciduous molar. At least 5% of routine tooth extractions result in an infection and the development of localised _____.	Osteitis, accidentally, communication, Primary haemorrhage

3. The surgical instrument used to raise a periosteal flap is a _____ elevator. A Hunt's syringe is used for _____ the surgical site. An Austin retractor is held by the dental nurse to _____ the patient's cheek and allow better visibility for the dentist. A Cryer's elevator is one of the many instruments used to _____ teeth.	retract, extract, periosteal, irrigating
4. Bone rongeurs are used during minor oral surgery to remove sharp bone spicules. Bone rongeurs are used after teeth have been extracted and _____ alveolar ridges are left. These may be very prominent and likely to be easily traumatised during the _____ _____. The most prominent edges are nibbled off with the _____ to produce a rounder ridge that will heal _____. Any small _____ instrument will lift out loose pieces of root. Bone is not usually prised away from retained roots; it is more likely to need to be _____ _____ to gain access to the roots.	uneventfully, rongeurs, sharp, drilled away, healing process, gripping
5. The surgical procedure carried out to amputate a root apex is called _____. _____ is a periodontal procedure designed to remove infected gingivae and allow the patient access to certain teeth for easier and more thorough cleaning of the area. _____ is a soft-tissue surgical procedure to relieve a tight or low-attached frenum. _____ is an endodontic procedure aimed at removing the full contents of the root canal.	Gingivectomy, Pulpectomy, Frenectomy, apicectomy

6. An oroantral fistula is most likely to develop following the attempted extraction of upper molar roots. An _____ _____ is an abnormal communication between the oral cavity and the maxillary antrum, usually produced when _____-_____ upper molar and premolar roots are being removed. Due to the close _____ of the antrum to the roots of these teeth, the antral lining is quite easily _____ during the extraction procedure, thereby producing the fistula. The antrum usually extends no further _____ than the first premolar tooth.	perforated, deep-seated, anteriorly, proximity, oroantral fistula
7. A gingivectomy is usually performed to remove gingivae to allow easier cleaning. Gingivectomy translates literally as '_____ the gingivae', so the procedure has nothing to do with _____ __ _____ of teeth. A biopsy procedure involves the _____ and microscopic study of the material removed for the determination of the presence or absence of any _____ in the sample taken.	preservation, pathology, treatment or removal, Cutting
8. The instrument used to _____ infected or cystic debris from a surgical site is a Mitchell's _____. A periosteal elevator is used to raise a _____ flap during oral surgery. A Coupland's chisel is used to _____ molar roots to allow their easier removal, as well as being used to help _____ sockets and loosen roots for their extraction.	trimmer, expand, curette, mucoperiosteal, split

9. Sedative _____ used after some surgical procedures are composed of zinc oxide/ eugenol cements. Eugenol is used throughout dentistry due to its superb _____ _____, as both a dressing internally and externally to the tooth. Carboxylate and _____ _____ cements are routinely used as _____ and _____ cements.	sedative properties, lining, dressing, luting, zinc phosphate
10. _____ that prevent the eruption of teeth are called dentigerous or follicular cysts. These form around the _____ of the unerupted tooth, and their presence prevents the tooth involved from _____ into the oral cavity. Apical cysts develop around the _____ of a tooth, usually after existing as a chronic apical abscess for some time. _____ cysts develop around the roots of erupted teeth.	Cysts, erupting, Radicular, crown, apex
11. A Blake's knife is used to perform a gingivectomy. This special gingivectomy knife holds a normal _____ _____ firmly at an _____ of 90° to the gingiva under treatment. A single cut can then be made at the same angle along the gingiva to remove a _____ of infected tissue. Normal scalpel blade handles are impossible to align at this angle, especially towards the_____ __ __ _____ where _____ is so restricted.	Strip, back of the mouth, space, scalpel blade, angle
12. A lower third molar tooth that is impacted at an acute angle into the lower second molar tooth is said to be mesially impacted.	on its side, horizontal, impaction, vertical

As the lower second molar tooth lies mesial to the third molar tooth, the _____ could only be described as mesial. _____ impactions occur into the ascending ramus of the mandible, while _____ impactions involve the third molar lying fully ___ ___ ___.	
13. The following patients should be referred to hospital for minor oral surgery: haemophiliacs, those taking anticoagulants, those taking high doses of _____, except diabetics. There is no _____ to diabetics receiving minor oral surgery in the practice as opposed to the hospital. All the other choices carry a high risk of _____ _____ during minor oral surgical procedures, and some patients should only ever be treated for these procedures at an ____ _____ department in a hospital.	severe haemorrhage, oral surgery, contraindication, aspirin
14. The flap of mucosa that lies over a partially erupted tooth is called operculum. The operculum especially lies over lower third molar teeth and is the soft tissue that _____ _____ when patients suffer from pericoronitis. The lingual frenum attaches the base of the _____ to the floor of the mouth, and the buccal mucosa is otherwise known as the _____. The _____ is the cartilage layer over the alveolar bone, which, with its overlayer of _____, forms the tough mucoperiosteum that has to be raised during surgical procedures.	periosteum, becomes inflamed, mucosa, cheek, tongue

Solution to Exercise 4

1k, 2d, 3e, 4g, 5f, 6a, 7i, 8j, 9m, 10b, 11l, 12c, 13h

Solution to Exercise 5

1j, 2a, 3f, 4h, 5m, 6g, 7k, 8e, 9i, 10b, 11d, 12d, 13n, 14o, 15c

Solution to Exercise 6

1e, 2i, 3d, 4a, 5f, 6n, 7b, 8g, 9j, 10k, 11m, 12l, 13c, 14h

Vocabulary

abscess /ˈæb.ses/ absces
absence /ˈæb.sᵊnts/ absence
absorb /əbˈzɔːb/ pohltit, absorbovat, vstřebat
access /ˈæk.ses/ přístup
accidentally /ˌæk.sɪˈden.tᵊl.i/ nešťastnou náhodou
according to /əˈkɔː.dɪŋ.tuː/ podle
acidic /ˈæs.ɪ.dɪk/ kyselý
acquire /əˈkwaɪəʳ/ získat
action /ˈæk.ʃən/ působení
adequate /ˈæd.ə.kwət/ adekvátní, přiměřený
administer /ədˈmɪn.ɪ.stəʳ/ podávat lék
advise /ədˈvaɪz/ poradit
affect /əˈfekt/ působit, ovlivňovat
aim /eɪm/ **at** /ət/ směřovat k
air /eəʳ/ **turbine** /ˈtɜː.baɪn/ vzduchová turbinka
air /eəʳ/ vzduch
align /əˈlaɪn/ vyrovnat se, zaměřit
allow /əˈlaʊ/ umožnit
alter /ˈɒl.təʳ/ upravit, změnit
alveolar /ˌæl.viˈəʊ.ləʳ/**bone** /bəʊn/ dásňová kost
alveolectomy /ˌale.viəˈlek.tə.mi/ alveolektomie, excise alveolárního výběžku čelisti
amalgam /əˈmæl.gəm/ amalgám

amount /əˈmaʊnt/ množství

amputate /ˈæm.pjʊ.teɪt/ amputovat

analgesia /ˌæn.əl.ˈdʒiː.zi.ə/ analgézie, snížená vnímavost bolesti

angle /ˈæŋ.gl̩/ úhel, roh

anteriorly /ænˈtɪə.ri.əʳ.li/ zepředu

anti- /æn.ti-/ proti

antibiotics /ˌæn.ti.baɪˈɒt.ɪks/ antibiotika

anticipate /ænˈtɪs.ɪ.peɪt/ anticipovat, očekávat

anticoagulant /ˌæn.ti.kəʊˈæg.jʊ.lənt/ antikoagulans, látka bránící srážení krve

antiseptic /ˌæn.tiˈsep.tɪk/ antiseptický, dezinfekční prostředek

antrum /ˈæn.trəm/ (pl. antra) antrum, dutina, předsíň

apex /ˈeɪ.peks/ (pl. apices) vrchol, hrot

apical /ˈeɪ.pɪ.kəl/ apikální, vrcholový, hrotový

appointment /əˈpɔɪnt.mənt/ schůzka, setkání

as /əz/ well /wel/ as /əz/ právě tak jako

ascend /əˈsend/ stoupat

aspiration /ˌæs.pɪˈreɪ.ʃən/ odsávání

assistance /əˈsɪs.tənt s/ asistence, pomoc

associated /əˈsəʊ.si.eɪ.tɪd/ spojený

attached /əˈtætʃt/ připojený

attempt /əˈtemp t/ pokusit se, pokus

autoclave /ˈɔː.təʊ.kleɪv/ autokláv, tlakový hrnec

avoid /əˈvɔɪd/ vyhýbat se

avulsion /æˈval.ʃ°n/ avulse, odtržení, vytržení

away /əˈweɪ/ pryč, daleko

back /bæk/ zadní část

bacterial /bækˈtɪə.ri.əl/ bakteriální

bare /beəʳ/ obnažený

base /beɪs/ základ, základna, opěrný bod

beaked /biːkt/ zobákovitý

bib /bɪb/ náprsenka zástěry

biopsy /ˈbaɪ.ɒp.si/ biopsie

bite /baɪt/ skus

blade /bleɪd/ čepel

bleeding /ˈbliː.dɪŋ/ krvácení

blood /blʌd/ clot /klɒt/ krevní sraženina

blood /blʌd/ clotting /klɒt.ɪŋ/ srážení krve

blood /blʌd/ disorder /dɪˈsɔː.dəʳ/ krevní porucha

braided /breɪd.ɪd/ silk /sɪlk/ opředené hedvábí

bronchus /ˈbrɒŋ.kəs/ průduška

bruised /bruːzd/ zhmožděný

bruising /ˈbruː.zɪŋ/ podlitina

bur /bɜːr/ vrtáček, fréza

burnisher /ˈbɜː.nɪʃ.əʳ/ leštič, hladítko

canine /ˈkeɪ.naɪn/ zub špičák

capsule /ˈkæp.sjuːl/ váček, pouzdro (anat.)

Carboxylate /kɑːˈbɒk.sɪl.eɪt/ karboxylát

carrier /ˈkær.i.əʳ/ nosič

carry /ˈkær.i/ nést

carry /ˈkær.i/ out /aʊt/ provést (realizovat)

cartilage /ˈkɑː.t°l.ɪdʒ/ chrupavka

catch /kætʃ/ zachytit

cavity /ˈkæv.ɪ.ti/ dutina, prohloubení

cease /siːs/ ustat

cellulose /ˈsel.jʊ.ləʊs/ celulóza, buničina

cement /sɪˈment/ cement

chair /tʃeəʳ/ křeslo

chairside /tʃeəʳ.saɪd/ vedle křesla

cheek /tʃiːk/ tvář

chew /tʃuː/ žvýkat

chisel /ˈtʃɪz.°l/ dlátko

choice /tʃɔɪs/ výběr

chronic /ˈkrɒn.ɪk/ chronický

clean /kliːn/ čistit

clearly /ˈklɪə.li/ jasně
close /kləʊz/ blízko
comfortably /ˈkʌmf.tə.bli/ pohodlně
communication /kə‚mjuː.nɪˈkeɪ.ʃ°n/
　spojení
completely /kəmˈpliːt.li/ úplně, zcela
complication /‚kɒm.plɪˈkeɪ.ʃ°n/
　komplikace, obtíž
composed /kəmˈpəʊzd/ složený
connection /kəˈnek.ʃən/ spojení
conservation /‚kɒnʃ.səˈveɪ.ʃ°n/
　zachování, udržování
considerable /kənˈsɪd.ər.ə.bl̩/ značný
content /ˈkɒn.tent/ obsah
continually /kənˈtɪn.ju.ə.li/ neustále
continue /kənˈtɪn.juː/ pokračovat
contraindication /
　ˈkɒn.trə‚ɪnd.ɪˈkeɪ.ʃ°n/
　kontraindikace
control /kənˈtrəʊl/ dohlížet na
corner /ˈkɔː.nəʳ/ cíp, růžek
correctly /kəˈrekʃ.li/ správně
cotton /ˈkɒt.°n/ wool /wʊl/ roll /rəʊl/
　svitek vaty
crush /krʌʃ/ rozdrtit
curette /kjʊəˈret/ kyreta
curvature /ˈkɜː.və.tʃəʳ/ zakřivení
curved /kɜːvd/ zakřivený, obloukový
cut /kʌt/ stříhat
cutting /ˈkʌt.ɪŋ/ řezací
cycle /ˈsaɪ.kl̩/ cyklus
cyst /sɪst/ cysta
cystic /‚sɪs.tɪk/ cystický
debris /ˈdeb.riː/, /ˈdeɪ.briː/ úlomky,
　zbytky
deciduous /dɪˈsɪd.ju.əs/ vypadavý
deep /diːp/ -seated /ˈsiː.tɪd/ hluboce
　uložený, mající hluboké kořeny
dentigerous /denˈtɪ.dʒə.rəs/
　obsahující zub
describe /dɪˈskraɪb/ popsat
destruction /dɪˈstrʌk.ʃən/ zničení, zánik

determination /dɪ‚tɜː.mɪˈneɪ.ʃ°n/
　určení
develop /dɪˈvel.əp/ radiograph /
　reɪ.di.ə.grɑːf/ vyvolat rentgenový
　snímek
dip /dɪp/ sklánět se
dirty /ˈdɜː.ti/ špinavý
displaced /dɪˈspleɪst/ fracture /
　ˈfræk.tʃəʳ/ dislokovaná zlomenina
displaced /dɪˈspleɪst/ posunutý
disposable /dɪˈspəʊ.zə.bl̩/ sloužící k
　jednomu použití
dispose /dɪˈspəʊz/ of /əv/ zbavit se
dissect /daɪˈsekt/ rozřezat, pitvat
dissection /daɪˈsek.ʃ°n/ oddělování
　tkání
distal /ˈdɪs.təl/ vzdálený, zadní (zuby)
disturb /dɪˈstɜːb/ vyrušovat
dose /dəʊs/ dávka
double /ˈdʌb.l̩/ dvojitý
dressing /ˈdres.ɪŋ/ obvaz
drill /drɪl/ vrtat, vyvrtat
drink /drɪŋk/ pít
dry /draɪ/ socket /ˈsɒk.ɪt/ suché zubní
　lůžko
dry /draɪ/ sušit
duration /djʊəˈreɪ.ʃ°n/ trvání
ease /iːz/ uvolnit
efficiently /ɪˈfɪʃ.°nt.li/ účinně
either /ˈaɪ.ðəʳ/ or /ɔːʳ/ buď anebo
elevate /ˈel.ɪ.veɪt/ zvednout
elevator /ˈel.ɪ.veɪ.təʳ/ zvedač, páka,
　zdviž
emergency /ɪˈmɜː.dʒənt.si/ naléhavá
　nutnost, pohotovost
emphysema /‚emp.fəˈsiː.mə/
　emfyzém, rozšíření tkání plynem
　nebo vzduchem
encourage /ɪnˈkʌr.ɪdʒ/ povzbuzovat
endodontics /‚en.dəˈdɒn.tɪks/
　prevence a léčení zubní dřeně
engage /ɪnˈgeɪdʒ/ zapadat, zajistit

ensuing /ɪn'sjuː.ɪŋ/ následující

ensure /ɪn'ʃɔːʳ/ zajistit

enucleate /ɪ'njuː.kli.əɪt/ enukleovat, odstranit celý orgán

equipment /ɪ'kwɪp.mənt/ vybavení

erupt /ɪ'rʌpt/ prořezávat se (zuby)

eugenol /juː'dʒen.ɒl/ eugenol

event /ɪ'vent/ jev, eventualita

excavator /'ek.skə.veɪ.təʳ/ excavátor

exercise /'ek.sə.saɪz/ cvičení

expand /ɪk'spænd/ rozšířit

expected /ɪk'spek.tɪd/ očekávaný

extend /ɪk'stend/ rozprostírat se

externally /ɪk'stɜː.nə.li/ zevně

extract /ɪk'strækt/ extrahovat, vytáhnout

extraction /ɪk'stræk.ʃ°n/ vytržení

fail /feɪl/ zanedbat

fall /fɔːl/ spadnout

fibrin /'fɪ.brɪn/ fibrin (biol.)

fiddle /'fɪd.l̩/ pohrávat si nervózně

file /faɪl/ pilník

filling /'fɪl.ɪŋ/ výplň, plnění

fine /faɪn/ jemný

firmly /'fɜːm.li/ pevně

fistula /'fɪs.tjʊ.lə/ fistula, píštěl

flap /flæp/ chlopeň, kousek volně visící kůže

flat /flæt/ plochý

floor /flɔːr/ dno

follicular /fə'lɪk.jʊ.ləʳ/ folikulární (anat.), váčkový

follow /'fɒl.əʊ/ instruction /ɪn'strʌk.ʃ°n/ plnit pokyn

following /'fɒl.əʊ.ɪŋ/ následující

food /fuːd/ potravina

force /fɔːs/ vyvíjet tlak na

forceps /'fɔː.seps/ kleště, pinzeta, nůžky, svorka

form /fɔːm/ utvářet

forwards /'fɔː.wədz/ kupředu (směřující)

fragment /'fræg.mənt/ část, úlomek

free /friː/ volný

frenectomy /frɪ'nɒ.tə.mi/ frenotomie, protětí uzdičky

frenum /friː.nəm/ frenum, uzdička

frequent /'friː.kwənt/ častý

full /fʊl/ plný, úplný

furcation /fɜː'keɪ.ʃ°n/ furkace, rozvětvení

further /'fɜː.ðəʳ/ dále, další, vzdálenější

gain /geɪn/ získat

gauze /gɔːz/ gáza

gelatine /'dʒel.ə.tiːn/ želatina

gingiva /ˌdʒɪn.dʒaɪ.və/ (pl. gingivae) dáseň

gingivectomy /ˌdʒɪn.dʒɪ'vekt.ə.mi/ gingivektomie, vynětí dásně nebo její části

give /gɪv/ advice /əd'vaɪs/ poradit

grip /grɪp/ pevně uchopit, uchytit

haemophiliac /ˌhiː.mə'fɪl.i.æk/ hemofilik, jedinec trpící hemofilií

haemorrhage /'hem.ᵊr.ɪdʒ/ krvácení

handle /'hæn.dl̩/ rukojeť, držátko

handpiece /hænd.piːs/ násadec vrtačky

hard /hɑːd/ palate /'pæl.ət/ tvrdé patro

healing /'hiː.lɪŋ/ hojení

held /held/ držený

high /haɪ/ pressure /'preʃ.əʳ/ vysoký tlak, vysokotlaký

high-speed /ˌhaɪ'spiːd/ vysokorychlostní

holding /'həʊl.dɪŋ/ držení

immediately /ɪ'miː.di.ət.li/ ihned

impacted /ɪm'pæk.tɪd/ vpáčený

impaction /ɪm'pæk.ʃ°n/ stlačení, zaklínění

importance /ɪm'pɔː.tᵊnts/ důležitost

impossible /ɪm'pɒs.ɪ.bl̩/ nemožný

207

in /ɪn/ line /laɪn/ v linii, řadový

inadequate /ɪˈnæd.ɪ.kwət/ nedostatečný

incidence /ˈɪnʧ.sɪ.dᵉnʧs/ výskyt

incisor /ɪnˈsaɪ.zəʳ/ řezák

inflammation /ˌɪn.fləˈmeɪ.ʃᵒn/ zánět

inhale /ɪnˈheɪl/ vdechnout

initially /ɪˈnɪʃ.ᵊl.i/ zpočátku, nejprve

intact /ɪnˈtækt/ nedotčený, neporušený

internal /ɪnˈtɜː.nəl/ vnitřní, interní

invasion /ɪnˈveɪ.ʒᵒn/ invaze, napadení

involve /ɪnˈvɒlv/ zahrnovat, znamenat, postihnout

irrigation /ˌɪr.ɪˈgeɪ.ʃᵒn/ výplach, zavlažení

irritate /ˈɪr.ɪ.teɪt/ dráždit

knife /naɪf/ nůž

labial /ˈleɪ.bi.əl/ labiální, retní

lay /leɪ/ out /aʊt/ vyložit

layer /ˈleɪ.əʳ/ vrstva, úroveň, poloha

lift /lɪft/ nadzvednout

likelihood /ˈlaɪ.kli.hʊd/ pravděpodobnost

likely /ˈlaɪ.kli/ pravděpodobný, pravděpodobně

lingual /ˈlɪŋ.gwᵊl/ jazykový

lining /ˈlaɪ.nɪŋ/ výstelka, vložka

lip /lɪp/ ret

literally /ˈlɪt.ᵊr.ᵊl.i/ doslova

load /ləʊd/ naplnit

lock /lɒk/ uzavřít

lodge /lɒdʒ/ ukládat, usazovat

loose /luːs/ uvolněný, uvolnit

loosen /ˈluː.sᵒn/ uvolnit, rozviklat

loss /lɒs/ ztráta

low /ləʊ/ nízký

lung /lʌŋ/ plíce

luting /ˈluːt.ɪŋ/ upnutí, sevření, upevnění, přitmelení, tmel

lying (inf. lie) /ˈlaɪ.ɪŋ/ ležící

material /məˈtɪə.ri.əl/ materiál

measure /ˈmeʒ.əʳ/ opatření

mesial /ˈmiː.zjəl/ střední

micro- /maɪ.krəʊ -/ mikro-

microscopic /ˌmaɪ.krəˈskɒp.ɪk/ mikroskopický

minor /ˈmaɪ.nəʳ/ malý

mix /mɪks/ míchat

mobility /məʊˈbɪl.ɪ.ti/ pohyblivost

molar /ˈməʊ.ləʳ/ stolička

mouthwash /ˈmaʊθ.wɒʃ/ ústní voda, kloktadlo

mucoperiosteum / ˈmjuː.kəˌper.ɪˈɒs.ti.əm/ mukoperiost, okostice mající mukózní povrch

mucosa /mjuːˈkəʊ.sə/ sliznice

nasal /ˈneɪ.zəl/ cavity /ˈkæv.ɪ.ti/ nosní dutina

necessity /nəˈses.ɪ.ti/ nutnost

needle /ˈniː.dl̩/ holder /ˈhəʊl.dəʳ/ držátko jehel

neglect /nɪˈglekt/ zanedbat

nibble /ˈnɪb.l̩/ oštipovat

numb /nʌm/ necitlivý

number /ˈnʌm.bəʳ/ počet

nursing /ˈnɜː.sɪŋ/ ošetřování

occur /əˈkɜːʳ/ nastat

operculum /əˈpɜːk.jʊ.ləm/ operculum, příklopka, víčko

opposed /əˈpəʊzd/ protikladný

order /ˈɔː.dəʳ/ pořadí

oroantral /ˌəʊ.rəʊˈæn.trəl/ oroantrální, týkající se úst a vedlejších nosních dutin

osteitis /ˌɒs.tiˈaɪ.tɪs/ osteitida, zánět kosti

over /ˈəʊ.vəʳ/ přes

overlying /ˌəʊ.vᵊlˈaɪ.ɪŋ/ ležící nad

oxidise /ˈɒk.sɪ.daɪz/ oxidovat, okysličovat

pack /pæk/ tampon, cpát, balit, ucpávat vatou

pad /pæd/ čtvereček, polštářek

pair /peəʳ/ of /əv/ pár, jedny

partial /ˈpɑː.ʃəl/ částečný, dílčí, neúplný

partially /ˈpɑː.ʃəl.i/ částečně

pass /pɑːs/ through /θruː/ procházet

pathology /pəˈθɒl.ə.dʒi/ patologie

peel /piːl/ oškrabat

penetrate /ˈpen.ɪ.treɪt/ proniknout

perforated /ˈpɜː.fʳr.eɪ.tɪd/ proražený

pericoronitis /ˌper.ɪ.kɒr.əˈnaɪ.tɪs/ perikoronitida, zánět kolem zubní korunky

periosteal /ˌper.ɪˈɒs.ti.əl/ elevator / ˈel.ɪ.veɪ.təʳ/ raspatorium

periosteal /ˌper.ɪˈɒs.ti.əl/ periosteální, okostiční

periosteum /ˌper.ɪˈɒs.ti.əm/ periost, okostice

phosphate /ˈfɒs.feɪt/ fosfát, fosforečnan

physically /ˈfɪz.ɪ.kli/ fyzicky

piece /piːs/ kus

place /pleɪs/ umístit

plastic /ˈplæs.tɪk/ plastový, plastický

platelet /ˈpleɪt.lət/ krevní destička

plugger /plʌg.əʳ/ cpátko

pocket /ˈpɒk.ɪt/ kapsa, chobot

poke /pəʊk/ šťourat se

position /pəˈzɪʃ.ən/ umístit

preference /ˈpref.ʳr.ʳnt s/ volba, větší záliba

premolar/ˌpriːˈməʊ.ləʳ/ třenový zub

prescribe /prɪˈskraɪb/ předepsat

presence /ˈprez.ʳnt s/ přítomnost osoby, věci

preservation /ˌprez.ə.veɪ.ʃən/ uchování

pressure /ˈpreʃ.əʳ/ tlak, stisk, napětí

prevent /prɪˈvent/ předejít, zajistit prevenci, zabránit čemu

preventive /prɪˈven.tɪv/ preventivní

primary /ˈpraɪ.mə.ri/ primární, první, základní

prior /ˈpraɪəʳ/ to /tʊ/ před, dříve než

prise /praɪz/ páčit

probe /prəʊb/ sonda

procedure /prəˈsiː.dʒəʳ/ procedura, postup

process /ˈprəʊ.ses/ proces, postup, průběh

produce /prəˈdjuːs/ vytvořit, produkt

projection /prəˈdʒek.ʃən/ výběžek, výstupek

prolonged /prəˈlɒŋd/ dlouhotrvající

prominent /ˈprɒm.ɪ.nənt/ vyčnívající

property /ˈprɒp.ə.ti/ kvalita, vlastnost

prosthesis /ˈprɒs.θiː.sɪs/ (pl. prostheses) protéza

provide /prəˈvaɪd/ poskytnout, připravit

proximity /prɒkˈsɪm.ɪ.ti/ blízkost

pulpectomy /pʌlˈpek.tə.mɪ/ pulpektomie, chirurg. vynětí dřeně

punch /pʌntʃ/ vytváření malých děr do tkáně

pus /pʌs/ hnis

put /pʊt/ umístit (kam)

radicular /ræˈdɪk.jʊ.ləʳ/ kořenový

radiograph /reɪ.di.ə.grɑːf/ rentgenový snímek

raise /reɪz/ zvednout, vytáhnout

rake /reɪk/ shrnovač

ramus /reɪ.məs/ rameno, větev

range /reɪndʒ/ rozsah, rozmezí

rare /reəʳ/ vzácný, zřídka

rat /ræt/ krysa

reactionary /riˈæk.ʃn.ʳr.i/ reakční

reassure /ˌriː.əˈʃɔːʳ/ uklidňovat

receive /rɪˈsiːv/ přijímat, získat

recommend /ˌrek.əˈmend/ doporučit

reduce /rɪˈdjuːs/ snížit, napravit, přemoct

remainder /rɪˈmeɪn.dəʳ/ zbytek

remodel /ˌriːˈmɒd.əl/ modelovat znovu

removal /rɪˈmuː.vᵊl/ odstranění

remove /rɪˈmuːv/ odstranit

reposition /rɪ.pəˈzɪʃ.ən/ opětné přiložení

request /rɪˈkwest/ požadavek, žádost

require /rɪˈkwaɪəʳ/ požadovat, chtít, být zapotřebí, vyžadovat

rest /rest/ zbytek

restrict /rɪˈstrɪkt/ omezit

retained /rɪˈteɪnd/ ponechaný

retract /rɪˈtrækt/ stáhnout zpět

retractor /rɪˈtræk.təʳ/ hák na rány, držák

retrieve /rɪˈtriːv/ vrátit, získat zpět

retrograde /ˈret.rəʊ.greɪd/ retrográdní, obrácený

ridge /rɪdʒ/ okraj

right- /raɪt/ **angle** /ˈæŋ.gl̩/ pravý úhel

risk /rɪsk/ riziko

rongeur /rɒːnˈʒeəʳ/ štípací kleště

root /ruːt/ **apex** /ˈeɪ.peks/ hrot kořene

rounder /ˈraʊn.dəʳ/ zaoblovací nástroj

safety /ˈseɪf.ti/ **glasses** /glɑː.sɪz/ bezpečnostní brýle

saline /ˈseɪ.laɪn/ fyziologický roztok

saltwater /sɒlt.ˈwɔː.təʳ/ slaná voda

same /seɪm/ tentýž, stejný

sample /ˈsɑːm.pl̩/ vzorek

scale /skeɪl/ odstranit zubní kámen

scalpel /ˈskæl.pᵊl/ skalpel

scissors /ˈsɪz.əz/ nůžky

scrape /skreɪp/ škrabat

seat /siːt/ usadit

secondary /ˈsek.ən.dri/ druhotný

sectioning /ˈsek.ʃᵊn.ɪŋ/ provádění řezů

sedative /ˈsed.ə.tɪv/ sedativum, uklidňující prostředek

separate /ˈsep.ᵊr.ət/ oddělovat

set /set/ **out** /aʊt/ vyložit (na prodej)

set /set/ souprava

sharp /ʃɑːp/ ostrý

single /ˈsɪŋ.gl̩/ jednotlivý

singly /ˈsɪŋ.gli/ po jednom, jednotlivě

slow /sləʊ/ **down** /daʊn/ zpomalovat

slow-speed /sləʊ.spiːd/ pomalý

socket /ˈsɒk.ɪt/ dutina, ložisko

solution /səˈluː.ʃᵊn/ roztok

sore /sɔːr/ bolavý

space /speɪs/ prostor

spicule /ˈspɪk.juːl/ úlomek, štěpina

spicy /ˈspaɪ.si/ kořeněný

split /splɪt/ rozštěpit, roztrhnout

spurt /spɜːt/ vytrysknout

square /skweəʳ/ čtverec

sterile /ˈster.aɪl/ sterilní

sterilise /ˈster.ɪ.laɪz/ sterilizovat

straight-bladed /streɪt.bleɪd.ɪd/ s rovnou čepelí

straight /streɪt/ rovný, přímý

stress /stres/ zdůraznit

strip /strɪp/ proužek

study /ˈstʌd.i/ rozbor

subsequent /ˈsʌb.sɪ.kwənt/ pozdější, následující

suction /ˈsʌk.ʃən/ **tip** /tɪp/ sací špička

superb /suːˈpɜːb/ znamenitý

surgical /ˈsɜː.dʒɪ.kᵊl/ **site** /saɪt/ operační místo

suture /ˈsuː.tʃəʳ/ **end** /end/ koneček stehů

suture /ˈsuː.tʃəʳ/ **removal** /rɪˈmuː.vᵊl/ odstranění stehů

swill /swɪl/ **out** /aʊt/ spláchnout, vymýt

swollen /ˈswəʊ.lən/ oteklý

syringe /sɪˈrɪndʒ/ stříkačka

thereby /ˌðeəˈbaɪ/ čímž, a tím

third /θɜːd/ **molar** /ˈməʊ.ləʳ/ zub moudrosti

third /θɜːd/ třetina

thorough /ˈθʌr.ə/ důkladný

throughout /θruːˈaʊt/ od počátku do konce, docela (veskrze)

tight /taɪt/ pevný, těsný

to /tʊ/ hand /hænd/ v dosahu, k ruce

tongue /tʌŋ/ jazyk

touch /tʌtʃ/ dotýkat se

tough /tʌf/ tuhý

towards /təˈwɔːdz/ směrem k

translate /trænsˈleɪt/ chápat, vysvětlit

traumatise /ˈtrɔː.mə.taɪz/ traumatizovat, poranit

tray /treɪ/ tácek, miska, lžíce

trim /trɪm/ odstřihnout, vyčistit

trimmer /ˈtrɪm.əʳ/ nůž, ořezávačka

troubled /ˈtrʌb.l̩d/ problémový

tweezers /ˈtwiː.zəz/ pinzeta

undercut /ˌʌn.dəˈkʌt/ vrub, zářez

undergo /ˌʌn.dəˈgəʊ/ podstoupit, snášet, přestát

underlying /ˌʌn.dəˈlaɪ.ɪŋ/ základní, ležící vespod

understand /ˌʌn.dəˈstænd/ pochopit

undiagnosed /ˌʌnˈdaɪ.əg.nəʊzd/ nediagnostikovaný

unerupted /ʌn.ɪrˈʌp.tᵊd/ neprořezaný

unevenness /ʌnˈiː.vᵊn.nəs/ nerovnost, nepravidelnost

uneventful /ˌʌn.ɪˈvent.fᵊl/ bez událostí

unnatural /ʌnˈnætʃ.ᵊr.ᵊl/ nepřirozený

upright /ˈʌp.raɪt/ position /pəˈzɪʃ.ᵊn/ ve vzpřímené poloze

vessel /ˈves.ᵊl/ céva

vision /ˈvɪʒ.ᵊn/ vidění

wall /wɑːl/ stěna

ward /wɔːd/ off /ɒf/ uchránit

warn /wɔːn/ varovat

water /ˈwɔː.təʳ/ syringe /sɪˈrɪndʒ/ vodní stříkačka

wax /wæks/ vosk

wear /weəʳ/ off /ɒf/ opotřebovat se

while /waɪl/ zatímco

wrapping /ˈræp.ɪŋ/ zabalení

zinc /zɪŋk/ zinek

Unit 15

Orthodontics

Risk/Benefit Considerations in Orthodontic Treatment. Classification and Occlusal Indices in Orthodontics. Patient Assessment and Examination. Cephalometrics. Principles of Treatment Planning. Management of the Developing Dentition. Removable Appliances. Fixed Appliances. Functional Appliances. Malocclusion. The Angle's Classification of Malocclusion. Instructions for Removable Appliance. Oral Hygiene Advice for Fixed Appliance. Needs for Orthodontic Treatment. Methods of Treating Malocclusion.

Text 1

Orthodontics is a branch of dentistry concerned with the growth of the face, development of the occlusion, and the **prevention and correction of occlusal anomalies**.

Malocclusion is an irregularity in the occlusion beyond the accepted range of normal. **Ideal** occlusion is a hypothetical concept based on the anatomy of the teeth. **Normal** occlusion is an occlusion within the accepted deviation from the ideal.

The general dental practitioner will often wish to refer patients for advice or treatment. If in doubt, refer sooner rather than later and before carrying out any intervention. The most difficult orthodontic problems are often those referred too late or have had previous unsuccessful or inappropriate orthodontic treatment.

Risk/Benefit Considerations in Orthodontic Treatment

Potential **benefits** can be categorised as: improved dental **health/function** improved **appearance**—malocclusion affecting appearance may also affect an individual's self-esteem, elicit an unfavourable social response, or provoke negative stereotyping

Potential **risks** can be categorised as: **tissue damage** during treatment (caries, periodontal disease, root resorption, pulp damage, ulceration, enamel damage at debond, headgear injury)
increased **susceptibility to dental disease**
effects of treatment **failure**—can be due to poor patient cooperation, underlying skeletal constrains, inappropriate treatment technique

Classification and Occlusal Indices in Orthodontics

An occlusal index is a rating or categorising system that assigns a numeric or alphanumeric label to an individual's occlusion.

Index of orthodontic treatment need has two components:

aesthetic component

dental **health** component—records the various aspects of malocclusion using the **MOCDO convention**, where:

M = missing teeth

O = overjet (relationship between incisors in the horizontal plane)

C = crossbite

D = displacement of contact points

O = overbite (relationship between incisors in the vertical plane)

This provides a reliable and rapid method of assessing the occlusion. A specifically **measuring ruler** is used and a grade awarded on the basis of the single most severe feature of the malocclusion.

The index has been validated as follows:

grades 1, 2 – no/slight need

grade 3 – borderline need

grades 4, 5 – need

Peer assessment rating index is used to determine orthodontic treatment **outcome**. It measures the following features of malocclusion: overjet, overbite, centreline relationship, buccal segment relationship, upper and lower anterior alignment.

Patient Assessment and Examination

Patient background—note:

age

relevant medical history

relevant dental history, e.g. attendance record, oral hygiene, caries rate, trauma social history—is there a complaint from the patient? Does the patient appreciate what orthodontic treatment involves? Level of parental support? Any friends/siblings having treatment?

Cephalometrics

Cephalometrics means the study of facial form as revealed in the analysis of lateral skull radiographs.

Exercise 1

1. What is orthodontics concerned with?
2. What is malocclusion?
3. Describe potential benefits and potential risks in orthodontic treatment.
4. Classification and occlusal indices in orthodontics.
5. What should a dentist know about the patient's background?

Translation 1

Růst obličeje, rozvoj okluze, prevence a korekce anomálií, normální okluze je okluze v mezích přijaté odchylky od ideálního stavu, praktický zubní lékař doporučí pacienty na radu nebo léčbu před vykonáním jakéhokoli zásahu, potenciální výhody, zlepšené zdraví zubů, funkce, vzhled, malokluze může vyvolat nepříznivou společenskou reakci, potenciální rizika, poškození tkání, kazy, onemocnění parodontu, resorpce kořene, poškození dřeně a skloviny, ulcerace, náchylnost k dentálnímu onemocnění, selhání léčby, slabá spolupráce pacienta, nevhodná technika, klasifikace a indexy okluze, systém přiřazuje okluzi jedince číselné a abecedně číselné označení, index ortodontické léčby, složka estetická, složka dentálního zdraví, konvence MOCDO, chybějící zuby, předkus, zkřížený skus, posunutí kontaktních míst, překus, spolehlivá a rychlá metoda posouzení okluze, specifické měřicí pravítko, index byl schválen, stupeň 1,2 žádná, mírná potřeba, stupeň 3 hraniční potřeba, určit výsledek léčby, měřit předkus, překus, vztah ke střední ose, vztahy v bukálním úseku, horní a dolní přední, posouzení, vyšetření, pacientovo zázemí, věk, lékařská anamnéza, dentální anamnéza, záznam návštěv, ústní hygiena, kazivost, úraz, sociální anamnéza, stížnost pacienta, ocenění ortodontické léčby, rodičovská podpora.

Text 2
Principles of Treatment Planning
The aim of treatment is to produce an **occlusion** that is **stable, functional, and acceptable in appearance**.
It must determine if treatment is indicated. If so, what are the goals of treatment—ideal or compromise result? The aims must be appropriate to the particular individual and must take account of likely compliance with treatment.
The prospective **patient must be fully aware** of the treatment plan, goals, and necessary implications for him or her in terms **of extraction, appliances, and cooperation**.

Management of the Developing Dentition
Awareness of the normal developmental pattern and sequence of eruption is

vital. It is crucial that, before extracting teeth for orthodontic purposes, **radiographs** are taken to **determine the presence/absence of suspected unerupted or missing teeth**.

Removable Appliances
Removable appliance is an orthodontic device which can be removed from the mouth by the patient for cleaning. It may be either passive or active:
active – designed to achieve **tooth movement** (tipping) by means of active components such as **wire springs and screws**
passive – appliance designed to **maintain teeth in their present position**, e.g. **space maintainers, retainers**

Appliance fitting
When fitting a removable appliance:
check whether the appliance provided complies with design
try the appliance in the mouth
ensure it is **comfortable**
adjust the appliance
take relevant measurements to **assess** progress and anchorage
give patient **instruction on insertion, removal, and care**, when to wear, what to expect, what to do if problems occur
arrange **next visit**

Appliance check visits
At each visit assess:
tooth movement
anchorage
cooperation
Ask the patient how he or she is coping. This will identify any specific

problems and allows an assessment of speech.

Examine the patient with the appliance in situ. Does it fit? Are the active components seating correctly? Are the teeth still free to move?

Ask the patient to remove the appliance. How does the patient handle the appliance? Does it look worn?

Check measurements – progress of tooth and anchorage

Adjust appliance: fixation, active components, baseplate

Check insertion and **removal**

Revise instructions to patient

Review in 4 weeks

Problems with removable appliance:
no tooth movement
incorrect tooth movement
anchorage loss

Advantages of removable appliances:
tip teeth efficiently
good overbite reduction
bite planes can eliminate displacements/occlusal interference
tooth movements usually few and simple
less chairside time needed than with fixed appliances
fewer inventory problems
can be removed for cleaning
good source of anchorage from baseplate

Disadvantages of removable appliances:
limited tooth movement available
limited scope in lower arch
affect speech
removable by the patient

Fixed Appliances

Fixed appliance is an orthodontic device in which attachments are fixed to the teeth and forces are applied by archwires or auxiliaries via these attachments.

Components are classified as:

attachments (brackets—fixed to the tooth by bonding, bands—cemented to the teeth)

archwires (the archwire is tied to the attachment)

auxiliaries (springs or elastics—used to apply force to the teeth)

Contraindications for fixed appliances:
poorly motivated patient
poor dental health
operator without appropriate training in use of fixed appliances
some malocclusions may not be amendable to fixed appliance treatment

Advantages of fixed appliance:
precise tooth control possible
multiple tooth movements can be made at once

Disadvantages of fixed appliances:
aesthetics
oral hygiene requirements
demanding in terms of material and operator time
anchorage control/treatment monitoring more difficult

Functional Appliances

The term functional appliance describes those appliances which engage both arches and act principally by holding the mandible away from its normal resting position and utilising the forces of the circumoral musculature.

Advantages of functional appliances: may utilise growth potential
can start treatment in the mixed dentition
effective vertical control of increased overbite
chairside adjustment is minimal

Disadvantages of functional appliances:

- precise tooth movement not possible
- very dependent on patient cooperation
- treatment duration is often prolonged

Exercise 2

o   Talk about principles of treatment planning.
o   What do we mean by active and passive removable appliance?
o   What must a dentist do when fitting a removable appliance?
o   What must a dentist assess when checking appliance?
o   Discuss the advantages and disadvantages of removable appliances.
o   Describe components of fixed appliances.
o   Discuss the contraindications for fixed appliances, advantages, and disadvantages.
o   Discuss the advantages and disadvantages of functional appliances.

Translation 2

Plánování léčby, cílem je okluze stabilní, funkční a vzhledově přijatelná, brát v úvahu pravděpodobnost dodržení léčby, být si plně vědom nutných extrakcí, ortodontických zařízení a spolupráce, vývoj dentice, pořadí prořezání, rentgenové snímky určí přítomnost, nepřítomnost suspektních neprořezaných či chybějících zubů, vyjmout z úst k vyčištění, dosáhnout pohybu zubu, aktivní složky, drátěné pružiny, šroubky, udržet zuby v jejich současné poloze, pomůcky na udržování mezery, napínače upevnění aparátu, zkontrolovat, vyzkoušet v ústech, zajistit aby byl pohodlný, upravit, zařídit další návštěvu instrukce o vložení, vyjmutí, péči, kdy nosit, co očekávat, co dělat když se objeví problémy, kontrolní návštěva, zhodnotit pohyb zubu, ukotvení, spolupráci, jak pacient zvládá situaci, problémy s řečí, upravit aparát, upevnění, aktivní součásti, základní destička, zkontrolovat vložení a vyjmutí, snímací ortodontický aparát, omezení předkusu, vyloučit posunutí, potřebovat méně času u křesla, než u pevných aparátů, nevýhody snímatelných aparátů, omezený pohyb zubu, omezený rozsah spodního oblouku, ovlivňují řeč, pevné aparáty, připojení upevněna k zubům, ortodontické zámky, tmelení, pásky, drátěné oblouky, pomocná zařízení, pružiny, pružné tkaniny, funkční aparáty, udržují spodní čelist mimo normální klidovou polohu, využívají svalstvo kolem úst, smíšená dentice, využít možnosti růstu, léčba velmi závislá na spolupráci pacienta, trvání často dlouhodobé.

Text 3
Malocclusion

There are three causes of malocclusion:
- localised **crowding**
- jaw-to-jaw **discrepancy/** jaw-to-tooth discrepancy
- **supernumeraries** or congenitally **absent teeth**

When a fixed appliance is fitted, the patient should be told to brush the teeth thoroughly, use interdental brushes under archwire and around metal components, and use good quality mouthwash.

The Angle's Classification of Malocclusion

This classification is based on a **description of the horizontal relationship of the jaws** and divides malocclusions into the following four types:

Class 1
- Mesiobuccal cusp of upper first molar bites into the buccal groove of the lower first molar
- Overjet is average at 2–4 mm
- Overbite is average at 50%

Angle's class 1 is considered normal—no treatment required.

Class 2 division 1
- Lower first molar is distal to normal position
- Overjet is increased
- Overbite may be average or reduced; there may even be no incisal contact—anterior open bite

Class 2 division 2
- Lower first molar is distal to normal position
- Overjet is increased
- Overbite is increased

Class 3
- Lower first molar is mesial to normal position
- Overjet may be zero or even reversed
- Overbite may be reduced to edge-to-edge incisally, or the patient may have anterior open bite.

Treatment methods
Class 2 division 1

The problem is due to the **lower jaw being too far back** and the **upper incisors being trapped outside the lower lip**.

Move the jaw forward with functional appliance, which uses the oral musculature to encourage growth of the mandible into a more forward position; retract upper incisors to a stable position inside the lower lip, using the same appliance or a separate upper removable appliance.

Accept lower jaw position, and extract upper teeth to create space to retract upper incisors, using upper removable appliance or upper fixed appliance.

Use upper and lower fixed appliances to pull upper teeth back and lower teeth forwards buccally, and retract upper incisors. Alternatively, accept malocclusion, and give no treatment, especially if the patient has poor oral hygiene or poor cooperation. Severe cases may require surgery to the jaws.

Class 2 division 2

The problem is due to **the mandible being too far back and the upper** incisors being trapped by the lower lip and retroclined. Correct buccal occlusion with fixed appliances and procline upper incisors.

Or accept buccal occlusion and procline upper incisors with upper removable appliance; bite plane anteriorly to reduce overbite too. Or accept malocclusion, as it is often the most difficult to treat and requires great cooperation on the patient's part.

Class 3

The problem is due to a short, narrow maxilla.

Expand upper arch, using upper removable appliance with an expansion screw or a fixed quadhelix device. Correct reverse overjet by moving upper incisors forward. Correct the buccal malocclusion with upper and lower fixed appliances and elastics to pull upper teeth forwards and lower teeth backwards.

Reverse overjet correction is often unstable, especially if there is a large jaw-size discrepancy. These patients often require jaw surgery (osteotomy) so that the mandible can be surgically shortened; sometimes, the maxilla is also surgically lengthened. Alternatively, accept malocclusion, especially in poorly motivated patients. Some patients will not accept surgery either.

Exercise 3

1. Give three causes of malocclusion.
2. Briefly explain the oral hygiene instructions that should be given to a patient when a fixed appliance is fitted.

3. Describe Angle's classification of malocclusion. Discuss the different methods of treating malocclusions.

Translation 3

Příčiny malokluze, městnání, nepoměr čelistí, zubů, nadpočetné zuby, vrozeně chybějící zuby, pevný aparát, důkladné čistění zubů, použít mezizubní kartáčky, pod drátěným obloukem, kolem kovových součástí, použít kvalitní ústní vodu, klasifikace založená na popisu horizontálního vztahu čelistí, meziobukální hrbolek, bukální rýha, vzdálený normální poloze, překus zvýšený, nulový, obrácený, předkus průměrný, snížený, žádný kontakt řezáků, funkční aparát, pohnout čelist dopředu, táhnout zuby dozadu, dopředu, závažné případy vyžadují chirurgický zásah do čelistí, přijmout malokluzi, nejobtížněji se léčí, vyžaduje velkou spolupráci ze strany pacienta, chirurgie čelistí, mandibula chirurgicky zkrácena, maxilla prodloužena.

Text 4

Instructions for Removable Appliance

The appliance is to be **worn for 24 hours a day** and should only need to be **removed after meals for cleaning**. All **sticky foods should be avoided** as they will stick to the appliance and be difficult to remove. **Sweets and fizzy pop should be avoided** during the course of the orthodontic treatment. The **appliance should be removed for all contact sports**. However, if such sports are played excessively, the dentist may advise **abstaining** from them during treatment, as the appliance may otherwise not be worn for long enough each day to actually move the teeth.

The teeth and the appliance should be **brushed thoroughly after every meal** so that debris is not likely to cause caries or gingival problems. Diet should be restricted to **three meals a day and no snacking**, or again the appliance may not be worn for long enough to actually move the teeth. **Full wear is necessary** to **achieve adequate tooth movement**, and holidays, days out, and meals out are not exceptions. All dental **appointments must be attended;** otherwise, the appliance will not work. Failure to comply with all the prefitting instructions will mean that the treatment may have to be stopped.

Oral Hygiene Advice for Fixed Appliance

Oral hygiene **must be excellent** while the fixed appliance is on the teeth; otherwise, the enamel may be damaged. Usual tooth brushing must be carried out after each meal as normal so that gingival margins are clean. Special **brushing around brackets and beneath archwire** is also recommended, using an **interspace brush. Diet should be modified** so that fizzy pop and sweets are not consumed during the course of orthodontic treatment. Other highly cariogenic foods should also be avoided.

Failure to comply with these rules means **the appliance** will have to be **removed by the dentist; otherwise,**

enamel damage will occur. It is advisable to use a weekly fluoride mouthwash so that no long-term damage will be done on the rare occasions when the oral hygiene methods are less than adequate. This is not an excuse, however, for poor oral hygiene methods.

Needs for Orthodontic Treatment

Poorly positioned teeth may be **exposed to abnormal trauma** by their positions, for example proclined incisors. **Crowded teeth** create food stagnation areas, which lead to carious attack or periodontal disease or both. **Malpositioned teeth or jaw discrepancies** may cause **difficulty in normal chewing** movements, such that **excess stresses** are put on the muscles of mastication and the temporomandibular joint, causing **facial pain in later life**.

Incompetent lip seals, common in severe class 2 division 1 malocclusion, allow the **gingivae to dry out** and lead to the onset of gingival problems, which may progress to **periodontal disease in later life**.

Severe malpositioning of teeth may lead to merciless teasing at school, as a result of which the patient develops great **anxiety about their appearance**. Vanity, the need for a 'perfect' smile.

Methods of Treating Malocclusion

Treating malocclusion means **selective extraction** of deciduous or permanent teeth or both, then **allowing spontaneous tooth movements** to correct the problem. This is especially useful when upper canine teeth are erupting buccally; first premolars can be extracted, and the canines should drop into position spontaneously. The extractions **need to be well timed**, though.

Removable appliances can be used to:
* **correct a single tooth or a few teeth movements**, using springs
* correct **reverse overjets**, using springs
* correct **buccal crossbites**, using expansion screws
* correct **proclination**, using retractors
* **reduce deep overbite**, using bite planes
* **retract canine** teeth, using retractors

For class 2 division 1 malocclusions, a functional appliance uses the oral musculature to improve jaw discrepancies.

Fixed appliances can be used to:
* **correct tooth rotations**
* correct **severe displacements of a single tooth or several teeth**
* correct **buccal crossbites**, using a quadhelix device
* correct **class 2 and class 3 jaw discrepancies**, using elastics between the two arches
* **close spaces in the arch**, using elastics in the arch
* correct **tipping of teeth in the labial segment**
* correct **intrusion** of teeth
* correct **extrusion** of teeth

Exercise 4
1. What instructions should be given to a patient before a removable appliance is fitted? What oral hygiene advice should be given to a patient with a fixed appliance?
2. Why might orthodontic treatment be necessary? By what methods may the dentist treat malocclusion?

Translation 4
Instrukce pro snímatelný aparát, nosit 24 hodin denně, vyjmout po jídle pro čistění, dieta, tři jídla denně, žádné svačení, vyhýbat se lepkavým jídlům, sladkostem a šumivým nápojům, vynechat kontaktní sporty během léčby, nepřetržité nošení je nezbytné, svátky, volné dny a jídla mimo domov nejsou výjimkou, dodržovat všechny pokyny, ústní hygiena u pevného aparátu musí být vynikající, jinak se poškodí sklovina, použít jednou za týden ústní vodu s fluoridem, potřeby ortodontické léčby, špatně postavené zuby, abnormální trauma, kaz, onemocnění parodontu, odchylky čelistí, obtíže při žvýkacích pohybech, nadměrný tlak na žvýkací svaly, nedostatečné uzavření rtů umožňuje vysychání dásní, metody léčení, selektivní extrakce vypadavých, stálých zubů, snímatelný aparát, pružiny, rozšiřovací šroubky, retraktory, nákusné desky, pevný aparát, opravit rotaci zubu, zkřížený skus, naklonění zubů, vtlačení, vytlačení zubů.

Exercise 5 / Homework
The sentences have been divided into separate halves. Match the

half-sentences in column A with the half-sentences in column B to make sentences which are complete and correct.

A

1. A class 1 malocclusion exists when the mesiobuccal cusp of the upper first molar lies . . .
2. Retention of an upper removable appliance is provided by . . .
3. In class 2 division 2 malocclusion, the upper central incisors are often . . .
4. A reverse overjet is often a feature of a . . .
5. When the posterior teeth are in contact but a gap exists between the anterior teeth, . . .
6. An operation to correct severe skeletal malocclusions is . . .
7. Buccally erupted upper canines can be retracted with . . .
8. A tooth is said to be in crossbite when . . .
9. Light-cured adhesives are used in orthodontics to . . .
10. Rotated teeth can only be corrected with . . .
11. Retainers are worn after orthodontic treatment . . .
12. Archwires used in fixed orthodontic treatment are made . . .
13. The usual cause of crowding in the mouth is . . .
14. Glass ionomer cements are used in orthodontics to . . .
15. A quadhelix device is used to . . .

B

a) *an osteotomy.*
b) *to provide maxillary expansion in patients who are to undergo*
   a course of fixed orthodontic treatment.
c) *a fixed appliance.*
d) *Adams clasps.*
e) *an anterior open bite is present.*
f) *buccal canine retractors.*
g) *adhere brackets onto the labial surfaces of teeth when performing fixed orthodontics.*
h) *of nickel-titanium or stainless steel.*
i) *a discrepancy between the size of the teeth in relation to the size of the jaws.*
j) *retroclined.*
k) *in the buccal groove of the lower first molar tooth.*
l) *the buccal cusps of an upper tooth occlude on the occlusal surface of the lower tooth.*
m) *a class 3 malocclusion.*
n) *to cement bands onto teeth.*
o) *hold the new tooth alignments stable and prevent relapse.*

Exercise 6 / Homework

Fill in the missing words. Choose the correct ones.

1. Angle's classification of occlusion is based on the position of the first molars and the canines. Angle's class 1 malocclusion, which is the _____, is when the upper canine tip lies between the lower canine and first premolar, and the mesiobuccal ____ of the upper first molar lies in the buccal _____ of the lower first molar. Class 2 malocclusion occurs when the lower canine and first molar lie _____ these ideal positions. Class 3 is when they lie __ _____ ____ them.	Behind, in front of, ideal, groove, cusp

2. Proclined upper incisors are usually a feature of class 2 division 1 malocclusion. In a class 2 division 1 malocclusion, the upper incisors are _____ so that there is an increase in _____. In a class 2 division 2 malocclusion, the upper incisors are not proclined, and there is an increased _____. In class 3 malocclusion, the lower teeth are in front of the upper teeth. In a class 1 malocclusion, class 1 incisors will have an _____ overjet of 2–4 mm.	average, overjet, overbite, proclined
3. The _____ between the upper incisal edge and the lower labial _____ of the central incisors is called overjet. Retroclination and proclination describe the _____ of the upper incisors, whereas the overbite is the amount of _____ of the lower incisors by the upper incisors.	angulations, coverage, distance, surface
4. The overjet may be zero or even a negative figure in class 3 malocclusion. In a class 3 _____, the lower teeth are in front of the uppers. The incisors may meet ____ __ ____, in which case the overjet is zero or the upper incisors may lie behind the lowers and there will be a _____ overjet.	Reverse, malocclusion edge to edge
5. _____ A crossbite exists when the upper teeth bite _____ the lower teeth. A term usually used to describe the _____ teeth. Ideally, the palatal cusps of the _____ should lie on the occlusal surfaces of the _____, but when a crossbite is present the buccal cusp of the uppers lies on the occlusal surface of the lowers. This is usually seen in patients with an upper arch.	Uppers, inside, lowers, buccal
6. A mesiodens is an example of a supernumerary tooth. This is the commonest _____ tooth seen, usually lying between the roots of the upper central incisors, in the midline—hence '_____'. A _____ upper lateral incisor is usually peg-shaped and therefore referred to as peg lateral. _____ teeth are not usually malformed, and first molar teeth do not have a pseudonym.	malformed, Premolar, mesiodens, supernumerary
7. A patient who sucks their thumb often has proclined incisors and an anterior open bite. The thumb in the patients' mouth prevents the incisor teeth _____ fully—an anterior open bite. The upper incisors may be proclined as the _____ prevents their growth at the correct _____. Continued _____ may constrict the upper arch and cause a _____.	Sucking, erupting, crossbite, angulation, thumb
8. Congenitally absent teeth are those which have been missing since birth. Anything _____ has a relationship to fetal development and _____. Thus any congenital defect is one that developed in the ____ and was present at birth. Teeth _____ after their usual eruption dates are merely late.	erupting, womb, congenital, birth
9. The usual retentive component of a removable appliance is an Adams crib. A _____ is the metal component adhering to individual teeth during _____ appliance therapy. A canine _____ and a finger spring are components of _____ appliances that actively move selected teeth.	removable, bracket, fixed, retractor

10. Good oral hygiene is important for those patients who are _____ orthodontic appliance. Even in the cleanest mouths, the presence of any type of _____ _____ will allow food trapping around and beneath it, so oral hygiene is of the utmost _____ of all orthodontic patients, whatever their appliance.	importance, orthodontic appliance, wearing
11. Which of the following should the dental nurse ___ ___ for a patient attending with a removable orthodontic appliance: Adams' universal or spring-forming pliers? Ligature cutters are used to cut _____ during fixed orthodontic therapy. A full _____ _____ is of little use to the dentist when treating a malocclusion. Adams' pliers and spring-forming pliers are the commonest instruments used to _____ removable appliances.	adjust, set out, ligatures, conservation tray
12. Functional appliances work by using muscular forces to move the jaws. They are so named because they rely on normal _____ function of the masticatory and expressive muscles around the oral cavity to _____ mandibular growth _____ to correct class 2 malocclusions. _____ are used in fixed appliance therapy. _____ are used in removable therapy, and no muscles could move the teeth in the alveolar bone.	encourage, forward, Springs, Archwires, muscular
13. Molar bands used in fixed appliance therapy are cemented with glass ionomer cement, zinc phosphate cement, polycarboxylate cement. All three give _____ _____ to enamel, being mixed to a creamy _____ and used as _____ cements.	consistency, luting, sufficient adhesion

14. The following should be set out for an orthodontic retention-check appointment: pre- and postoperative study models, _____ _____, radiographs, except the completed orthodontic claim form. The completed orthodontic _____ _____ must be sent to the Business Services Agency as soon as the active phase of treatment has been completed. There is a time limit six months from _____ of treatment for the forms to be submitted to _____.	Claim form, payment, clinical records, completion
15. The following radiographs may be required before considering orthodontic treatment: a cephalometric radiograph, left and right bitewing radiographs, an anterior occclusal radiograph, except an orthopantomograph. An _____ is essential to determine the presence and positions of any unerupted teeth, as well as any unexpected _____ of the jaws. An _____ ____ is required to determine the presence of supernumerary teeth and the positions of canines. A _____ radiograph is only required in difficult cases and is usually taken by a hospital or a specialist orthodontic practice. Bitewing radiographs have no value in orthodontic treatment planning.	Orthopan-tomograph, occlusal view, cephalometric, pathology
16. Included in the instructions given to patients who have had a fixed appliance fitted is to expect some tooth _____ initially. Chewing gum and sweets are ___ _____ during fixed appliance work. The former will be impossible to _____ from the metal work and the latter will cause _____	devastating, not allowed, remove, discomfort

223

caries unless the oral hygiene of the patient is absolutely perfect. The teeth must be brushed after every meal.	
17. Practice patients' pre- and postoperative _____ must be stored for at least two years at the practice. Patients who have undergone orthodontic treatment in the _____ can be called for random _____ by the Business Services Agency at any time up to two years after the _____ of treatment, so the model must be kept for at least this length of time. If given to the patient, they are very likely to be broken or discarded. Under no circumstances should they be disposed of from the practice.	Study models, assessment, completion, practice
18. A _____ occurring between erupted teeth in either arch is called diastema. The overjet is the _____ between the upper and the labial surface of the lower incisors, while the overbite is the _____ labial coverage of the lower incisors by the upper incisors. An anterior open bite describes the space present between the incisors when the _____ teeth are fully closed and is often a _____ of thumb-suckers.	percentage, posterior, feature, natural space, distance
19. When teeth are described as proclined, they _____ forwards. Proclined teeth are a feature of class 2 division 1 malocclusions, where the _____ lies further back than normal and the upper incisors have developed _____ the force of the lower lip. In class 2 division 2 malocclusions, the upper incisors tend to be held upright or even forced to slope backwards, and this is called _____.	protrude, mandible, palatally, retroclination, outside

Teeth lying inside the upper arch are closed _____, and those with a reverse overjet are a feature of class 3 malocclusions, where the mandible lies too far forwards of normal.	

Solution to Exercise 5
1k, 2d, 3j, 4m, 5e, 6a, 7f, 8l, 9g, 10c, 11o, 12h, 13i, 14n, 15b

Vocabulary

absent /ˈæb.sənt/ nepřítomný
abstain /æbˈsteɪn/ from /frɒm/ zdržovat se (čeho)
accept /əkˈsept/ přijmout
acceptable /əkˈsept.ə.bl̩/ přijatelný
accepted /əkˈsep.tɪd/ přijatý
achieve /əˈtʃiːv/ dosáhnout
active /ˈæk.tɪv/ aktivní
actually /ˈæk.tʃu.ə.li/ vlastně, ve skutečnosti
adequate /ˈæd.ə.kwət/ adekvátní, odpovídající
adhesion /ədˈhiː.ʒən/ adhese, přilnavost
adjust /əˈdʒʌst/ upravit
adjustment /əˈdʒʌst.mənt/ nastavení, seřizování
advantage /ədˈvɑːn.tɪdʒ/ výhoda
advisable /ədˈvaɪ.zə.bl̩/ vhodný, doporučeníhodný
advise /ədˈvaɪz/ poradit
affect /əˈfekt/ ovlivnit, postihnout
aim /eɪm/ záměr, cíl
alignment /əˈlaɪn.mənt/ seřazení, uspořádání
alphanumeric /ˌæl.fə.njuːˈmer.ɪk/ abecedně číselný
alternatively /ɒlˈtɜː.nə.tɪv.li/ alternativně, eventuálně
alveolar /ˌæl.viˈəʊ.ləʳ/ bone /bəʊn/ dásňová kost

amend /əˈmend/ zlepšit, pozměnit

amount /əˈmaʊnt/ množství

anchorage /ˈæŋ.kər.ɪdʒ/ ukotvení, úchyt

angulation /ˌæŋ.gjʊˈleɪ.ʃⁿn/ úhel

anomaly /əˈnɒm.ə.li/ anomálie, odchylka

anterior /ænˈtɪə.ri.əʳ/ přední

anxiety /æŋˈzaɪ.ə.ti/ úzkost

appearance /əˈpɪə.rənts/ vzhled

appliance /əˈplaɪ.ənts/ zařízení, aparát

appointment /əˈpɔɪnt.mənt/ schůzka, sjednané vyšetření

appreciate /əˈpriː.ʃi.eɪt/ ocenit

appropriate /əˈprəʊ.pri.ət/ vhodný

arch /ɑːtʃ/ oblouk

archwire /ɑːtʃ.waɪəʳ/ drátěný oblouk

arrange /əˈreɪndʒ/ zařídit

assess /əˈses/ zhodnotit, určit

assessment /əˈses.mənt/ stanovení, posouzení, určení

assign /əˈsaɪn/ přiřadit, stanovit

at /ət/ once /wʌnts/ ihned

attachment /əˈtætʃ.mənt/ připojení, upevnění, spoj, vazivo

attack /əˈtæk/ útok, záchvat

attend /əˈtend/ navštěvovat

attendance /əˈten.dənts/ record / ˈrek.ɔːd/ záznam o návštěvách

auxiliary /ɔːgˈzɪl.i.ər.i/ pomocné zařízení, příslušenství

average /ˈæv.ᵊr.ɪdʒ/ průměrný

avoid /əˈvɔɪd/ vyhnout se

award /əˈwɔːd/ přisoudit

aware /əˈweəʳ/ být si vědom

awareness /əˈweə.nəs/ informovanost

away /əˈweɪ/ pryč

background /ˈbæk.graʊnd/ zázemí, pozadí

backwards /ˈbæk.wədz/ směrem dozadu

hand /bænd/ páska, kroužek

based /beɪst/ on /ɒn/ založený na

baseplate /beɪs.pleɪt/ bazální deska

basis /ˈbeɪ.sɪs/ základ, báze

benefit /ˈben.ɪ.fɪt/ výhoda, prospěch

beyond /biˈjɒnd/ za, dále než

birth /bɜːθ/ narození

bite /baɪt/ plane /pleɪn/ nákusná deska

bitewing /baɪt.wɪŋ/ bitewing

bond /bɒnd/ tmelit, spojit

borderline /bɔː.dəʳ.laɪn/ hraniční, sporný

bracket /ˈbræk.ɪt/ ortodontický zámek

broken /brəʊ.kⁿn/ rozbitý, prasklý

buccal /bʌk.l/ tvářový

care /keəʳ/ péče

caries /ˈkeə.riːz/ rate /reɪt/ kazivost

cariogenic /ˌkeə.ri.əˈdʒen.ɪk/ kazový

carry /ˈkær.i/ out /aʊt/ vykonávat

case /keɪs/ případ

categorise /ˈkæt̮.ə.gə.raɪz/ vytvářet kategorie

cement /sɪˈment/ cement, tmel, pojivo, stmelit

centreline /sen.trə.laɪn/ střednice, osa

cephalometric /ˌse.fəˈlom.ɪt.rɪk/ cefalometrický, měřící lebku

chairside /tʃeəʳ.saɪd/ u křesla

check /tʃek/ kontrolovat

chew /tʃuː/ žvýkat

chewing /tʃuː.ɪŋ/ gum /gʌm/ žvýkačka

chickenpox /ˈtʃɪk.ɪn.pɒks/ plané neštovice

circumoral /ˈsɜː.kəm.ˈɔː.rəl/ okolo úst

claim /kleɪm/ žádost

clasp /klɑːsp/ spona, připnout

cline /klaɪn/ klín

clinical /ˈklɪn.ɪ.kᵊl/ klinický

comfortable /ˈkʌmp.fə.tə.bl̩/ pohodlný

complaint /kəmˈpleɪnt/ stížnost, potíž

complete /kəmˈpliːt/ skončit, doplnit

completion /kəmˈpliː.ʃən/ dokončení

compliance /kəmˈplaɪ.ənts/ spolupráce, dodržení

comply /kəmˈplaɪ/ with /wɪð/ dodržet (co), vyhovovat

component /kəmˈpəʊ.nənt/ složka

compromise /ˈkɒm.prə.maɪz/ oslabit

concept /ˈkɒn.sept/ představa

congenital /kənˈdʒen.ɪ.təl/ vrozený

conservation /ˌkɒnt.səˈveɪ.ʃən/ uchování

consideration /kənˌsɪd.əˈreɪ.ʃən/ úvaha

consistency /kənˈsɪs.tənt.si/ konzistence, hutnost

constrain /kənˈstreɪn/ omezení, omezovat, škrtit

constrict /kənˈstrɪkt/ stáhnout, stisknout

consume /kənˈsjuːm/ konzumovat, sníst

contraindication /ˈkɒn.trə.ˌɪnd.ɪ.ˈkeɪ.ʃən/ kontraindikace

convention /kənˈvent.ʃən/ pravidlo

cooperation /kəʊˌɒp.əˈreɪ.ʃən/ spolupráce

cope /kəʊp/ zvládat

correct /kəˈrekt/ správný

correction /kəˈrek.ʃən/ oprava

correctly /kəˈrekt.li/ správně

corrosive /kəˈrəʊ.sɪv/ žíravina

course /kɔːs/ průběh

coverage /ˈkʌv.ər.ɪdʒ/ pokrytí

creamy /ˈkriː.mi/ krémový

create /kriˈeɪt/ vytvořit

crib /krɪb/ kotevní spona

crossbite /krɒs.baɪt/ zkřížený skus

crowding /kraʊd.ɪŋ/ městnání

crucial /ˈkruː.ʃəl/ rozhodující, klíčový

cusp /kʌsp/ vrchol

cutter /ˈkʌt.əʳ/ dláto, fréza

damage /ˈdæm.ɪdʒ/ poškození

debond /dɪ.ˈbɒnd/ zeslabit spojení

debris /ˈdeb.riː/, /ˈdeɪ.briː/ zbytky, úlomky

demanding /dɪˈmɑːn.dɪŋ/ náročný

dental /ˈden.təl/ history /ˈhɪs.tər.i/ dentální anamnéza

dentition /denˈtɪʃ.ən/ dentice, chrup

dependent /dɪˈpen.dənt/ on /ɒn/ závislý

description /dɪˈskrɪp.ʃən/ popis

determine /dɪˈtɜː.mɪn/ určit

devastating /ˈdev.ə.steɪ.tɪŋ/ zničující

development /dɪˈvel.əp.mənt/ rozvoj

deviation /ˌdiː.viˈeɪ.ʃən/ odchylka

device /dɪˈvaɪs/ zařízení

diastema /ˌdaɪ.əsˈtiːm.ə/ diastéma, mezera mezi středními řezáky

disadvantage /ˌdɪs.ədˈvɑːn.tɪdʒ/ nevýhoda

discard /dɪˈskɑːd/ vyřadit

discomfort /dɪˈskʌmp.fət/ nepohoda

discrepancy /dɪˈskrep.ənt.si/ nepoměrnost, odchylka

displacement /dɪˈspleɪs.mənt/ posunutí, chybné postavení zubu, vytlačení

dispose /dɪˈspəʊz/ zbavit se, vyhodit

distal /dɪˈstəl/ vzdálený

distance /ˈdɪs.tənts/ vzdálenost

drop /drɒp/ klesnout

dry /draɪ/ out /aʊt/ vyschnout

duration /djʊəˈreɪ.ʃən/ trvání

edge /edʒ/ okraj, hrana

efficiently /ɪˈfɪʃ.ənt.li/ účinně

either /ˈaɪ.ðəʳ/ buď

elastic /ɪˈlæs.tɪk/ elastický, pružná tkanina, guma

elicit /ɪˈlɪs.ɪt/ vyvolat

encourage /ɪnˈkʌr.ɪdʒ/ povzbudit

engage /ɪnˈgeɪdʒ/ obsadit, zaměstnávat

ensure /ɪnˈʃɔːʳ/ zajistit

eruption /ɪˈrʌp.ʃən/ prořezání

even /'iː.vᵊn/ stejný

examine /ɪg'zæm.ɪn/ vyšetřit, prohlídka

excellent /'ek.səl.ənt/ vynikající

exception /ɪk'sep.ʃᵊn/ výjimka

excess /ek'ses/ nadměrný

excessively /ek'ses.ɪv.li/ nepřiměřeně

excuse /ɪk'skjuːs/ omluva, výmluva

expand /ɪk'spænd/ rozšířit se

expansion /ɪk'spæn.tʃᵊn/ expanze, rozšíření

expect /ɪk'spekt/ očekávat

exposed /ɪk'spəʊzd/ vystavený

expressive /ɪk'spres.ɪv/ výrazový

extrusion /ɪk'struː.ʒᵊn/ vystrčení, vypuzení

facial /'feɪ.ʃᵊl/ obličejový

failure /'feɪ.ljᵊr/ selhání, chyba

far /fɑːʳ/ daleko

feature /'fiː.tʃəʳ/ rys

few /fjuː/ málo

finger /'fɪŋ.gəʳ/ prst

fit /fɪt/ padnout

fitting /'fɪt.ɪŋ/ montování, úprava

fixation /fɪk'seɪ.ʃᵊn/ upevnění

fixed /fɪkst/ pevný, nepohyblivý, stálý

fizzy /'fɪz.i/ pop /pɒp/ šumivý nápoj (šampaňské apod.)

force /fɔːs/ síla, účinnost

form /fɔːm/ tvar, podoba

former /'fɔː.məʳ/ the latter /'læt.əʳ/ první - druhý

forward /'fɔː.wəd/ přední, posunout dopředu

forwards /'fɔː.wədz/ směrem dopředu

free /friː/ volný

full /fʊl/ zcela, úplný

functional /'fʌŋk.ʃᵊn.ᵊl/ funkční

gap /gæp/ mezera

gingival /dʒɪn'dʒaɪ.vᵊl/ dásňový

glass /glɑːs/ ionomer /aɪ'ɒn.ə.məʳ/ sklo ionomer

goal /gəʊl/ cíl

grade /greɪd/ stupeň

groove /gruːv/ rýha, žlábek

growth /grəʊθ/ růst

handle /'hæn.dl̩/ zacházet, rukojeť

headgear /'hed.gɪəʳ/ extraorálné kotvení, zevní tah

hold /həʊld/ držet

horizontal /ˌhɒr.ɪ'zɒn.tᵊl/ plane / pleɪn/ vodorovná plocha

hypothetical /ˌhaɪ.pə'θet.ɪ.kᵊl/ hypotetický

identify /aɪ'den.tɪ.faɪ/ identifikovat

implication /ˌɪm.plɪ'keɪ.ʃən/ důsledek

improve /ɪm'pruːv/ zlepšit

in situ /ˌɪn'sɪt.juː/ na místě

in /ɪn/ doubt /daʊt/ na pochybách, nejistý

inappropriate /ˌɪn.ə'prəʊ.pri.ət/ nevhodný, neúčelný

incisal /ɪn'sɪ.zᵊl/ řezný

incisor /ɪn'saɪ.zəʳ/ řezák

included /ɪn'kluː.dɪd/ obsažený, zahrnutý

incompetent /ɪn'kɒm.pɪ.tᵊnt/ slabý

index /'ɪn.deks/ (pl. indices /'ɪn. dɪ.siːz/)index, ukazatel, seznam

indicate/'ɪn.dɪ.keɪt/ indikovat, označit

individual /ˌɪn.dɪ'vɪd.ju.əl/ jednotlivec

initially /ɪ'nɪʃ.ᵊl.i/ z počátku

insertion /ɪn's3ː.ʃᵊn/ vložení

inside /ɪn'saɪd/ uvnitř

interference /ˌɪn.tə'fɪə.rᵊnts/ překážení, porucha

interspace /'ɪn.tə.speɪs/ mezera

intervention /ˌɪn.tə'ven.ʃᵊn/ zásah

intrusion /ɪn'truː.ʒᵊn/ intruse, vnikání, vtlačení

inventory /'ɪn.vᵊn.tri/ inventář (věcí)

involve /ɪn'vɒlv/ zahrnovat

irregularity /ɪˌreg.jə'lær.ə.ti/ nepravidelnost

joint /dʒɔɪnt/ kloub

label /'leɪ.bəl/ nálepka, označení

labial /'leɪ.bi.əl/ retný

later /'leɪ.təʳ/ později, pozdější

lateral /'læt.rəl/ postranní

lengthen /'leŋk.θən/ prodloužit

level /'lev.əl/ úroveň, hladina

lie /laɪ/ ležet

ligature /'lɪg.ə.tʃəʳ/ ligatura, podvázání

likely /'laɪ.kli/ pravděpodobně

limited /'lɪm.ɪ.tɪd/ omezený

lip /lɪp/ ret

long-term /ˌlɒŋ't3ːm/ dlouhodobý

look /lʊk/ vypadat

loss /lɒs/ ztráta

lower /'ləʊ.əʳ/ spodní

luting /luːt.ɪŋ/ upevnění, sevření, přitmelení, tmel

maintain /meɪn'teɪn/ udržet

malformed /ˌmæl'fɔːmd/ chybně vytvořený

malocclusion/ˌmæl.ə'kluː.ʒᵊn/ chybný skus

management /'mæn.ɪdʒ.mənt/ ovládání, řízení

mandible /'mæn.dɪ.bəl/ mandibula, dolní čelist

margin /'mɑː.dʒɪn/ okraj

mastication /ˌmæs.tɪ'keɪ.ʃᵊn/ žvýkání

masticatory /ˌmæs.tɪ'keɪ.tᵊr.i/ žvýkací

maxilla /mæ'ksɪ.lə/ maxilla, horní čelist

measure /'meʒ.əʳ/ měřit

measurement /'meʒ.ə.mənt/ opatření

medical /'med.ɪ.kᵊl/ history /'hɪs.tər.i/ lékařská anamnéza

merciless /'m3ː.sɪ.ləs/ nelítostný

merely /'mɪə.li/ pouze

mesiodens /ˌmiː.zɪə.'denz/ přespočetný zub, ve střední čáře horní čelisti

metal /'met.əl/ kov, kovový

midline /'mɪd.laɪn/ střednice

missing /'mɪs.ɪŋ/ chybějící

mixed /mɪkst/ smíchaný

model /'mɒd.əl/ model

modify /'mɒd.ɪ.faɪ/ upravit, modifikovat

monitor /'mɒn.ɪ.tər/ monitorovat, sledovat

movement /'muːv.mənt/ pohyb

multiple /'mʌl.tɪ.pl̩/ mnohačetný

muscle /'mʌs.l̩/ sval

muscular /'mʌs.kjʊ.lᵊr/ svalový

musculature /'mʌs.kjʊ.lə.tʃəʳ/ svalstvo

narrow /'nær.əʊ/ úzký

natural /'nætʃ.ᵊr.əl/ přirozený

numeric /njuː'mer.ɪk/ číselný

occlude /ə'kluːd/ uzavřít

occlusal /ɒkluː.zl/ skusový

occlusion /ə'kluː.ʒən/ skus, okluze

on /ɒn/ the part /pɑːt/ na straně (koho)

orthopantomograph /ˌɔːr.θoʊ'pæn.taʊ.mə.grɑːf/ panoramatický snímek

osteotomy /ˌɒs.ti'ɒ.tə.mi/ osteotomie, protětí kosti

outcome /'aʊt.kʌm/ výsledek

outside /ˌaʊt'saɪd/ vně

overbite /ˌəʊ.və.baɪt/ překus (vertikální)

overjet /'əʊ.və.dʒet/ předkus (horizontální)

pain /peɪn/ bolest

palatal /pæ.lə.tl/ patrový

parental /pə'ren.tᵊl/ rodičovský

particular /pə'tɪk.jʊ.ləʳ/ konkrétní

passive /'pæs.ɪv/ pasivní

pathology /pə'θɒl.ə.dʒi/ patologie, choroba

pattern /'pæt.ən/ vzor, model

payment /'peɪ.mənt/ platba

peer /pɪəʳ/ vrstevník

peg-shaped /peg.ʃeɪpt/ čípkovitý

percentage /pəˈsen.tɪdʒ/ procento

perforation /ˌpɜː.fʳrˈeɪ.ʃən/ proniknutí, propíchnutí

phase /feɪz/ fáze

plane /pleɪn/ rovina

pliers /ˈplaɪ.əz/ kleště, klíšťky, pinzeta

polycarboxylate /pɒl.i.kɑːˈbɒk.sɪl.eɪt/ polykarboxylát

position /pəˈzɪʃ.ən/ poloha,. místo, umístit

potential /pəʊˈten.tʃʳl/ potenciál, potenciální, možný, možnost

practitioner /prækˈtɪʃ.ʳn.ʳr/ praktický lékař

precise /prɪˈsaɪs/ přesný

present /ˈprez.ʳnt/ přítomný

present /prɪˈz.ent/ představit se

prevention /prɪˈventʃ.ʃən/ ochrana, prevence

previous /ˈpriː.vi.əs/ dosavadní, před, předešlý, předchozí, překotný

principally /ˈprɪntʃ.sɪ.pli/ hlavně

principle /ˈprɪntʃ.sɪ.pl̩/ zásada, princip

procline /prəʊˈklaɪn/ naklonit dopředu

progress /ˈprəʊ.gres/ pokrok, postup

prospective /prəˈspek.tɪv/ předpokládaný, případný

provoke /prəˈvəʊk/ vyvolat

pseudonym /ˈsuː.də.nɪm/ pseudonym

pull /pʊl/ táhnout

quadhelix /kwɒdˈhiː.lɪks/ čtvercová šroubovice

radiograph /reɪ.di.ə.grɑːf/ rentgenový snímek

random /ˈræn.dəm/ namátkou

range /reɪndʒ/ rozsah

rapid /ˈræp.ɪd/ rychlý

rate /reɪt/ rychlost

rather /ˈrɑː.ðəʳ/ than /ðən/ spíše než

rating /ˈreɪ.tɪŋ/ ohodnocení

record /ˈrek.ɔːd/ záznam

reduce /rɪˈdjuːs/ snížit, omezit

reduction /rɪˈdʌk.ʃən/ omezení

relapse /rɪˈlæps/ recidiva

relationship /rɪˈleɪ.ʃən.ʃɪp/ vztah, příbuzenství

reliable /rɪˈlaɪə.bl̩/ spolehlivý

rely /rɪˈlaɪ/ on /ɒn/ spolehnout se na

removable /rɪˈmuː.və.bl̩/ vyjímatelný

removal /rɪˈmuː.vʳl/ odstranění

remove /rɪˈmuːv/ odstranit, vyjmout

require /rɪˈkwaɪəʳ/ vyžadovat

requirement /rɪˈkwaɪə.mənt/ požadavek

resorption /rɪˈsɔːp.ʃən/ chřadnutí, vstřebání

response /rɪˈspɒntʃs/ reakce

resting /ˈrest.ɪŋ/ klidový

restricted /rɪˈstrɪk.tɪd/ omezený

retainer /rɪˈteɪ.nəʳ/ napínač, držák, retenční přístroj

retention /rɪˈten.tʃən/ zadržení

retract /rɪˈtrækt/ stáhnout

retractor /rɪˈtræk.təʳ/ retraktor, háček, držák

retrocline /ˌret.rəʊˈklaɪn/ naklonit dozadu

reveal /rɪˈviːl/ odhalit

reverse /rɪˈvɜːs/ obrácený

review /rɪˈvjuː/ prohlédnout opět, překontrolování

revise /rɪˈvaɪz/ zopakovat

rotation /rəʊˈteɪ.ʃən/ rotace, otočení

ruler /ˈruː.ləʳ/ měřítko, pravítko

same /seɪm/ tentýž

scope /skəʊp/ rozsah

screw /skruː/ spirála, šroubek, šroubovat

seal /siːl/ utěsnění

seat /siːt/ dosedat

segment /ˈseg.mənt/ úsek, segment

selective /sɪˈlek.tɪv/ výběrový

self-esteem /ˌself.ɪˈstiːm/ sebe-ocenění

separate /ˈsep.ᵊr.ət/ oddělený

sequence /ˈsiː.kwənts/ pořadí, postup

severe /sɪˈvɪəʳ/ závažný

shorten /ˈʃɔː.tᵊn/ zkrátit

sibling /ˈsɪb.lɪŋ/ vrstevník, sourozenec

single /ˈsɪŋ.gl̩/ jediný

size /saɪz/ velikost

skeletal /ˈskel.ɪ.tᵊl/ kosterní

skull /skʌl/ lebka

slight /slaɪt/ mírný

slope /sləʊp/ sklánět se, naklonění

snack /snæk/ svačit, pojídat malá jídla

social /ˈsəʊ.ʃᵊl/ history /ˈhɪs.tər.i/ sociální anamnéza

soon /suːn/ dříve, brzy

source /sɔːs/ zdroj

space /speɪs/ maintainer /meɪnˈteɪn.əʳ/ mezerník

speech /spiːtʃ/ řeč

spontaneous /spɒnˈteɪ.ni.əs/ spontánní

spring /sprɪŋ/ pero, pružina

stable /ˈsteɪ.bl̩/ stabilní, stálý

stagnation /stægˈneɪ.ʃᵊn/ stagnace, váznutí

stainless /ˌsteɪn.ləs/ nerezavící

steel /stiːl/ ocel

sticky /ˈstɪk.i/ lepkavý

store /stɔːʳ/ uložit

stress /stres/ namáhat, tlačit

study /ˈstʌd.i/ studijní

submit /səbˈmɪt/ předložit

suck /sʌk/ cucat, sát

sufficient /səˈfɪʃ.ᵊnt/ dostatečný

supernumerary /ˌsuː.pəˈnjuː.mᵊr.ᵊr.i/ nadpočetný

support /səˈpɔːt/ podporovat

surface /ˈsɜː.fɪs/ povrch

surgery /ˈsɜː.dʒᵊr.i/ ordinace, chirurgie

surgically /ˈsɜː.dʒɪ.kli/ chirurgicky

susceptibility /səˌsep.tɪˈbɪl.ɪ.ti/ náchylnost, vnímavost

suspected /səˈspek.tɪd/ předpokládaný

sweets /swiːts/ sladkosti

take /teɪk/ account /əˈkaʊnt/ of /əv/ počítat s (čím), přihlížet (k)

tease /tiːz/ škádlit

temporomandibular /ˌtem. pər.ə.mænˈdɪ.bjʊ.ləʳ/ temporomandibulární

thoroughly /ˈθʌr.ə.li/ důkladně

thumb /θʌm/ palec

thus /ðʌs/ takto, tudíž

tie /taɪ/ svázat, zavázat

time /taɪm/ doba

tip /tɪp/ hrot, špička, naklonit, sklopit

tissue /ˈtɪʃ.uː/, /ˈtɪs.juː/ tkáň

trap /træp/ zachycovat

trauma /ˈtrɔː.mə/, /ˈtraʊ-/ trauma, úraz

tray /treɪ/ tác

try /traɪ/ zkusit

undergo /ˌʌn.dəˈgəʊ/ podstoupit

underlying /ˌʌn.dəˈlaɪ.ɪŋ/ ležící pod, základní

unerupted /ʌn.ɪrˈʌp.tᵊd/ neprořezaný

unexpected /ˌʌn.ɪkˈspek.tɪd/ neočekávaný

unfavourable /ʌnˈfeɪ.vᵊr.ə.bl̩/ nepříznivý

unstable /ʌnˈsteɪ.bl̩/ nestálý

unsuccessful /ˌʌn.səkˈses.fᵊl/ neúspěšný

upright /ˈʌp.raɪt/ vzpřímený

utilise /ˈjuː.tɪ.laɪz/ využít

validate /ˈvæl.ɪ.deɪt/ uznat platnost, schválit

value /ˈvæl.juː/ hodnota, ocenit

vanity /ˈvæn.ɪ.ti/ marnivost

vertical /ˈvɜː.tɪ.kᵊl/ vertikální, kolmý

wear /weəʳ/ nosit na sobě

weekly /ˈwiː.kli/ týdně

well timed /ˌwelˈtaɪmd/ dobře
    načasovaný
whatever /wɒtˈev.əʳ/ kterýkoliv
wire /waɪəʳ/ drát
womb /wuːm/ děloha

work /wɜːk/ fungovat
worn /wɔːn/ opotřebovaný
zinc /zɪŋk/ phosphate /ˈfɒs.feɪt/
    fosforečnan zinečnatý

Unit 16

Text 1

Treatment Planning

Obtaining a comprehensive history is critical to prescription of appropriate prosthodontic treatment (patient's complaint, denture history, general dental history, medical history, social history).

Diagnosis in edentulous patients

Good denture wearers require replacement because they are worn, lost, broken, aesthetically poor, or loose.

Good denture wearers with poor denture—their present denture has a major fault.

Poor denture wearers who, if provided with very well designed and constructed dentures, may tolerate their dentures, often have different dentists, never being totally satisfied.

Poor denture wearers who do not tolerate dentures despite their very well design and construction.

Changes Following Extraction of Teeth

facial changes

intraoral changes

psychological changes – some patients find edentulousness difficult to accept, perhaps as a sign of growing old. Consequently, some patients despise the thought of dentures and require careful management.

Complete Dentures

Features—these comprise good retention, good support, good muscle balance, good occlusal balance, and stability.

retention is the resistance to displacement of a denture away from the ridge

support is the resistance of vertical movement of a denture towards the ridge

muscle balance is achieved when the muscular forces of tongue, lips, and cheeks do not dislodge a denture

232

during functional movements of the mouth with the teeth out of contact
occlusal balance is achieved when the forces of one denture on another do not dislodge either denture during functional jaw movements with the teeth in contact
stability is the ability of a denture to resist displacement by functional stresses

Stages in complete denture construction are examination, diagnosis, and treatment plan.
primary impressions
master impressions
jaw registration
trial of teeth
insertion of prosthesis
review

Common denture problems:
inadequate support, inadequate retention, muscle balance problem, occlusal problem, appearance problems, speech problems, retching, acrylic allergy

Exercise 1
What is important for right treatment planning?
How are edentulous patients diagnosed?
Talk about changes following extraction of teeth.
Describe the features of complete dentures and stages in their construction.
Which are the common denture problems?

Translation 1
Získání komplexní anamnézy, předepsání vhodné protetické léčby, pacientovy obtíže, vývoj změn protézy, dentální anamnéza, lékařská anamnéza, sociální anamnéza, diagnóza u bezzubého pacienta, protézy opotřebované, ztracené, rozbité, esteticky slabé, uvolněné, mají velkou vadu, poskytnout dobře navržené a konstruované protézy, tolerovat protézy, být spokojen, změny po extrakci, obličejové, uvnitř úst, psychologické, charakteristické znaky úplných protéz, dobrá retence, podpora, svalová rovnováha, okluzní rovnováha a stabilita, retence, odolnost vůči posunutí protézy od okraje, podpora, odolnost proti kolmému posunutí, svalová rovnováha, síly jazyka, rtů a tváří, nepohybují protézou, okluzní rovnováha, síla jedné protézy na druhou protézu neposunuje ani jednu z nich, zuby v kontaktu, stabilita, schopnost protézy odolat posunování způsobenému funkčními tlaky, stádia konstrukce úplné protézy, vyšetření, diagnóza, plán léčby, prvotní otisky, hlavní otisky, registrace čelistí, zkouška zubů, vložení protézy, opětovná prohlídka, běžné problémy s protézami, nedostatečná podpora, nedostatečná retence, problém se svalovou rovnováhou, problém skusu, vzhledu, řeči, mimovolný pocit na zvracení, alergie na akrylát.

Text 2
Partial Dentures
A partial denture is a prosthesis which replaces one or more but less than all of the natural teeth and is removable by the patient.

Precision Attachments
Precision attachments are used in removable prosthetics to provide additional retention. Consider only in well-motivated patients with good oral hygiene and controlled caries.

Copy Dentures
Copy dentures (also known as replica dentures) are a method of producing replacement dentures that are similar in shape and dimension to the patient's existing dentures.

Overdentures
An overdenture is a prosthesis that gains support from one or more abutment teeth by enclosing them beneath its fitting surface.

Care of abutments:
tooth brushing with a **fluoride-containing toothpaste**
denture hygiene, including **removal of prosthesis at night**
self-application of **topical fluoride**
dietary advice regarding reduction of sugar in diet
frequent **recall visits** to check status of abutment teeth

Immediate Dentures
An immediate denture is a prosthesis used to replace one or more teeth and inserted on the day of extraction of the tooth or teeth.

Other Prosthetic Appliances
gingival veneers, useful to mask recession following periodontal disease
palatal lift appliances, used to improve speech
gumshields are an essential feature of trauma protection in contact sports
antisnoring appliances, may be useful in reducing snoring
mouthpieces for diving and wind instrument playing, highly specialised appliances but essential for these activities

Repairs, Relines, and Additions
repairs – denture fractures are quite common. If persistent denture fracture occurs, re-evaluate the treatment plan. Often a replacement denture of a different design is common.
relines – a reline of a denture involves placing new material on the fitting surface.
additions – describes the placing of an additional tooth or part of a denture to an existing prosthesis.

Exercise 2

Give the main features of partial dentures, precision attachments, copy dentures, and overdentures.
Describe principles of good care of abutments.
Talk about other prosthetic appliances and their use.
What are repairs, relines, and additions?

Translation 2

Částečné protézy nahrazují jeden nebo více přirozených zubů a jsou vyjímatelné pacientem, přesné upevnění, poskytnout dodatečné upevnění, kopie zubních protéz, repliky, podobné tvarem a rozměry, hybridní protézy získávají podporu z pilířových zubů, péče o pilířové zuby, čistění pastou obsahující fluorid, hygiena protézy, vyjmutí protézy na noc, místní aplikace fluoridu, omezení cukru, časté kontrolní návštěvy, okamžité protézy, vložené v den extrakce, protetická zařízení, obložení dásní, maskovat ústup dásně po onemocnění parodontu, zařízení k zvednutí patra, zlepšit řeč, chrániče dásní, ochrana před úrazem při kontaktních sportech, náustky pro potápění, hraní na dechové nástroje, opravy, zlomení protézy je docela běžné, nahrazení protézou odlišného designu, podložení vnitřní strany protézy, umístění nového materiálu k přiléhajícímu povrchu, dodatky, umístění dalšího zubu nebo části protézy na existující protézu.

Text 3
Craniomandibular Disorders
Craniomandibular disorders are a range of musculoskeletal disorders affecting the temporomandibular joint complex. Pain history is most important. Features often include **pain on waking**, pain **radiating** to temporal region of head. Pain is often **chronic** and **recurrent**.
Symptoms and signs:
pain on function
limited jaw **opening**
audible joint **click**
signs of tooth wear or denture **wear**

Management options
patient education and palliative home care – this involves patient reassurance, avoidance of heavy mastication, yawning, sighing, singing, object biting, home therapeutic exercises, application of heat or cold by patients to muscle
behaviour modification – by methods such as progressive relaxation, hypnosis, lifestyle counselling, and biofeedback
drug therapy – this may relieve symptoms by reducing pain, inflammation, muscle hyperactivity, anxiety, and depression
exercise therapy – repetitive exercises, isotonic exercises, isometric exercises
mobilisation – repeated joint manipulation
physical therapy (electrotherapy, ultrasound, vapocoolants, local anaesthetic injections, acupuncture
splint therapy – stabilisation splints, repositioning splints, provisional splints
occlusal therapy – this should be considered only by a specialist practitioner
other therapy – include acupuncture, orthodontics, orthognathic surgery, and joint surgery

With the vast range of potential management options available CMD can appear most confusing. In general, patient education and home care is a useful start, with perhaps progression to stabilisation splints. In cases that do not respond to these treatment modalities, specialist help should be sought.

Implant-Borne Prostheses
Osseointegrated titanium implants are most common.
Uses of implants:
complete **overdentures**

full arch fixed **bridges**
partial fixed bridges
partial overdentures
single tooth replacement
orbital, nasal, auricular, and hearing aid prostheses

Osseointegration is a **direct structural and functional connection** between ordered, **living bone,** and the surface of a load-carrying **implant**. Osseointegrated implants are not a panacea. They are a well-recognised form of prosthetic rehabilitation which is of great benefit in individuals with poor neuromuscular control and retention difficulties. Implants are costly and complex, and good case selection is absolutely critical to success.

Advice to Patients
Patients should usually be informed of the following:
Coping with new dentures - to get used to new dentures they should be worn as much as possible. Dentures should not be worn overnight.
Eating with new dentures - initially food should be cut into small pieces. Food often goes under the denture at first. The patient should attempt to chew on both sides at the same time.
Speaking with new dentures - speech is often a little difficult for the first few days. This usually improves relatively quickly.
Discomfort with new dentures - it is quite normal to experience some discomfort after the dentures are fitted. If the discomfort is minor, the patient should persevere with it until he or she sees the dentist again.

Exercise 3

Talk about craniomandibular disorders: features, symptoms, and signs.
Talk about management options in craniomandibular disorders.
Which are the uses of titanium implants?
What is osseointegration?
What would be your advice concerning new dentures?

Translation 3

Kraniomandibulární poruchy, muskuloskeletální poruchy, postihující temporomandibulární kloub, bolest při probouzení, bolest vystřelující do spánkové oblasti, chronická, vracející se, omezené otevření úst, slyšitelné lupnutí kloubu, známky opotřebení zubů, protéz, útěcha pacienta, vyloučení namáhavého žvýkání, zívání, vzdychání, zpívání, okusování předmětů, domácí léčebná cvičení, aplikace tepla či chladu na sval, modifikace chování, postupná relaxace, hypnóza, poradenství o životním stylu, biologická zpětná vazba, léková terapie, snížení bolesti, zánětu, nadměrné aktivity svalů, úzkosti, deprese, léčba cvičením, manipulace s kloubem, cvičení opakovaná, izotonická, izometrická, elektroléčba, ultrazvuk, akupunktura, léčba pomocí dlah, ortodoncie, ortognátní chirurgie, protézy nesené implantátem, titanové implantáty vhojené do kosti, hybridní protézy úplné, částečné, pevné můstky, náhrada jednotlivých zubů, protézy očnicové, nosní, boltcové, sluchových pomůcek, vhojení do kosti, přímé strukturální a funkční spojení mezi živou kostí a implantátem, implantáty

jsou nákladné a složité, ale mohou
být velkým přínosem u některých
jednotlivců, zacházení s novými
protézami,
zvyknout si na nové protézy, nenosit
přes noc, nakrájet jídlo na malé kousky,
žvýkat na obou stranách současně, řeč
je často trochu obtížná prvních několik
dnů, nepohodlí u nových protéz je
docela normální, je-li nepohodlí malé,
pacient by je měl vydržet do další
návštěvy zubního lékaře.

Vocabulary

achieve /əˈtʃiːv/ dosáhnout
acrylic /əˈkrɪl.ɪk/ akrylový,
　pryskyřičný
acupuncture /ˈæk.jʊ.pʌŋk.tʃəʳ/
　akupunktura
addition /əˈdɪʃ.ᵊn/ dodatek
additional /əˈdɪʃ.ən.əl/ dodatečný,
　další, doplňkový
advice /ˈæd.vɜːs/ rada
aesthetically /esˈθet.ɪ.kli/ esteticky
affect /əˈfekt/ ovlivnit
aid /eɪd/ pomůcka
allergy /ˈæl.ə.dʒi/ alergie
anti- /æn.ti-/ proti
appear /əˈpɪəʳ/ objevit se
appliance /əˈplaɪ.ənts/ zařízení, aparát
application /ˌæp.lɪˈkeɪ.ʃən/ aplikace
appropriate /əˈprəʊ.pri.ət/ vhodný
arch /ɑːtʃ/ oblouk, klenout
at /ət/ **the same** /seɪm/ **time** /taɪm/
　současně
attachment /əˈtætʃ.mənt/ attachment,
　připojení
attempt /əˈtempt/ pokoušet se
audible /ˈɔː.dɪ.bl̩/ slyšitelný
auricular /ɔːˈrɪ.kjʊ.ləʳ/ ušní, boltcovitý
avoidance /əˈvɔɪ.dənts/ vyvarování se
away /əˈweɪ/ **from** /frɒm/ pryč od

balance /ˈbæl.ənts/ rovnováha
behaviour /bɪˈheɪ.vjər/ chování
beneath /bɪˈniːθ/ pod
benefit /ˈben.ɪ.fɪt/ prospěch, užitek
bio- /baɪ.əʊ-/ **feedback** /ˈfiːd.bæk/
　biologická zpětná vazba
biting /baɪ.tɪŋ/ kousání
bone /bəʊn/ kost
borne /bɔː.ʳn/ nesený
both /bəʊθ/ oba
broken /brəʊ.kᵊn/ zlomený, rozbitý
careful /ˈkeə.fəl/ pečlivý, opatrný
caries /ˈkeə.riːz/ kaz
case /keɪs/ případ
cavernous /ˈkæv.ən.əs/ porézní,
　sklípkový
check /tʃek/ kontrolovat
cheek /tʃiːk/ tvář
chew /tʃuː/ žvýkat
chronic /ˈkrɒn.ɪk/ chronický
click /klɪk/ kliknutí, klapnutí
cold /kəʊld/ chlad, studený
common /ˈkɒm.ən/ běžný
complaint /kəmˈpleɪnt/ stížnost
complete /kəmˈpliːt/ úplný
complex /ˈkɒm.pleks/ komplex,
　složitý
comprehensive /ˌkɒm.prɪˈhent.sɪv/
　komplexní, obsáhlý
comprise /kəmˈpraɪz/ zahrnovat,
　obsahovat
confusing /kənˈfjuː.zɪŋ/ matoucí
connection /kəˈnek.ʃən/ spojení
consequently /ˈkɒnt.sɪ.kwənt.li/
　následně
consider /kənˈsɪd.əʳ/ uvážit
construct /kənˈstrʌkt/ vytvořit,
　sestavit
construction /kənˈstrʌk.ʃən/
　konstrukce
contain /kənˈteɪn/ obsahovat
control /kənˈtrəʊl/ kontrolovat, řídit

237

cope /kəʊp/ zvládnout

copy /ˈkɒp.i/ kopie

costly /ˈkɒst.li/ nákladný

counselling /ˈkaʊnt.səl.ɪŋ/
poradenství

craniomandibular/
ˈkreɪ.ni.əˌmæn.ˈdɪ.bjʊ.ləʳ/
kraniomandibulární, týkající se
lebky a dolní čelisti

critical /ˈkrɪt.ɪ.kᵊl/ kritický, velmi
důležitý

denture /ˈden.tʃə/ zubní náhrada

depression /dɪˈpreʃ.ən/ deprese

design /dɪˈzaɪn/ návrh

despise /dɪˈspaɪz/ ignorovat,
opovrhovat

despite /dɪˈspaɪt/ navzdory

diagnosis /ˌdaɪ.əgˈnəʊ.sɪs/ diagnóza

dietary /ˈdaɪ.ə.tər.i/ dietní

difficulty /ˈdɪf.ɪ.kəl.ti/ obtíž

dimension /ˌdaɪˈmen.tʃᵊn/ rozměr

direct /daɪˈrekt/ přímý

discharge /dɪsˈtʃɑːdʒ/ výtok

discomfort /dɪˈskʌmp.fət/ nepohoda

disease /dɪˈziːz/ nemoc

dislodge /dɪˈslɒdʒ/ vypudit, vyplavit,
vyjmout, přemístit, pohybovat se

disorder /dɪˈsɔː.dəʳ/ porucha (zdraví)

displacement /dɪˈspleɪs.mənt/
posunutí

diving /ˈdaɪ.vɪŋ/ potápění

eat /iːt/ jíst

edentulous /əˈden.tju.ləs/ bez zubů,
bezzubý

edentulousness /əˈden.tju.ləs.nəs/
bezzubost

electrotherapy /ɪˌlek.trəʊˈθer.ə.pi/
elektroléčba

enclose /ɪnˈkləʊz/ uzavřít

essential /ɪˈsen.tʃəl/ základní, důležitý

examination /ɪgˌzæm.ɪˈneɪ.ʃᵊn/
vyšetření

exercise /ˈek.sə.saɪz/ cvičení

experience /ɪkˈspɪə.ri.ᵊnts/ prožívat

extraction /ɪkˈstræk.ʃən/ extrakce,
vytržení

facial /ˈfeɪ.ʃᵊl/ obličejový

fault /fɒlt/ vada, chyba

feature /ˈfiː.tʃəʳ/ rys, znak

fit /fɪt/ upevnit

fitting /ˈfɪt.ɪŋ/ přiléhající

fixed /fɪkst/ bridge /brɪdʒ/ pevný
můstek

fluoride /ˈflʊə.raɪd/ fluorid, s
fluoridem

following /ˈfɒl.əʊ.ɪŋ/ následující

force /fɔːs/ síla

fracture /ˈfræk.tʃəʳ/ fraktura,
zlomenina

frequent /ˈfriː.kwənt/ častý

full /fʊl/ plný, úplný

function /ˈfʌŋk.ʃᵊn/ funkce, fungování

functional /ˈfʌŋk.ʃn.ᵊl/ funkční

gain /geɪn/ získat

general /ˈdʒen.ᵊr.ᵊl/ celkový

get /get/ used /juːst/ to /tʊ/ zvyknout
si na

gingival /ˌdʒɪn.dʒɪ.val/ gingivální,
dásňový

growing /ˈgrəʊ.ɪŋ/ old /əʊld/ stárnutí

gumshield /gʌm.ʃiːld/ ochrana zubů
(boxera)

hearing /ˈhɪə.rɪŋ/ sluch

heat /hiːt/ teplo

heavy /ˈhev.i/ obtížný

history /ˈhɪs.tᵊr.i/ anamnéza, vývoj
změn

home /həʊm/ care /keəʳ/ domácí péče

hygiene /ˈhaɪ.dʒiːn/ hygiena,
zdravověda

hyper-/ˈhaɪ.pəʳ-/ activity /ækˈtɪv.ɪ.ti/
nadměrná aktivita

hypnosis /hɪpˈnəʊ.sɪs/ hypnóza

immediate /ɪˈmiː.di.ət/ okamžitý

implant /ɪmˈplɑːnt/ implantát

impression /ɪmˈpreʃ.ən/ otisk

improve /ɪmˈpruːv/ zlepšit

in /ɪn/ general /ˈdʒen.ər.əl/ všeobecně

inadequate /ɪˈnæd.ɪ.kwət/ nepřiměřený

individual /ˌɪn.dɪˈvɪd.ju.əl/ jednotlivec

inflammation /ˌɪn.fləˈmeɪ.ʃᵊn/ zánět

initially /ɪˈnɪʃ.əl.i/ zpočátku

injection /ɪnˈdʒek.ʃᵊn/ injekce

input /ˈɪn.pʊt/ přísun, vstup

insertion /ɪnˈsɜː.ʃᵊn/ vložení

intraoral /ɪn.trəˈɔː.rəl/ intraorální, uvnitř úst

involve /ɪnˈvɒlv/ zahrnovat

isometric /aɪ.səʊ ˈmet.rɪk/ izometrický, mající stejné rozměry

isotonic /aɪ.səʊ ˈtɒn.ɪk/ izotonický, se stejným osmotickým tlakem

jaw /dʒɔː/ čelist

joint /dʒɔɪnt/ kloub

less /les/ than /ðən/ méně než

lifestyle /ˈlaɪf.staɪl/ životní styl

lift /lɪft/ zvednutí

limit /ˈlɪm.ɪt/ omezit

lip /lɪp/ ret

living /ˈlɪv.ɪŋ/ živý

load-carrying /ləʊd.kær.i.ɪŋ/ nesoucí váhu

local /ˈləʊ.kəl/ anaesthetic / ˌæn.əsˈθet.ɪk/ místní anestetikum

loose /luːs/ uvolněný, viklající se

lost /lɒst/ ztracený

major /ˈmeɪ.dʒəʳ/ velký, důležitý

management /ˈmæn.ɪdʒ.mənt/ péče, snaha o zvládnutí

manipulation /məˌnɪp.juˈleɪ.ʃᵊn/ manipulace

mask /mɑːsk/ zakrýt

master /ˈmɑː.stəʳ/ hlavní, originální

mastication /ˌmæs.tɪˈkeɪ.ʃᵊn/ mastikace, žvýkání

medical /ˈmed.ɪ.kᵊl/ history /ˈhɪs.tər.i/ lékařská anamnéza

mobilisation /ˌməʊ.bɪ.lɑ ɪˈzeɪ.ʃᵊn/ uvolnění

modification /ˌmɒd.ɪ.fɪˈkeɪ.ʃᵊn/ modifikace, obměna

mouthpiece /ˈmaʊθ.piːs/ náustek

movement /ˈmuːv.mənt/ pohyb

muscle /ˈmʌs.l̩/ sval

musculoskeletal /ˈmʌs.kjʊ. ləˈskel.ɪ.tᵊl/ muskuloskeletární, skládající se ze svalů a kostí

nasal /ˈneɪ.zəl/ nosní

natural /ˈnætʃ.ᵊr.ᵊl/ přírodní

neuromuscular /ˌnjʊəˈrə.mæsk.jʊ.ləʳ/ neuromuskulární, nervosvalový

object /ˈɒb.dʒɪkt/ předmět

obtain /əbˈteɪn/ získat, dostat (obdržet)

occlusal /ɒklʊː.zl/ okluzní

on /ɒn/ waking /ˈweɪ.kɪŋ/ při probuzení

opening /ˈəʊ.pᵊn.ɪŋ/ otevření

option /ˈɒp.ʃən/ volba

orbital /ˈɔː.bɪ.tᵊl/ orbitální, očnicový

ordered /ˈɔː.dəd/ napravovaný

orthodontics /ˌɔː.θəʊ ˈdɒn.tɪks/ ortodoncie

orthognathic /ˌɔː.θəʊ.ˈnæː.θɪk/ ortognátní, správný skus

osseointegration /ɒs.i.əˌɪn.tɪˈgreɪ.ʃᵊn/ vhojení do kosti

out /aʊt/ of /əv/ bez

overdentures /ˈəʊ.və.ˈden.t ʃəz/ hybridní protézy

overnight /ˌəʊ.vəˈnaɪt/ přes noc

palatal /ˈpæ.lə.tl/ patrový

palliative /ˈpæl.i.ə.tɪv/ paliativní, utišující

panacea /ˌpæn.əˈsiː.ə/ všelék (univerzální lék)

part /pɑːt/ část

partial /ˈpɑː.ʃᵊl/ částečný

239

periodontal /ˌper.i.əˈdɒn.tl/ periodontální

persevere /ˌpɜː.sɪˈvɪəʳ/ vytrvat

persistent /pəˈsɪs.tᵊnt/ ustavičný, neustálý

physical /ˈfɪz.ɪ.kᵊl/ fyzikální

piece /piːs/ kousek

place /pleɪs/ umístit

poor /pɔːʳ/ chybný, špatný

potential /pəʊˈten.tʃᵊl/ možný, potenciální

precision /prɪˈsɪʒ.ᵊn/ **attachment** / əˈtætʃ.mənt/ přesné upevnění

prescription /prɪˈskrɪp.ʃᵊn/ lékařský předpis

present /ˈprez.ᵊnt/ přítomný

primary /ˈpraɪ.mə.ri/ prvotní, primární

produce /prəˈdjuːs/ vytvářet, produkovat

progression /prəˈgreʃ.ᵊn/ pokrok, postup

progressive /prəˈgres.ɪv/ postupný

prosthesis /ˈprɒs.θiː.sɪs/ (pl. **prostheses**) protéza, náhrada

prosthodontics /ˌprɒs.θəˈdɒnt.ɪks/ protetická stomatologie

protection /prəˈtek.ʃᵊn/ ochrana

provide /prəˈvaɪd/ poskytovat

provisional /prəˈvɪʒ.ᵊn.ᵊl/ provizorní, dočasný, prozatímní

psychological /ˌsaɪ.kᵊlˈɒdʒ.ɪ.kᵊl/ psychologický

radiate /ˈreɪ.di.eɪt/ vyzařovat

range /reɪndʒ/ rozsah, řada

reassurance /ˌriː.əˈʃɔː.rənts/ uklidnění, útěcha

recall /rɪˈkɔːl/ opětné pozvání pacienta

recession /rɪˈseʃ.ᵊn/ odstoupení, ústup

recognise /ˈrek.əg.naɪz/ rozpoznat

recurrent /rɪˈkʌr.ᵊnt/ opakující se

reduce /rɪˈdjuːs/ snížit, zmenšit

reduction /rɪˈdʌk.ʃᵊn/ snížení

re-evaluate /ˌriː.ɪˈvæl.ju.eɪt/ přehodnotit

regarding /rɪˈgɑː.dɪŋ/ týkající se, s ohledem na

registration /ˌredʒ.ɪˈstreɪ.ʃᵊn/ registrace

rehabilitation /ˌriː.həˌbɪl.ɪˈteɪ.ʃᵊn/ rehabilitace

relaxation /ˌriː.lækˈseɪ.ʃᵊn/ uvolnění

relieve /rɪˈliːv/ vykrýt, ulevit

reline /riːˈlaɪn/ podložit vnitřní stranu protézy

removable /rɪˈmuː.və.bl̩/ snímatelný

repair /rɪˈpeəʳ/ oprava

repeat /rɪˈpiːt/ opakovat

repetitive /rɪˈpet.ə.tɪv/ opakovaný, opakující se

replace /rɪˈpleɪs/ dát zpět

replacement /rɪˈpleɪs.mənt/ znovudosazení, nahrazení

replica /ˈrep.lɪ.kə/ replika, duplikát

reposition /rɪ.pəˈzɪʃ.ən/ repozice, nové upevnění

resist /rɪˈzɪst/ odolat

resistance /rɪˈzɪs.tᵊnts/ odolnost

respond /rɪˈspɒnd/ reagovat (odpovídat)

retch /retʃ/ říhat, mít mimovolní pocit na zvracení

review /rɪˈvjuː/ prohlédnout opět

ridge /rɪdʒ/ okraj, lišta, rýha, hřeben

satisfied /ˈsæt.ɪs.faɪd/ spokojený

selection /sɪˈlek.ʃᵊn/ výběr

self-/self/ sebe

shape /ʃeɪp/ tvar

side /saɪd/ strana

sigh /saɪ/ vzdychat, naříkat

sign /saɪn/ znak, příznak

similar /ˈsɪm.ɪ.lər/ podobný

singing /ˈsɪŋ.ɪŋ/ zpívání

single /ˈsɪŋ.gl̩/ jediný

snore /snɔːʳ/ chrápat

social /ˈsəʊ.ʃəl/ history /ˈhɪs.tər.i/ sociální anamnéza

speaking /spiː.kɪŋ/ mluvení

specialised /ˈspeʃ.əl.aɪzd/ specializovaný

speech /spiːtʃ/ řeč

splint /splɪnt/ dlaha, klínek, štěpina

stability /stəˈbɪl.ɪ.ti/ stabilita

stabilization /ˌsteɪ.bɪ.laɪˈzeɪ.ʃən/ stabilizace

stable /ˈsteɪ.bl̩/ stabilní, stálý

stage /steɪdʒ/ stádium, stupeň

stress /stres/ tlak, stlačení

structural /ˈstrʌk.tʃər.əl/ strukturální

success /səkˈses/ úspěch

support /səˈpɔːt/ podpora

surface /ˈsɜː.fɪs/ povrch, plocha

surgery /ˈsɜː.dʒər.i/ chirurgie

symptom /ˈsɪmp.təm/ symptom

temporal /ˈtem.pər.əl/ temporální, skráňový (na spáncích)

temporomandibular /ˌtem.pər.ə.mænˈdɪ.bjʊ.ləʳ/ joint /dʒɔɪnt/ kloub spánkový a dolní čelisti

therapeutic /ˌθer.əˈpjuː.tɪk/ terapeutický (léčebný), lék

therapy /ˈθer.ə.pi/ terapie, léčba

thought /θɔːt/ myšlenka

titanium /tɪˈteɪ.ni.əm/ titan

tolerate /ˈtɒl.ər.eɪt/ tolerovat

tongue /tʌŋ/ jazyk, špice

topical /ˈtɒp.ɪ.kəl/ místní

totally /ˈtəʊ.təl.i/ úplně

trauma /ˈtrɔː.mə/, /ˈtraʊ-/ trauma, úraz

treatment /ˈtriːt.mənt/ modality / məˈdæl.ə.ti/ varianta léčby

trial /traɪəl/ zkouška

ultrasound /ˈʌl.trə.saʊnd/ ultrazvukový, sonogram

useful /ˈjuːs.fəl/ užitečný

vapocoolant /ˈveɪ.pə.ˈkuː.lənt/ chladicí prostředek s použitím odpařování

vast /vɑːst/ rozsáhlý

veneer /vəˈnɪəʳ/ obložení

vertical /ˈvɜː.tɪ.kəl/ vertikální, kolmý

wear /weəʳ/ nosit na sobě, oblékat si

wearer /weə.rəʳ/ nositel, kdo nosí

wind /wɪnd/ instrument / ˈɪn.strə.mənt/ dechový nástroj

worn /wɔːn/ opotřebovaný

yawning /ˈjɔː.nɪŋ/ zívání

Unit 17

Dental Materials and Conservation Instruments

Properties of Materials. Dental Amalgam. Resin Composites. Glass Ionomers. Cermets, Resin-Modified Glass Ionomers, and Similar Materials. Adhesion and Bonding Agents. Luting Cements, Linings, and Bases. Temporary Cements and Restorations. Impression Materials. Porcelain and Ceramics. Casting and Wrought Alloys. Denture Base Material. Polymer Denture Base Materials. Endodontic Materials. Implant Materials. Waxes. Fissure Sealants. Periodontal Materials. Investment Materials. Temporary Crown Materials. Materials and Principles of Cavity Design.

Text 1

Properties of Materials

Dental materials can also be defined by their molecular form: **metals, polymers, ceramics, and composites**.

The properties of dental materials can be classified as:

mechanical (e.g. strength, stress, strain, elastic deformation, plastic deformation, brittleness, ductility, hardness, fatigue)

physical (e.g. thermal expansion, electrical conductivity, thermal conductivity, radiopacity, optical properties)

chemical (e.g. corrosion, solubility, formation of oxide layer)

biocompatibility (ideally dental materials should produce no adverse effects on the oral tissues)

Dental amalgam is an alloy of mercury with silver and tin.

Basic properties:

very strong restorative material

composite nature

corrodes

brittle

no adhesion to enamel or dentine

dimensional changes on setting

cheap

simple to use

some concerns about biocompatibility and toxicity

creeps

much higher thermal conductivity than tooth tissue

similar proportional limit to enamel

double the thermal expansion of tooth

Resin composites are based on BIS-GMA resin and glass fillers.

Basic properties:

no inherent adhesion to enamel or dentine
tensile and compressive strength comparable to tooth
lower elastic modulus than tooth
higher thermal expansion and contraction than tooth
cheap
curing shrinkage

Glass Ionomers
Basic properties:
hard and brittle
chemical adhesion to tooth (adversely affected by salivary contamination)
susceptible to erosion in first few minutes
increase in surface roughness in mouth over time
low translucency (aesthetics not as good as composite)
low abrasion wear resistance
release fluoride ions (some anticariogenic effect)
biocompatible

Cermets, Resin-Modified Glass Ionomers, and Similar Materials
A cermet is a ceramic metal glass. Cermets were developed to combat the wear resistance problems of glass ionomers by reinforcing them with metal.

Adhesion and Bonding Agents
Adhesion occurs when two surfaces are held together by interfacial forces; these can be molecular attraction or mechanical forces.

Luting Cements, Linings, and Bases
Luting cements are setting pastes which retain indirect restorations in tooth.

Linings provide a bland thermal barrier.
Bases provide a strong barrier, structural lining.
They are used to give a thermal, mechanical, and chemical barrier to dentine and be compatible.

Temporary Cements and Restorations
Cements must be strong enough for short-term retention of a restoration but weak enough for easy removal. Restorations must be bland, withstand occlusal forces for several weeks, easy to remove, and have low thermal conductivity.

Impression materials are classified as rigid, elastic, hydrocolloids, elastomeric.
Impression materials should be:
accurate
dimensionally stable
biocompatible
easy to mix
have short working and setting times

Porcelain and Ceramics
Porcelains are inorganic salts which fuse when heated. Ceramics have a composite-like structure—hard brittle particles between fused glass.
Properties of dental porcelain:
hard
biocompatible
good aesthetics
brittle
good compressive strength
good abrasion resistance (can be a problem as unpolished porcelain can abrade enamel)

Uses of dental porcelain: crowns and bridges, veneers, adhesive crowns, inlays and onlays, inserts within direct composites, denture teeth. Crowns and bridges are individually made in a laboratory.

Casting and Wrought Alloys
Alloys are combinations of metals in solid solutions. Alloy metals can combine by precipitation, crystallisation, or immiscibility in solid solution, depending on the metals involved: dental gold alloys, cobalt-chromium alloys, nickel-chromium alloys, steel alloys.

Denture Base Material - metal based, polymer based

Polymer Denture Base Materials
Properties:
poor impact resistance
moderate strength
generally nontoxic
low density
cheap
easy to process
not radio-opaque
poor thermal conductivity
weak in thin section
poor wear resistance
easy to add to, permitting ease of repair, reline, or addition
Uses: dentures, orthodontic appliances, individual impression trays

Endodontic Materials
Materials used in endodontics **can be classified as**:
root canal cleansers
preformed root canal fillings

root canal sealers
retrograde root-filling materials
intracanal medicaments

Implant Materials
Types of implant materials: subperiosteal, transmandibular, osseointegrated.

Miscellaneous
Waxes occur naturally from animal, mineral, and plant sources. Some distillation products of petroleum exist as a wax (e.g. paraffin wax). Addition of natural gums and resins may give wax adhesive properties.

Fissure Sealants
Properties of ideal sealant:
adhesion between enamel and sealant
need flow of sealant into pits and fissures
sufficient strength and wear resistance to withstand occlusal forces

Periodontal Materials
Periodontal pack or dressing—two-paste zinc oxide-eugenol system uses:
postsurgery, protects wound surface from mechanical trauma
prevents excessive granulation tissue formation
provides a physical barrier to bacterial contamination
used mainly after gingivectomy, apically repositioned flaps, and free gingival grafts

Investment Materials
These are used in lost wax processes, e.g. metal casting, denture bases.

Properties:
withstand high temperature
set at room temperature
expand slightly to compensate for
casting shrinkage
reproduce detail
porous to let gases escape
strong

Polishing
Polishing involves surface restructuring
and surface loss or abrasion.

Temporary Crown Materials
Properties:
cheap
moderate strength
reasonable aesthetics
set easily and quickly
nonadhesive to tooth
often use cartridge mixing systems

Although there is active research in
all areas of dental materials, much
attention surrounds the following:
Adhesion
Current trends involve the development
of multipurpose adhesives that can
bond enamel, dentine, composites,
amalgams, and ceramics rather than
individual kits of separate materials.

Casting
The 'lost wax' technique remains
the main method of casting. There is
currently some interest in spark erosion
as an alternative method.

Posterior composites
Direct resin composites, which are
packable in a similar manner to
amalgam, are showing some early

signs of promise for use in posterior
teeth.

**Hydrophilic silicone impression
materials**
Hydrophilic silicone impression
materials are being developed for use
in situations where moisture control is
a problem.

Amalgam
There appears to be a very slow
progression to an amalgam-free
mouth due to patient pressure and
environmental concerns regarding
mercury. There are satisfactory
alternatives, e.g. gallium.

Exercise 1
1. List the dental materials by their
   molecular form.
2. Talk about the classification of
   their properties.
3. Describe amalgam, resin
   composites, and glass ionomers.
4. What are adhesion and bonding
   agents, impression materials,
   casting and wrought alloys?
5. Give the properties and the use of
   dental porcelain and ceramics.
6. What is the use of denture base
   material? And the properties?
7. Which endodontic materials do
   you know?
8. Talk about periodontal and
   investment materials.

Translation 1
Vlastnosti materiálů, síla, tlak,
napětí, křehkost, kujnost, tvrdost,
únava materiálu, tepelné rozpínání,
elektrická vodivost, nepropustnost

záření, koroze, tavitelnost, nevytvářet nepříznivé účinky, amalgám, slitina rtuti stříbra a cínu, rozměrové změny při tuhnutí, plnící nástroj, plnivo, síla tahu a stlačení, smrštění při tuhnutí, náchylné k erozi, hrubost povrchu, průsvitnost, cermety a pryskyřicí upravené sklo-ionomery, pojivové a spojovací materiály, dočasné náhrady, otiskovací materiály pevné, pružné, stabilní, snadné míchání, krátká doba zpracování a usazení, roztavit se při zahřátí, korunky a můstky, fazety, vložky, zuby protézy, litiny a kujné slitiny, tuhé roztoky, srážení, krystalizace, nemísitelnost, základna zubní protézy, malá odolnost proti nárazům, individuální otiskovací lžíce, čističe kořenových kanálků, předem utvořené výplně, utěsňovací materiály, materiál na implantáty, vosky, přírodní gumy a pryskyřice, pečetidla, jamky a rýhy, vydržet sílu skusu, dásňový lalok, dásňový štěp, formovací hmota, porézní, umožňuje únik plynů, leštění, jednotlivé soupravy, obavy o životní prostředí týkající se rtuti, uspokojivé alternativy.

Text 2

General dental materials used daily and the routine conservation instruments required

Dental materials and its uses
a)   **Zinc phosphate cement**
Zinc phosphate cement is **adhesive** in dry cavities to dentine and **sets quickly** to a hard set. It is **mixed stiffly** as a **lining cement** for cavities, although it needs a **sublining** in deep cavities as the phosphoric acid content is **irritant**

to the pulp. Mixed to a **thin creamy** consistency, however, it is used as a **luting cement** to place **inlays and crowns**.

b)   **Alginate impression material**
Alginate impression material **sets quickly** and is relatively **pleasant tasting** but has **poor tear resistance** and **low dimensional stability**. It is therefore useful for impressions whose surface accuracy is not critical, for example:
- **study models**
- **prosthetic appliances**
- **orthodontic** appliances
- **opposing jaw impressions** during crown and bridge work

c)   **Glass ionomer cement**
Glass ionomer cement is **adhesive to dentine and enamel** and **releases fluoride** in cavities on setting. It is used:
- for **class 5 cavities** where minimal tooth preparation is required
- for other minimal **tooth preparation cavities** anywhere, except where maximum occlusal forces will occur
- as **a temporary filling** material where no time for cavity preparation is available
- as a **filling material for deciduous teeth**
- mixed to a **creamy** consistency, as a **luting cement** for the placement of **crowns, bridges, inlays, and veneers**
- mixed **stiffly**, as a **lining cement**, especially **under composite restorations**, but it must have a

sublining of calcium hydroxide in deep cavities
- as a **fissure sealant** to prevent occlusal caries

Light-cured varieties are available nowadays; these **set quicker** once placed than the chemically set type and, therefore, offer **less chance of moisture contamination. Reinforced types** are also available, with **silver particles** incorporated into the powder component; these are stronger than the usual glass ionomers and can be used for **core build-ups beneath the crowns.** It can also be used as a **luting cement** to place **orthodontic bands,** usually on molar teeth.

d) **Gutta-percha**
Flexible preformed and colour-coded points for **endodontic use to obturate root canals.** It can be supplied **in tubes** with a **plasticiser** added so that the material is **runny on heating** and can be **spun into root canals** to give a more **accurate seal.** It is also supplied **in sticks** that can be **heated directly** and used as **temporary fillings,** especially during the construction of indirect inlays.
It is **easily removed by inserting a warmed instrument** into the filling mass. Portions can be heated and used **to test the vitality of teeth** or to diagnose which tooth is **hypersensitive** to heat and suffering from **pulpitis.** Whole sticks can be heated and used as a **border moulding material** during **denture construction.** Applied to the borders of an existing denture or at the try-in stage of a new denture, the material **moulds itself** during normal muscle movements **in the mouth.**

Exercise 2
1. Describe how the following materials can be used in the dental surgery
a) Zinc phosphate cement
b) Zinc alginate impression material
c) Glass ionomer cement
d) Gutta-percha

Translation 2
Zink-fosfátový cement, přilnavý k dentinu, rychle tuhne, míchá se ztuha potřebuje podložit, dráždí zubní dřeň, řídká krémová konzistence, přitmelení, otisk, příjemná chuť, odolnost proti natržení, rozměrová stálost, přesnost není rozhodující, uvolňuje fluorid, při tuhnutí, vyžaduje se příprava zubu, síla skusu, prozatímní výplň, umístění korunek, můstků, litých výplní a fazet, výplně, náhrady, hydroxid vápenatý, těsnicí materiál na praskliny, druhy tvrzené světlem, kontaminace vlhkostí, zesílené typy, částečky stříbra, vmíchat do práškové složky, střed, výstavba, obroučka, špička, pracovní konec nástroje, ucpat kořenové kanálky, dodávaný v tubách se změkčovačem, materiál je tekutý při zahřátí, být roztočen, vtlačen, dodávaný v tyčinkách, odstranit, vložit ohřátý nástroj, testovat vitalitu zubů, trpět zánětem zubní dřeně, materiál na modelování okraje, stádium, zkouška nové protézy.

Text 3
Restorative techniques and properties of different types of impression material

Replacement of a missing tooth
By partial denture

An impression of the lower jaw is taken in alginate, as surface accuracy is not critical. An impression of the upper jaw is also taken in alginate so that opposing models can be put into occlusion. The denture is then constructed through bite, try-in, and fit stages, as usual. A special tray may be made from the original lower model so that a second, more accurate, working model can be produced. A second impression is taken in alginate again.

By resin-bonded bridge

The upper model is taken in alginate for occlusal record. The lower model is taken after tooth preparation has been completed; it must be very accurate in order to record the preparation fully as well as being dimensionally stable with good tear resistance. Elastomer material is used, which can be either silicone putty and wash paste or a polyether putty and paste-type material.

By fixed bridge/cantilever bridge

Again, tooth preparation will have been carried out, so the impression material required for the lower jaw impression must be accurate, dimensionally stable, and with good tear resistance. Elastomers—either silicones or polyethers—are the material of choice. Both can be taken in a single-stage or in a two-stage technique, with the putty component being taken first, then the wash material placed on this and the impression reinserted into the patient's mouth until setting is complete. The upper jaw is recorded in alginate, for occlusal registration purposes.

By single-unit titanium implant

It is used where good bone support is available and in cases where, because adjacent teeth are sound, bridge preparation would be quite destructive. Surgery is carried out first to insert the titanium implant.
This is left to allow osseointegration to occur and then an elastomeric impression material is used to record the implant head as a core for a conventional bonded crown. The upper jaw is recorded in alginate.

Dealing with the replacement—prevention of cross-infection

Once the impressions have set and have been removed from the patient's mouth, they will ultimately be sent to a laboratory for denture, bridge, or crown construction.
They must, at least, be disinfected first to limit the risk of cross-infection occurring, and it is the dental nurse's duty to perform this task. Immediately on removal from the mouth, the alginate and elastomer impressions should be run under the cold water tap to remove any particulate debris and strings of saliva from their surfaces.
Alginate impressions should then be immersed in a 10% solution of sodium hypochlorite for ten minutes, which, because it is a good disinfectant, will kill all bacteria, fungi, and most viruses.

Then **elastomeric** impression can also be dealt with as above, but ideally it should be immersed in one of the **aldehyde-type cold sterilising solutions** for up to 30 minutes, as these act as sterilisers rather than just disinfectants. The risk of **cross-infection** is thus **eliminated**. After immersion, the impressions should be washed again.

The **alginates** should then be covered in **wet gauze and sealed** in an **airtight bag**. The **elastomer** impressions should be **rinsed and blown dry**, then sealed in a **separate bag**.

Exercise 3

1. Which impression materials and techniques might the dentist use when providing treatment to replace a missing lower incisor tooth?
2. How should these materials be dealt with by the dental nurse after the impression has set?

Translation 3

Konzervační techniky, materiál na otisky, zabránění šíření infekce, náhrada chybějícího zubu, částečná protéza, upevnit, spojený pryskyřicí, záznam skusu, pevný můstek, konzolový můstek, na výběr, jednostupňová technika, tmelová složka, sousední zuby jsou zdravé, vložit implantát, dovolit vhojení do kosti, tradiční korunka, zacházení s, znovu umístit, poslat do laboratoře, sestrojení protézy, být nejprve dezinfikován, dát pod kohoutek se studenou vodou, odstranit zbytky a praménky slin, ponořit do roztoku chlornanu sodného, usmrtit

všechny baktérie, plísně a většinu virů, pokrýt vlhkou gázou, uzavřít do vzduchotěsného obalu, opláchnout a vysušit.

Text 4

Materials and Principles of Cavity Design

a) **Glass ionomer cement in a class 5 cavity**

A class 5 cavity is one at the **gingival one-third of any tooth** on the **buccal surface**. There is **little enamel** in this situation, and the **nerve is not too deep**, so **minimal cavity preparation** is essential to avoid exposure of the pulp. Hence, a **material** is required that is **adhesive to dentine** and which can **easily be placed** in such a cavity. Glass ionomer meets these requirements. A **surface set** is achieved **relatively quickly,** but the **restoration** must be **coated immediately** with **varnish** to allow full setting without **saliva contamination** occurring. Class 5 cavities are often due to toothbrush abrasion and can sometimes be dislodged, so the use of glass ionomers with minimal, if any, tooth preparation is ideal.

b) **Amalgam in a class 2 cavity**

A class 2 cavity is one which **involves two surfaces of a posterior tooth** (premolar or molar). Hence, any filling **material** used here will have to be **strong enough to withstand** normal **occlusal forces**. Except for gold, which is expensive and difficult to use due to the **accuracy required, amalgam** is **the strongest restorative material** available.

An **undercut**, keyhole shaped cavity is required **since amalgam is not adhesive to enamel or dentine**, and a **matrix band has to be used** while the amalgam is packed into the cavity **to prevent it being squashed out** mesially or distally. **A lining** must also be placed beneath the filling to **prevent thermal conduction to the pulp**.

c)   **Zinc polycarboxylate as a luting cement**

A luting cement is one that is mixed to a **creamy consistency** for **cementing crowns, bridges, and inlays**. The material used must also be **adhesive to dentine** in order to actually **cement the restoration** to the prepared tooth. Zinc polycarboxylate is **the most adhesive** of the luting cements and is **easily mixed** to a creamy consistency for this purpose. It is also relatively **cheap to use** and relatively **easy to clean instruments** after use. It is mixed on a **glass slab** with a **metal spatula**.

d)   **Composite in a class 3 cavity**

A class 3 cavity is one **involving the mesial or distal aspect of an incisor or canine tooth**. Hence, **aesthetics are of paramount importance**, but the material used must also be able to **withstand** normal **incisal forces**. **Composite appears more likely enamel when set** than glass ionomer cement does, especially when a **celluloid matrix strip** has been used to adapt the restoration correctly into the cavity, as a **shiny set surface** is produced.

With the availability of composites in **compound form for easy application**, the technique is an **easy** one, especially using **light-cured materials** that do **not set until the dentist is ready** for them to do so.

A calcium hydroxide lining must be used **before the enamel margins of the cavity are acid-etched**.

Exercise 4

Explain how the properties of the following materials make them best suited for the uses given:

1.   Glass ionomer cement in a class 5 cavity
2.   Amalgam in a class 2 cavity
3.   Zinc polycarboxylate as a luting cement
4.   Composite in a class 3 cavity

Translation 4

Zásady konstrukce, nerv není příliš hluboko, co nejmenší preparace je velmi důležitá, vyhnout se vystavení dřeně, snadno se umístí, splnit tyto požadavky, pokrýt okamžitě lakem, kvůli odírání kartáčkem, zadní zub (třenový či stolička), vydržet sílu skusu, řezací sílu, spodní řez, dutina ve tvaru klíčové dírky, matricová páska, nacpat do dutiny, být vytlačen, pod výplň, umístit vyložení, tmelící cement, relativně levný, nástroje se po použití snadno čistí, skleněná destička a kovová lopatka, střední či vzdálená poloha, řezák nebo špičák, estetický vzhled je nesmírně důležitý, správně přizpůsobit náhradu, zářivý povrch, snadná aplikace, nejlépe vyhovující.

Exercise 5 / Homework

The sentences have been divided into separate halves. Match the half-sentences in column A with the half-sentences in column B to make sentences which are complete and correct.

A

1. Besides preventing the progression of caries to the pulp, fillings are required to . . .
2. Spoon excavators are used to . . .
3. Cavities to be filled with composite materials need not to be undercut because . . .
4. The alloy powder of amalgam contains silver, . . .
5. Four examples of temporary filling materials are . . .
6. Mercury should be handled with care because . . .
7. Enamel chisels are hand instruments used to . . .
8. Zinc oxide/eugenol cements cannot be used as linings beneath . . .
9. Impressions taken in alginate should be cast the same day because . . .
10. Moisture contamination whilst placing an amalgam filling will result in . . .
11. Calcium hydroxide is the best lining to use in very deep cavities because the calcium . . .
12. Two types of impression material commonly used for crown and bridge preparations are . . .
13. Ball-ended and pear-shaped burnishers are used to . . .
14. If alloy powder and mercury are overmixed, the resulting amalgam filling . . .
15. Luting cements are . . .
16. Glass ionomer cements consist of . . .
17. Besides its use as a root-filling material, gutta-percha can be used to . . .

B

a. *the material becomes mechanically locked into enamel prisms after acid etching.*
b. *zinc oxid/eugenol cement, zinc phosphate cement, gutta-percha, zinc polycarboxylate cement (also calcium hydroxide).*
c. *alginate has poor dimensional stability and soon dries out.*
d. *prevent food stagnation in the cavity and to restore the function of the tooth.*
e. *composite filling materials.*
f. *those mixed to a creamy consistency to cement crowns, bridges, and inlays.*
g. *will contract and allow marginal leakage to occur.*
h. *can be used by odontoblasts to form secondary dentine and so protect the pulp.*
i. *remove unsupported enamel at the edges of cavities, before filling commences.*
j. *expansion of the filling.*
k. *elastomers and silicone putty and paste.*
l. *its vapours are poisonous, and it can enter the body through the skin and cause poisoning in this way too.*
m. *copper, zinc, and tin.*
n. *powder containing polyacrylate, quartz, alumina, and fluoride mixed with pure water.*

o.   *adapt metal filling margins closely to the cavity edges.*

p.   *to test tooth vitality and as a temporary filling material.*

q.   *hand-excavate very deep cavities where the risk of pulp exposure is high.*

14. The hand instrument used to pack amalgam fillings is . . .

15. Gold, porcelain, and composites can all be used to make . . .

16. Ceramic-tipped hand instruments should be used with . . .

17. Chrome-cobalt is used in dentistry to . . .

Exercise 6/ Homework

The sentences have been divided into separate halves. Match the half-sentences in column A with the half-sentences in column B to make sentences which are complete and correct.

A

1.   Reinforced glass ionomer cements contain . . .

2.   Cavity varnish is used to . . .

3.   Enamel is chemically roughened using . . .

4.   Celluloid matrix strips are used when placing composite fillings because . . .

5.   Glass ionomers are wiped with varnish after setting to . . .

6.   Siqveland matrix bands are used with amalgam in . . .

7.   Tungsten carbide burs are used to . . .

8.   Three examples of permanent plastic filling materials are . . .

9.   Slow-speed handpieces are used to remove deep caries because . . .

10. Glass ionomer cements do not require undercut cavities because . . .

11. Eugenol-containing materials should be handled with care because . . .

12. Some special glass ionomer materials can be used as luting cements because they contain . . .

13. Polishing discs are used to . . .

B

a.   *light curing can occur through the strip, which it cannot if metal matrix bands are used.*

b.   *the dentist has better tactile sensation with these, rather than with air turbine handpieces.*

c.   *class 2 cavities and can be adapted interproximally using wooden wedges.*

d.   *silver particles to give increased strength and are especially useful during crown preparations to help form the tooth core.*

e.   *an amalgam plugger.*

f.   *indirect inlays.*

g.   *polish composite fillings.*

h.   *finer filler particles than normal glass ionomer cements.*

i.   *seal their surfaces and prevent moisture contamination whilst they set fully within.*

j.   *smooth composite filling materials.*

k.   *amalgam, composite, and glass ionomer cement.*

l.   *form a partial denture bases with clasps or as the base of a full upper denture.*

m.   *33% phosphoric acid before a composite filling is placed.*

n.   *eugenol burns soft tissues.*

o.   *composite filling materials to prevent streaking of the composite with metal.*

p. *they are adhesive to dentine,
    enamel, and cementum.*

q. *help seal the cut dentinal tubules
    and minimise thermal irritation
    after filling.*

Exercise 7/ Homework

Fill in the missing words. Choose the
correct ones.

1. Cavities need to be undercut when they are to be filled with amalgam. Composite and glass ionomer are _____ to enamel and dentine, respectively, so _____ cavities to be filled with these materials is not imperative. Gold castings are constructed at the laboratory and cannot be _____ if the cavity walls are undercut. Ideally, the cavity should have parallel sides to allow the _____ to be fully inserted and to give maximum _____.	seated, undercutting, casting, retention, adhesive
2. Very deep _____ can be carefully removed by hand using spoon excavators. Ball-ended _____ are used to adapt filling margins to the cavity walls, and flat plastic instruments are used to place plastic filling materials (except amalgam) into the _____ cavity. _____ _____ are used to remove unsupported enamel from cavity margins before restoration commences.	Spoon chisels, burnishers, caries, repaired
3. The dental material best _____ to the restoration of a class 5 cavity is glass ionomer cement. Although ____ and amalgam can be used to restore class 5 cavities, they are both quite unsightly compared to the _____-_____ materials available now.	of choice, gold, suited, tooth-coloured, lack

Both require certain cavity shapes to be produced because of their ____ of adhesiveness. At the gingival margin, the enamel is quite thin but dentine is in abundance, so glass ionomers, which are adhesive to dentine, are the material __ _____ with the highest chance of success. Composites can also be used but are only adhesive to enamel.	
4. The main constituent of the alloy powder used when mixing amalgam is silver. The alloy powder does not contain mercury but is mixed with it to _____ amalgam. Both zinc and copper are _____ of the alloy, but their amounts are far surpassed by _____, which accounts for __ __ 75% of the _____ powder.	alloy, up to, produce, silver, constituents
5. Which dental material has _____ properties: glass ionomer cements. Glass ionomer cements _____ fluoride, which they release into the _____ after the material has been mixed and _____ into the tooth. No other dental _____ _____ has this property.	cavity, filling material, placed, contain, cariostatic
6. All of the following dental materials can be used to construct indirect inlays: porcelain, light-cured composite, gold, except glass ionomer cements. Porcelain, composite, and gold can all be used in the _____ to form indirect _____ using models of the patient's prepared inlay cavity. The materials can be _____ constructed, set in the laboratory and _____ whole to the surgery for seating and cementation. Glass ionomers _____ be used in this way.	Inlays, transferred, individually, cannot, laboratory

7. The following are plastic materials: amalgam, composite, glass ionomer cement. A _____ material is defined as one which is placed in a cavity in a plastic (mouldable) _____, where it can be _____ to fit the cavity _____ before setting. All three choices are examples of materials abiding by this _____.	accurately, state, adapted, plastic, definition

Phosphoric acid is used to etch cavity _____ before the placement of _____ restorations. Cavity varnish is wiped in a thin _____ around the cavity walls before the _____ of an amalgam filling to seal dentinal tubules and reduce thermal irrigation to the pulp. Its use during filling with glass ionomer cements would prevent their adhesion to the dentine and cause _____ of the restoration.	

8. All of the following are examples of dental impression materials: silicone, elastomer, zinc oxide/eugenol, except calcium hydroxide _____ _____ is a thin lining material especially useful in _____ cavities, where its calcium content is taken up by odontoblasts and used to form a protective _____ of secondary dentine between the _____ and the overlying filling. Its presence in these situations is often enough to prevent the _____ of irreversible pulpitis in the tooth.	Barrier, onset, calcium hydroxide, pulp, deep

11. Composite dental materials are mechanically adhesive after acid etching to enamel. The phosphoric acid of the _____ microscopically roughens the enamel prisms so that the _____ and resin can mechanically lock into the prism's _____. This does not occur with dentine because of its hollow _____ structure.	Tubular, ends, etchant, composite

12. A shiny surface can be achieved on glass ionomer fillings by using a foil matrix. Special cervical margin _____ _____ are available for class 5 cavities, when pressed against the placed glass ionomer during _____. They will produce a _____ surface. Wiping with saliva will contaminate the glass ionomer and prevent its proper setting. Polishing with any bur will produce a chalky surface. The set restoration should be coated with _____ to prevent _____ moisture contamination, but this will not itself produce a shiny surface.	Further, shiny, foil matrices, varnish, setting

9. Composite filling materials contain powdered glass. The _____ appearance of a well-finished composite filling is due to its powdered-glass _____, which reflects _____ in a similar manner to enamel and thus mimics it well. Glass ionomer cements contain polyacrylate and _____. Reinforced glass ionomers are so named because of their silver particle content. Calcium hydroxide is a _____ filing material.	quartz, content, light, excellent, temporary

10. Cavities should be conditioned before the placement of glass ionomer cements, using polyacrylate.	layer, packing, failure, composite, margins

13. Amongst the _____ of alginate is poor tear resistance.	dimensional, tearing, pulled out, disadvantages, same day

Alginate is renowned for _____ easily, especially when _____ ___ of deep undercuts. It also has a low _____ stability, which is why models should be cast from alginate impressions on the ____ ___, the impression being sterilised and then wrapped in wet gauze until casting is possible.	

| 14. Zinc oxide/eugenol materials can be used for a sedative dressing, an impression material, a surgical dressing.
Zinc oxide/eugenol cement is routinely used as a _____ _____ for deep cavities and in _____ teeth. As a plasticized _____, it can be used as a wash _____ material for relining dentures. A similar material is available as a surgical dressing following periodontal surgery, such as _____ . | Hypersensitive, impression, gingivectomy, paste, sedative dressing |

| 15. Silver has all of the following dental uses: a root-filling material, a component of some glass ionomers, a component of amalgam, except denture construction.
Silver points are still available as a ____ filling material; silver particles give added _____ to glass ionomer cements to form _____ glass ionomer materials, and silver powder accounts for up to 75% of the alloy _____ which is mixed with mercury to form amalgam. _____ and chrome-cobalt alloys are those commonly used in denture construction. | stainless steel, strength, root, powder, reinforced |

| 16. Zinc phosphate cements can be used to permanently place crowns and bridges because they are adhesive to dentine. | Luting cement, fully, moisture control, irritant, crown |

Zinc phosphate cement is very _____ to the pulp because of its acid contents. It cannot be used on wet preparations as good _____ _____ is important to the success of the _____ cementation. A _____ _____ should not set quickly otherwise the crown will not be seated _____ before the cement has set.	

| 17. The aim of good _____ when mixing dental materials is to _____ air bubbles.
All the constituents must be mixed completely together to produce a material with predictable _____ qualities and _____. If this were not the case there would be no need for accurate measurement of the material's components before _____ . | properties, remove, mixing, setting, spatulation |

Solution to Exercise 5

1d, 2q, 3a, 4m, 5b, 6l,7i,8e, 9c, 10j, 11h, 12k, 13o,14g, 15f, 16n, 17p

Solution to Exercise 6

1d, 2q, 3m, 4a, 5i, 6c, 7j, 8k, 9b, 10p, 11n, 12h, 13g, 14e, 15f, 16o, 17l

Vocabulary

abide /əˈbaɪd/ trvat, dodržovat
above /əˈbʌv/ nahoře shora (v citaci)
abrasion /əˈbreɪ.ʒən/ **resistance** / rɪˈzɪs.tənɟs/ otěruvzdornost
abundance /əˈbʌn.dənɟs/ velké množství
account /əˈkaʊnt/ **for** /fɔːʳ/ odpovídat za, vysvětlit fakt
accuracy /ˈæk.jʊ.rə.si/ přesnost, správnost věci
acid-etch /ˈæs.ɪd/ /ˈetʃ/ leptat kyselinou

adapt /ə'dæpt/ přizpůsobit

adapted /ə'dæp.tɪd/ přizpůsobený

add /æd/ přidávat, doplnit

adhesion /əd'hiː.ʒən/ přilnavost

adhesive /əd'hiː.sɪv/ přilnavý, lepivý, lepicí páska

adjacent /ə'dʒeɪ.sənt/ sousední, hraničící

adverse /'æd.vɜːs/ effect /ɪ'fekt/ nepříznivý účinek

adversely /'æd.vɜː.sli/ nepříznivě, příčně

aesthetics /es'θet.ɪks/ estetika

affected /ə'fek.tɪd/ ovlivněný, napadený

agent /'eɪ.dʒənt/ činitel

aid /eɪd/ pomoc, pomáhat

air /eəʳ/ turbine /'tɜː.baɪn/ vzduchová turbinka

airtight /'eə.taɪt/ vzduchotěsný, neprodyšný

aldehyde /'æl.dɪ.haɪd/ aldehyd

alginate /æ'ldʒɪ.neɪt/ alginát

alloy /'æl.ɔɪ/ slitina, směs

alumina /ə'luː.mɪ.nə/ kysličník hlinitý

amongst /ə'mʌŋst/ mezi

appearance /ə'pɪə.rənts/ vzhled, objevení se

around /ə'raʊnd/ okolo, přibližně

aspect /'æs.pekt/ poloha

attach /ə'tætʃ/ připojit

attraction /ə'træk.ʃən/ přitažlivost

ball-ended /bɔːl.en.dɪd/ kulatě zakončený

band /bænd/ obroučka, proužek, spojit

barrier /'bær.i.əʳ/ bariéra, zábrana, překážka

base /beɪs/ základna, podklad

beneath /bɪ'niːθ/ pod, vespod

bland /blænd/ jemný, nedráždivý

blow /bləʊ/ foukat

bond /bɒnd/ tmelit, spojit

bonding /'bɒnd.ɪŋ/ agent /'eɪ.dʒənt/ pojivo, tmel, lepidlo

bone /bəʊn/ kost

border /bɔː.dəʳ/ hranice, okraj, rámeček, lemovat

brittle /'brɪt.l̩/ křehký

bubble /'bʌb.l̩/ bublinka

build /ˌbɪld/ up /ʌp/ výstavba, zvyšování

bur /bɜːr/ vrtáček

burnisher /'bɜː.nɪʃ.əʳ/ leštítko, hladítko, cpátko

calcium hydroxide / ˌkæl.si.əm.haɪ'drɒk.saɪd/ hydroxid vápenatý

cantilever /'kæn.ti.liː.vəʳ/ bridge / brɪdʒ/ samonosný můstek

carbide /'kɑː.baɪd/ karbid, tvrdý kov

carboxylate /kɑː'bɒk.sɪl.eɪt/ karboxylát

cariostatic /ˌkeər.i.ə 'stæt.ɪk/ působící zastavení kazu

carry /'kær.i/ nést

cartridge /'kɑː.trɪdʒ/ karpule, kapsle, typ balení, výměnný zásobník

casting /kɑːst.ɪŋ/ alloy /'æl.ɔɪ/ slévárenská slitina

casting /kɑːst.ɪŋ/ odlévání, odlitek

cavity /'kæv.ɪ.ti/ dutina

celluloid /'sel.ju.lɒɪd/ celuloid, film, buničina

cementation /ˌsiː.men'teɪ.ʃᵊn/ tmelení, zalévání cementem

ceramics /sɪ'ræm.ɪks/ keramický materiál

chalky /'tʃɔː.ki/ křídovitý

chisel /'tʃɪz.ᵊl/ dláto, sekáč

choice /tʃɔɪs/ volba, výběr

chrome /krəʊm/ chrom

chromium /'krəʊ.mi.əm/ chrom, chromový

clasp /klɑːsp/ spona, háček

cleanser /ˈklen.zəʳ/ čisticí prostředek

coated /ˈkəʊ.tɪd/ pokrytý, povlečený, potažený

cobalt /ˈkəʊ.bɒlt/ kobalt

commence /kəˈmenʦ/ otevřít, začínat

compatible /kəmˈpæt.ɪ.bl̩/ slučitelný, zaměnitelný

compensate /ˈkɒm.pən.seɪt/ vyrovnat, vynahradit, vyvážit

complete /kəmˈpliːt/ dokončit, hotový

composite /ˈkɒm.pə.zɪt/ kompozitní výplňový materiál

compound /ˈkɒm.paʊnd/ sloučenina, směs

compress /kəmˈpres/ působit tlakem

concern /kənˈsɜːn/ týkat se, zájem, znepokojení

conditioned /kənˈdɪʃ.ənd/ podmíněný, upravený, určený

conductivity /ˌkɒn.dʌkˈtɪv.ɪ.ti/ vodivost (tepelná)

consistency /kənˈsɪs.tᵊnʦ.si/ hustota, tuhost, shoda, důslednost

constituent /kənˈstɪt.ju.ənt/ prvek (složka, člen, součást)

construct /kənˈstrʌkt/ postavit, vybudovat

content /ˈkɒn.tent/ obsah, objem, kapacita, spokojený, ochoten

contract /ˈkɒn.trækt/ uzavřít smlouvu, chytit (nemoc), smrštit se

contraction /kənˈtræk.ʃən/ tažení, zmenšení

copper /ˈkɒp.əʳ/ měď

core /kɔːʳ/ hlavní, střed

corner /ˈkɔː.nəʳ/ cíp, růžek

corrode /kəˈrəʊd/ rezavět

corrosion /kəˈrəʊ.ʒᵊn/ rozežírání, leptání

cover /ˈkʌv.əʳ/ pokrýt, kryt

creamy /ˈkriː.mi/ bělavý

creep /kriːp/ roztahovat se, tečení

critical /ˈkrɪt.ɪ.kᵊl/ rozhodující

crown /kraʊn/ korunka

crystallisation /ˌkrɪs.təl.aɪˈzeɪ.ʃᵊn/ tvoření krystalů

curing /kjʊər.ɪŋ/ ošetřování, vytvrzení (lepidla, plastu)

deal /dɪəl/ with /wɪð/ jednat, zacházet, týkat se

debris /ˈdeb.riː/, /ˈdeɪ.briː/ úlomky, pozůstatky, poškozená tkáň

density /ˈden.ʦ.sɪ.ti/ denzita, objemová hmotnost, hutnost

dentine /ˈden.tiːn/ dentin, zubovina

denture /ˈden.tʃə/ base /beɪs/ základna protézy

denture /ˈden.tʃə/ zubní protéza

depth /depθ/ hloubka

design /dɪˈzaɪn/ návrh, nákres, schéma

destructive /dɪˈstrʌk.tɪv/ ničící, rušivý

detection /dɪˈtek.ʃən/ odhalení, vypátrání

dimensional /daɪ.menʦ.ʃən.ᵊl/ objemový rozměrový

disadvantage /ˌdɪs.ədˈvɑːn.tɪdʒ/ nevýhoda, nedostatek

disinfectant /ˌdɪs.ɪnˈfek.tᵊnt/ dezinfekční prostředek

dislodge /dɪˈslɒdʒ/ vytlačit

distal /ˈdɪs.təl/ vzdálený

distillation /ˌdɪs.tɪˈleɪ.ʃən/ destilace, překapávání

double /ˈdʌb.l̩/ dvojitý, dvojnásobný

dressing /ˈdres.ɪŋ/ obvaz, desinfekční vložka

drill /drɪl/ vrták, vrtačka

dry /draɪ/ out /aʊt/ vysušit se, vysychat

dry /draɪ/ suchý

ductility /dʌkˈtɪl.ɪ.ti/ kujnost, tažnost, poddajnost

due /djuː/ to /tʊ/ následkem, v důsledku, díky

edge /edʒ/ okraj

elastic /ɪˈlæs.tɪk/ pružný, pružná tkanina

elastomer /ɪˈlæs.tə.məʳ/ elastomer, pružný kaučuk, gumovitý polymer

elastomeric /ɪˈlæs.təˈmer.ɪk/ elastomerní

elevator /ˈel.ɪ.veɪ.təʳ/ zdvihák, elevátor

enamel /ɪˈnæm.ᵉl/ sklovina

environmental /ɪnˌvaɪəˈrən.ˈmen.tᵊl/ vnější, týkající se okolí, životního prostředí

erosion /ɪˈrəʊ.ʒən/ odírání, mechanické opotřebení

escape /ɪˈskeɪp/ uniknutí, otvor, výlevka

essential /ɪˈsen.t ʃəl/ základní, nezbytný

etch /etʃ/ leptat, vyrýt

etchant /etʃ.ᵊnt/ leptadlo

eugenol /juːˈdʒen.ɒl/ eugenol

expand /ɪkˈspænd/ rozpínat se, šířit se

expansion /ɪkˈspæn.t ʃᵊn/ expanze

exposure /ɪkˈspəʊ.ʒəʳ/ obnažení

failure /ˈfeɪ.ljəʳ/ selhání, porucha, nedostatek

fatigue /fəˈtiːg/ únava (též materiálu)

filler /ˈfɪl.əʳ/ plnící nástroj, plnivo

filling /ˈfɪl.ɪŋ/ výplň, plnění

firmly /ˈfɜːm.li/ pevně

fissure /ˈfɪʃ.əʳ/ rýha

fit /fɪt/ upravit, vhodný, nával

flap /flæp/ chlopeň, lalok

flat /flæt/ plochý, rovný

flexible /ˈflek.sɪ.bl̩/ flexibilní, pružný

flow /fləʊ/ proud (vzduchu), tok, prýštit (krev)

fluoride /ˈflʊə.raɪd/ fluorid

foil /fɔɪl/ folie

force /fɔːs/ síla, účinnost, nutit, vyvíjet tlak

forceps /ˈfɔː.seps/ kleště

full /fʊl/ plný, úplný

fully /ˈfʊl.i/ zcela, v hojné míře

further /ˈfɜː.ðəʳ/ dále, další, kromě toho

fuse /fjuːz/ roztavit, slit, sloučit se

gallium /ˈgæl.ɪ.əm/ gallium, síran galitý

gas /gæs/ plyn

gauze /gɔːz/ gáza, mul

gingival /ˌdʒɪn.dʒɪ.val/ gingivální, dásňový

gingivectomy /ˌdʒɪn.dʒɪˈvect.ə.mi/ gingivektomie

gold /gəʊld/ zlato, zlatý

graft /grɑːft/ štěp, transplantovat

gum /gʌm/ guma

gutta-percha /ˌgʌt.əˈpɜː.tʃə/ gutaperča

handle /ˈhæn.dl̩/ ovládat

handpiece /ˈhænd.piːs/ držadlo, rukojeť, násadec

hard /hɑːd/ tvrdý, pevný

hardness /ˈhɑːd.nəs/ odolnost, tvrdost

heat /hiːt/ zahřát, rozžhavit

hence /hentʃ/ odtud, z toho důvodu, a proto

hollow /ˈhɒl.əʊ/ dutý, dutina, vykotlaný (zub)

hydrocolloid /ˈhaɪ.drəʊˈkɒl.ɒid/ hydrokoloid

hydrophilic /ˌhaɪ.drəˈfɪl.ɪk/ smáčivý

immerse /ɪˈmɜːs/ ponořit

immiscibility /ɪˌmɪs.əˈbɪl.ɪ.ti/ nemísivost

impact /ˈɪm.pækt/ **resistance** /rɪˈzɪs. tᵊntʃ/ odolnost proti nárazu

imperative /ɪmˈper.ə.tɪv/ pravidlo, nevyhnutelný (nutný)

impression /ɪmˈpreʃ.ən/ **tray** /treɪ/ otiskovací lžíce

in /ɪn/ **order** /ˈɔː.dəʳ/ **to** /tʊ/ aby mohl, za účelem

incorporated /ɪnˈkɔː.pᵊr.eɪ.tɪd/ vmíchaný, začleněný

indirect /ˌɪn.dɑ ɪ'rekt/ nepřímý, vedlejší

inherent /ɪn'her.ᵊnt/ inherentní, vnitřní

inlay /'ɪn.leɪ/ inlej, litá výplň

insert /ɪn's3ːt/ vsunout, vložka, příloha

interfacial /ˌɪn.tə'feɪ.ʃᵊl/ meziplošný

investment /ɪn'vest.mənt/ formovací hmota

irreversible /ˌɪr.ɪ'v3ː.sɪ.bl̩/ nezvratný, nevyléčitelný

irrigate /'ɪr.ɪ.geɪt/ zavlažovat

irrigation /ˌɪr.ɪ'geɪ.ʃᵊn/ syringe / sɪ'rɪndʒ/ stříkačka pro výplach

irritant /'ɪr.ɪ.tᵊnt/ dráždidlo, dráždící

irritation /ˌɪr.ɪ'teɪ.ʃᵊn/ dráždění

keyhole /'kiː.həʊl/ klíčová dírka

kit /kɪt/ výbava, sada nástrojů

LA local /'ləʊ.kəl/ anaesthesia /ˌæn.əs'θiː.zi.ə/ místní anestezie

lack /læk/ of /əv/ nedostatek

layer /'leɪ.ər/ vrstva, úroveň

leakage /'liː.kɪdʒ/ netěsnost, vytékání, unikání

light /laɪt/ světlo, osvětlit, lehký

light-cured /laɪt.kjʊəʳ.d/ tvrzený světlem

limit /'lɪm.ɪt/ hranice (omezení)

liner /'laɪ.nəʳ/ podložka, vložka, izolační materiál

lining /'laɪ.nɪŋ/ obložení, výstelka

load /ləʊd/ zatížení, plnit

lock /lɒk/ zámek, zamknout, uzavřít

low /ləʊ/ nízký

luting /luːt.ɪŋ/ přitmelení, tmel

manner /'mæn.əʳ/ způsob, metoda

margin /'mɑː.dʒɪn/ okraj

marginal /'mɑː.dʒɪ.nəl/ okrajový, mezní, krajní

matrix /'meɪ.trɪks/ band /bænd/ matriční páska, otiskovací kroužek

matrix /'meɪ.trɪks/ matice, matrice, základní hmota

measure /'meʒ.əʳ/ měřit

measurement /'meʒ.ə.mənt/ měření, velikost

mercury /'m3ː.kjʊ.ri/ rtuť

metal /'met.əl/ kov, potáhnout kovem

mimic /'mɪm.ɪk/ napodobit

miscellaneous /ˌmɪs.əl'eɪ.ni.əs/ rozmanitý

missing /'mɪs.ɪŋ/ chybějící, nepřítomný

mix /mɪks/ míchat

moderate /'mɒd.ər.ət/ mírný, zmírňovat

modulus /'mɒd.jə.ləs/ modul

moisture /'mɔɪs.tʃəʳ/ vlhkost

mould /məʊld/ forma, tvar, modelovat

moulding /məʊld.ɪŋ/ tváření, výlisek

multipurpose /ˌmʌl.tɪ'p3ː.pəs/ víceúčelový

natural /'nætʃ.ᵊr.ᵊl/ přírodní

nature /'neɪ.tʃəʳ/ povaha, přirozená vlastnost

nickel-chromium /'nɪk.ᵊl.krəʊ.mi.əm/ steel /stiːl/ niklochromová ocel

obturate /'ɒb.tjʊə.reɪt/ ucpat

odontoblast /əʊ'dɒn.tə.blaːst/ odontoblast, buňka dentinu tvořící zubovinu

onlay /'ɒn.leɪ/ onlej, štěp aplikovaný na povrch tkáně

onset /'ɒn.set/ příchod (počátek, nástup)

opacity /əʊ'pæs.ə.ti/ neprůhlednost, temnost, matnost

osseointegration /ɒs.i.ə.ˌɪn.tɪ'greɪ.ʃᵊn/ vhojení do kosti

over /'əʊ.vəʳ/ nad, přes, příliš

overhang /ˌəʊ.və'hæŋ/ přečnívat, odstávat, viset přes

overlay /ˌəʊ.və'leɪ/ potažení, překrytí

oxide /'ɒk.saɪd/ layer /'leɪ.əʳ/ oxidová vrstva

pack /pæk/ tamponovat, ucpávka, balení

parallel /ˈpær.ə.lel/ souběžný, shodný

paramount /ˈpær.ə.maʊnt/ nejdůležitější, hlavní

partial /ˈpɑː.ʃəl/ částečný, neúplný

particle /ˈpɑː.tɪ.kl̩/ částečka, zrnko

paste /peɪst/ pasta, lepit, keramická směs

paste /peɪst/ zinkoxid-eugenolová pasta

pear-shaped /ˈpeə.ʃeɪpt/ ve tvaru hrušky

permit /pəˈmɪt/ dovolit

petroleum /pəˈtrəʊ.li.əm/ ropa, nafta

phosphoric /fɒsˈfɒr.ɪk/ **acid** /ˈæs.ɪd/ kyselina fosforečná

pit /pɪt/ jamka

placement /ˈpleɪs.mənt/ uspořádání, kladení, poloha

plastic /ˈplæs.tɪk/ pružná hmota, plast

plasticiser /ˈplæs.tɪ.saɪz.əʳ/ změkčovadlo

plugger /plʌg.əʳ/ zátka, cpátko

pocket /ˈpɒk.ɪt/ kapsa, chobot, váček

point /pɔɪnt/ bod, špička, pracovní konec nástroje

poisonous /ˈpɔɪ.zən.əs/ jedovatý, škodlivý

polish /ˈpɒl.ɪʃ/ leštit

polishing /ˈpɒl.ɪʃ.ɪŋ/ **disc** /dɪsk/ lešticí kotouč

polyacrylate /pɒl.i.æˈkrɪ.leɪt/ polyakrylan, polyakrylát

polymer /ˈpɒl.ɪ.mər/ polymer

porous /ˈpɔː.rəs/ porézní, propustný

posterior /pɒsˈtɪə.ri.əʳ/ pozdější, zadní část

powder /ˈpaʊ.dər/ rozdrtit na prášek, posypat

powdered /ˈpaʊ.dəd/ **glass** /glɑːs/ práškové sklo

precipitation /prɪˌsɪp.ɪˈteɪ.ʃən/ srážení, vylučování

predictable /prɪˈdɪk.tə.bl̩/ předvídatelný

preparation /ˌprep.əˈreɪ.ʃən/ preparace, příprava

prevention /prɪˈvent.ʃən/ zabránění, ochrana

prism /ˈprɪz.əm/ prizma, hranol

product /ˈprɒd.ʌkt/ produkt

progression /prəˈgreʃ.ən/ postup (pokrok), průběh

property /ˈprɒp.ə.ti/ vlastnost, charakteristika

proportional /prəˈpɔː.ʃən.əl/ poměrný, přiměřený

pull /pʊl/ **out** /aʊt/ vytáhnout

pulpitis /pʌlˈaɪ.tɪs/ pulpitida, zánět zubní dřeně

pure /pjʊəʳ/ čistý, pouhý

push /pʊʃ/ tlačit, pohánět

putty /ˈpʌt.i/ tmel (sklenářský), stmelit

quartz /ˈkwɔːts/ krystal, křemen, křemenný

radio/ˈreɪ.di.əʊ/ **-opaque** /əʊˈpeɪk/ nepropustný, radiopakní

raise /reɪz/ zvednout, vytáhnout

reflect /rɪˈflekt/ odrážet (světlo), uvažovat

reinforce /ˌriː.ɪnˈfɔːs/ posílit, zesílit, zpevnit

reinsert /riː.ɪnˈsɜːt/ znovu vložit

release /rɪˈliːs/ uvolnit, pustit, spustit

reline /riːˈlaɪn/ podložit vnitřní stranu protézy

relining /riːˈlaɪn.ɪŋ/ obnova vnitřní strany protézy

renowned /rɪˈnaʊnd/ renomovaný, chvalně známý

replacement /rɪˈpleɪs.mənt/ nahrazení, přeložení, znovudosažení reposition /rɪ.pəˈzɪʃ.ən/ repozice, nové upevnění

requirement /rɪˈkwaɪə.mənt/ požadavek, potřeba

residual /rɪˈzɪd.ju.əl/ zbytkový

resin /ˈrez.ɪn/ pryskyřice

resin /ˈrez.ɪn/ composite /ˈkɒm.pə.zɪt/ kompozitní pryskyřice

resin-bonded /ˈrez.ɪn.bɒnd.ɪd/ pojený pryskyřicí

resistance /rɪˈzɪs.tᵊnt s/ odolnost, stálost, vzdor, odpor, pevnost

respectively /rɪˈspek.tɪv.li/ co se každého týče

restoration /ˌres.tᵊrˈeɪ.ʃᵊn/ výplň, obnova, oprava, náhrada

restorative /rɪˈstɒr.ə.tɪv/ obnovený, opravený, konzervační

restore /rɪˈstɔːʳ/ obnovit, opravit, navrátit do původního stavu

retain /rɪˈteɪn/ ponechat, zachytit, zadržet, zachovat

retention /rɪˈten.tʃᵊn/ upevnění, zadržení, uchování, retence (zubů)

retract /rɪˈtrækt/ odtáhnout

retrograde /ˈret.rəʊ.greɪd/ retrográdní, obrácený

rigid /ˈrɪdʒ.ɪd/ pevný, neohebný, tuhý

rinse /rɪnts/ vypláchnout, propláchnout

roughen /ˈrʌf.ᵊn/ zdrsnit

runny /ˈrʌn.i/ tekutý

saline /ˈseɪ.laɪn/ fyziologický roztok

salivary /səˈlaɪ.vᵊr.i/ slinný

satisfactory /ˌsæt.ɪsˈfæk.tᵊr.i/ uspokojivý, splňující všechny podmínky

scale /skeɪl/ odstranit zubní kámen

scaler /skeɪl.əʳ/ škrabka

scalpel /ˈskæl.pᵊl/ blade /bleɪd/ čepelka skalpelu

seal /siːl/ zaplombovat, plomba, uzávěr

sealant /ˈsiː.lənt/ tmel, těsnicí materiál

sealer /ˈsiː.ləʳ/ pečetidlo, prostředek pro utěsnění

seat /siːt/ umístit, usadit

secondary /ˈsek.ən.dri/ sekundární, druhotný

section /ˈsek.ʃᵊn/ průřez, odříznutí, pitva

sedative /ˈsed.ə.tɪv/ uklidňující, bolesti utišující lék

sensation /senˈseɪ.ʃᵊn/ pocit, vnímání, dojem

set /set/ sada, umístění, tuhnutí, nastavit

setting /ˈset.ɪŋ/ time /taɪm/ doba tuhnutí

setting /ˈset.ɪŋ/ tuhnutí, nasazení, nastavení

shaped /ʃeɪpt/ ve tvaru

shiny /ˈʃaɪ.ni/ lesklý, jasný

shrinkage /ˈʃrɪŋ.kɪdʒ/ smrštění, srážení

sickle /ˈsɪk.ḷ/ srpek

silicone /ˈsɪl.ɪ.kəʊn/ silikon

single-stage /ˈsɪŋ.gḷ.steɪdʒ/ jednostupňový

slab /slæb/ destička

smooth /smuːð/ jemný, hladký, vyhladit

sodium /ˈsəʊ.di.əm/ hypochlorite / haɪ.pəʊˈklɔː.raɪt/ chlornan sodný

solid /ˈsɒl.ɪd/ pevný, tuhá hmota

solubility /ˌsɒl.juˈbɪl.ɪ.ti/ rozpustnost, tavitelnost

sound /saʊnd/ zdravý, sonda

source /sɔːs/ zdroj

spark /spɑːk/ erosion /ɪˈrəʊ.ʒᵊn/ elektrojiskrové obrábění

spatula /ˈspæt.jʊ.lə/ třecí lopatka, špachtle, stěrka

spatulation /ˌspæt.jəˈleɪ.ʃᵊn/ míchání, tření

spoon /spuːn/ excavator /
'ek.skə.veɪ.təʳ/ exkavační lžička
spun /spʌn/ roztočen, vtlačen
squash /skwɒʃ/ rozmačkat, kašovitá
hmota
stable /'steɪ.bl̩/ stabilní, stálý
stage /steɪdʒ/ stav, stupeň, stádium
stagnation /stæg'neɪ.ʃ°n/ stagnace
(váznutí), hniloba
state /steɪt/ stav, skupenství
steel /stiːl/ ocel
steriliser /'ster.°l.aɪz.əʳ/ sterilizační
zařízení
stick /stɪk/ tyčinka (vosku apod.)
stiffly /'stɪf.li/ ztuha
strain /streɪn/ napětí
streak /striːk/ tvořit proužky,
pruhovat, čmouha
strength /streŋθ/ síla, houževnatost,
mez pevnosti
stress /stres/ tlak, napětí, namáhání
string /strɪŋ/ provázek, zde: pramének
strip /strɪp/ pásek, proužek
sublining /sʌb.'laɪ.nɪŋ/ podložení
subperiosteal /sʌb,per.ɪ'ɒs.ti.əl/
subperiostální, ležící pod okosticí
suited /'sjuː.tɪd/ to /tʊ/ vhodný k
surface /'sɜː.fɪs/ povrch, stěna,
opracovat povrch
surgical /'sɜː.dʒɪ.k°l/ chirurgický
surpass /sə'pɑːs/ překonat
susceptible /sə'sep.tɪ.bl̩/ náchylný k
suture /'suː.tʃəʳ/ needle /'niː.dl̩/ šicí
jehla s vláknem
system /'sɪs.təm/ systém
tactile /'tæk.taɪl/ taktilní, dotekový
tasting /-teɪ.stɪŋ/ chutnající
tear /teəʳ/ resistance /rɪ'zɪs.t°n*t* s/
pevnost proti natržení
temporary /'tem.p°r.°r.i/ prozatímní,
dočasný
tensile /'ten.saɪl/ tažný (síla)

thermal /'θɜː.məl/ expansion /
ɪk'spæn.t*ʃ°*n/ tepelná rozpínavost
thin /θɪn/ tenký, řídký, zeslabit
thread /θred/ niť
time /taɪm/ doba
tin /tɪn/ cín
tip /tɪp/ špička, zahrocení
towel /taʊəl/ ručník, utěrka
transfer /træns'fɜːʳ/ přenést
translucence /trænz'luː.sənt s/
průsvitnost
tray /treɪ/ otiskovací lžíce, miska,
destička
trimmer /'trɪm.əʳ/ nůž, ořezávačka
try /traɪ/ zkouška, vyzkoušet
tubular /'tjuː.bjʊ.ləʳ/ tubulární,
trubicovitý
tubule /'tjuː.bjuːl/ tubulus, kanálek
tungsten /'tʌŋ.stən/ wolfram
ultimately /'ʌl.tɪ.mət.li/ nakonec,
skutečně
ultrasonic /,ʌl.trə'sɒn.ɪk/
ultrazvukový
undercut /,ʌn.də'kʌt/ podebrat,
spodní zářez, odkrojit spodní část
unpolished /ʌn'pɒl.ɪʃt/ nevyleštěný
unsightly /ʌn'saɪt.li/ nevzhledný
unsupported /,ʌn.sə'pɔː.tɪd/ bez
podpory
up /ʌp/ to /tʊ/ až do, do výše
use /juːs/ použití
use /juːz/ použít
vapour /'veɪ.pəʳ/ výpary
variety /və'raɪə.ti/ druh, odrůda
varnish /'vɑː.nɪʃ/ lak, lesk
veneer /və'nɪəʳ/ dýha, fazeta, obložení
visibility /,vɪz.ɪ'bɪl.ɪ.ti/ viditelnost
wax /wæks/ vosk
wear /weəʳ/ resistance /rɪ'zɪs.t°n*t* s/
otěruvzdornost
wedge /wedʒ/ klínek, vklínit
wet /wet/ mokrý, vlhký

whilst /waɪl.st/ zatímco, kdežto

wipe /waɪp/ utřít, otřít

withstand /wɪð'stænd/ vydržet

wooden /'wʊd.ᵊn/ dřevěný

working /'wɜː.kɪŋ/ pracovní

wrapped /ræpt/ zabalený

wrought /rɔːt/ alloy /'æl.ɔɪ/ tvářecí
slitina, kujná slitina

zinc /zɪŋk/ oxide /'ɒk.saɪd/ /eugenol
/juː'dʒen.ɒl/ zinkoxid-eugenolová
pasta

zinc /zɪŋk/ phosphate /'fɒs.feɪt/
cement /sɪ'ment/ zink-fosfátový
cement

Key to Translations

Preventive and Community Dental Practice

Translation 1

1. Čerstvé ovoce je vhodnější než čokoládové tyčinky: **fresh fruit is preferable to chocolate bars**
2. čistěte si zuby dvakrát denně: **brush teeth twice daily**
3. faktory prostředí, faktory sociální, životní styl: **environmental, social, and lifestyle factors**
4. navštěvujte pravidelně zubního lékaře: **attend the dentist regularly**
5. obnovit funkci, vyhnout se dalším epizodám: **to restore function and avoid further episodes**
6. omezte příjem jídla a pití s obsahem cukru: **reduce the intake of sugar-containing food and drink**
7. preventivní opatření, fluorizace vody, kampaně propagující zdraví: **preventive measures, water fluoridation, and health-promoting campaigns**
8. rentgenová diagnóza, prosvícení skleněným optickým vláknem, elektronický detektor kazů, barviva: **radiographic diagnosis, fibre-optic transillumination, electronic caries detector, dyes**
9. ústní onemocnění, zubní kazy, onemocnění parodontu, rakovina: **oral diseases, dental caries, periodontal disease, oral cancer**
10. utěsnění prasklin, dietní poradenství: **fissure sealants, diet counselling**
11. včasný zásah: **early intervention**
12. zubní kaz, kaz skloviny, fisurální kaz, kaz zuboviny, skrytý kaz, kaz kořene, recidivující kaz, sekundární kaz, akutní kaz, kaz způsobený dětskou lahvičkou, zastavený zubní kaz: **dental caries, enamel caries, fissure caries, dentine caries, occult caries, root caries, recurrent caries, secondary caries, rampant caries, nursing bottle caries, arrested caries**
13. zuby zkažené, chybějící, vyplněné: **decayed, missing, filled teeth**

Translation 2

1. bílé fleky, hnědé skvrny v závažnějších případech: **white flecks, brown stains in more severe cases**
2. dávat přednost mrkvi a jablkům před svačinou s vysokým obsahem

cukru: **prefer carrots and apples to high-sugar snacks**

3. faktory komplikující prevenci: **factors complicating prevention**

4. fluoridové doplňky, tablety, kapky, sůl, mléko, pasty s obsahem fluoridu: **fluoride supplements, tablets, drops, salt, milk, fluoride-containing toothpastes**

5. fluoróza vzniká kvůli nadměrnému příjmu fluoridu: **fluorosis occurs due to the excessive intake of fluoride**

6. chabý zrak a snížená zručnost: **poor eyesight and reduced dexterity**

7. jezte méně cukru, jezte cukr méně často: **eat less sugar, eat sugar less often**

8. každoroční prohlídky u bezzubých pacientů, včasné objevení onemocnění sliznic: **annual dental examinations in edentulous patients, early detection of mucosal disease**

9. kontrola diety a užití fluoridu: **dietary control and use of fluoride**

10. kontrola plaku, ústup dásní, vyviklané a skloněné zuby, částečné protézy: **plaque control, gingival recession, migrated and tilted teeth, partial dentures**

11. konzumace cukru, frekvence, množství: **sugar consumption frequency, amount**

12. mírné formy se časem zmenší: **mild forms diminish with time**

13. možné vedlejší účinky na zažívací systém: **possible side effects on the gastrointestinal system**

14. nadměrné užívání léčiv je běžné, některé léky snižují tok slin: **polypharmacy is common; some drugs reduce salivary flow**

15. náhražky cukru: **sugar substitutes**

16. náchylní k opakujícím se kazům, kazům kořenů: **prone to recurrent caries and root caries**

17. nechte pomalu rozpustit v ústech: **allow to dissolve slowly in the mouth**

18. období tvoření zubu: **the period of tooth formation**

19. odstraňování plaku: **plaque removal**

20. omezte množství pasty s fluoridem u dětí: **restrict the amount of fluoride toothpaste used by children**

21. péče o protézy, vyjímání protéz na noc, dobrá hygiena: **denture care, removal of dentures at night, good hygiene**

22. péče o starší lidi: **care of elderly people**

23. perlivé nápoje způsobují znatelnou ztrátu zubní struktury erozí: **carbonated beverages cause marked loss of tooth structure via erosion**

24. přidávání fluoridu do vody: **addition of fluoride to the water**

25. příchuť máty peprné odradí děti od požívání pasty: **mint flavours discourage children eating the paste**

26. sladidla bez cukru udržují touhu po sladkém: **nonsugar sweeteners perpetuate the craving for sweet foods**

27. účinný v prevenci kazů: **effective in caries prevention**

28. ukládat mimo dosah dětí: **store out of the reach of children**
29. výskyt a závažnost zubních kazů: **the prevalence and severity of dental caries**
30. zlepšit leptáním, leštěním: **improve by etching and polishing**
31. zubní kaz se nerozvine při nepřítomnosti zubního plaku: **dental caries will not develop in the absence of dental plaque**
32. žvýkačka bez cukru stimuluje tvorbu slin: **sugar-free chewing gum stimulates saliva**

Unit 2
History Taking and Examination
Translation 1

1. bolest tupá, ostrá, škubavá, vystřelující, způsobující nespavost, zklidněná mírnými analgetiky: **pain dull, sharp, throbbing, shooting, causing sleep loss, relieved by mild analgesics**
2. bolest v určitém zubu, celková, šíření, vyzařování: **pain in specific tooth or generalised, spread, radiation**
3. bolest, nepohoda, abnormální pocit: **pain, discomfort, an abnormal feeling**
4. dělat jednoduché náhrady, trhat první zuby: **do simple restorations, extract primary teeth**
5. estetický problém, zhoršená funkce: **aesthetic problem, altered function**
6. je problém stálý nebo přerušovaný, jak často se objevuje: **is the problem continuous or**

intermittent? How frequently does it occur?
7. konstruovat pevné a vyjímatelné náhrady: **construct fixed and removable prostheses**
8. krvácení, výpotek, otok, zápach z úst: **bleeding, exudates, swelling, halitosis**
9. obtíž, kde přesně, kdy byla poprvé zaznamenána: **complaint, where exactly, when was it first noticed?**
10. odstraňování zubního kamene, leštění, aplikace profylaktických materiálů, včetně pečetidla fisur: **scaling, polishing, application of prophylactic materials including fissure sealants**
11. podávat místní anestesii injekčně: **administer local anaesthesia by infiltration**
12. pracovat dle psaných pokynů lékaře: **work to the written prescription of a dentist**
13. práh bolesti se u jednotlivců velice liší: **pain thresholds vary greatly between individuals**
14. role sestry, vzdělávání pacientů, asistovat u křesla: **role of the dental nurse, education of patients, assist at the chairside**
15. schopnost vytvořit správnou anamnézu: **the ability to take a good history**
16. spouštějící nebo ulevující faktory: **initiating or relieving factors**
17. teplo, chlad, zhoršující se při kousání, při předklonu: **hot, cold, worse on biting, on bending forwards**
18. vykonávat administrativní a recepční práce: **undertake**

receptionist and administrative
duties

19. zlepšuje se zhoršuje, je stejný:
    becoming better, worse, is the
    same

Translation 2

1. „Berete nebo jste v posledních
   dvou letech bral steroidy? " : 'Are
   you taking or have you taken
   steroids in the last two years?'

2. „Byl jste někdy hospitalizován?
   Pokud ano, z jakého důvodu
   a kdy? ": 'Have you been
   hospitalised? If yes, what for and
   when?'

3. „Cítíte se celkově zdráv? ": 'Do
   you feel generally healthy?'

4. „Dostáváte nějaké tabletky, krémy,
   masti od Vašeho lékaře? ": 'Are
   you receiving any tablets, creams
   or ointments from your doctor?'

5. „Jste alergický na nějaké léky,
   potraviny, látky? ": 'Are you
   allergic to any medicines, food,
   or material?'

6. „Jste celkově zdráv a v pořádku?":
   'Are you generally fit and well?'

7. „Jste nastávající matka? Jste
   těhotná? ": 'Are you an expectant
   mother? Are you pregnant?'

8. „Kdo je Vaším lékařem? ": 'Who
   is your doctor?'

9. „Krvácel jste někdy nadměrně
   po říznutí či vytržení zubu? ":
   'Have you ever bled excessively
   following a cut or tooth
   extraction?'

10. „Máte cukrovku? " : 'Do you have
    diabetes?'

11. „Máte nějaké problémy se srdcem
    jako je srdeční angína, srdeční

šelest, náhrada chlopně, utrpěl jste
někdy srdeční záchvat? " : 'Do
you have any heart problems
such as angina, heart murmur,
replacement valve, or have you
suffered a heart attack?'

12. „Máte vysoký krevní tlak? " : 'Do
    you have high blood pressure?'

13. „Máte zánět kloubů? " : 'Do you
    have arthritis?'

14. „Měl jste někdy revmatickou
    horečku? " : 'Have you had
    rheumatic fever?'

15. „Měl jste někdy zánět jater nebo
    žloutenku? " : 'Have you had
    hepatitis or jaundice?'

16. „Navštěvujete jinou nemocnici,
    kliniku či specialisty? " : 'Are
    you attending any other hospital
    clinics or specialists?'

17. „Navštěvujete nějaké lékaře či
    střediska, užíváte nějaké léky či
    tabletky?" : 'Are you attending
    any doctors or clinics or taking
    any medicines or tablets?'

18. „Používáte nějaké tabletky, krémy,
    masti, prášky, nebo léky koupené
    bez receptu v lékárně či obchodě?
    " : 'Are you using any tablets,
    creams, ointments, powders,
    or medicines bought over the
    counter in a pharmacy or shop?'

19. „Trpíte epilepsií, jste náchylný k
    záchvatům mdloby? " : 'Do you
    suffer from epilepsy, or are you
    prone to fainting attacks?'

20. „Trpíte zánětem průdušek,
    astmatem, nebo jinými hrudními
    obtížemi? " : 'Do you suffer from
    bronchitis, asthma, or any other
    chest condition?'

21. kdy byl pacient naposledy ošetřen: **when the patient last received dental treatment**
22. návštěvy pravidelné, nepravidelné: **regular, irregular attendee**
23. obecné otázky: **general questions**
24. pacientův věk, povolání, okolnosti manželství, vyživované osoby, návyk kouření, požívání alkoholu: **patient's age, occupation, marital circumstances, dependants, smoking habit, alcohol consumption**
25. postoj k ošetření, úzkostný, klidný: **attitude to dental treatment, anxious, relaxed**
26. předchozí anamnéza dentální, lékařská, sociální: **previous dental history, medical, social**
27. relevantní dotazy v lékařské diagnóze: **relevant questions in a medical history**

Translation 3
1. celkový stav chrupu, stav ústní hygieny, přítomnost a umístění oprav a kazů, přítomnost a stáří protéz, stav parodontu: **general state of the dentition, oral hygiene status, presence and site of restorations and carious lesions, presence and age of dentures, periodontal condition**
2. diagnóza, plán léčby: **diagnosis, treatment planning**
3. dostupnost plánovaných postupů v rámci systému zdravotnické péče nebo systému pojištění, který kryje pacientovu léčbu: **availability of planned procedures under the health-care system or insurance** scheme covering patient's treatment
4. endodoncie, korunky, můstky, částečné protézy: **endodontics, crowns, bridges, partial dentures**
5. faktory ovlivňující léčbu, komplikující lékařská anamnéza, úzkost pacienta, neschopnost či neochota udržovat adekvátní úroveň kontroly plaku: **factors influencing treatment, complicating medical history, patient anxiety, inability, unwillingness to maintain adequate standards of plaque control**
6. faktory týkající se nákladů, co si pacient může dovolit: **cost-related factors, what patient can afford**
7. otoky na obličeji a krku, celistvost rtů: **swellings of the face and neck, lip competence**
8. plán léčby, zásada, zmírnit bolest, vytrhnout zuby s beznadějnou prognózou: **treatment planning, principle, to relieve pain, extract teeth of hopeless prognosis**
9. poskytnout poradenství o prevenci, zlepšit stav parodontu, opravit zkažené zuby: **provide preventive advice, improve periodontal condition, restore carious teeth**
10. prohmatejte lymfatické uzliny, temporo-mandibulární oblast, žvýkací svaly: **palpate lymph nodes, TMJ area, muscles of mastication**
11. rentgenové snímky, testy citlivosti, studijní modely, biopsie: **radiographs, sensitivity tests, study models, biopsy**

12. sledujte celkový vzhled pacienta: **look for general appearance of the patient**
13. vyšetření vně úst, v ústech: **extraoral examination, intraoral examination**
14. zaznamenejte stav měkkých tkání, přítomné, chybějící a neprořezané zuby: **note condition of soft tissues, teeth present, missing, unerupted**

Unit 3

Dental Radiology

Translation 1
1. CT ukazuje jak měkké tkáně tak kost: **CT shows both soft tissues and bone**
2. digitální údaje uložené v počítači: **the digital data stored on a computer**
3. digitální zobrazování, konvenční rentgenové přístroje: **digital imaging, conventional X-ray machines**
4. kontraindikován u pacientů s feromagnetickými chirurgickými svorkami, srdečními stimulátory, kochleárními implantáty a v prvních třech měsících těhotenství: **contraindicated in patients with ferromagnetic surgical clips, pacemakers, choclear implants, and in the first three months of pregnancy**
5. konvenční tomografie, tenké plátky znázorněné na průřezu: **conventional tomography, cross-sectional slices**
6. plánování implantátů, zhodnocení rozsahu patologie tváří a jazyka: **implant planning, assessing**

the buccolingual extension of pathology
7. počítačová tomografie: **computer tomography (CT)**
8. pokročilé techniky zobrazování: **advanced imaging techniques**
9. povrchové měkké části jako slinné žlázy, lymfatické uzliny a štítná žláza: **superficial soft-tissue structures such as salivary glands, lymph nodes, and the thyroid**
10. protony vodíku v tělesné tekutině převezmou energii ze signálu: **hydrogen protons in body fluid take up energy from the signal**
11. protony vydávají radiový signál, který je zachycen a zpracován počítačem: **the protons emit a radio signal which is picked up and processed by a computer**
12. předvedení tumoru, zhodnocení nitrolebečního onemocnění: **tumour staging, the assessment of intracranial disease**
13. přístroje vypadají podobně jako panoramatické jednotky, mají větší rozsah pohybu, umožňují vytvářet průřezy čelistmi téměř v jakékoli poloze: **the machines look similar to panoramic units, have a greater range of movement, allow slices to be made through the jaws in almost any position**
14. receptory obrazu, převést získanou informaci do digitální formy: **image receptors, convert the information received into digital form**
15. senzor, fosforová destička citlivá na světlo: **sensor, photostimulable phosphor plate**

16. skenování pacienta čidlem, které vydává vysokofrekvenční zvukové vlny, zjišťuje vlny odražené od různých styčných ploch uvnitř tkání: **scanning the patient with a transducer that emits high-frequency sound waves, detects the waves reflected from various interfaces within the tissues**

17. spočítat hloubku částí a vytvořit obraz: **to calculate the depth of the structures and create a picture**

18. škálový obraz ukazující se na monitoru: **scale image displayed on a monitor**

19. trubice rentgenu prochází v kruhu kolem těla, řada detektorů měří v každém bodu blokování paprsku: **X-ray tube passes in a circle around the body, series of detectors measure the blocking of the beam at each point**

20. umístit pacienta do silného magnetického pole, použít ráz radiových vln, vybrat frekvenci: **place the patient into a strong magnetic field, apply a pulse of these waves, choose frequency**

21. zhodnocení závažného traumatu střední části obličeje nebo onemocnění zahrnujícího kost: **assessing serious midfacial trauma or disease involving bone**

22. zobrazování pomocí magnetické resonance: **magnetic resonance imaging (MRI)**

23. zobrazování pomocí ultrazvuku: **ultrasonography**

Unit 4
Psychological Aspects of Dental Care
Translation 1

1. akceptovat občasnou bolest: **accept intermittent pain**

2. časová tíseň, informace předávané příliš rychle: **time pressures information presented too quickly**

3. etiologie je ovlivněna chováním a životním stylem: **the aetiology is influenced by behavioural and lifestyle factors**

4. finanční náklady mohou být překážkou: **financial cost may be a barrier**

5. komunikovat efektivně se členy personálu: **to communicate effectively with members of the practice staff**

6. motivovat pacienty a ovlivnit změnu chování: **motivate patients and influence behaviour change**

7. možnost zdraví úst ovlivnit: **ability to influence oral health**

8. nemoc, nepohoda či překážka: **disease, discomfort, or embarrassment**

9. pacienti nerozumí technickým výrazům: **technical language is not understood by patients**

10. pochopit povahu bolesti: **understand the nature of pain**

11. postoje, gestikulace a výraz lékaře, reakce pacienta: **postures, gestures, and expressions of the clinician, the patient's reaction**

12. povzbudit nebo odradit od návštěvy: **encourage or discourage attendance**

13. povzbuzení ke změně chování: **encouraging behaviour change**

14. praxe zubního lékařství zahrnuje práci s lidmi: **the practice of dentistry involves working with people**
15. priority se mohou lišit: **priorities may differ**
16. předpokládaná závažnost onemocnění: **perceived seriousness of a disease**
17. příjmy, vzdělání, životní a pracovní podmínky: **income, education, living and working conditions**
18. přispívat k celkovému pocitu zdraví: **contribute to general well-being**
19. rozhodnutí navštívit zubního lékaře: **the decision to attend a dentist**
20. rozumět příčinám úzkosti: **understand causes of anxiety**
21. schopnost efektivně komunikovat: **the ability to communicate effectively**
22. sociální a psychologické vlivy na dentální péči: **social and psychological influences on dental care**
23. umístění ordinace, dostupnost veřejné dopravy: **location of the office, availability of public transport**
24. umožňuje jedinci jíst, mluvit a společensky žít: **it enables an individual to eat, speak, and socialise**
25. úzkost brání schopnosti informace vstřebat: **anxiety hinders ability to absorb information**
26. vyhledávat péči až když se bolest stane stálou nebo nesnesitelnou: **seek care only when pain becomes constant or intolerable**
27. vysvětlování navrhované léčby: **explaining proposed treatment**
28. vzít si volno z práce, zařídit hlídání dítěte: **take time off work, arrange a babysitter**
29. zdraví úst, normální stav tkání úst a okolních tkání: **oral health, a standard of health of the oral and related tissues**
30. zhoršení symptomů: **worsening of symptoms**
31. získávání anamnézy pacienta: **eliciting a history from a patient**
32. zubní zdravotní sestra, hygienistka, recepční, technik: **dental nurse, hygienist, receptionist, technician**
33. zvládání úzkostných pacientů: **managing anxious patients**

Unit 5
Paediatric Dentistry
Translation 1
1. bolest je běžným symptomem, vede pacienty k vyhledání péče: **pain is a common symptom, leads patients to seek care**
2. cíle změny chování by měly být dosažitelné, realistické, pro pacienta důležité, měřitelné, pozitivní, časově vymezené, přesně stanovené: **targets for behaviour change should be achievable, realistic, important to the patient, measurable, positive, time related, specific**
3. hypnóza může být užitečná u některých pacientů: **in some patients hypnosis can be useful**

4. konečným cílem je integrovat pozitivní chování do pacientova každodenního životního stylu: **the ultimate aim is to integrate positive behaviour into patient's everyday lifestyles**
5. mít znalosti a dovednosti dovolující změnu: **have the knowledge and skills to permit change**
6. písemné pokyny (letáček) mohou být užitečné: **written information (a leaflet) may be helpful**
7. poskytnutí informace je často nedostatečné: **providing information is frequently insufficient**
8. procedura možná bude trochu nepříjemná: **the procedure may be slightly uncomfortable**
9. přátelský a chápavý postoj, příjemné prostředí: **friendly and understanding attitude, welcoming environment**
10. příčiny úzkosti: **causes of anxiety**
11. reakce na bolest je ovlivněna kulturními a emočními faktory: **reaction to pain is influenced by cultural and emotional factors**
12. rozptýlení, odvrácení pacientovy pozornosti: **distraction, shifting the patient's attention**
13. strach z bolesti může zabránit pacientům vyhledat ošetření: **fear of pain may prevent patients from seeking treatment**
14. strach z bolesti, nejistota, předchozí zkušenosti, připravenost: **fear of pain, uncertainty, previous experience, preparedness**

15. účinná komunikace: **effective communication**
16. udržení změny, opětné zhoršení: **maintaining change, relapse**
17. varujte pacienta než skloníte křeslo, pustíte vzduch ze stříkačky: **warn patients before reclining chair, blowing air from 3-in-1 syringe**
18. Vědí pacienti jak zuby čistit? Jak často si je čistí?: **Do the patients know how to brush? How frequently do they brush?**
19. věnujte dost času rozhovoru a vysvětlování: **take time to discuss and explain**
20. věřit, že změna bude mít žádaný účinek: **believe change will have the desired effect**
21. vyhnout se přemíře informací: **avoid information overload**
22. změna chování: **behaviour change**
23. zmírnit úzkost: **alleviate anxiety**
24. zvedněte ruku pokud si budete přát, abych přestal: **raise your hand if you want me to stop**
25. zvládnutí bolesti: **pain control**
26. zvukové nahrávky, obrázky na stropě: **audiotapes, pictures on the ceiling**

Translation 2
1. demonstrujte, potom proveďte: **demonstrate, then do**
2. dětem přátelské prostředí, plakáty, hračky: **child-friendly environment, posters, toys**
3. děti jsou velmi citlivé na prostředí a neverbální komunikaci: **children are very sensitive to environment and nonverbal communication**

4. dětské zubní lékařství: **paediatric dentistry**
5. dovednosti nezbytné pro přijetí zubního ošetření: **the appropriate skills to cope with dental treatment**
6. jednoduché pokyny pro prevenci: **simple preventive messages**
7. malé děti by měly být pod dohledem: **young children should be supervised**
8. nálepky, odznaky a pochvala působí pozitivní posílení: **stickers, badges, and praise act as positive reinforcers**
9. netraumatizující přijetí: **atraumatic introduction**
10. omezit množství spolknuté pasty: **limit amount of toothpaste consumed**
11. oslovujte dítě jeho správným jménem, usmívejte se: **call child by his or her correct name, smile**
12. ovládání chování u dětí, praktické otázky: **managing behaviour in children, practical points**
13. po čistění vyplivnout, nikoli vypláchnout: **spit, not rinse after brushing**
14. poskytnout nutnou opravnou péči: **provide any necessary restorative care**
15. postoje dítěte a jeho chování jsou ovlivněny mnoha faktory: **the child's attitude and behaviour will be influenced by many factors**
16. postrádat dostatečnou manuální zručnost: **lack sufficient manual dexterity**

17. předchozí zkušenost s lékaři, se zubními lékaři: **previous medical experience, dental experience**
18. přístup personálu, prostředí ordinace, přístup rodičů: **attitude of dental staff, environs of surgery, attitude of parents**
19. rozsah pozornosti je malý: **attention span is short**
20. řekněte dítěti co se chystáte udělat: **tell the child what you are going to do**
21. věk, zralost, osobnost: **age, maturity, personality**
22. zavést dobrou prevenci: **institute good preventive practice**

Translation 3
1. běžný výskyt: **a common occurrence**
2. cíle dlouhodobé, korunky, náhrada ztracených zubů, ortodontická léčba, snímatelná pevná protéza: **long-term aims, crown, replacement of lost teeth, orthodontic therapy, removable/ fixed prosthodontics**
3. cíle okamžité, uklidnění pacienta a rodiče, úleva od bolesti, ochrana dřeně, sešití lacerací měkké tkáně, zpevnění zlomených a pohyblivých zubů: **immediate aims, reassurance of patient and parent, relieve of pain, protection of pulp, suture of soft-tissue lacerations, stabilisation of fractured or mobile teeth**
4. cíle střednědobé, léčba dřeně, polotrvalé náhrady: **intermediate aims, pulp therapy, semipermanent restoration**

5. děti se zvláštními potřebami: **children with special needs**

6. dietní doporučení určené rodičům, fluoridové doplňky, vhodná opatření pro dentální hygienu: **dietary advice to parents, fluoride supplements, appropriate arrangements for oral hygiene**

7. dosáhnout a udržet ústní zdraví: **to attain and maintain oral health**

8. fyzické poškození zahrnuje mozkovou obrnu, zadní rozštěp páteře, svalovou dystrofii: **physical disability includes cerebral palsy, spina bifida, muscular dystrophy**

9. izolace zubu během operačních postupů: **isolation of the tooth during the operative procedures**

10. jeden z opravdu naléhavých případů: **one of the true emergencies**

11. klasifikace úrazu, léčebné cíle: **classification of trauma, objectives of treatment**

12. maximální účinek: **maximum benefit**

13. neschopnost učení vrozená (Downův syndrom), získaná, např. jako důsledek poškození mozku před porodem, při porodu či po porodu: **learning disability congenital (Down's syndrome), acquired (e.g. as a result of brain damage pre-, peri-, or postnatally)**

14. neúplné vyvrácení (zub je rozviklán v chobotu, ale není odstraněný): **subluxation, tooth loosened in the pocket but not displaced**

15. obvyklé příčiny zahrnují: batolata – zakopnutí a pády, starší děti – nehody na kole, dospívající – kontaktní sporty, rvačky, alkohol: **common causes include: toddlers – trips and falls, older children – bicycle accidents, teenagers – contact sports, fights, alcohol**

16. odtržení, zub úplně odstraněn z chobotu: **avulsion, tooth totally displaced from the socket**

17. pohmoždění, zub je poraněný, ale není uvolněný: **concussion, tooth traumatised but not loosened**

18. posunutí do strany (zub je zatlačen do strany, směrem k tváři či směrem k patru): **lateral displacement, tooth pushed laterally, buccally, or palatally**

19. retraktor, odsavač slin, vysoko- a nízko-objemový odsávací přístroj, vatové svitky, absorpční tampony, gumová blána: **retractor, saliva ejector, high- and low-volume aspirators, cotton-wool rolls, absorbent pads, rubber dam**

20. smyslové poškození, slepota, hluchota: **sensory disability, blindness, deafness**

21. udržování operačního pole: **maintenance of the operating field**

22. vtlačení, zub je posunutý v chobotu směrem ke kořenovému hrotu: **intrusion, tooth displaced apically into socket**

23. vyčnívání, zub je posunutý ve směru kousání: **extrusion, tooth displaced in occlusal direction**

24. vytváření vzorů – dítě se učí pozorováním ostatních:

modelling—child learns by watching others

25. vyžadovat zvláštní ošetření či speciální vybavení: **require extra attention or special facilities**

26. zdravotně oslabení, srdeční poruchy, hemofilie: **medically compromised, cardiac disorders, haemophilia**

27. zlomeniny, sklovina, zubovina, dřeň, kořen: **fractures, enamel, dentine, pulp, root**

28. zvážit možnost závažnějšího základního poranění, např. otřes mozku: **to consider the possibility of more serious underlying injury, e.g. concussion**

Unit 6
General Medicine of Relevance to Dentistry
Translation 1

1. astma: **asthma**
2. cukrovka: **diabetes mellitus**
3. epilepsie: **epilepsy**
4. choroby ledvin: **renal disease**
5. nenoci: **illnesses**
6. infarkt myokardu, srdeční angína: **myocardial infarction, angina**
7. lékařská a léková anamnéza: **medical and drug history**
8. léky užívané v současnosti a minulosti: **medications taken currently and in the past**
9. mrtvice: **stroke**
10. onemocnění jater, zánět jater: **hepatic disease, hepatitis**
11. poruchy s krvácením: **bleeding disorders**
12. přijetí do nemocnice, operace: **hospital admissions, operative procedures**

13. revmatická horečka: **rheumatic fever**
14. srdeční selhání, hypertenze: **heart failure, hypertension**
15. stimulátory: **pacemakers**
16. určení anamnézy: **history taking**
17. všeobecná medicína ve vztahu ke stomatologii: **general medicine of relevance to dentistry**
18. zánět kloubů: **arthritis**

Translation 2

1. dermatologické, změny týkající se vlasů a nehtů, olupování kůže, suchost, pigmentace, zažloutnutí, svědění, poranění, biopsie: **dermatological, hair, or nail changes, scaling, dryness, pigmentation, jaundice, itching, lesions, biopsy**

2. endokrinní, struma, nesnášenlivost tepla/chladu, změny hlasu, struktury vlasů, zvýšená žízeň, zvýšená tvorba moči, vývoj prsů a pohlavních znaků: **endocrine, goitre, hot/cold intolerance, voice changes, hair pattern, increased thirst, increased production of urine, development of breasts and sexual characteristics**

3. hematologické, zhmožděniny, krvácení, uzliny, bulky, anémie: **haematological, bruising, bleeding, nodes, lumps, anaemia**

4. neurologické, bolest hlavy, mdloby, nevolnost, zvracení, závratě, bolesti, ztráta čichu, chuti nebo zraku, svalová slabost, nebo ochabování, změny pocitů, ztráta smyslového vnímání, ztráta koordinace, třes, záchvaty, brýle, dvojité vidění, slepé

skvrny, tunelové vidění, bolest,
otok, začervenání, suchost očí,
snížené slyšení, zvonění v uších:
**neurological, headache, fainting,
nausea, vomiting, vertigo,
dizziness, pains, loss of smell,
taste, or vision, muscle weakness
or wasting, change in sensation,
loss of sensation, loss of
coordination, tremors, seizures,
spectacles, double vision, blind
spots, tunnel vision, pain,
swelling, redness or dryness
of the eyes, decreased hearing,
ringing in the ears**
5. obecné údaje, váhový úbytek
či přibývání na váze, anorexie,
hladina energie, horečky a noční
pocení: **general, weight loss or
gain, anorexia, energy level,
fevers and night sweats**
6. údaje o dýchání, epistaxe
(krvácení z nosu), rinorea (vodnatý
výtok z nosu), kašel, vytváření
hlenu, dyspnoe (dušnost), sípání,
cyanóza (promodrání kůže),
bolesti pohrudnice: **respiratory,
epistaxis, rhinorrhoea, cough,
sputum production, dyspnoea,
wheezing, cyanosis, pleuritic
pain**
7. úplný přehled bude zahrnovat
následující: **a full review will
include following**

Translation 3
1. gastrointestinální systém, chuť
k jídlu, snášenlivost potravin,
flatulence (nadýmání), špatné
trávení, bolest břicha, nevolnost,
zvracení, zvracení krve, zácpa
či průjem, barva stolice,

konzistence a vlastnosti, hlen,
hemeroidy, zánět jater a žloutenka,
zneužívání alkoholu, problémy
v ústech, na sliznici a se zuby:
**gastrointestinal, appetite,
food tolerance, flatulence,
indigestion, abdominal pain,
nausea, vomiting, vomiting
blood, constipation or diarrhoea,
stool colour, consistency and
quality, mucus, haemorrhoids,
hepatitis, and jaundice, alcohol
abuse, oral, mucosal, and dental
problems**
2. kardiovaskulární systém, palpitace
(bušení), vyzařování bolesti
na hrudi, počet používaných
polštářů, hypertenze, cyanóza,
hemoptýza (vykašlávání krve),
edém (otok), křečové žíly a
flebitida (zánět žil), vrozené
či získané srdeční anomálie,
šelesty, tolerance tělesné námahy:
**cardiovascular, palpitations,
chest pain radiations, number
of pillows used, hypertension,
cyanosis, haemoptysis (coughing
up blood), oedema, varicose
veins, and phlebitis, congenital
or acquired cardiac anomalies,
murmurs, exercise tolerance**
3. pohlavní a vylučovací systém,
frekvence močení, prodlévání,
změny v proudu, obtíže při
zahájení a zastavení, infekce
močového traktu, impotence,
sexuálně přenosné nemoci:
**genitourinary, urinary
frequency, hesitancy, changes in
stream, difficulties starting or
stopping stream, urinary tract**

infections, impotence, sexually transmitted diseases

4. porodnictví/gynekologie, komplikace v těhotenství, potrat a spontánní potrat, průběh menstruace, před menstruační syndrom, dysmenorea (bolestivá menstruace), menoragie (silné menstruační krvácení), datum posledních měsíčků, menopauza, krvácení po menopauze: **obstetric/ gynaecology, complications of pregnancy, abortion, or miscarriages, menstrual history, premenstrual syndrome, dysmenorrhoea, menorrhagia, date of last menstrual period, menopause, postmenopausal bleeding**

5. psychiatrické okolnosti, nálada a vzhled, úzkost, deprese, poruchy osobnosti, nespavost, časné probouzení, halucinace, bludy: **psychiatric, mood and appearance, anxiety, depression, and personality disorders, insomnia, early morning wakening, hallucinations, delusions**

6. svalový a kosterní systém, zlomeniny, artritida, bolest a otok kloubů, bolest a slabost svalů, omezení hybnosti a deformita: **musculoskeletal, fractures, arthritis, joint pain, and swelling, muscle pain and weakness, limitation of movement and deformity**

Translation 4

1. akutní virový zánět jater, chronický zánět jater, chronická jaterní choroba: **acute viral hepatitis, chronic hepatitis, chronic liver disease**

2. astma, infekce a chronické obstrukční onemocnění plic: **asthma, infections, and chronic obstructive pulmonary disease**

3. bronchiální karcinom, cystická fibróza: **bronchial carcinoma, cystic fibrosis**

4. celiakie, průjem, steatorea (tuková stolice), úbytek váhy a u dětí nemožnost správně prospívat: **coeliac disease, diarrhoea, steatorrhoea, weight loss, and failure to thrive normally in children**

5. Crohnova choroba, chronický zánět: **Crohn's disease, a chronic inflammation**

6. druhotné ústní projevy: **secondary oral manifestations**

7. dysfagie (obtížné polykání) : **dysphagia (difficulty in swallowing)**

8. ezofagitida (zánět jícnu), pálení žáhy: **oesophagitis, heartburn**

9. gastrointestinální systém: **gastrointestinal system**

10. hypertenze: **hypertension**

11. chronická ztráta krve, způsobující nedostatek železa: **chronic blood loss, causing iron deficiency**

12. chronické zánětlivé onemocnění tlustého střeva: **a chronic inflammatory disease of the colon**

13. ischemická choroba srdeční: **ischaemic heart disease**

14. jaterní onemocnění: **hepatic disease**

15. krví přenášené virové infekce jsou velmi důležité pro zubní obory: **blood-borne viral infections are of great concern to the dental professions**

16. nedostatek železa s výslednými problémy ústní sliznice, opakující se aftózní stomatitida: **iron deficiency with resultant oral mucosal problems, recurrent aphthous stomatitis**

17. onemocnění slinivky, zánět pankreatu, akutní. chronický: **pancreatic disease, inflammation of the pancreas, acute, chronic**

18. otok rtu při Crohnově nemoci: **lip swelling in Crohn's disease**

19. peptický vřed, žaludeční, dvanáctníkový: **peptic ulceration, gastric, duodenal**

20. predisponujícími faktory jsou výhřez v otvoru jícnu, těhotenství, obezita, kouření: **predisposing factors include hiatus hernia, pregnancy, obesity, smoking**

21. rakovina tlustého střeva: **colonic cancer**

22. reflux návykový, bulimie: **reflux habitual, bulimia nervosa**

23. respirační systém: **respiratory system**

24. slinění při anorexii: **sialosis in anorexia nervosa**

25. srdečně cévní systém: **cardiovascular system**

26. srdeční selhání: **cardiac failure**

27. srdeční šelest: **cardiac murmurs**

28. strava chudá na vlákninu, psychologické faktory: **a diet deficient in fibre, psychological factors**

29. syndrom dráždivého střeva, symptomy zhoršeného stavu střev, bolesti břicha, nadmutí břicha: **irritable bowel syndrome, symptoms of altered bowel habit, abdominal pain, bloating**

30. ústní projevy, primární, sekundární: **oral manifestations, primary, secondary**

31. vředovitá kolitida: **ulcerative colitis**

32. zpětný tok žaludečních kyselin: **gastric acid reflux**

33. žaludeční karcinom (rakovinný nádor) : **gastric carcinoma**

34. žloutenka, žluté zbarvení skléry (oční bělimy), kůže a sliznice úst: **jaundice, yellow discolouration of the sclera, the skin, and oral mucous membranes**

Translation 5

1. Anémie, koncentrace hemoglobinu, udávaný rozsah, věk a pohlaví pacienta: **anaemia, haemoglobin concentration, reference range, age, and gender of patient**

2. cukrovka, hypertenze: **diabetes mellitus, hypertension**

3. endokrinní poruchy: **endocrine disorders**

4. glomerulonefritida (zánět ledvin spojený se zánětem glomerulů) : **glomerulonephritis**

5. hyperglykemie (zvýšené množství cukru v krvi) kvůli nedostatku (Typ 1) nebo sníženému účinku (Typ 2) insulinu: **hyperglycaemia due to deficiency (Type 1) or reduced effectiveness (Type 2) of insulin**

6. chronické selhání ledvin: **chronic renal failure**

7. infekce, pyelonefritida (postihující ledvinu), cystitida (postihující močový měchýř): **infections, pyelonephritis (affecting the kidney), cystitis (affecting the bladder)**

8. krevní systém: **haematological system**

9. menopauza je obdobím velké fyziologické a psychologické proměny: **menopause is a time of great physiological and psychological change**

10. onemocnění ledvin: **renal disease**

11. onemocnění štítné žlázy a příštitných tělísek: **thyroid and parathyroid disease**

12. poruchy hypofýzy (podvěsek mozkový) a poruchy žlázy nadledvin: **pituitary and adrenal gland disorders**

13. poruchy krvácení, defekty krevních cév, defekty krevních destiček, defekty koagulace (dědičné a získané): **bleeding disorders, blood vessel defects, platelet defects, coagulation defects (hereditary and acquired)**

14. postupující poškození ledvin: **progressive kidney damage**

15. pyelonefritida (současný zánět ledvinné pánvičky a ledviny): **pyelonephritis**

16. rutinní dentální ošetření by měla být prováděna krátce po jídle: **routine dentistry should be performed soon after mealtimes**

17. symptomy, časté močení, nutkání, dysurie (bolest při močení)

a inkontinence, zadržování: **symptoms, frequency, urgency, dysuria (pain on micturition), incontinence, retention**

18. symptomy, polyurie (nadměrné močení), nokturie (noční močení), anorexie, zvracení a svědivost kůže: **symptoms, polyuria, nocturia, anorexia, vomiting, and itchiness of the skin**

19. menopauza, syndromy bolesti úst a obličeje psychického původu, syndrom pálení v ústech jsou v této době relativně běžné: **menopause, psychogenic orofacial pain syndromes such as burning mouth syndrome are relatively common at this time**

20. těhotenství, zhoršení zánětu dásní, rozvoj zánětlivých nádorků dásně: **pregnancy, worsening of gingivitis, development of inflammatory epulides**

21. vyhýbat se rentgenu, celkové anestézii a lékům, pokud nejsou nezbytné: **to avoid radiographs, general anaesthesia, and drugs, except if essential**

22. zvýšená činnost příštitných tělísek, snížená činnost příštitných tělísek: **hyperparathyroidism, hypoparathyroidism**

23. zvýšená činnost štítné žlázy, snížená činnost štítné žlázy: **hyperthyroidism, hypothyroidism**

24. zvýšená hladina obíhající močoviny (urémie): **increased levels of circulating urea (uraemia)**

Translation 6

1. anorexie, malátnost, letargie, myalgie (bolest svalů): **anorexia, malaise, lethargy, myalgia**

2. bolest a ztuhlost, zejména kloubů nesoucích váhu: **pain and stiffness, particularly of weight-bearing joints**

3. cévní léze (např. infarkt nehtových lůžek): **vasculitic lesions (e.g. nail bed infarcts)**

4. epilepsie, klasifikována dle typu záchvatu, částečná (částečné záchvaty) a celková (záchvaty s bezvědomím): **epilepsy, classified according to seizure type, partial (partial seizures) and generalised (absence seizures)**

5. charakteristickými rysy jsou bolest kosti, bolest zad, zlomeniny obratlů, zlomeniny periferní kosti vřetenní a krčku kosti stehenní: **features are bone pain, backache, and fractures of vertebrae, distal radius, and neck of femur**

6. metabolické onemocnění kosti (např. osteoporóza, definovaná jako snížení hmoty kosti): **metabolic bone disease (e.g. osteoporosis, defined as a reduction in bone mass)**

7. migréna, smíšená bolest hlavy a bolest hlavy spojená s tlakem: **migraine, mixed headache, tension headache**

8. nervové poruchy: **neurological disorders**

9. neuropatie (onemocnění nervů): **neuropathies**

10. ochrnutí a neuropatie: **palsy and neuropathy**

11. onemocnění kloubů (např. osteoartritida) je běžnou nemocí kloubů související s věkem: **joint disease (e.g. osteoarthritis) is a common age-related disease of joints**

12. onemocnění pohybového ústrojí: **locomotor system disease**

13. onemocnění vývoje kosti: **developmental bone disease**

14. pankarditida (zánět všech vrstev srdeční stěny) a poranění plic: **pancarditis and lung lesions**

15. Parkinsonova nemoc, způsobená degenerací neuronů v CNS: **Parkinson's disease, caused by degeneration of neurons in the CNS**

16. projevy systémové (týkající se těla jako celku): **the systemic manifestations**

17. příčinami jsou stavy po menopauze, endokrinní, výživové a iatrogenní (lékařem vyvolané): **causes include postmenopausal, endocrine, nutritional, and iatrogenic**

18. přítomností cirkulujících antigenů působících proti vlastnímu organismu (revmatický faktor): **presence of circulating autoantibodies (rheumatoid factor)**

19. revmatická artritida je chronické, zánětlivé, ničící a deformující onemocnění více kloubů s mimo-kloubními systémovými projevy: **rheumatoid arthritis is a chronic inflammatory, destructive, and deforming polyarthropathy with**

extra-articular systemic manifestations

20. roztroušená skleróza, zánětlivá porucha s demyelinizací (zničení myelinu v nervových vláknech): **multiple sclerosis, an inflammatory, demyelinating disorder**

21. složitá porucha, charakteristická malátností: **a complex disorder characterised by lassitude**

22. syndrom chronické únavy: **chronic fatigue syndrome**

23. třes, ztuhlost, bradykineze (extrémní zpomalení pohybu) a porušené postojové reflexy: **tremor, rigidity, bradykinesia, and disturbed postural reflexes**

24. vyšetření nervového systému je složitý a časově náročný proces: **examination of the nervous system is a complex and time-consuming process**

25. znalost lebečních nervů může být užitečná při rozlišení onemocnění organického od psychosomatického: **knowledge of the cranial nerves may be useful in discriminating organic disease from the psychosomatic**

Translation 7

1. Dát podporu a porozumění: **be supportive and understanding**

2. dermatologie: **dermatology**

3. hlavní skutečností je HIV a AIDS : **the major entity is HIV and AIDS**

4. chronická aktivní hepatitida: **chronic active hepatitis**

5. imunitní nedostatečnost vrozená (primární), získaná (sekundární), související s nemocemi nebo terapií, která potlačuje imunitu: **congenital (primary) immunodeficiency, acquired (secondary), related to diseases, or immunosuppressive therapy**

6. léčba poruch pojivové tkáně kožní onemocnění, onemocnění sliznice: **management of connective tissue disorders, dermatological diseases, mucosal disease**

7. léčba, která má imunosupresivní účinky (snížení schopnosti organismu reagovat na cizí látky) je nyní velice běžná: **immunosuppresive therapy is now extremely common**

8. leukémie a lymfomy (maligní tumor lymfatické tkáně): **leukaemias and lymphomas**

9. obličejové a periorální (kolem úst) projevy stavů kůže jako je lupénka a dermatitida (zánět kůže): **the facial and perioral manifestations of skin conditions such as psoriasis and dermatitis**

10. odmítnout ošetření, které není nezbytné a dlouho trvající ošetření: **resist unnecessary and prolonged treatment**

11. pacient by měl být převeden k lékaři, zabývajícímu se těmito poruchami: **the patient should be referred to a physician with an interest in such disorders**

12. po chirurgických transplantacích (např. srdce/plíce, ledviny, jater, slinivky): **following organ transplant surgery (e.g. heart/ lung, kidney, liver, pancreas)**

13. poruchy imunitního systému: **immune system disorders**

14. poruchy osobnosti, neurózy a psychózy: **personality disorders, neuroses, and psychoses**
15. pravděpodobnost infekce, dispozice ke krvácení, profylaxe steroidy: **likelihood of infection, bleeding diathesis, steroid prophylaxis**
16. psychiatrické poruchy: **psychiatric disorders**
17. revmatická artritida: **rheumatoid arthritis**
18. součást etiologie určitých stavů (např. chronické bolesti úst a obličeje): **part of the aetiology of certain conditions (e.g. chronic orofacial pain disorders)**
19. špatná výživa: **malnutrition**
20. vyloučit přispívající dentální onemocnění (jako třeba zánět zubní dřeně): **exclude contributory dental disease (such as pulpitis)**
21. zvýšená náchylnost k infekci: **increased susceptibility to infection**

Unit 7
Emergencies in Dental Practice.
Medical Emergencies and Drugs
Translation 1
1. aerosolový sprej nitroglycerinu: **glyceryl trinitrate aerosol spray**
2. ambu vak, samonafukovací s ventilem a maskou: **Ambu bag, self-inflating with valve and mask**
3. antihistaminika, injekce a tablety: **antihistamine, injections, and tablets**
4. emulze diazepamu: **diazepam emulsion**

5. glukóza injekční a prášek pro ústní užití: **glucose for injection and powder for oral use**
6. inhalátor salbutamolu: **salbutamol inhaler**
7. injekce adrenalinu, injekce hydrokortisonu: **epinephrine (adrenaline) injection, hydrocortisone injection**
8. injekce glukagonu: **glucagon injection**
9. jehly a motýlky: **needles and butterflies**
10. kanyly na venózní přístup (venózní kanyly): **venous access cannulae**
11. koloidní roztok pro infuze: **colloid solution for infusion**
12. koncepce týmové péče: **the concept of team care**
13. krikotyreoidní punkční jehly: **cricothyroid puncture needles**
14. kyslík, oxid dusný (rajský plyn): **oxygen, nitrous oxide**
15. lékař, sestra, hygienista, recepční, technik: **surgeon, nurse, hygienist, receptionist, technician**
16. naléhavé případy v dentální praxi: **emergencies in dental practice**
17. nezbytný pro spolehlivé a kompetentní zvládání naléhavých případů: **essential in dealing with emergencies confidently and competently**
18. orofaryngeální průchody: **oropharyngeal airways**
19. procvičovat pravidelně záchranné postupy: **practise emergency procedures regularly**
20. předem určené úlohy, otvírání pohotovostních lékárniček, telefonování pro pomoc:

predeterminated roles, opening
emergency kit, telephoning for
help

21. přenosný defibrilátor (s možností
záznamu EKG): **portable
defibrillator (incorporating ECG
printout)**

22. přenosný kyslíkový přístroj:
portable oxygen delivery system

23. sety na intravenózní infuse IV: **IV
infusion sets**

24. stříkačky na jedno použití:
disposable syringes

25. škrtidlo, přístroj na měření tepu
a krevních plynů, stetoskop:
**tourniquet, sphygmomanometer,
stethoscope**

26. tyčinky na rychlé určení úrovně
cukru v krvi: **sticks for rapid
assessment of blood sugar levels**

27. vybavení a léky pro první pomoc:
emergency equipment and drugs

28. vysoko-objemové odsávání se
sacími katétry: **high-volume
aspiration with suction catheters**

Translation 2

1. infarkt myokardu, bolest
doprovázena dušností, nevolností,
zvracením, ztrátou vědomí, slabý,
nepravidelný puls, snížený tlak:
**myocardial infarction, pain
accompanied by breathlessness,
nausea, vomiting, loss of
consciousness, weak, irregular
pulse, hypotension**

2. mdloby kvůli strachu, bolesti,
nezvyklé podívané, pachům,
úzkosti, slabosti, hladovění:
**fainting due to fear, pain,
unusual sights, smells, anxiety,
fatigue, fasting**

3. náhlá bolest na hrudi, krutá drtivá
bolest za hrudní kostí, vyzařování
do paže, krku nebo čelisti: **acute
chest pain, severe crushing
retrosternal pain, radiations to
arm, neck, or jaw**

4. naléhavý převoz do nemocnice:
urgent transfer to hospital

5. nepokládejte pacienta dolů,
zvyšuje to pocity dušnosti a
paniky: **do not lie flat, it increases
feelings of breathlessness and
panic**

6. odložte ošetření úst, není-li
naléhavé: **delay dental treatment
unless urgent**

7. pacient nedýchá, poskytněte dva
pomalé, účinné záchranné vdechy,
kontrolujte známky cirkulace
na pulsu karotidy, pokračujte
se záchrannými vdechy, dokud
pacient není schopen dýchat
bez pomoci: **the patient is
not breathing, give two slow,
effective rescue breaths, check
for signs of a circulation at the
carotid pulse, continue rescue
breaths until the patient is able
to breathe unaided**

8. pátrejte zrakem, sluchem a
hmatem po normálním dýchání:
**look, listen, and feel for normal
breathing**

9. pocit závrati, pocit horka, pocení,
nadměrná bledost, pokožka
na dotek chladná a vlhká,
bradykardie, ztráta vědomí a
zhroucení s následným rychlým
a silným pulsem: **light-headed
feeling, warm, sweaty feeling,
pallor, skin cool and moist to
touch, bradycardia, loss of**

consciousness and collapse with resultant rapid, full pulse

10. podejte pacientovi jeho vlastní léky: **give patient's own medication**

11. podejte ústy jednu tabletu aspirinu proti srážlivosti krve: **administer oral aspirin (one tablet) as antiplatelet agent**

12. položte pacienta na podlahu rovně na záda, otevřete dýchací cesty jemným zakloněním hlavy a vytáhnutím čelisti: **lie patient flat on the floor on his or her back, open the airway with a gentle head tilt and chin lift**

13. položte pacienta rovně, hlava je níže než srdce, změřte puls na hlavní cévě, rozhodněte, zda jde o bradykardii: **lie patient flat with head bellow heart, take pulse at major vessel, determine bradycardia**

14. pošlete pro pomoc: **send for help**

15. uvolněte oděv a otevřete okna: **loosen clothing and open windows**

16. zahajte slovní povzbuzování pacienta a podejte glukózu: **establish verbal encouragement of patient and administer glucose**

17. zástava srdeční a dechová, ztráta vědomí, absence pulsu na hlavních tepnách, absence zvuků dechu a pohybů hrudníku: **cardiorespiratory arrest, loss of consciousness, absence of central arterial pulses, absence of breath sounds and chest movement**

18. zatřeste lehce pacientem a zavolejte "Jste v pořádku?": **gently shake the patient and shout 'Are you all right?'**

19. známky cirkulace chybí, zahajte stlačování hrudníku v rytmu 100 za minutu, po 15 stlačeních dejte dva účinné vdechy a pokračujte ve stlačování a dýchání v poměru 15:2: **no evidence of a circulation, start chest compressions at a rate 100 per minute, after 15 compressions, give two effective breaths and continue compressions and breaths in a ratio 15:2**

20. známky zotavení, uložit do stabilizované polohy: **evidence of recovery, turn to the recovery position**

Translation 3

1. anafylaktický šok, zrudnutí obličeje, svědění pokožky, poruchy citlivosti, zejména na končetinách, obličeji a rtech, otok, sípání, bolest břicha, nevolnost, zvracení, panika se ztrátou vědomí, nadměrná bledost, promodrání, chladná, vlhce lepkavá pokožka, puls je slabý, nehmatný, rychlý, krevní tlak nízký, nelze zaznamenat: **facial flushing, itching of the skin, paraesthesia, particularly of the extremities, face, and lips, oedema, wheezing, abdominal pain, nausea, and vomiting, panic with loss of consciousness, pallor, cyanosis, cold and clammy skin, pulse is weak, impalpable, rapid, blood pressure low, unrecordable**

2. astma, základním problémem je nadměrná aktivita respiračního

traktu s výsledným bronchiálním spasmem, dušnost, sípání, panika, strach, neschopnost mluvit: **asthma, the underlying problem is that of respiratory tract hyperactivity with resultant bronchospasm, breathlessness, wheezing, panic, and fear, inability to speak**

3. cerebrovaskulární příhody, mrtvice, v dentální praxi neobvyklé, udržet dýchací cesty, naléhavý převoz do nemocnice: **cerebrovascular accidents, stroke, uncommon dental emergencies, maintain the airway, urgent transfer to hospital**

4. epilepsie, stres, hladovění, hypoglykémie, mdloba mohou způsobit záchvat v ordinaci: **epilepsy, stress, fasting, hypoglycaemia, fainting can cause a fit in the surgery**

5. po záchvatu ospalost a touha spát, většina záchvatů netrvá déle než 5 minut a nevyžaduje jiný zásah než ochranu pacienta před sebepoškozením: **postictal drowsiness and the desire to sleep, most fits last less than 5 minutes and require no intervention except protecting the patient from self-inflicted damage**

6. položte pacienta na záda a zvedněte mu nohy: **lay patient flat and raise the legs**

7. provést Heimlichův manévr, zezadu obemkněte pacienta rukama, dolní hranice hrudního koše, ruce míří nahoru směrem k hrudníku, náhlé prudké stlačení: **perform the Heimlich manoeuvre, encircle the patient by your arms from behind, the lower border of the rib cage, the hands are directed upwards towards the chest, a sudden forceful squeeze**

8. srdeční a dechová zástava, kardiopulmonární resuscitace: **cardiorespiratory arrest, CPR**

9. vdechnutí cizího tělíska, kašlání neodstraní obtěžující předmět, dejte až pět ostrých plesknutí mezi lopatky: **inhaled foreign bodies, coughing does not dislodge the offending article, give up to five sharp slaps between the shoulder blades**

10. záchvaty jsou často předcházeny aurou, ztráta vědomí, tělo ztuhlé a napjaté (tonická fáze), pohyby trhavé nebo ochromené (klonická fáze): **seizures are often preceded by an aura, followed rapidly by loss of consciousness and a rigid, extended body (tonic phase) and jerking or flailing movements (clonic phase)**

Translation 4

1. Abnormální elektrické impulsy v mozku: **abnormal electrical impulses in the brain**

2. bolest nastává ihned po námaze, sednout si a odpočinout: **the pain occurs immediately after exertion, sit down and rest**

3. bolest není zmírněna odpočinkem, trvá víc než 30 minut, srdeční selhání, srdeční arytmie: **the pain is not relieved by rest, lasts for**

more than 30 minutes, heart failure, cardiac arrhythmias

4. dát tabletku pod jazyk, podat ústní sprej: **place a tablet under their tongue, administer an oral spray**

5. dýchání ustává, modré rty, život ohrožující situace: **respiration ceases, blue lips, the life-threatening situation**

6. infarkt myocardu, následující po náhlé ztrátě okysličené krve v srdečním svalu s odumřením příslušné části: **myocardial infarction, following a sudden loss of oxygenated blood to the heart muscle with death of that part**

7. kašlat nezvladatelně, překrvený obličej, dojde ke ztrátě vědomí: **to cough uncontrollably, congested face, consciousness will be lost**

8. krutá bolest na hrudi s náhlým nástupem, předpokládaná příčina je buď angína pectoris nebo srdeční záchvat: **severe chest pain of sudden onset assumed cause is either angina or a heart attack**

9. náhlá ztráta vědomí, možná inkontinence: **sudden loss of consciousness, possible incontinence**

10. nechte pacienta sedět zpříma, dejte aspirin, kyslíkovou terapii: **keep the patient sitting upright, give aspirin, give oxygen therapy**

11. nenechávejte pacienta bez dozoru za žádných okolností: **under no circumstances leave the patient unattended**

12. neporanit se během záchvatu: **not to injure during the fit**

13. nevkládat žádnou podporu do úst: **not to insert any kind of mouth prop**

14. pacient má strach, je úzkostný: **the patient is fearful, anxious**

15. pacient se zdá bledý, náhle kolabuje, puls je slabý, rychlý: **patient appears pale, suddenly collapses, pulse is weak, rapid**

16. pacient se zdá netečný, zraková, čichová aura (předzvěst): **the patient appears vacant, a visible, olfactory aura**

17. poškodit dýchací cesty pacienta nebo si nechat pokousat prsty: **compromise the patient's airway or to get their own fingers bitten**

18. přístroj na vysoko-rychlostní odsávání: **high-speed suction apparatus**

19. rozvázat těsný oděv u krku: **undo tight neck clothing**

20. uchopte a vytáhněte jazyk dopředu, pokud zapadl do hrdla, často dýchání může začít samovolně: **grasp and pull the tongue forwards if it has fallen into the throat, respiration may often commence spontaneously**

21. uklidňovat pacienta, když se zotaví: **reassure the patient as they recover**

22. velký epileptický záchvat: **a grand mal epileptic fit**

23. vyčistit zjevnou překážku v ústech: **clear any obvious oral blockage in the mouth**

24. vzít pacienta do nemocnice sanitkou: **take a patient to hospital by ambulance**

25. zásoba čerstvého vzduchu, léčba kyslíkem: **supply of fresh air, oxygen therapy**
26. zástava dechu kvůli ucpání cizím tělískem: **respiratory arrest due to obstruction with a foreign body**
27. zlepšení oběhu: **improving the circulation**
28. zotavit se úplně, jít domů s doprovodem: **make a full recovery, to go home with an escort**

Translation 5

1. Cirkulace, zahájit vnější masáž srdce, zmáčknutí srdce mezi hrudní kostí a páteří: **circulation, begin external heart massage, squeezing the heart between the sternum and the spine**
2. dýchací cesty zkontrolovat zrakem překážky, zvratky, kousky zlomeného zubu, a jiné zbytky: **airway, check visibly for blockages, vomit, pieces of fractured tooth, or other debris**
3. dýchání abnormální, chybí po 10 vteřinách, volejte pohotovostní službu: **breathing abnormal, absent after 10 seconds, call the emergency services**
4. dýchání pomocí masky, foukat do masky přes ventil rychlostí 20 dechů za minutu v případě zástavy dechu, u kardiopulmonární resuscitace 30 stlačení s rychlostí 100 za minutu po 2 vdechnutích: **mouth-to-mask ventilation, blow into the mask through the valve, at a rate of 20 breaths a minute in respiratory arrest, in**

cardiopulmonary resuscitation 30 chest compressions at a rate of 100 per minute to 2 breaths

5. dýchání, podívat se, zda se hruď zvedá, poslouchat zvuky dechu, pocítit přiložením tváře blízko úst a nosu postiženého: **breathing, look to see if the chest rises, listen for breath sounds, feel for any breath by placing the cheek close to the casualty's nose and mouth**
6. hlava je skloněna dozadu, dýchací cesty se otevřou přirozeně: **head is tilted right back, the airway opens naturally**
7. kontrolovat puls: **check a pulse**
8. lékárna první pomoci, sterilní obvazy, čtverce, náplasti, sáčky s fyziologickým roztokem na jedno použití: **a first-aid kit, sterile dressings, pads, plasters, and disposable sachets of sterile saline**
9. nebezpečí, rozlití chemických látek, elektřina: **dangers, chemical spillages, electrical supplies**
10. odstranit zbytky: **remove any debris**
11. pokud jde o velkou ránu, přidržte okraje rány k sobě: **if a large wound is involved, hold the edges of the wound together**
12. položení postiženého na záda: **lying the casualty on their back**
13. použít prsty, ne palec: **use fingers, not a thumb**
14. použít přímý tlak na místo krvácení, sterilní čtverec: **apply direct pressure to the bleeding site, sterile pad**
15. požadavky na první pomoc: **first-aid requirements**

16. puls na karotidě, na krku, radiální puls, na zápěstí: **the carotid pulse in the neck, the radial pulse in the wrist**

17. reakce, při vědomí úplně, napolo, možná dezorientovaný, v bezvědomí, bez reakce: **responsiveness, fully conscious, semiconscious, possibly disorientated, unconscious, unresponsive**

18. ruční odsávací jednotka: **mains-operated suction unit**

19. souprava léků pro naléhavé případy, kyslíkový přístroj, všechny věci v platné době použití: **emergency drugs kit, oxygen cylinder, all items within their shelf-life dates**

20. udržet naživu: **maintain life**

21. vyčistit, a otevřít dýchací cesty: **clear and open an airway**

22. vykonat malý tlak, cítit puls pod prostředníčkem: **exert a little pressure, feel the pulse under your middle finger**

23. základní postupy první pomoci: **basic first-aid procedures**

24. zastavit žilní krvácení, vytékání z rány: **stop venous bleeding, gushing from a wound**

25. zaznamenat všechny nehody: **record all accidents**

26. zkratka Doktor ABC, stanovit pořadí, přístup, zhodnocení, pomoc: **abbreviation Doctor ABC, set out the sequence, approach, assess, help**

27. zvednout končetinu, omezit tok krve: **elevate the limb, reduce blood flow**

Translation 6

1. dát pod studenou vodu, osušit, použít antiseptický krém, krýt nepromokavou náplastí: **run under a cold tap, dry and apply an antiseptic cream, cover with a waterproof plaster**

2. mdloba, zhroutit se na židli, upadnout na zem: **fainting, slump in the chair, fall to the floor**

3. nosit rukavice, bezpečnostní brýle: **wear gloves, safety glasses**

4. oblečení může být přichycené ke kůži, poškození tkáně: **clothing may be stuck to the skin, tissue damage**

5. odstranit šperky než nastane otok: **remove jewellery before swelling occurs**

6. odstranit zrnko, ujistit se, že vidění postiženého není zasaženo: **remove the speck, ensure the casualty's vision is unaffected**

7. okamžitě zastavit zubní ošetření: **stop all dental treatment immediately**

8. opaření parou z autoklávu nebo horkou tekutinou: **scald from autoclave steam or hot liquid**

9. pokrýt nepřilnavým obvazem: **cover with a nonadhesive dressing**

10. ponořit do studené vody nejméně na 10 minut: **immerse in cold water for a minimum of 10 minutes**

11. poranění čistou jehlou, žádné riziko přenosu infekce: **clean needlestick injury, no risk of cross-infection**

12. poranění oka úlomkem amalgámu: **eye injury from a speck of amalgam**

13. použít sáčky z lékárničky první pomoci: **use the sachets from the first-aid kit**
14. rychlé, bolestivé vytvoření puchýřů: **rapid and painful blistering**
15. vyhledat lékařskou pomoc: **seek medical attention**
16. vypláchnout postižené oko velkým množstvím fyziologického roztoku: **irrigate the affected eye with copious amounts of saline**
17. zabránit opakovanému výskytu: **prevent recurrences**
18. zavolat pomoc, odstranit přihlížející, zachovat pacientovu důstojnost: **summon help, clear away onlookers, maintain the patient's dignity**

Translation 7
1. anafylaktický šok nastává jako závažná reakce na alergen, zčervenání kůže, otok obličeje, bledost, cyanóza, kolaps, ztráta vědomí, srdeční zástava, změněná citlivost, mravenčení končetin, obtíže s dýcháním: **anaphylactic shock occurs as a severe reaction to an allergen, skin flushing, facial swelling, pallor, cyanosis, collapse, loss of consciousness, cardiac arrest, paraesthesia, tingling of the extremities, difficulty in breathing**
2. cirkulace, udržet tok krve do hlavních orgánů a mozku: **circulation, maintain blood flow to the major organs and brain**
3. cítit nevolnost, lehká závrať, závrať, tunelové vidění: **feel unwell, light-headed, dizziness, tunnel vision**
4. dýchací cesty, vyčistit prstem, když odsávací zařízení není po ruce: **airway, clear by finger sweep, if suction equipment is not at hand**
5. dýchání, dívat se, poslouchat, procítit zvuky dechu, pozorovat pohyb hrudníku: **breathing, look, listen, and feel for breath sounds observe the chest movement**
6. epileptický záchvat, mírný, denní snění, nepozorný, oči nezaostřené, zírající, krátce v bezvědomí, zřídka zmatený při zotavení: **epileptic fit, mild, daydreaming, inattentive, eyes unfocused, staring, unconscious briefly, rarely confused on recovery**
7. epileptický záchvat, závažný, náhlá ztráta vědomí, svalová ztuhlost, trhavé pohyby, tonicko-klonické záchvaty, inkontinence, zmatený během zotavování: **epileptic fit, severe, sudden loss of consciousness, muscle rigidity, jerking movements, tonic-clonic seizures, incontinence, confused during recovery**
8. hlava zakloněná, brada zvednutá: **head tilted back, the chin lifted**
9. kontrolovat puls na karotidě každou minutu, pokračovat CPR bez přestávek, dokud pacient není oživen, zachránce vyčerpán, nebo nepřijede pomoc: **check the carotid pulse every minute, continue CPR with no breaks until the patient revived, the**

first-aider exhausted, or help
arrived

10. léky uložené v pohotovostní
lékárničce, adrenalin k podání
do svalu během anafylaktického
šoku, GTN sprej k použití
ústně při podezření na záchvat
angíny pectoris, inhalátor
Salbutamolu k ústnímu použití
během astmatického záchvatu:
**drugs kept in the emergency
drug box, adrenaline to be
given intramuscularly during
anaphylactic shock, GTN
spray to be used orally during
a suspected angina attack,
Salbutamol inhaler to be used
orally during an asthma attack**

11. mdloba, dočasné omezení toku
okysličené krve do mozku,
bledost a lepkavost kůže, na
obočí a horním rtu, krátká ztráta
vědomí, puls slabý, nitkovitý,
před zhroucením opakovaně
zívat: **simple faint, temporary
reduction in oxygenated blood
flow to the brain, skin pallor
and clamminess, sweat on the
brow and upper lip, a brief loss
of consciousness, the pulse weak
and thready, yawn repeatedly
before collapsing**

12. rychlé zotavení, poskytnout kyslík,
nápoj s glukózou či tabletku:
**rapid recovery, provide oxygen,
a glucose drink or tablet**

13. symptomy, to co postižený
pociťuje: **the symptoms, what the
casualty actually feels**

14. určit úroveň vědomí, volat
o pomoc, vyvolat poplach:
determine their level of

consciousness, shout for help,
raise the alarm

15. ventilace, ambu vak, technika z úst
do úst: **ventilation, Ambu bag,
the mouth-to-mouth technique**

16. vnější příčiny, úraz elektrickým
proudem, nadýchání jedovatých
výparů: **external causes,
electrocution, inhalation of
poisonous vapours**

17. zástava srdce, kolaps, není puls:
cardiac arrest, collapse, no pulse

18. znaky, to co vidíme: **the signs,
what we see**

Unit 8
Analgesia, Sedation, and General Anaesthesia
Translation 1

1. analgetika a nesteroidní
protizánětlivé léky: **analgesics and
nonsteroidal anti-inflammatory
drugs**

2. antibiotika působí odumření
mikroorganismu: **antibiotics cause
the death of microorganism**

3. anxiolitika snižují úzkost, napětí
či strach: **anxiolytics reduce
anxiety, tension, or fear**

4. baktericidní lék ničí citlivé
organismy, bakteriostatický lék
brání úspěšnému rozmnožení
baktérií: **a bactericidal drug
kills sensitive organisms, a
bacteriostatic drug prevents
successful reproduction of
bacteria**

5. benzodiazepiny, nejběžnější
skupinou léků: **the
benzodiazepines, the most
common group of drugs**

6. brát lék v doporučený čas a dokončit předepsanou dobu léčby: **take the drug at the recommended time and finish the prescribed course of treatment**
7. děti, dávky zmenšené dle věku nebo tělesné váhy: **children, doses reduced by age or body weight**
8. generické jméno léku, forma a síla: **the generic name of the drug, its form, and strength**
9. hypnotika navozují spánek: **hypnotics induce sleep**
10. chlorhexidin přilne k zubní sklovině, povlaku a plaku, působí dramatický pokles počtu baktérií ve slinách: **chlorhexidine adheres to tooth enamel, pellicle, and plaque, it causes a dramatic fall in bacterial count in saliva**
11. jaterní onemocnění, určité léky mohou dále poškodit orgán: **liver disease, certain drugs may further damage the organ**
12. jméno a adresa, věk pacienta, celkový počet dnů léčby: **name and address, age of patient, total number of days treatment**
13. kojení, některé léky přecházejí do mléka, což může být nebezpečné pro dítě: **breast feeding, some drugs pass into the milk, which is potentially dangerous for the baby**
14. ledviny, špatná funkce, zvýšená hladina léků v plasmě, rostoucí citlivost na určité léky, špatná snášenlivost vedlejších účinků: **increased drug levels in the plasma, rising sensitivity to**

certain drugs, poor tolerance to side effects
15. místní užití v ústech: **topical use in the mouth**
16. nadměrné užívání léků je běžné, identifikovat možné vzájemné působení: **polypharmacy is common, identify possible interactions**
17. nepříznivá reakce, vyrážka kůže, závažný průjem: **untoward reaction, skin rash, severe diarrhoea**
18. nežádoucí účinky: **unwanted effects**
19. předávkování, potlačené dýchání, hypotenze: **overdosage, depressed respiration, hypotension**
20. odolnost baktérií na antibiotika je vzrůstající problém na celém světě: **bacterial resistance to antibiotics is an increasing problem worldwide**
21. onemocnění ledvin, mnohé léky jsou vylučovány ledvinami: **kidney disease, many drugs are excreted through the kidney**
22. pacienti obzvláště ohrožení: **patients at particular risk**
23. pokyny jak a kdy se má lék brát: **instruction as to how and when drug is to be taken**
24. použití antibiotik v zubním lékařství, profylaktické, prevence infekce, léčebné, ošetření existující infekce: **use of antibiotics in dentistry, prophylactic, prevention of infection, therapeutic treatment of existing infection**
25. premedikace, uvolnění svalů, nitrožilní sedace, antikonvulzívum:

premedication, muscle
relaxation, intravenous sedation,
anticonvulsant

26. předepisování léku, psaní receptu:
**drug prescribing, prescription
writing**

27. starší lidé, nadměrné reakce
na léky: **elderly, exaggerated
reactions to drugs**

28. těhotenství, předepisovat pouze
léky nezbytně nutné: **pregnancy,
prescribe only drugs absolutely
essential**

29. ukládat léky bezpečně z dosahu
dětí: **keep medicines safely out of
the reach of children**

30. uklidňující účinky, ospalost,
ataxie, zejména u starších lidí:
**sedative effects, drowsiness,
ataxia, particularly in elderly
people**

31. ústní voda, výplach, gel, ústní
sprej: **dental mouthwash,
irrigant, gel, oral spray**

32. varování pro pacienty: **warnings
to patients**

33. vysvětlit pozitivní vlastnosti léku
ve vztahu k pacientovi: **explain
the positive qualities of the drug
in the patient's context**

34. závislost jak fyzická, tak psychická
při dlouhodobém užívání,
při vysazení závažná úzkost,
nervozita, třes: **dependence both
physical and psychological on
prolonged use, on withdrawal
severe anxiety, nervousness,
tremor**

35. zhoršená funkce jater může
ovlivnit rozkládáni léků: **impaired
liver function may affect the
breakdown of drugs**

36. známé vedlejší účinky, interakce:
known side effects, interactions

37. žádné zkratky, smazat volný
prostor na formuláři, datum a
podpis: **no abbreviations, delete
any space remaining on the
form, date and signature**

Translation 2

1. bez doprovodu, není platný
souhlas: **unaccompanied, no
valid consent**

2. být podán místně, infiltrací, do
regionálního bloku, injekcí do
vaziva: **be administered topically,
by infiltration, by regional block,
by intraligament injection**

3. celková anestesie, je vytvořen stav
bezvědomí: **general anaesthesia,
a state of unconsciousness is
produced**

4. dentální a chirurgické procedury
jsou vykonávány bez bolesti,
uvědomění, pohybu, nadměrného
krvácení: **dental and oral surgical
procedures are performed
without pain, awareness,
movement, excessive bleeding**

5. hladovět alespoň čtyři hodiny je
nezbytně nutné: **to starve at least
4 hours is essential**

6. intravenózní sedace: **intravenous
sedation**

7. kardiovaskulární a respirační
problémy: **cardiovascular and
respiratory problems**

8. kontraindikace celkové anestézie
u ambulantních pacientů:
contraindications to outpatient GA

9. kontrola bolestivosti u chronické
bolesti obličeje: **pain control in
chronic facial pain**

10. léky, které se mohou vzájemně ovlivňovat: **medication which may interact**

11. letargie, zpoždění či zpomalení reakce na prosbu: **lethargy, delay or slowing of reaction to request**

12. mírná intoxikace: **mild intoxication**

13. místní anestetika: **local anaesthetic agents**

14. nedávná expozice infekcím: **recent exposure to infections**

15. nejběžněji používané léky: **the most commonly used drugs**

16. odlišení mezi bolestí pocházející z horních či dolních zubů: **differentiation between pains arising from upper or lower tooth**

17. orální premedikace, inhalace, intravenózní sedace: **oral premedication, inhalation, intravenous sedation**

18. pacient bude reagovat na pokyn: **the patient will respond to command**

19. pacienti by měli mít doprovod domů, neměli by řídit motorové vozidlo či používat složité domácí přístroje: **patients should be escorted home, should not drive a motor vehicle or use complicated domestic appliances**

20. pohodlí během operačních procedur: **comfort during operative procedures**

21. pochopitelná úzkost: **understandable anxiety**

22. poškození funkce centrálního nervového systému při zotavení: **detriment to central nervous system function on recovery**

23. potlačení centrálního nervového systému: **depression of the central nervous system**

24. potřebovat další pomoc: **need additional help**

25. přerušit přenos nervových impulsů: **interrupt the transmission of nerve impulses**

26. reakce na bolest, dotek, tlak a stimulaci teplem: **response to pain, to touch, pressure, and thermal stimulation**

27. skřípání zuby by vyžadovalo vybavení lůžkového zařízení: **trismus would require inpatient facilities**

28. smyslové poruchy, pocit mravenčení v prstech nohou a rukou, rtů, jazyka, hučení, zvonění v uších: **sensory disturbances, tingling sensation (pins and needles) in fingers, toes, lips, tongue, tinnitus, ringing noise in ears**

29. snížení hloubky celkové anestézie: **reduction of the depth of general anaesthesia**

30. snížení krvácení: **reduction of bleeding**

31. těhotenství: **pregnancy**

32. technika je bezpečná, malé množství pacientů může projevovat snížený tlak, deprese dýchání: **the technique is safe, a small number of patients may exhibit hypotension, respiratory depression**

33. udržovat komunikaci během ošetření: **maintain communication during the treatment**

34. uklidnění při vědomí: **conscious sedation**
35. uklidňovat pacienta: **reassure the patient**
36. vdechování oxidu dusíku podávaného s kyslíkem: **nitrous oxide inhalation administered with oxygen**
37. závažné problémy zneužívání alkoholu a drog: **severe alcohol or drug abuse problems**

Translation 3
1. analgetika a nesteroidní protizánětlivé léky: **analgesics and nonsteroidal anti-inflammatory drugs**
2. antibiotika působí odumření mikroorganismu: **antibiotics cause the death of microorganism**
3. anxiolitika snižují úzkost, napětí či strach: **anxiolytics reduce anxiety, tension, or fear**
4. baktericidní lék ničí citlivé organismy, bakteriostatický lék brání úspěšnému rozmnožení baktérií: **a bactericidal drug kills sensitive organisms, a bacteriostatic drug prevents successful reproduction of bacteria**
5. benzodiazepiny, nejběžnější skupinou léků: **the benzodiazepines, the most common group of drugs**
6. brát lék v doporučený čas a dokončit předepsanou dobu léčby: **take the drug at the recommended time and finish the prescribed course of treatment**
7. děti, dávky zmenšené dle věku nebo tělesné váhy: **children, doses reduced by age or body weight**
8. generické jméno léku, forma a síla: **the generic name of the drug, its form, and strength**
9. hypnotika navozují spánek: **hypnotics induce sleep**
10. chlorhexidin přilne k zubní sklovině, povlaku a plaku, působí dramatický pokles počtu baktérií ve slinách: **chlorhexidine adheres to tooth enamel, pellicle, and plaque, it causes a dramatic fall in bacterial count in saliva**
11. jaterní onemocnění, určité léky mohou dále poškodit orgán: **liver disease, certain drugs may further damage the organ**
12. jméno a adresa, věk pacienta, celkový počet dnů léčby: **name and address, age of patient, total number of days treatment**
13. kojení, některé léky přecházejí do mléka, což může být nebezpečné pro dítě: **breast feeding, some drugs pass into the milk, which is potentially dangerous for the baby**
14. ledviny, špatná funkce, zvýšená hladina léků v plasmě, rostoucí citlivost na určité léky, špatná snášenlivost vedlejších účinků: **increased drug levels in the plasma, rising sensitivity to certain drugs, poor tolerance to side effects**
15. místní užití v ústech: **topical use in the mouth**
16. nadměrné užívání léků je běžné, identifikovat možné vzájemné působení: **polypharmacy is**

common, identify possible
interactions

17. nepříznivá reakce, vyrážka kůže, závažný průjem: **untoward reaction, skin rash, severe diarrhoea**

18. nežádoucí účinky: **unwanted effects**

19. předávkování, potlačené dýchání, hypotenze: **overdosage, depressed respiration, hypotension**

20. odolnost baktérií na antibiotika je vzrůstající problém na celém světě: **bacterial resistance to antibiotics is an increasing problem worldwide**

21. onemocnění ledvin, mnohé léky jsou vylučovány ledvinami: **kidney disease, many drugs are excreted through the kidney**

22. pacienti obzvláště ohrožení: **patients at particular risk**

23. pokyny jak a kdy se má lék brát: **instruction as to how and when drug is to be taken**

24. použití antibiotik v zubním lékařství, profylaktické, prevence infekce, léčebné, ošetření existující infekce: **use of antibiotics in dentistry, prophylactic, prevention of infection, therapeutic treatment of existing infection**

25. premedikace, uvolnění svalů, nitrožilní sedace, antikonvulzívum: **premedication, muscle relaxation, intravenous sedation, anticonvulsant**

26. předepisování léku, psaní receptu: **drug prescribing, prescription writing**

27. starší lidé, nadměrné reakce na léky: **elderly, exaggerated reactions to drugs**

28. těhotenství, předepisovat pouze léky nezbytně nutné: **pregnancy, prescribe only drugs absolutely essential**

29. ukládat léky bezpečně z dosahu dětí: **keep medicines safely out of the reach of children**

30. uklidňující účinky, ospalost, ataxie, zejména u starších lidí: **sedative effects, drowsiness, ataxia, particularly in elderly people**

31. ústní voda, výplach, gel, ústní sprej: **dental mouthwash, irrigant, gel, oral spray**

32. varování pro pacienty: **warnings to patients**

33. vysvětlit pozitivní vlastnosti léku ve vztahu k pacientovi: **explain the positive qualities of the drug in the patient's context**

34. závislost jak fyzická, tak psychická při dlouhodobém užívání, při vysazení závažná úzkost, nervozita, třes: **dependence both physical and psychological on prolonged use, on withdrawal severe anxiety, nervousness, tremor**

35. zhoršená funkce jater může ovlivnit rozkládáni léků: **impaired liver function may affect the breakdown of drugs**

36. známé vedlejší účinky, interakce: **known side effects, interactions**

37. žádné zkratky, smazat volný prostor na formuláři, datum a podpis: **no abbreviations, delete**

any space remaining on the form, date and signature

Translation 4

1. bez doprovodu, není platný souhlas: **unaccompanied, no valid consent**
2. být podán místně, infiltrací, do regionálního bloku, injekcí do vaziva: **be administered topically, by infiltration, by regional block, by intraligament injection**
3. celková anestesie, je vytvořen stav bezvědomí: **general anaesthesia, a state of unconsciousness is produced**
4. dentální a chirurgické procedury jsou vykonávány bez bolesti, uvědomění, pohybu, nadměrného krvácení: **dental and oral surgical procedures are performed without pain, awareness, movement, excessive bleeding**
5. hladovět alespoň čtyři hodiny je nezbytně nutné: **to starve at least 4 hours is essential**
6. intravenózní sedace: **intravenous sedation**
7. kardiovaskulární a respirační problémy: **cardiovascular and respiratory problems**
8. kontraindikace celkové anestézie u ambulantních pacientů: **contraindications to outpatient GA**
9. kontrola bolestivosti u chronické bolesti obličeje: **pain control in chronic facial pain**
10. léky, které se mohou vzájemně ovlivňovat: **medication which may interact**
11. letargie, zpoždění či zpomalení reakce na prosbu: **lethargy, delay or slowing of reaction to request**
12. mírná intoxikace: **mild intoxication**
13. místní anestetika: **local anaesthetic agents**
14. nedávná expozice infekcím: **recent exposure to infections**
15. nejběžněji používané léky: **the most commonly used drugs**
16. odlišení mezi bolestí pocházející z horních či dolních zubů: **differentiation between pains arising from upper or lower tooth**
17. orální premedikace, inhalace, intravenózní sedace: **oral premedication, inhalation, intravenous sedation**
18. pacient bude reagovat na pokyn: **the patient will respond to command**
19. pacienti by měli mít doprovod domů, neměli by řídit motorové vozidlo či používat složité domácí přístroje: **patients should be escorted home, should not drive a motor vehicle or use complicated domestic appliances**
20. pohodlí během operačních procedur: **comfort during operative procedures**
21. pochopitelná úzkost: **understandable anxiety**
22. poškození funkce centrálního nervového systému při zotavení: **detriment to central nervous system function on recovery**
23. potlačení centrálního nervového systému: **depression of the central nervous system**

24. potřebovat další pomoc: **need additional help**
25. přerušit přenos nervových impulsů: **interrupt the transmission of nerve impulses**
26. reakce na bolest, dotek, tlak a stimulaci teplem: **response to pain, to touch, pressure, and thermal stimulation**
27. skřípání zuby by vyžadovalo vybavení lůžkového zařízení: **trismus would require inpatient facilities**
28. smyslové poruchy, pocit mravenčení v prstech nohou a rukou, rtů, jazyka, hučení, zvonění v uších: **sensory disturbances, tingling sensation (pins and needles) in fingers, toes, lips, tongue, tinnitus, ringing noise in ears**
29. snížení hloubky celkové anestézie: **reduction of the depth of general anaesthesia**
30. snížení krvácení: **reduction of bleeding**
31. těhotenství: **pregnancy**
32. technika je bezpečná, malé množství pacientů může projevovat snížený tlak, deprese dýchání: **the technique is safe, a small number of patients may exhibit hypotension, respiratory depression**
33. udržovat komunikaci během ošetření: **maintain communication during the treatment**
34. uklidnění při vědomí: **conscious sedation**
35. uklidňovat pacienta: **reassure the patient**

36. vdechování oxidu dusíku podávaného s kyslíkem: **nitrous oxide inhalation administered with oxygen**
37. závažné problémy zneužívání alkoholu a drog: **severe alcohol or drug abuse problems**

Translation 5

1. dát bezbolestně, vpíchnout pomalu zahřátý roztok, jehla s úzkým kalibrem, okolní měkké tkáně viditelně zblednou: **give painlessly, inject slowly a warmed solution, a narrow-bore needle, surrounding soft tissues will be seen to blanch**
2. oblast se bude zdát necitlivá a oteklá, dokud roztok nezačne vyprchávat, pocit mravenčení: **the area will feel numb and swollen until the solution begins to wear off, tingling sensation**
3. otvírání úst může způsobit citlivost, dásně mohou být bolestivé: **opening the mouth may cause tenderness, gingivae may be sore**
4. rady po anestézii: **postanaesthetic advice**
5. speciální stříkačky a náplně pro místní anestézii: **special local anaesthetic syringes and cartridges**
6. technika aspirace zajistí, že sousední krevní cévy nejsou proniknuty: **aspirating technique will ensure that the nearby blood vessels are not penetrated**
7. technika do kosti, roztok anestetika je uložen přímo kolem kořenů vybraného zubu: **intraosseous**

technique, the anaesthetic solution is deposited directly around the roots of the chosen tooth

8. technika do vaziva, pomáhá znecitlivět jednotlivé zuby, dásně obklopující aktuální zub: **intraligamentary technique helps to anaesthetise individual teeth, gingivae surrounding the actual tooth**

9. technika infiltrace: **infiltration technique**

10. technika zablokování nervu: **nerve block technique**

11. techniky místní anestézie: **local anaesthetic techniques**

12. účinky budou trvat několik hodin: **the effects will last for several hours**

13. uložení roztoku anestetika do nervových ukončení, ležících pod povrchem dásňové kosti: **depositing anaesthetic solution at nerve endings lying beneath the alveolar bone surface**

14. vynikající výsledky, méně bolestivé: **excellent results, less painful**

15. vyvarovat se zraňování měkkých tkání, horkých tekutin: **beware of traumatising the soft tissues, hot fluids**

16. znecitlivění hlavního nervového kmene než vstoupí do kosti různými otvory: **anaesthetising the main nerve trunk before it enters the bone through the various foramina**

Translation 6
1. být přenesen k srdci oběhovým systémem: **be carried to the heart via the circulatory system**

2. hrot jehly může být znovu umístěn a aspirace opakována, dokud krev už není nasávána, roztok anestetika může být pak vpíchnut bezpečně: **the needle tip can be repositioned and the aspirating technique repeated until blood is not aspired, the anaesthetic solution can then be injected safely**

3. místní anestézie mléčných zubů, podání anestetik je pro pacienty přijatelnější: **local anaesthesia of deciduous teeth, anaesthetic administration is more acceptable to the patients**

4. místo hrotu jehly leží blízko velkých krevních cév nebo uvnitř neurovaskulárního svazku: **the site of the needle tip will lie close to large blood vessels or within a neurovascular bundle**

5. podání místního anestetika: **administering a local anaesthetic**

6. použití adrenalinu je kontraindikováno u pacientů se srdečním onemocněním, hypertenzí, starších pacientů, diabetiků, pacientů se zvýšenou činností štítné žlázy, pacientů, kteří užívají léky proti depresi, pacientů s komplikovanou lékařskou anamnézou: **the use of adrenaline is contraindicated in patients with heart disease, hypertension, elderly patients, diabetic patients, patients with hyperthyroidism, patients taking drugs for depression, patients with complicated medical histories**

7. použití vybavení pro aspiraci: **use of aspirating equipment**
8. přímo do periodontálního vaziva u zubu, který je dosud citlivý na stimulaci, u pacientů s anatomickým odchylkami od normy: **directly into the periodontal ligament of a tooth which is still sensitive to stimulation, in patients with anatomical variations to the norm**
9. riziko vpíchnutí roztoku místního anestetika do krevní cévy: **a risk of the local anaesthetic solution being deposited into a blood vessel**
10. srdeční stimulace, arytmie: **cardiac stimulation, arrhythmias**
11. umožnit vyhlazení stěn kořene bez nežádoucích účinků na měkké tkáně: **to allow root planing with no unwanted soft-tissue effects**
12. zánět dřeně, zub je nadměrně citlivý: **pulpitis, the tooth becomes hypersensitive**

Translation 7
1. Ambulantní extrakce v celkové anestézii: **outpatient GA extraction**
2. injekce do vaziva může způsobit bolestivost dásní postiženého zubu během následujícího dne: **any intraligamentary injection may cause soreness in the gums of the affected tooth for a day afterwards**
3. intravenózní sedace: **intravenous sedation**
4. nahlaste jakékoli infekce dýchacího traktu, včetně běžného nachlazení: **report any respiratory tract infections, including the common cold**
5. nahlaste předem jakékoli předchozí nežádoucí reakce na lokální anestézii lékaři: **report any previous adverse reactions to local anaesthesia to the dentist beforehand**
6. nejezte ani nepijte horké tekutiny: **do not eat or drink hot fluids**
7. několik hodin předem si dejte lehkou přesnídávku, jinak vám může být špatně od žaludku: **have a light snack a few hours before, otherwise you may become nauseous**
8. neoblékejte si oblečení těsné kolem krku: **do not wear restrictive clothing around the neck**
9. neoblékejte si oblečení těsné na pažích, nepoužívejte lak na nehty: **do not wear tight clothing on arms, do not wear nail varnish**
10. nepijte 6 hodin před operací: **do not drink for 6 hours preoperatively**
11. nepijte alkohol 24 hodin před procedurou a po proceduře: **do not drink alcohol for 24 hours before and after the procedure**
12. nepokoušejte se řídit vozidlo nebo obsluhovat stroje či elektrická zařízení, do následujícího dne: **do not attempt to drive a vehicle or operate machinery or electrical appliances until the following day**
13. nepoužívejte ústní vody po zbytek dne: **do not use mouthwashes for the remainder of the day**

14. obujte si boty bez podpatku: **wear flat shoes**
15. oznamte jakoukoli nedávnou celkovou anestézii: **declare any recent experience of general anaesthesia**
16. po příjezdu domů jděte do postele, účinky léku budou přítomny několik hodin po operaci: **go to bed on arriving home, as the effects of the drug will be present for several hours postoperatively**
17. pocit hlubokého znecitlivění okolních měkkých tkání, oblast se cítí jako oteklá: **the sensation of a profound numbness of the surrounding soft tissues, the area will feel swollen**
18. pocit pichlavosti: **a pins-and-needles sensation**
19. podání zahrnuje injekci v ústech, na požádání může lékař použít předtím místní anestetikum: **administration involves an intraoral injection, the dentist can use a topical anaesthetic beforehand if requested**
20. ponechte tampon na místě skusu alespoň 30 minut: **keep the bite pack in place at least 30 minutes**
21. poučení před operací a po operaci: **preoperative and postoperative instructions**
22. přijďte se zodpovědným dospělým, aby Vás doprovodil do ordinace a domů: **come with a responsible adult to escort you to the dental surgery and home**
23. rady o místní anestézii: **advice on local anaesthesia**
24. řiďte se radami o braní léků proti bolesti: **follow the advice issued on taking painkillers**
25. snězte lehké jídlo asi tři hodiny před procedurou: **eat a light meal about 3 hours before the procedure**
26. účinky budou trvat přibližně 2 hodiny po podání: **the effects will last for approximately 2 hours after administration**
27. vezměte léky jako obvykle, pokud lékař nenařídil jinak: **take normal medications as usual, unless the dentist has instructed otherwise**
28. vyplňte a aktualizujte formulář pro anamnézu: **complete and up-to-date medical history form**
29. zajistěte si vhodně soukromou dopravu domů: **make suitable arrangements for private transport home**

Unit 9
Oral Medicine

Translation 1
1. Idiopatické, nezávisle vzniklé, opakovaná aftózní stomatitida: **idiopathic, recurrent aphthous stomatitis**
2. infekce virové, bakteriální, plísňové: **infection viral, bacterial, fungal**
3. kožní choroby, lišej, poruchy s tvořením puchýřků a puchýřů: **dermatological diseases, lichen planus, vesiculobullous disorders**
4. léky způsobené, cytotoxické činitele (škodlivé pro buňky): **drug induced, cytotoxic agents**
5. místní a systemické faktory, předcházející infekci kandidózy:

local and systemic factors predisposing to candidal infection

6. místní faktory, úraz, nošení protéz, chabá hygiena protéz, xerostomie: **local factors, trauma, denture wearing, poor denture hygiene, xerostomia**

7. novotvary, karcinom (rakovinný nádor plochých buněk) a jiné tumory: **neoplastic, squamous cell carcinoma, and other tumours**

8. opakované herpetické infekce: **recurrent herpetic infections**

9. opakující se tvoření vředů v ústech: **recurrent oral ulceration**

10. pocit pálení, píchání: **burning, prickling sensation**

11. poměrně neobvyklé (tuberkulóza, kapavka, syfilis): **relatively uncommon (tuberculosis, gonorrhoea, syphilis)**

12. potlačení imunity, kouření cigaret, výživa s vysokou spotřebou uhlovodanů: **immunosuppression, cigarette smoking, high-carbohydrate diet**

13. strupy, samovolně se hojí: **crusts heal spontaneously**

14. systemické faktory, radioterapie, léčba antibiotiky, léčba kortikosteroidy, dětství, stáří, cukrovka, nedostatky ve výživě: **systemic factors, radiotherapy, antibiotic therapy, corticosteroid therapy, infancy, old age, diabetes mellitus, nutritional deficiency**

15. systemické onemocnění (krevní onemocnění, Crohnova choroba, vředová kolitida – zánět tlustého střeva): **systemic disease (haematological disorders, Crohn's disease, ulcerative colitis)**

16. úrazové, mechanické, chemické, tepelné, zářením: **traumatic, mechanical, chemical, thermal, radiation**

17. ústní infekce: **oral infection**

18. ústní sliznice mohou být zasaženy rozmanitými plísňovými chorobami, kandidóza: **the oral mucosa may be affected by a variety of fungal diseases, candidosis**

19. virus setrvává v klidovém stadium a je reaktivován rozmanitými urychlujícími faktory: **the virus lies dormant and is reactivated by a variety of precipitating factors**

20. viry, způsobující ústní poranění, opar rtu, pásový opar, lidské papilom viry: **viruses responsible for causing oral lesions, herpes simplex, herpes zoster, human papilloma viruses**

21. vředovatění, porušení celistvosti epitelové výstelky: **ulceration, breaking in the continuity of an epithelial lining**

22. vytvoření malých puchýřků, které se zvětšují a pak prasknou: **formation of small vesicles which enlarge and then rupture**

23. zranění, vystavení slunečnímu světlu, stress, menstruace, potlačení imunity: **trauma, exposure to sunlight, stress, menstruation, immunosupression**

24. zubní kazy, nemoc parodontu: **dental caries, periodontal disease**

Translation 2

1. Alkohol, zvýšené riziko v souvislosti s požíváním alkoholu, zvyšuje účinek tabáku a znásobuje riziko: **alcohol, increased risk in association with alcohol consumption, acts synergistically with tobacco, multiplies the risk**
2. dehydratace, např. cukrovka, selhání ledvin, ztráta tekutin: **dehydration, e.g. diabetes mellitus, renal failure, fluid loss**
3. etiologické (příčinné) faktory rakoviny úst: **aetiological factors of oral cancer**
4. chronická infekce kandidy je považována za předrakovinný stav: **chronic candida infection is considered to be a premalignant condition**
5. chronické trauma, mechanické trauma ze špatně upevněných protéz, špatně udržovaný chrup, chabá ústní hygiena: **chronic trauma, mechanical trauma from ill-fitting dentures, a poorly maintained dentition, poor oral hygiene**
6. klinické a histologické rysy, spojeny se zvýšeným rizikem maligních přeměn: **clinical and histological features associated with an increased risk of malignant transformation**
7. náchylnost ke kandidóze: **predisposition to oral candidosis**
8. onemocnění slinné žlázy při HIV: **HIV salivary gland disease**
9. po ozáření: **postirradiation**

10. poruchy slinné žlázy: **salivary gland disorders**
11. potenciálně maligní poškození a stavy, významně zvýšené riziko rakoviny: **potentially malignant lesions and conditions, significantly increased risk of cancer**
12. rakovina úst většinou vzniká nově, bez poznatelných předcházejících předrakovinných stavů: **most oral cancers arise de novo with no recognisable preceding premalignant state**
13. rostoucí bakteriální sialoadenitida (zánět slinné žlázy): **ascending bacterial sialadenitis**
14. Sjögrenův syndrom, chronické zánětlivé onemocnění, pravděpodobně na autoimunitním základě: **Sjögren's syndrome, chronic inflammatory disease with probable autoimmune basis**
15. strava a výživa, zvýšené riziko nádorů jícnu a nosohltanu u pacientů s prvotní anémií z nedostatku železa: **diet and nutrition, increased risk of oesophageal and oropharyngeal tumours in patients with primary sideropenic anaemia**
16. tabák, kouření cigaret, doutníků, dýmky, šňupání a žvýkání tabáku: **tobacco, smoking cigarettes, cigars, pipe smoking, the use of snuff, and chewing tobacco**
17. ultrafialové záření, důležitý rizikový faktor karcinomu rtu: **ultraviolet light, important risk factor for carcinoma of the lip**
18. xerostomie (suchost úst), možné příčiny, psychogenní

(úzkost, deprese, hypochondrie): **xerostomia, possible causes, psychogenic (anxiety, depression, hypochondria)**

19. způsobený léky, atropin, léky proti vysokému tlaku, antihistaminika: **drug-induced, atropine, antihypertensive agents, antihistamines**

20. zvýšený výskyt lymfonu (maligní nádor lymfatické tkáně): **an increased incidence of lymphoma**

21. zvýšený výskyt zubních kazů: **increased incidence of dental caries**

Translation 3

1. Alergie, materiály protéz, přídavky do jídla: **allergy, denture base materials, food additives**

2. atypická bolest obličeje: **atypical facial pain**

3. atypická bolest zubů, považována za variantu atypické bolesti obličeje: **atypical odontalgia, considered to be a variant of atypical facial pain**

4. bolest dostatečně vážná, aby pacienta vzbudila: **pain sufficiently severe to waken patient**

5. bolest je často popisována jako podobná elektrickému šoku, povahou řezavá, bodavá, pronikavá: **pain is often described as like an electric shock, lancinating, stabbing, or piercing in nature**

6. bolest jednostranná, převážně zasahující oblast očí, čela a spánků: **unilateral pain predominantly affecting the ocular, frontal, and temporal regions**

7. bolest obecně není dostatečně silná, aby rušila spánek, pacienti mohou hlásit časné ranní probouzení: **the pain is generally not sufficiently severe to disturb sleep, patients may report early morning wakening**

8. bolest trojklanného nervu: **trigeminal neuralgia**

9. bolest v obličeji, syndrom pálení v ústech, postihující ústní měkké tkáně, nepřítomnost klinicky prokázaného onemocnění sliznice: **facial pain, burning mouth syndrome, affecting the oral soft tissues in the absence of clinically evident mucosal disease**

10. epizody často doprovází rinorea, slzení a infekce spojivek: **episodes are often accompanied by rhinorrhoea, lacrimation, and conjunctival infection**

11. faktory spojené s protézou, nedostatek prostoru pro jazyk, nestabilní protézy, nedostatek volného místa, přecitlivělost: **denture factors, inadequate tongue space, unstable dentures, inadequate freeway space, hypersensitivity**

12. infekce sliznice, kandidóza: **mucosal infections, candidosis**

13. muži jsou postiženi častěji: **males are more commonly affected**

14. nediagnostikovaná či špatně léčená cukrovka: **undiagnosed or poorly controlled diabetes mellitus**

15. nedostatky ve výživě: **nutritional deficiencies**
16. nefunkční činnosti, vystrkování jazyka, svírání, skřípání zuby: **parafunctional activity, tongue thrusting, clenching, bruxism**
17. nepřetržitá, hluboká, difuzní bolest proměnlivé intenzity a závažnosti, bez zjevné organické patologie v postižené oblasti: **continuous, deep, diffuse pain of variable intensity and severity with no obvious organic pathology in the affected area**
18. oční symptomy: **ocular symptoms**
19. opakovaně nebo stále oteklé slinné žlázy: **recurrently or persistently swollen salivary glands**
20. pacienti odmítají umývání a holení určitého místa na obličeji ze strachu z vyvolání záchvatu bolesti: **patients may avoid washing or shaving a particular area on the face for fear of precipitating an attack of pain**
21. periodická migrenózní neuralgie, bolest hlavy podobná migréně: **periodic migrainous neuralgia, cluster headache**
22. pít často tekutiny na pomoc při polykání suché potravy: **frequently drink liquids to aid swallowing dry food**
23. pocit písku nebo štěrku v očích: **sensation of sand or gravel in the eyes**
24. postihuje ženy mezi 40 a 50 lety: **affects females in the fourth or fifth decade of life**
25. příčinné faktory při ústní dyzestezii (abnormální pocity na kůži jako pálení, píchání, svědění):

aetiological factors in oral dysaesthesia
26. psychologické faktory, úzkost, deprese, zveličený strach z rakoviny: **psychological factors, anxiety, depression, cancerphobia**
27. suché oči, každý den, trvale, nepříjemně, po dobu nejméně 3 měsíců: **dry eyes, daily, persistent, troublesome, for at least 3 months**
28. ústní poranění se objevuje běžně u HIV-séropozitivních pacientů, odráží stav zhoršené imunity: **oral lesions occur commonly in HIV-seropositive patients, reflect the immunocompromised state**
29. ústní symptomy, každodenní pocit suchých úst po dobu delší 3 dnů: **oral symptoms, a daily feeling of a dry mouth for more than 3 days**
30. užívat léky zvlhčující oči víc než třikrát denně: **use tear substitutes more than 3 times daily**
31. výskyt se snižuje vysoce účinnou anti-retrovirální léčbou: **the prevalence is reduced by highly active antiretroviral therapy**
32. záchvaty, mohou trvat několik dnů i týdnů, následovány různě dlouhou dobou remise (vymizení příznaků): **bouts can last for several days or weeks, followed by variable period of remission**

Unit 10
Oral and Maxillofacial Surgery
Translation 1
1. biopsie, vyříznutí tkáně pro histologické vyšetření, malý

okraj zdravé tkáně, obklopující
ránu, u potenciálně maligní
léze výrazná dysplazie: **biopsy,
excision of tissue for histological
examination, a small margin of
healthy tissue surrounding the
lesion, significant dysplasia in
potentially malignant lesions**

2. faktory ovlivňující hojení ran:
**factors influencing wound
healing**

3. fáze zánětlivá, fáze bujení
a nového modelování:
**inflammatory phase,
proliferative, and remodelling
phase**

4. chirurgické odstranění hrotu
kořene: **surgical removal of the
root apex**

5. krevní zásobení, lymfatické a žilní
odčerpání, výživa: **blood supply,
venous and lymphatic drainage,
nutrition**

6. možné komplikace extrakce,
selhání místní anestézie, poranění
měkkých tkání, nervu, zlomený
zub, kost, ztracený zub, krvácení,
suché lůžko, komplikace
temporomandibulárního kloubu,
otok: **potential complications
of extraction, failed local
anaesthesia, soft-tissue injuries,
nerve injuries, fractured tooth,
bone, lost tooth, haemorrhage,
dry socket, TMJ complications,
swelling**

7. oslabený, starší pacient, nepříznivé
fyzické faktory, imunitní reakce
snížená: **debilitated, elderly
patient, adverse physical factors,
immune response reduced**

8. šití, stehy, usnadnit hojení ran,
odstranění stehů, nevstřebatelné
stehy uvnitř úst, uchopit zavázané
konce, pinzeta, nůžky, nůžky
na stehy, vložit pod uzlík,
ustřihnout, jemně zatáhnout:
**suturing, sutures, to facilitate
wound healing, suture removal,
nonresorbable intraoral sutures,
grasp the tied ends, forceps,
scissors, stitch cutter, inserted
under the knot, cut, pull gently**

9. tkáň netknutá, zjizvená: **intact
tissue, scar tissue**

Translation 2

1. Nasát jehlou, zkušební vzorek,
sterilní kelímek, vata na špejli:
**aspirate with a needle, specimen,
sterile pot, swab**

2. otoky úst, obličeje a krku, trvání,
povaha bolesti, postižení nervů:
**swellings of mouth, face, and
neck, duration, nature of pain,
neurological involvement**

3. pohled, místo, velikost, tvar,
povrch, barva otoku: **look, site,
size, shape, surface, colour of the
swelling**

4. pohmat, konsistence otoku,
naplněný tekutinou, měkký, pevný,
tvrdý: **feel, consistency of the
swelling, fluid filled, soft, firm,
hard**

5. pokročilé zobrazovací metody,
počítačová tomografie,
skenování, zobrazování pomocí
magnetické rezonance: **advanced
imaging techniques, computer
tomography, scanning, magnetic
resonance imaging**

6. šíření infekce, hnis z infikovaného zubu, cestou nejmenšího odporu, závažné, život ohrožující systémové infekce: **spreading infection, pus from an infected tooth, along the path of least resistance, severe, life-threatening systemic infections**

7. zaznamenat rychlost nástupu, malátnost, zimnici, účinek na dýchání a polykání, léky, teplotu, srdeční rytmus, křeč žvýkacího svalstva, onemocnění mízních uzlin: **record speed of onset, malaise, rigors, effect on breathing and swallowing, drugs, temperature, heart rate, trismus, lymphadenopathy**

Translation 3

1. Abnormální tkáňová hmota, nekoordinovaný růst: **abnormal mass of tissue, uncoordinated growth**

2. cestou krevní, lymfatickou, tělními dutinami: **via blood, lymphatics, body cavities**

3. cysta na čelisti, patologická dutina s tekutým či polotekutým obsahem, která není vytvořena nahromaděním hnisu: **a cyst of the jaw, a pathological cavity having fluid or semifluid contents, which has not been created by the accumulation of pus**

4. karcinomy, zhoubné nádory epitelové tkáně, karcinom dlaždicových buněk: **carcinomas, malignant tumours of epithelial tissue, squamous cell carcinoma**

5. nezhoubné invazivní tumory, napadení okolních tkání, ameloblastom, hlodavý vřed: **locally invasive tumours, invasion into surrounding tissues, ameloblastoma, rodent ulcer**

6. nezhoubné tumory, zůstávají na původním místě, lipom, neurom, papilom: **benign tumours remain at their site of origin, lipoma, neuroma, papilloma**

7. potřeba včasné diagnózy, pečlivé prohlížení ústní sliznice: **the need for early diagnosis, careful screening of the oral mucosa**

8. připravit pacienta duševně, fyzicky, příbuzní, součástí procesu rozhodování: **prepare the patient mentally, physically, relatives, part of the decision-making process**

9. rakovina úst, primární poranění, obvykle vřed, speciální testy, úplný krevní obraz, funkce jater, analýza kalcia a fosforečnanu, rentgen čelistí a hrudníku, biopsie: **oral cancer, the primary lesion, usually an ulcer, special tests, full blood count, liver function, calcium and phosphate analysis, radiography of jaws and chest, biopsy**

10. sarkomy, zhoubné nádory pojivové tkáně, liposarkom, osteosarkom: **sarcomas, malignant tumours of connective tissue, liposarcoma, osteosarcoma**

11. tumory nezhoubné, zhoubné: **tumours benign, malignant**

12. zhoubné tumory, abnormální růst, místní invaze, vzdálené metastázy:

307

malignant tumours, abnormal growth, local invasion, distant metastases

Translation 4

1. Krvácení, skryté krvácení ze zranění uvnitř břišní dutiny, zlomená pánev, stehenní kost, poranění hlavy, porucha úrovně vědomí: **bleeding, hidden haemorrhage from intra-abdominal injury, fractured pelvis, femur, head injury, deterioration in the level of consciousness**

2. naléhavý příjem: **emergency receiving**

3. oči otevřené samovolně, na mluvení, na bolest, neotvírají se: **eyes open, spontaneously, to speech, to pain, do not open**

4. ošetření, redukce, fixace, znehybnění, prevence infekce, návrat k funkčnosti: **treatment, reduction, fixation, immobilisation, prevention of infection, return to function**

5. podezření na poranění krční páteře, znehybnění pomocí límce: **suspicion of cervical spine injury, immobilisation with collar**

6. pohotovostní akce, mít přednost, zjevná dechová tíseň, řinoucí se krvácení: **emergency action, take precedence, obvious respiratory distress, torrential haemorrhage**

7. pohybová reakce, je poslušný pokynů, lokalizuje bolest, ohnutí, natažení na bolest: **motor response, obeys commands,** localises pain, flexion, extension to pain

8. poranění horní čelisti a obličeje: **maxillofacial trauma**

9. posuzovat společně krční páteř, dýchací cesty, krvácení: **consider together cervical spine, airway, bleeding**

10. pozorování, Glasgow škála komatu: **observation, Glasgow Coma Scale**

11. slovní reakce, orientovaná, zmatená konverzace, nepatřičná slova, nesrozumitelná, žádná: **verbal response, orientated, confused conversation, inappropriate words, incomprehensible, none**

12. tržné rány, odřeniny, čistící roztoky, použít na neporušenou pokožku, v samotné ráně použít fyziologický roztok: **lacerations, abrasions, cleaning solutions, use on the intact skin, use saline in the wound itself**

13. ucpání horních cest dýchacích, cizí tělíska, zuby, úlomky protéz, zvratky, krev: **upper airway obstruction, foreign bodies, teeth, denture fragments, vomit, blood**

14. zkontrolovat prevenci proti tetanu: **to check tetanus prophylaxis**

15. zlomeniny dolní, horní čelisti, lícního komplexu, nosní: **mandibular fractures, maxillary, zygomatic complex fractures, nasal fractures**

16. zlomeniny v obličeji, uzavřené, otevřené, roztříštěné, částečné, patologické: **facial fractures**

simple, compound, comminuted, greenstick, pathological

Unit 11
Periodontology
Translation 1

1. absence odpovídající ústní hygieny: **the absence of adequate oral hygiene**
2. akumulace plaku vede vždy k zánětu dásní, ale nevede nutně k zánětu parodontu: **plaque accumulation always leads to gingivitis, but it does not invariably lead to periodontitis**
3. dentální plak se hromadí, za tři týdny se objeví zánět dásní: **dental plaque accumulates, gingivitis occurs over a 3-week period**
4. fáze hygieny obsahuje: **hygiene phase comprises**
5. klinické rysy zánětu dásní, rudá barva, oteklý vzhled, dolíčky se ztratí, při sondování ihned krvácí: **clinical features of gingivitis, red in colour, swollen appearance, stippling is lost, bleed readily on probing**
6. korektivní fáze, onemocnění je léčeno: **corrective phase, disease is treated**
7. monitorovat orální hygienu, včasné rozpoznání nového výskytu nemoci: **to monitor oral hygiene, early detection of recurrent disease**
8. nechirurgické odstranění zubního kamene pod dásněmi a vyhlazení kořenů: **nonsurgical subgingival scaling and root planing**
9. nové posouzení provedené 4–6 týdnů po dokončení fáze hygieny:

reassessment conducted 4–6 weeks after the completion of hygiene phase

10. poučení o dentálním zdraví a kontrole plaku: **dental health education and instruction in plaque control**
11. stádia léčby parodontu: **stages in periodontal therapy**
12. struktura tkání parodontu, dásně, periodontální vazivo: **structure of the periodontal tissues, gingiva and periodontal ligament**
13. tkáně obklopují a podporují zuby: **the tissues surround and support the teeth**
14. udržovací fáze, pacienti jsou prohlíženi v pravidelných intervalech: **maintenance/recall phase, patients are reviewed at regular intervals**
15. vyloučení překážek efektivní orální hygieny: **elimination of obstacles to effective oral hygiene**
16. vyšetření a diagnóza: **examination and diagnosis**
17. zánětlivá onemocnění vyvolaná plakem, gingivitida, periodontitida: **inflammatory diseases, plaque-induced, gingivitis, periodontitis**
18. zdravé dásně, bledě růžová barva, vzhled s dolíčky, dobře patrný okraj, vroubkovaný obrys, při jemném použití sondy nekrvácí: **healthy gingivae, pale pink in colour, a stippled appearance, a well-defined margin, scalloped outline, do not bleed on gently probing**

19. zdůraznit specifické problémy
či oblasti vyžadující další léčbu:
**highlight specific problems or
areas requiring further therapy**
20. zničení vaziva parodontu a rozvoj
chobotu: **breakdown of the
periodontal ligament and the
development of a periodontal
pocket**

Translation 2
1. elektrické kartáčky, prospěšné pro
pacienty s omezenou manuální
zručností: **electric toothbrushes,
of benefit in patients with
reduced manual dexterity**
2. chladicí prostředek, jemný trysk
vody směrovaný na vibrující
hrot: **a coolant, a fine water jet
directed onto the vibrating tip**
3. kartáčky s jedním chomáčkem
pro čistění kolem osamocených
nebo částečně prořezaných
zubů: **single-tufted brushes for
cleaning around alone-standing
or partially erupted teeth**
4. kartáčky, velikost hlavy, střední
struktura vlákna, kulaté konce
štětin: **toothbrushes, the size
of the head, medium texture
filaments, rounded ends to the
bristles**
5. mezizubní kartáčky dostupné v
řadě velikostí: **interproximal
brushes available in a range of
sizes**
6. naklonit hlavu kartáčku, vlákna
jsou ve 45 stupních k dlouhé
ose zubu: **angle the head of the
toothbrush, the filaments are at
45 degrees to the long axis of the
tooth**

7. násadec a vložka s pracovním
hrotem: **handpiece and an insert
with a working tip**
8. nit voskovaná, nevoskovaná: **floss,
waxed, unwaxed**
9. odstraňování zubního kamene a
leštění kořenů: **scaling and root
planing**
10. páska, širší než nit, snadněji
prochází mezi zuby: **tape, broader
than floss, it passes between
teeth more easily**
11. pohyb dozadu a dopředu: **a
back-and-forth movement**
12. pomůcky pro mezizubní čistění:
aids for between-tooth cleaning
13. ruční nástroje, dlátka, srpky,
motyčky a kyrety: **hand
instruments, chisels, sickles,
hoes, and curettes**
14. technika čistění zubů,
modifikovaná Bassova technika
je nejjednodušší a nejúčinnější:
**tooth-brushing technique,
modified Bass technique is the
simplest and most effective**
15. ultrazvukové odstraňovače
zubního kamene: **ultrasonic
scalers**
16. umístit k dásňovému okraji,
umožnit špičkám vláken vstoupit
do dásňové skuliny: **to place at
the gingival margin, to allow the
tips of the filaments to enter the
gingival crevice**
17. vyhnout se technikám drhnutí
a kartáčkům s tvrdými vlákny,
které způsobují ústup dásní:
**avoid scrub techniques and
toothbrushes with hard
filaments which cause gingival
recession**

18. vysvětlit povahu nemoci parodontu, úlohu dentálního plaku: **explain the nature of periodontal disease, the role of dental plaque**
19. zlepšit čistění, modely, informační letáky: **improve cleaning, models, and information leaflets**
20. zviditelnění plaku, odhalující prostředky, rukou držené zrcadlo: **visualisation of plaque, disclosing agents, a handheld mirror**

Unit 12
Restorative Dentistry
Translation 1
1. amalgam zvětšuje objem: **amalgam expands**
2. cementy nedrží: **cements do not adhere**
3. držet na místě: **hold in place**
4. držet pod jazykem: **hold beneath the tongue**
5. fyziologický dásňový chobot: **gingival crevice of the tooth**
6. izolace ošetřovaného zubu: **isolation of the tooth undergoing treatment**
7. kontrola vlhkosti: **moisture control**
8. náhrady se uvolňují: **restorations become loose**
9. nasáknout hromadící se vlhkost: **soak up pooling moisture**
10. nepřesné otisky a odlitky: **inaccurate impressions and casts**
11. nepříjemné pro pacienta: **uncomfortable for the patient**
12. nitrožilní injekce: **an intravenous injection**
13. odsavač slin: **saliva ejector**

14. okamžité a rychlé odstranění vlhkosti: **immediate and fast moisture removal**
15. plynové bubliny: **gas bubbles**
16. polknout, vyplivnout: **to swallow, spit out**
17. poloha vleže: **the supine position**
18. pomalé odsávání, vysokorychlostní odsávání: **slow-speed aspiration, high-speed aspiration**
19. použít vzduchovou turbínku: **use an air turbine**
20. provést zubní ošetření: **perform dental treatment**
21. přerušit ošetření: **interrupt the treatment**
22. svitky vaty: **cotton-wool rolls**
23. šňůrka na odtažení dásně: **gingival retraction cord**
24. špatná viditelnost: **poor visibility**
25. špička savky: **suction tip**
26. tuhnout správně: **set correctly**
27. uchopené v kleštích: **held in forceps**
28. umístěný do tvářové rýhy: **placed in the buccal sulcus**
29. užití gumové blány: **the use of rubber dam**
30. v extrémních případech: **in extreme cases**
31. vyfoukat trojitou stříkačkou: **blow dry using the triple syringe**
32. výplň je slabá: **filling is weak**
33. vysušit vatovými tamponky: **wipe dry by cotton wool pledgets**
34. zabránit krvácení v místě: **to prevent bleeding at the site**

Translation 2
1. během úpravy a umístění náhrady: **during any adjustment and placement of the restoration**

2. být k dispozici: **be available**
3. dezinfikovat otisky: **disinfect all impressions**
4. dohlédnout, aby nástroje byly po použití vyčištěny a sterilizovány: **see that the used instruments are cleaned and sterilised after use**
5. dolní stoličky: **lower molar teeth**
6. kontrola vlhkosti: **moisture control**
7. konzervační techniky: **restorative techniques**
8. míchat a pomáhat umístit dočasné výplně či pokrytí: **mix and help place any temporary filling or covering**
9. odtažení měkké tkáně: **soft-tissue retraction**
10. ordinace je uklizena a připravena pro dalšího pacienta: **the surgery is tidied and made ready for the next patient**
11. podávat nástroje lékaři: **pass instruments to the dentist**
12. postižení tváře: **the buccal involvement**
13. použitý výplňový materiál: **employed filling material**
14. preparace zubu: **tooth preparation**
15. předat připravené k použití: **to hand ready for use**
16. silné žvýkání: **heavy mastication**
17. úloha zubní sestry: **role of the dental nurse**
18. umístění dočasné výplně: **placement of a temporary filling**
19. vrátit zubu úplnou funkčnost: **return the tooth to its full function**
20. všechny nepoužité materiály jsou odklizeny: **all unused materials are disposed of**
21. vydržet velkou zátěž skusu: **withstand heavy occlusal loads**
22. vyplněné stvrzenky: **completed dockets**
23. vytvořený v laboratoři: **formed at the laboratory**
24. vytvořit a umístit u křesla: **form and place at the chairside**
25. vzít otisk dutiny: **take an impression of the cavity**
26. zabalit a připravit pro převoz do laboratoře: **pack and make ready for transportation to the laboratory**
27. zahrnovat postup dvou návštěv: **involve a two-visit procedure**
28. zajistit správně odsávání: **provide good aspiration**

Translation 3
1. akrylátová náhrada: **acrylic denture**
2. artikulační papír: **articulating paper**
3. bezzubý pacient: **edentulous patient**
4. čistý papírový čtverec: **a clean paper pad**
5. držet pacientovi zrcátko: **hold a mirror for the patient**
6. fréza na pryskyřici: **denture trimming bur**
7. hlásit jakékoli problémy s novou protézou: **to report any problems with the new dentures**
8. kontaktovat ordinaci: **to contact the surgery**
9. míchat důkladně: **mix thoroughly**
10. naplnit každou lžíci: **load each tray**
11. nerez ocel: **stainless steel**

12. než pacient odejde z ordinace: **before the patient leaves the surgery**
13. odevzdat vzorník odstínů zubaři: **hand the shade guide to the dentist**
14. omytí náhrady pod studenou vodou z kohoutku: **running the denture under the cold tap**
15. pacient je spokojen: **the patient is satisfied**
16. písemné instrukce o dentální péči: **written denture-care instructions**
17. po každém setkání: **after each appointment**
18. podat lékaři: **present to the dentist**
19. podrobnosti o pacientech a nezbytné pokyny: **patient's details and the necessary instructions**
20. ponoření do roztoku chlornanu sodného na 10 minut: **immersing in a solution of sodium hypochlorite for 10 minutes**
21. poskytnout kapesníčky a výplach úst: **provide tissues and mouthwash**
22. propláchnout v desinfekčním roztoku: **rinse in disinfectant solution**
23. protézy musí být znovu vyzkoušeny: **the prostheses have to be retried**
24. přijmout pacienty: **receive the patients**
25. přikrýt vlhkým kouskem gázy: **cover with a wet piece of gauze**
26. připraven na převoz do laboratoře: **ready for transport to the laboratory**
27. připravit k použití: **place ready for use**
28. připravit k vyzvednutí balíček otisků a dokumentů: **place the package of impressions and sheets ready for collection**
29. registrační pasta: **registration paste**
30. rovný násadec: **straight handpiece**
31. sterilizovat otisky: **sterilise impressions**
32. umístit ochranou náprsenku: **put a protective bib in place**
33. upevnění dokončených protéz: **fitting of completed dentures**
34. usadit je pohodlně: **seat them comfortably**
35. uzavřít do neprodyšného vaku: **seal in an airtight bag**
36. vybrat správné otiskovací lžíce: **choose the correct impression trays**
37. vyčistit důkladně míchací misky a lopatky: **clean mixing bowls and spatulas thoroughly**
38. vyplnit záznam pro laboratoř: **fill in the laboratory sheet**
39. vzhled a upevnění: **appearance and fit**
40. záznam skusu: **bite record**
41. zaznamenat vybraný odstín: **record the chosen shade**

Translation 4
1. apikální absces, devitalizovaný zub: **apical abscess, nonvital tooth**
2. cpátko na amalgam, hladítko: **amalgam plugger, burnisher**
3. dočasný výplňový materiál: **temporary filling material**

4. držák můstku, pilíř náhrady: **bridge retainer, denture abutment**

5. fraktura korunky, odumření zubu: **crown fracture, death of the tooth**

6. gumová blána, dírkovač kofferdamu: **rubber dam sheet, rubber dam punch**

7. kaz, dráždivá hluboká výplň: **caries, irritant deep filling**

8. kontraindikace vytržení, porucha krvácení: **contraindicated extraction, bleeding disorder**

9. léčba kořene: root treatment

10. malý a velký lžícový exkavátor: **small and large spoon excavators**

11. miska na nástroje: **tray for instruments**

12. naplněná stříkačka: **loaded syringe**

13. násadce a doplňky: **handpieces and attachments**

14. nástroje a materiály: **instruments and materials**

15. pinzeta, svorka, dezinfekční roztok: **forceps, clamp, disinfectant wash**

16. plochý plastový nástroj: **flat plastic instrument**

17. pulpextraktor, pilníky, papírové čípky: **barbed broach, files, paper points**

18. registrovaný antiseptický výplach, antiseptický obvaz: **proprietary antiseptic mouthwash, antiseptic dressing**

19. traumatické obnažení, poranění: **traumatic exposure, injury**

20. vzduchová turbinka, diamantový brousek, rozšiřovač: **air turbine, diamond bur, reamer**

21. zachránit zub: **to save a tooth**

22. zánět dřeně: **pulpitis**

23. zavlažovací stříkačky, zavlažovací roztok: **irrigation syringes, irrigation solution**

24. zrcátko, sonda, kleště: **mirror, probe, forceps**

Translation 5

1. Být namočen do roztoku chlornanu sodného přes noc: **be soaked in a sodium hypochlorite solution overnight**

2. čekat, než se vyrobí protéza: **to wait before a denture is constructed**

3. čistit celá ústa jako obvykle: **brush all the mouth as normal**

4. čistit protézu i vaše vlastní zuby kartáčkem a pastou: **brush the denture and your own teeth with a toothbrush and toothpaste**

5. další léčba: **further treatment**

6. infekce kandidózy pod protézou: **Candidal infection under dentures**

7. je třeba učinit rozhodnutí: **decision has to be made**

8. mimo ústa: **out of the mouth**

9. navštěvovat pravidelně: **to attend on a regular basis**

10. nechat náhradu v ústech 24 hodin: **keep the denture in the mouth 24 hours**

11. nechat protézu v ordinaci: **to leave the denture at the surgery**

12. nestabilní v ústech: **unstable in the mouth**

13. neuhodit se do jamky po vytržení: **not to knock the extraction socket**

14. obnova vnitřní strany protézy: **relining of the denture**

15. odstranit zbytky: **to remove debris**
16. ohlásit co nejdříve silnou bolest či krvácení: **report any severe pain or bleeding as soon as possible**
17. ochránit krevní sraženinu a zabránit infekci: **protect the blood clots and avoid an infection**
18. okamžitá náhrada: **immediate replacement**
19. padnutí a vzhled: **fit and appearance**
20. podporovat hojení: **to promote healing**
21. podstoupit chirurgickou proceduru: **undergo a surgical procedure**
22. pokračovat do 12 měsíců po extrakci: **continue until 12 months postextraction**
23. pokyny pro ústní hygienu: **oral hygiene instructions**
24. ponořit do studené vody, ústní vody, čističe na protézy: **immerse it in cold water, mouthwash, denture cleanser**
25. poradit pacientovi: **advise the patient**
26. potrava se hromadí pod protézou: **food collects beneath the denture**
27. požadovat umělou náhradu: **request an artificial replacement**
28. protéza se uvolní: **the prosthesis will become loose-fitting**
29. přední zub potřebuje vytrhnout: **an anterior tooth requires extraction**
30. příliš silná koncentrace: **too strong a concentration**
31. resorpce okolní dásňové kosti: **surrounding alveolar bone resorption**

32. spoléhat na lepidla na protézy: **rely on denture adhesives**
33. udržovat protézu vlhkou: **keep the denture moist**
34. upevnit protézu: **fit the prosthesis**
35. vrátit do laboratoře: **return to the laboratory**
36. vybělit do světlejšího odstínu: **bleach to a lighter shade**
37. vyjmout protézu a propláchnout pod studenou vodou: **remove the denture and rinse it under the cold tap**
38. vypláchnout teplou slanou vodou: **rinse with hot, saltwater**
39. vytrhnout zbývající zuby: **extract remaining teeth**
40. vytvořit úplně novou náhradu: **construct completely new appliance**

Translation 6
1. asistence zubní sestry: **dental nurse assistance**
2. být dán do autoklávu: **be autoclaved**
3. dostupné pacientovi k použití: **available for patient use**
4. držet ochranný štít: **hold the protective shield**
5. jakmile pacient opustil ordinaci: **once the patient has left the surgery**
6. leštit a dokončit: **polish and complete**
7. mít připravené výplňové materiály: **have the filling materials ready**
8. naplněná stříkačka: **a loaded syringe**
9. naplnit do aplikátoru: **load into the applicator**

10. nezakrývat lékaři výhled: **not to obscure the dentist's vision**
11. obsluhovat polymerační lampu na tuhnutí kompozit: **to operate the curing lamp**
12. ochranná náprsenka a bezpečnostní brýle: **protective bib and safety glasses**
13. po celou dobu procedury: **throughout the procedure**
14. podávat lékaři podle potřeby: **hand to the dentist as required**
15. pojivová pryskyřice s vhodným aplikátorem: **bonding resin with its appropriate applicator**
16. pomůcky na jedno použití: **disposables**
17. poskytnout vhodné odsávání: **provide adequate aspiration**
18. poznámky a diagramy: **notes and charting**
19. přetřít všechny pracovní povrchy dezinfekcí: **wipe over all work surfaces with disinfectant**
20. přijmout dalšího pacienta: **admit the next patient**
21. připravit k použití: **set out ready for use**
22. připravit pro lékaře k použití: **lay out ready for use by the dentist**
23. pytel na klinický odpad: **the clinical waste bag**
24. rozdělit na papírový čtverec: **dispense onto a paper pad**
25. spojit násadce s vrtáčky: **connect handpieces with the burs**
26. správně držet a podat: **hold and pass correctly**
27. sterilní vybavení: **sterile equipment**
28. světlem tvrzený materiál: **light-cured material**

29. upevnit jehlu: **fit with needle**
30. upravovat pojivo do zubu: **adapt the matrix strip to the tooth**
31. usadit pacienta do křesla: **seat the patient in the dental chair**
32. vatové tampóny, celuloidová páska: **cotton wool rolls, celluloid matrix strip**
33. vybraná náplň: **the cartridge of choice**
34. vydrhnout všechny nástroje: **scrub clean all instruments**
35. vyhodit do nádoby na ostré předměty: **discard in the sharps bin**
36. vyložení, leptání skloviny: **a lining, enamel etching**
37. vypláchnout leptadlo, vysušit zub: **wash the etchant off, dry the tooth**
38. vypláchnutí úst a ubrousky: **mouthwash and tissues**
39. vzorník odstínů kompozitních výplňových materiálů: **the composite shade guide**

Translation 7
1. aluminosilikát (hlinito-křemičitan) : **aluminosilicate**
2. artikulační papír, držáky, zubní nit: **articulating paper, holders, dental floss**
3. během tuhnutí: **during setting**
4. cement sklo-ionomerní cement: **glass monomer cement**
5. čistá voda, čtverec voskového papíru: **pure water, waxed paper pad**
6. dočasná korunka, stálá korunka: **temporary crown, permanent crown**

7. doprovodit pacienta z ordinace: **escort the patient from the surgery**
8. dvojitě vytvrzované kompozity: **dual-cure composites**
9. jemné částice: **fine particles**
10. krémová konsistence: **creamy consistency**
11. kyselina polyakrylová: **polyacrylic acid**
12. nezbytné úpravy skusu: **necessary occlusal adjustments**
13. odstranit nadbytečný cement: **remove excess cement**
14. polyakrylát: **polyacrylate**
15. prášek zinkové běloby a kyselina fosforečná: **zinc oxide powder and phosphoric acid**
16. roztírat po částech: **spatulate by portions**
17. smíchat důkladně tmelící cement: **mix the luting cement thoroughly**
18. stroje na samočinné míchání: **self-mix machines**
19. umožnit přesné umístění: **allow the accurate placement**
20. upevnění korunky: **the fitting of a crown**
21. vhodná místní anestézie: **suitable local anaesthesia**
22. vyčistit a sterilizovat použité nástroje: **clean and sterilise the used instruments**
23. vyzkoušet zapadnutí a skus: **try for fit and occlusion**
24. zchlazená skleněná destička, kovová třecí lopatka: **a cooled glass slab, a metal spatula**

Translation 8
1. aplikace matriční pásky: **application of a matrix band**
2. aplikovat kompozit: **apply the composite**
3. celuloidová páska kolem zubu: **a celluloid matrix strip around the tooth**
4. čepová korunka: **a post crown**
5. dráždivý pro dřeň: **irritant to the pulp**
6. dutina je obložena: **the cavity is lined with**
7. dutina je vyčištěna od kazů: **the cavity is cleared of all caries**
8. fraktura v dásňovém okraji: **fracture at the gingival margin**
9. funkční obnova: **a functional restoration**
10. hodit se k barvě zubu: **to match to the colour of the tooth**
11. horní střední řezák: **an upper central incisor**
12. indikovat korunku: **indicate a crown**
13. izolovat zub: **to isolate the tooth**
14. když pacient mluví a usmívá se: **when the patient talks and smiles**
15. kontrola vlhkosti musí být důkladná během plnění: **moisture control must be thorough during filling**
16. lak na povrch: **surface varnish**
17. materiál pro výplň kořene: **a root-filling material**
18. návyk skřípat zuby: **grinding habits**
19. nebezpečí odhalení dřeně: **a danger of pulp exposure**
20. nezůstává korunka: **no crown remains**
21. odhalit sklovinu co nejvíce: **expose as much enamel as possible**

22. okraje skloviny mohou být leptány, vypláchnuty a vysušeny: **the enamel margins can be acid-etched, washed, and dried**

23. opravit amalgámovou výplní: **to restore with an amalgam filling**

24. podpěra v kořenovém kanálku: **a post in the root canal**

25. porcelánová fazeta: **porcelain veneer**

26. poskytnout adekvátní podporu: **to provide adequate support**

27. potáhnout leptanou sklovinu pryskyřicí: **coat resin over the etched enamel**

28. premoláry mohu být vidět: **premolars may be visible**

29. přední zub, zadní zub: **an anterior tooth, posterior tooth**

30. přijatelný vzhled: **an acceptable appearance**

31. připravit kořenovou frézu: **to prepare root face**

32. připravit otvor pro čep: **prepare a post hole**

33. přístup je obtížný: **the access is difficult**

34. řezák s vyplněným kořenem: **a root-filled incisor**

35. řezáková hrana: **an incisal edge**

36. sklo-ionomerní cement: **glass ionomer cement**

37. sklo-ionomery jsou přilnavé k dentinu i sklovině: **glass ionomers are adhesive to dentine and enamel**

38. sousední zuby: **the adjacent teeth**

39. střed pro korunku: **a core for the crown**

40. světlem tvrzené varianty: **light-cured varieties**

41. šablona na korunku: **a crown former**

42. tuhnutí povrchu: **surface setting**

43. umístit výplň: **to place a filling**

44. utrpět další úraz: **to suffer further trauma**

45. vrtačka, vyvrtat: **a drill, drill out**

46. vyčistit (oříznout) a vyleštit: **trim and polish**

47. vydržet sílu při kousání: **to withstand biting forces**

48. vzduchová turbinka, diamantový brousek, kulatý vrtáček: **the air turbine diamond bur, round bur**

49. vzít otisky: **to take impressions**

50. zabránit styčnému předávkování: **to prevent overspill interproximally**

51. zatmelit čep do kořenového kanálku: **to cement a post into the root canal**

52. zlatá výplň je velmi nákladná, nemá žádnou výhodu proti ostatním technikám: **gold inlay is very costly, has no benefit over the other techniques**

53. znát šířku a hloubku: **to know width and depth**

54. zub se pravděpodobně bude dále lámat: **the tooth is likely to continue to fracture**

Unit 13
Operative Dentistry
Translation 1

1. Anamnéza lékařská, sociální, obtíže pacienta: **medical history, social history, patient complaints**

2. bolest zubů, kazy, opotřebení zubů, onemocnění parodontu: **dental pain, caries, tooth wear, periodontal disease**

3. diagnóza dřeňové bolesti, ostrá, tupá, tepající, stálá, místo a vyzařování: **diagnosis of pulpal pain, sharp, dull, throbbing, constant, site and radiation**

4. endotontická léčba, zhotovení korunek a můstků, vyjímatelných náhrad, implantátů: **endodontic treatment, crown and bridgework, removable prosthesis construction, implants**

5. klinické vyšetření, zrakem, sondou, poklepem, testováním citlivosti, pomocí laseru, rentgenových snímků, prosvícení: **clinical examination, visual, probing, percussion, sensibility testing, with the help of laser, radiographs, transillumination**

6. kontrola, problém estetický, okluze, funkční, traumatický: **check-up, problem aesthetics, occlusal, functional, traumatic**

7. okluze, hroty, žvýkací povrchy, zuby horní a dolní čelisti: **occlusion, the cusps, masticating surfaces, maxillary and mandibular teeth**

8. okluzní harmonie, pohyb dolní čelisti ve všech směrech, žádné nepohodlí, napětí, či poškození zubů ani žvýkacího aparátu: **occlusal harmony, mandibular movement in all excursions, no discomfort, strain, or harm to the teeth or masticatory apparatus**

9. reakce na teplo, chlad, tlak, na sladké podněty: **reaction to heat, cold, pressure, sweet stimuli**

Translation 2

1. Cíle preparace kavity, odstranění zubní tkáně, sekundární prevence, minimalizovat poškození: **objectives of cavity preparation, removal of tooth tissue, secondary prevention, minimise damage**

2. fazetovaná korunka, zhodnocení zubu pro korunky, vitalita zubu, stav dásní, ústní hygiena, kontrola kazu, okluze, vzhled na rentgenu, estetika, sousední zuby: **crown veneer, assessment of teeth for crowns, tooth vitality, gingival condition, oral hygiene, caries control, occlusion, radiographic appearance, aesthetics, adjacent teeth**

3. fixní pohyblivé můstky, spojení umožňující omezený pohyb: **fixed-movable bridges, a joint allowing limited movement**

4. hluboké poškození kazem: **deep carious lesion**

5. inleje, vyrobené v laboratoři, zlaté, kompozitní, porcelánové: **inlays, manufactured in the laboratory, gold, composite, porcelain**

6. jamka, fisura: **pit, fissure**

7. klasifikace kavit: **classification of cavities**

8. klinická stádia, příprava, otisky, vyčkání, přitmelení: **clinical stages, preparation, impressions, temporisation, cementation**

9. moderní adhesivní můstky, mikromechanické připojení, k leptané sklovině: **modern adhesive bridges, micromechanical bonding to etched enamel**

10. obrys, tvar zajišťující odolnost výplně, retenční tvar: **outline form, resistance form, retention form**

11. onleje, na okluzním povrchu zubu: **onlays, on the occlusal surface of a tooth**

12. ošetření zbylých kazů, dokončení okraje skloviny, toaleta kavity: **management of remaining caries, enamel margin finishing, cavity toilet**

13. pevné můstky, nahrazují chybějící zub, připojeny nastálo: **fixed bridges, replace a missing tooth, attached permanently**

14. pilíř, držák, umělý zub na můstku, pilířový zub, krakorcový můstek: **abutment tooth, retainer, pontic, pier, cantilever bridge**

15. stoličky, třenové zuby, řezáky, špičáky: **molar, premolar teeth, incisors, canines**

16. strana lícní, jazyková, patrová: **buccal, lingual, palatal aspects**

17. výplně, amalgám, pryskyřičný kompozit, sklo ionomer: **restorations, amalgam, resin composite, glass ionomer**

Translation 3

1. chirurgická endodoncie, resekce kořenového hrotu, amputace kořene, hemisekce, reimplantace zubů, rozříznutí a drenáž: **surgical endodontics, apicectomy, root amputation, hemisection, reimplantation of teeth, incision, and drainage**

2. obrušování, agresivní čistění, kartáček, pasta, mezizubní čistění, zlozvyk okusování, nehty, skořápky ořechů: **abrasion, aggressive brushing, toothbrush, toothpaste, interdental cleaning, habitual chewing, fingernails, nut shells**

3. odírání, ztráta tvrdých tkání, sycené nápoje, ovocné džusy, citrusové ovoce, potraviny v kyselém nálevu, ústní vody, opakované zvracení, bulimie, gastrointestinální problémy, alkoholismus, ranní nevolnost: **erosion, loss of hard dental tissues, carbonated drinks, fruit juices, citrus fruits, pickled foods, mouthwashes, regurgitation, bulimia nervosa, gastrointestinal problems, alcoholism, morning sickness**

4. opětovná kontrola, určit, zda opotřebování pokračuje, provizorní zásah, definitivní výplně, náhrady: **review, to determine if wear is progressing, provisional intervention, definitive restorations, dentures**

5. opotřebování zubů: **tooth wear**

6. ošetření kořenových kanálků, nástroje, pilník, násadec, kořenová jehla, pulpextraktor, vrtáček, plnič, pečetidlo, cpátko pro kořenové kanálky, ucpání kořenových kanálků: **root canal treatment, instruments, file, handpiece, broach, barbed broach, bur, filler, sealer, spreader, root canal obturation**

7. otírání, bruxismus, skřípání, svírání, nedostatek podpory, kolaps okluze, tok slin, složení, struktura zubu: **attrition, bruxism, grinding, clenching, lack of**

support, occlusal collapse, salivary flow, composition, tooth structure

Unit 14
Minor Oral Surgery
Translation 1

1. Analgesie, oblast necitlivá několik hodin, nežvýkat, nepít alkohol, horké nápoje, necvičit po zbytek dne: **analgesia, area numb for several hours, not to chew, drink alcohol, hot drinks, not to exercise for the remainder of the day**

2. mít všechny nástroje a vybavení připravené k použití: **have all instruments and equipment ready for use**

3. nástroje chirurgické, čepel skalpelu, rukojeť, ořezávací nůž, raspatorium, držáky, držátka na jehly, šití, kleště na oddělování tkání, chirurgický násadec a vrtáčky, vodní stříkačka, sada pák, sací špičky, nůžky: **surgical instruments, scalpel blade, handle, Mitchell's trimmer, periosteal elevator, retractors, needle holders, suture, dissecting forceps, surgical handpiece, burs, water syringe, set of elevators, suction tips, scissors**

4. nástroje konzervační, miska, zrcadélko, sonda, pinzeta, exkavátory, cpátko na amalgam, hladítko, plochý tvárlivý nástroj: **conservation instruments, tray, mirror, probe, tweezers, excavators, amalgam plugger, burnisher, flat plastic instrument**

5. ošetřování u křesla, podávat a brát zpět nástroje, pomoci vypláchnout: **chairside nursing, pass and retrieve instruments, help to swill out**

6. pomoci pacientovi z ordinace, vyčistit a sterilizovat nástroje, vyhodit pomůcky na jedno použití, připravit ordinaci pro dalšího pacienta: **help patient from surgery, clean and sterilise instruments, dispose of disposables, prepare surgery for next patient**

7. pooperační pokyny, oblast může být bolestivá, zhmožděná, oteklá: **postoperative instructions, area may be sore, bruised, and swollen**

8. usadit pacienta do křesla, náprsenka, ochranné brýle: **seat the patient in the chair, bib, safety glasses**

9. výplach teplou slanou vodou, do vyjmutí stehů: **hot, saltwater mouthwash, until suture removal**

10. zajistit dostatečné odsávání, odtahovat měkké tkáně, mít nástroje po ruce, nerušit lékaře, odstraňovat patologické úlomky, vyvolat rentgenové snímky: **ensure adequate aspiration, retract soft tissues, have the instruments to hand, not to disturb the dentist, remove pathological debris, mix materials, develop radiographs**

Translation 2

1. Druhotné krvácení do 7 dnů od procedury, infekce v místě vytržení: **secondary haemorrhage**

within 7 days of the procedure, an infection at the site of the extraction

2. extrakce obtížné, značný tlak na stěny lůžka, konce krevních cév jsou rozdrcené: **difficult extractions, considerable pressure put on the socket walls, the end blood vessels are crushed**

3. komplikace po extrakci: **complications following extraction**

4. nejíst kořeněné a kyselé potraviny, které mohou dráždit jamku: **not to eat any spicy or acidic foods which may irritate the socket**

5. osteitida, obnažené lůžko, ztráta krevní sraženiny z jamky, odhalená dásňová kost, napadení bakteriemi, akutní zánět: **osteitis, dry socket, the loss of the blood clot from the socket, bare alveolar bone, bacterial invasion, acute inflammation**

6. reakční krvácení, do 24 hodin po proceduře, nediagnostikovaná porucha srážlivosti krve: **reactionary haemorrhage, within 24 hours after the procedure, undiagnosed blood clotting disorder**

7. vyhnutí se pooperativním komplikacím, důležitost dodržení pokynů: **avoiding postoperative complications, the importance of following the instructions**

8. zanedbaná ústní hygiena, odstranění zubního kamene, preventivní opatření, umístění antiseptických obvazů, uvážit léčbu antibiotiky: **neglected oral hygiene, tooth scaling, preventive measures, placing antiseptic dressings, consider antibiotic therapy**

9. zůstat sedět zpříma, vyhýbat se dotýkání, šťourání či nervózního pohrávání v místě po vytržení: **stay sitting upright, avoid touching, poking, or fiddling with the extraction site**

Translation 3

1. Couplandovo dlátko, oddělit kořeny po vrtání: **Coupland's chisel, to split the roots following drilling**

2. čepel skalpelu a rukojeť, odříznutí útržku okostice: **scalpel blade and handle, cutting the periosteal flap**

3. disekční kleště, držet koutky chlopně při procházení jehly během šití: **dissecting forceps, to hold the corners of the flap while passing the needle through during suturing**

4. držátko jehel, držení jehly během šití po úplném odstranění zubů: **needle holder, holding the needle during suturing following the complete tooth removal**

5. Huntova vodní stříkačka, pro zavlažení při užití pomalé vrtačky: **Hunt's water syringe, for irrigation while using the slow handpiece**

6. chirurgický jemný sací hrot, odstraňování krve a zavlažovacího roztoku v operačním místě: **surgical fine suction tip, blood and irrigation solution removal at the surgical site**

7. kleště na horní moláry, odstranění zubu, jakmile je proveden chirurgický zákrok a odstraněna kost: **upper molar forceps, removal of tooth once surgery has been performed and bone removed**
8. Mitchellův ořezávací nůž, nejprve zvednout koutek útržku: **Mitchell's trimmer, to raise the corner of the flap initially**
9. násadec s pomalou rychlosti a vrtáčky, odstranění kosti: **slow-speed handpiece and burs, bone removal**
10. nůžky, ustřihnout konce stehů: **scissors, to cut the suture ends**
11. raspatorium, úplně zvednout útržek, umožnit přístup pro odstranění kosti: **periosteal elevator, to raise the flap completely, allow access for bone removal**
12. seznam nástrojů a jejich užití: **list of instruments and their uses**
13. sonda, pinzety, testování anestézie, odstraňování úlomků zubu a výplní: **probe, tweezers, testing for anaesthesia, removing tooth and filling spicules**
14. šití, černé opředené hedvábí na zahnuté 3.0 jehle, opětné přiložení a držení chlopně po chirurgickém zákroku: **suture, black braided silk on a curved 3.0 needle, repositioning and holding the flap after surgery**
15. tvářové a tkáňové držáky: **cheek and tissue retractors**
16. ústní zrcadélko, prohlédnutí operačního místa: **mouth mirror, viewing the surgical area**

17. vysoko-rychlostní sací hrot, nezbytný při provádění průřezu zubu: **high-speed suction tip, necessary if tooth sectioning is carried out**
18. vzduchová turbinka a vrtáčky, oddělení kořenů jednotlivě: **air turbine and burs, separating the roots singly**
19. zvedače, uvolnit a zvednout kořeny, jestliže jsou odděleny: **elevators, to loosen and elevate roots if they are separated**

Unit 15
Orthodontics
Translation 1
1. Index byl schválen, stupeň 1,2 žádná, mírná potřeba, stupeň 3 hraniční potřeba: **the index has been validated, grades 1, 2 no, slight need, grade 3, borderline need**
2. index ortodontické léčby, složka estetická, složka dentálního zdraví: **index of orthodontic treatment, aesthetic component, dental health component**
3. klasifikace a indexy okluze: **classification and occlusal indices**
4. konvence MOCDO, chybějící zuby, předkus, zkřížený skus, posunutí kontaktních míst, překus: **the MOCDO convention, M = missing teeth, O = overjet, C = crossbite, D = displacement of contact points, O = overbite**
5. malokluze může vyvolat nepříznivou společenskou reakci: **malocclusion may elicit an unfavourable social response**

6. normální okluze je okluze v mezích přijaté odchylky od ideálního stavu: **normal occlusion is an occlusion within the accepted deviation from the ideal state**

7. pacientovo zázemí, věk, lékařská anamnéza, dentální anamnéza, záznam návštěv, ústní hygiena, kazivost, úraz: **patient background, age, medical history, dental history, attendance record, oral hygiene, caries rate, trauma**

8. posouzení, vyšetření: **assessment, examination**

9. potenciální rizika, poškození tkání, kazy, onemocnění parodontu, resorpce kořene, poškození dřeně a skloviny, ulcerace, náchylnost k dentálnímu onemocnění: **potential risks, tissue damage, caries, periodontal disease, root resorption, pulp and enamel damage, ulceration, susceptibility to dental disease**

10. potenciální výhody, zlepšené zdraví zubů, funkce, vzhled: **potential benefits, improved dental health, function, appearance**

11. praktický zubní lékař doporučí pacienty na radu nebo léčbu před vykonáním jakéhokoli zásahu: **the dental practitioner will refer patients for advice or treatment before carrying out any intervention**

12. růst obličeje, rozvoj okluze, prevence a korekce anomálií: **growth of the face, development of the occlusion, and the prevention and correction of anomalies**

13. selhání léčby, slabá spolupráce pacienta, nevhodná technika: **treatment failure, poor patient cooperation, inappropriate technique**

14. sociální anamnéza, stížnost pacienta, ocenění ortodontické léčby, rodičovská podpora: **social history, a complaint from the patient, appreciation of orthodontic treatment, parental support**

15. specifické měřicí pravítko: **a specifically measuring ruler**

16. spolehlivá a rychlá metoda posouzení okluze: **a reliable and rapid method of assessing the occlusion**

17. systém přiřazuje okluzi jedince číselné a abecedně číselné označení: **system assigns a numeric or alphanumeric label to an individual's occlusion**

18. určit výsledek léčby, měřit předkus, překus, vztah ke střední ose, vztahy v bukálním úseku, horní a dolní přední uspořádání: **to determine orthodontic treatment outcome, measure overjet, overbite, centreline relationship, buccal segment relationship, upper and lower anterior alignment**

Translation 2

1. Brát v úvahu pravděpodobnost dodržení léčby: **take account of likely compliance with treatment**

2. být si plně vědom nutných extrakcí, ortodontických zařízení

a spolupráce: **be fully aware of the necessary extractions, orthodontic appliances, and cooperation**

3. dosáhnout pohybu zubu, aktivní složky, drátěné pružiny, šroubky: **to achieve tooth movement, active components, wire springs, screws**

4. funkční aparáty, udržují spodní čelist mimo normální klidovou polohu, využívají svalstvo kolem úst: **functional appliances, hold the mandible away from its normal resting position, utilise the circumoral musculature**

5. instrukce o vložení, vyjmutí, péči, kdy nosit, co očekávat, co dělat když se objeví problémy: **instruction on insertion, removal, care, when to wear, what to expect, what to do if problems occur**

6. kontrolní návštěva, zhodnotit pohyb zubu, ukotvení, spolupráci, jak pacient zvládá situaci, problémy s řečí: **check visit, assess tooth movement, anchorage, cooperation, how the patient is coping with the situation, problems of speech**

7. nevýhody snímatelných aparátů, omezený pohyb zubu, omezený rozsah spodního oblouku, ovlivňují řeč: **disadvantages of removable appliances, limited tooth movement, limited scope in lower arch, affect speech**

8. omezení předkusu, vyloučit posunutí: **overbite reduction, eliminate displacements**

9. plánování léčby, cílem je okluze stabilní, funkční a vzhledově přijatelná: **treatment planning, the aim is an occlusion that is stable, functional, and acceptable in appearance**

10. potřebovat méně času u křesla, než u pevných aparátů: **less chairside time needed than with fixed appliances**

11. rentgenové snímky určí přítomnost, nepřítomnost suspektních neprořezaných či chybějících zubů: **radiographs will determine the presence, absence of suspected unerupted or missing teeth**

12. smíšená dentice, využít možnosti růstu, léčba velmi závislá na spolupráci pacienta, trvání často dlouhodobé: **mixed dentition, utilise growth potential, treatment very dependent on patient cooperation, duration is often prolonged**

13. snímací ortodontický aparát: **removable appliance**

14. pevné aparáty, připojení jsou upevněna k zubům, ortodontické zámky, tmelení, pásky, drátěné oblouky, pomocná zařízení, pružiny, pružné tkaniny: **fixed appliances, attachments are fixed to the teeth, brackets, bonding, bands, archwires, auxiliaries, springs, elastics**

15. udržet zuby v jejich současné poloze, pomůcky na udržování mezery, napínače: **maintain teeth in their present position, space maintainers, retainers**

16. upevnění aparátu, zkontrolovat, vyzkoušet v ústech, zajistit aby byl pohodlný, upravit, zařídit další návštěvu: **appliance fitting, check, try in the mouth, ensure it is comfortable, adjust, arrange next visit**

17. upravit aparát, upevnění, aktivní součásti, základní destičku, zkontrolovat vložení a vyjmutí: **adjust appliance, fixation, active components, baseplate, check insertion and removal**

18. vyjmout z úst k vyčištění: **remove from the mouth for cleaning**

19. vývoj dentice, pořadí prořezání: **development of dentition, sequence of eruption**

Translation 3

1. funkční aparát, pohnout čelist dopředu: **functional appliance, move the jaw forward**

2. chirurgie čelistí, osteotomie, mandibula chirurgicky zkrácena, maxilla prodloužena: **jaw surgery (osteotomy), the mandible surgically shortened, the maxilla surgically lengthened**

3. klasifikace založená na popisu horizontálního vztahu čelistí: **classification based on a description of the horizontal relationship of jaws**

4. meziobukální hrbolek, bukální rýha, vzdálený normální poloze: **mesiobuccal cusp, buccal groove, distal to normal position**

5. pevný aparát, důkladné čistění zubů, použít mezizubní kartáčky, pod drátěným obloukem, kolem kovových součástí, použít kvalitní ústní vodu: **a fixed appliance, brushing the teeth thoroughly, use interdental brushes under archwire and around metal components and use good quality mouthwash**

6. předkus průměrný, snížený, žádný kontakt řezáků: **overbite average, reduced, no incisal contact**

7. překus zvýšený, nulový, obrácený: **overjet increased, zero, reversed**

8. příčiny malokluze, městnání, nepoměr čelistí, zubů, nadpočetné zuby, vrozeně chybějící zuby: **causes of malocclusion, crowding, discrepancy of jaws, teeth, supernumeraries, congenitally absent teeth**

9. přijmout malokluzi, nejobtížněji se léčí, vyžaduje velkou spolupráci ze strany pacienta: **accept malocclusion, the most difficult to treat, requires great cooperation on the patient's part**

10. táhnout zuby dozadu, dopředu, závažné případy vyžadují chirurgický zásah do čelistí: **to pull teeth back, forwards, severe cases require surgery to the jaws**

Translation 4

1. Dieta, tři jídla denně, žádné svačení, vyhýbat se lepkavým jídlům, sladkostem a šumivým nápojům: **diet, three meals a day, no snacking, avoid sticky foods, sweets, and fizzy pop**

2. dodržovat všechny pokyny: **to comply with all the instructions**

3. instrukce pro snímatelný aparát: **instructions for removable appliance**

4. metody léčení malokluze: **methods of treating malocclusion**
5. nedostatečné uzavření rtů umožňuje vysychání dásní: **incompetent lip seal will allow the gingivae to dry out**
6. nepřetržité nošení je nezbytné, svátky, volné dny a jídla mimo domov nejsou výjimkou: **full wear is necessary, holidays, days out, and meals out are not exceptions**
7. nosit 24 hodin denně, vyjmout po jídle pro čistění: **wear the appliance for 24 hours a day, remove after meals for cleaning**
8. odchylky čelistí, obtíže při žvýkacích pohybech, nadměrný tlak na žvýkací svaly a temporomandibulární kloub, bolest v obličeji: **jaw discrepancies, difficulty in chewing movements, excess stress on the muscles of mastication and the temporomandibular joint, facial pain**
9. pevný aparát, opravit rotaci zubu, zkřížený skus, naklonění zubů, vtlačení, vytlačení zubů: **fixed appliances correct tooth rotation, crossbite, tipping of teeth, intrusion, extrusion of teeth**
10. potřeby ortodontické léčby: **needs for orthodontic treatment**
11. použít jednou za týden ústní vodu s fluoridem: **to use a weekly fluoride mouthwash**
12. selektivní extrakce vypadavých, stálých zubů: **selective extraction of deciduous, permanent teeth**
13. snímatelný aparát, pružiny, rozšiřovací šroubky, retraktory,

nákusné desky: **removable appliances, springs, expansion screws, retractors, bite planes**
14. špatně postavené zuby, abnormální trauma, kaz, onemocnění parodontu: **poorly positioned teeth, abnormal trauma, carious attack, periodontal disease**
15. ústní hygiena u pevného aparátu musí být vynikající, jinak se poškodí sklovina: **oral hygiene advice for fixed appliance must be excellent otherwise the enamel will be damaged**
16. vynechat kontaktní sporty během léčby: **abstain from contact sports during treatment**

Unit 16
Removable Prosthodontics
Translation 1
1. běžné problémy s protézami, nedostatečná podpora, nedostatečná retence, problém se svalovou rovnováhou, problém skusu, vzhledu, řeči, mimovolný pocit na zvracení, alergie na akrylát: **common denture problems, inadequate support, inadequate retention, muscle balance problem, occlusal problem, appearance, speech, retching, acrylic allergy**
2. diagnóza u bezzubého pacienta: **diagnosis in edentulous patients**
3. charakteristické znaky úplných protéz, dobrá retence, podpora, svalová rovnováha, okluzní rovnováha a stabilita: **features of complete dentures, good retention, support, muscle**

balance, occlusal balance, and
stability

4. okluzní rovnováha, síla jedné
protézy na druhou neposunuje ani
jednu z nich, zuby v kontaktu:
occlusal balance, forces of one
denture on another do not
dislodge either denture, the teeth
in contact

5. pacientovy obtíže, vývoj změn
protézy, dentální anamnéza,
lékařská anamnéza, sociální
anamnéza: patient's complaint,
denture history, general dental
history, medical history, social
history

6. podpora, odolnost proti kolmému
posunutí: support, the resistance
of vertical movement

7. poskytnout dobře navržené a
konstruované protézy: provide
with well-designed and
constructed dentures

8. protézy jsou opotřebované,
ztracené, rozbité, esteticky slabé,
uvolněné, mají velkou vadu:
dentures are worn, lost, broken,
aesthetically poor, loose, have a
major fault

9. retence, odolnost vůči posunutí
protézy od okraje: retention,
resistance to displacement of a
denture away from the ridge

10. stabilita, schopnost protézy
odolat posunování způsobenému
funkčními tlaky: stability, the
ability of a denture to resist
displacement by functional
stresses

11. stádia konstrukce úplné
protézy, vyšetření, diagnóza,
plán léčby, prvotní otisky,

hlavní otisky, registrace čelistí,
zkouška zubů, vložení protézy,
opětovná prohlídka: stages in
complete denture construction,
examination, diagnosis,
treatment plan, primary
impressions, master impressions,
jaw registration, trial of teeth,
insertion of prosthesis, review

12. svalová rovnováha, síly jazyka,
rtů a tváří nepohybují protézou:
muscle balance, the forces of
tongue, lips, and cheeks do not
dislodge a denture

13. tolerovat protézy, být spokojen:
tolerate dentures, be satisfied

14. získání komplexní anamnézy,
předepsání vhodné protetické
léčby: obtaining a comprehensive
history, prescription of
appropriate prosthodontic
treatment

15. změny po extrakci, obličejové,
uvnitř úst, psychologické: changes
following extraction of teeth,
facial, intraoral, psychological

Translation 2

1. Částečné protézy nahrazují jeden
nebo více přirozených zubů a jsou
vyjímatelné pacientem: partial
dentures replace one or more
of the natural teeth and are
removable by the patient

2. dodatky, umístění dalšího zubu
nebo části protézy na existující
protézu: additions, the placing of
an additional tooth or part of a
denture to an existing prosthesis

3. hybridní protézy získávají podporu
z pilířových zubů: overdentures

gain support from abutment teeth

4. chrániče dásní, ochrana před úrazem při kontaktních sportech: **gumshields, trauma protection in contact sports**

5. kopie zubních protéz, repliky, podobné tvarem a rozměry: **copy dentures, replica dentures, similar in shape and dimension**

6. náustky pro potápění, hraní na dechových nástrojích: **mouthpieces for diving, wind instrument playing**

7. obložení dásní, maskovat ústup dásně po onemocnění parodontu: **gingival veneers mask recession following periodontal disease**

8. okamžité protézy, vložené v den extrakce: **immediate dentures, inserted on the day of extraction**

9. opravy, zlomení protézy je docela běžné, nahrazení protézou odlišného designu: **repairs, denture fracture is quite common, replacement denture of a different design**

10. péče o pilířové zuby, čistění pastou obsahující fluorid, hygiena protézy, vyjmutí protézy na noc, místní aplikace fluoridu, omezení cukru, časté kontrolní návštěvy: **care of abutments, tooth brushing with a fluoride-containing toothpaste, denture hygiene, removal of prosthesis at night, application of topical fluoride, reduction of sugar, frequent recall visits**

11. podložení vnitřní strany protézy, umístění nového materiálu k přiléhajícímu povrchu: **relines, placing new material on the fitting surface**

12. protetická zařízení: **prosthetic appliances**

13. přesné upevnění, poskytnout dodatečné upevnění: **precision attachments, to provide additional retention**

14. zařízení k zvednutí patra, zlepšit řeč: **palatal lift appliances, improve speech**

15. zařízení proti chrápání: **antisnoring appliances**

Translation 3

1. Bolest při probouzení, bolest vystřelující do spánkové oblasti, chronická, vracející se: **pain on waking, pain radiating to temporal region, chronic, recurrent**

2. domácí léčebná cvičení, aplikace tepla či chladu na sval: **home therapeutic exercises, application of heat or cold to muscle**

3. elektroléčba, ultrazvuk, akupunktura: **electrotherapy, ultrasound, acupuncture**

4. hybridní protézy úplné, částečné, pevné můstky, náhrada jednotlivých zubů: **complete overdentures full, partial, fixed bridges, single tooth replacement**

5. implantáty jsou nákladné a složité, ale mohou být velkým přínosem u některých jednotlivců: **implants are costly and complex but may be of great benefit in some individuals**

6. kraniomandibulární poruchy, muskuloskeletální poruchy,

postihující temporomandibulární kloub: **craniomandibular disorders, musculoskeletal disorders affecting the temporomandibular joint**

7. léčba cvičením, manipulace s kloubem, cvičení opakovaná, izotonická, izometrická: **exercise therapy, joint manipulation, repetitive exercises, isotonic exercises, isometric exercises**

8. léčba pomocí dlah: **splint therapy**

9. léková terapie, snížení bolesti, zánětu, nadměrné aktivity svalů, úzkosti, deprese: **drug therapy, reducing pain, inflammation, muscle hyperactivity, anxiety, depression**

10. modifikace chování, postupná relaxace, hypnóza, poradenství o životním stylu, biologická zpětná vazba: **behaviour modification, progressive relaxation, hypnosis, lifestyle counselling, biofeedback**

11. nepohodlí u nových protéz je docela normální, je-li nepohodlí malé, pacient by je měl vydržet do další návštěvy zubního lékaře: **discomfort with new dentures is quite normal, if the discomfort is minor, the patient should persevere with it until he or she sees the dentist again**

12. omezené otevření úst, slyšitelné lupnutí kloubu, známky opotřebení zubů, protéz: **limited jaw opening, audible joint click, signs of tooth wear, denture wear**

13. ortodoncie, ortognátní chirurgie: **orthodontics, orthognathic surgery**

14. protézy nesené implantátem: **implant-borne prostheses**

15. protézy očnicové, nosní, boltcové, sluchových pomůcek: **orbital, nasal, auricular, and hearing-aid prostheses**

16. řeč je často trochu obtížná prvních několik dní: **speech is often a little difficult for the first few days**

17. titanové implantáty vhojené do kosti: **osseointegrated titanium implants**

18. útěcha pacienta, vyloučení namáhavého žvýkání, zívání, vzdychání, zpívání, okusování předmětů: **patient reassurance, avoidance of heavy mastication, yawning, sighing, singing, object biting**

19. vhojení do kosti, přímé strukturální a funkční spojení mezi živou kostí a implantátem: **osseointegration, a direct structural and functional connection between living bone and the implant**

20. zacházení s novými protézami: **coping with new dentures**

21. zvyknout si na nové protézy, nenosit přes noc, nakrájet jídlo na malé kousky, žvýkat na obou stranách současně: **to get used to new dentures, not to wear overnight, cut food into small pieces, to chew on both sides at the same time**

Unit 17
Dental Materials and Conservation Instruments

Translation 1

1. amalgám, slitina rtuti stříbra a cínu: **amalgam, an alloy of mercury with silver and tin**

2. cermety a pryskyřicí upravené skloionomery: **cermets and resin-modified glass ionomers**
3. čističe kořenových kanálků, předem utvořené výplně, utěsňovací materiály: **root canal cleansers, preformed fillings, sealers**
4. dásňový lalok, dásňový štěp: **gingival flap, gingival graft**
5. dočasné náhrady: **temporary restorations**
6. formovací hmota: **investment**
7. hrubost povrchu: **surface roughness**
8. individuální otiskovací lžíce: **individual impression trays**
9. jamky a rýhy: **pits and fissures**
10. jednotlivé soupravy: **individual kits**
11. koroze, tavitelnost, vytvoření vrstvy oxidu: **corrosion, solubility, formation of oxide layer**
12. korunky a můstky, fazety, vložky, zuby protézy: **crowns and bridges, veneers, inserts, denture teeth**
13. leštění: **polishing**
14. litiny a kujné slitiny, tuhé roztoky: **casting and wrought alloys, solid solutions**
15. malá odolnost proti nárazům: **poor impact resistance**
16. materiál na implantáty: **implant material**
17. náchylné k erozi: **susceptible to erosion**
18. nevytvářet nepříznivé účinky: **produce no adverse effects**
19. obavy o životní prostředí týkající se rtuti: **environmental concerns regarding mercury**
20. otiskové materiály pevné, pružné: **impression materials rigid, elastic**
21. pečetidla: **sealants**
22. plnící nástroj, plnivo: **filler**
23. pojivové a spojovací materiály: **adhesion and bonding agents**
24. porézní, umožňuje únik plynů: **porous to let gases escape**
25. průsvitnost: **translucency**
26. rozměrové změny při tuhnutí: **dimensional changes on setting**
27. roztavit se při zahřátí: **fuse when heated**
28. síla tahu a stlačení: **tensile and compressive strength**
29. síla, tlak, napětí, křehkost, kujnost, tvrdost, únava materiálu: **strength, stress, strain, brittleness, ductility, hardness, fatigue**
30. smrštění při tuhnutí: **curing shrinkage**
31. srážení, krystalizace, nemísitelnost: **precipitation, crystallisation, immiscibility**
32. stabilní, snadné míchání, krátká doba zpracování a usazení: **stable, easy to mix, short working and setting times**
33. tepelné rozpínání, elektrická vodivost, nepropustnost záření: **thermal expansion, electrical conductivity, radiopacity**
34. uspokojivé alternativy: **satisfactory alternatives**
35. vlastnosti materiálů: **properties of materials**
36. vosky, přírodní gumy a pryskyřice: **waxes, natural gums, and resins**
37. vydržet sílu skusu: **withstand occlusal forces**

38. základna zubní protézy: **denture base**

Translation 2
1. být roztočen, vtlačen: **be spun**
2. částečky stříbra: **silver particles**
3. dodávaný v tubách se změkčovačem: **supplied in tubes with a plasticiser**
4. dodávaný v tyčinkách: **supplied in sticks**
5. dráždí zubní dřeň: **irritant to the pulp**
6. druhy tvrzené světlem: **light-cured varieties**
7. hydroxid vápenatý: **calcium hydroxide**
8. kontaminace vlhkostí: **moisture contamination**
9. materiál je tekutý při zahřátí: **the material is runny on heating**
10. materiál na modelování okraje: **border moulding material**
11. míchá se ztuha: **it is mixed stiffly**
12. obroučka: **band**
13. odolnost proti natržení: **tear resistance**
14. odstranit: **remove**
15. otisk: **impression**
16. potřebuje podložit: **it needs a sublining**
17. prozatímní výplň: **temporary filling**
18. přesnost není rozhodující: **accuracy is not critical**
19. při tuhnutí: **on setting**
20. příjemná chuť: **pleasant tasting**
21. přilnavý k dentinu: **adhesive to dentine**
22. přitmelení: **luting**
23. rozměrová stálost: **dimensional stability**

24. rychle tuhne: **it sets quickly**
25. řídká krémová konzistence: **thin creamy consistency**
26. síla skusu: **occlusal forces**
27. stádium: **stage**
28. střed: **core**
29. špička, pracovní konec nástroje: **point**
30. těsnicí materiál na praskliny: **fissure sealant**
31. testovat vitalitu zubů: **to test the vitality of teeth**
32. trpět zánětem zubní dřeně: **suffer from pulpitis**
33. ucpat kořenové kanálky: **obturate root canals**
34. umístění korunek, můstků, litých výplní a fazet: **placement of crowns, bridges, inlays, and veneers**
35. uvolňuje fluorid: **it releases fluoride**
36. vložit ohřátý nástroj: **insert a warmed instrument**
37. vmíchat do práškové složky: **incorporate into the powder component**
38. výplně, náhrady: **restorations**
39. výstavba: **build-up**
40. vyžaduje se příprava zubu: **tooth preparation is required**
41. zesílené typy: **reinforced types**
42. zink-fosfátový cement: **zinc phosphate cement**
43. zkouška nové protézy: **try-in of a new denture**

Translation 3
1. být nejprve dezinfikován: **be disinfected first**
2. částečná protéza: **partial denture**

3. dát pod kohoutek se studenou vodou: **run under the cold water tap**
4. dovolit vhojení do kosti: **allow osseointegration**
5. jednostupňová technika: **a single-stage technique**
6. konzervační techniky: **restorative techniques**
7. konzolový můstek: **cantilever bridge**
8. materiál na otisky: **impression material**
9. na výběr: **of choice**
10. náhrada chybějícího zubu: **replacement of a missing tooth**
11. odstranit zbytky a pramínky slin: **remove any debris and strings of saliva**
12. opláchnout a vysušit: **rinse and blow dry**
13. pevný můstek: **fixed bridge**
14. pokrýt vlhkou gázou: **cover in wet gauze**
15. ponořit do roztoku chlornanu sodného: **immerse in a solution of sodium hypochlorite**
16. poslat do laboratoře: **send to a laboratory**
17. sestrojení protézy: **denture construction**
18. sousední zuby jsou zdravé: **adjacent teeth are sound**
19. spojený pryskyřicí: **resin-bonded**
20. tmelová složka: **putty component**
21. tradiční korunka: **conventional crown**
22. upevnit: **fit**
23. usmrtit všechny baktérie, plísně a většinu virů: **kill all bacteria, fungi, and most viruses**

24. uzavřít do vzduchotěsného obalu: **seal in an airtight bag**
25. vložit implantát: **insert the implant**
26. zabránění šíření infekce: **prevention of cross-infection**
27. zacházení s: **dealing with**
28. záznam skusu: **occlusal record**
29. znovu umístit: **replace**

Translation 4
1. být vytlačen: **be squashed out**
2. co nejmenší preparace je velmi důležitá: **minimal preparation is essential**
3. dutina ve tvaru klíčové dírky: **keyhole shaped cavity**
4. estetický vzhled je nesmírně důležitý: **aesthetics are of paramount importance**
5. kvůli odírání kartáčkem: **due to toothbrush abrasion**
6. matricová páska: **a matrix band**
7. nacpat do dutiny: **pack into the cavity**
8. nástroje se po použití snadno čistí: **instruments are easy to clean after use**
9. nejlépe vyhovující: **best suited**
10. nerv není příliš hluboko: **the nerve is not too deep**
11. pod výplň: **beneath the filling**
12. pokrýt okamžitě lakem: **coat immediately with varnish**
13. relativně levný: **relatively cheap**
14. řezák nebo špičák: **incisor or canine tooth**
15. skleněná destička a kovová lopatka: **a glass slab with a metal spatula**
16. snadná aplikace: **easy application**

17. snadno se umístí: **it is easily placed**
18. splnit tyto požadavky: **meet these requirements**
19. spodní řez: **an undercut**
20. správně přizpůsobit náhradu: **to adapt the restoration correctly**
21. střední či vzdálená poloha: **the mesial or distal aspect**
22. tmelící cement: **a luting cement**
23. umístit vyložení: **place lining**
24. vydržet sílu skusu, řezací sílu: **withstand occlusal forces, incisal forces**
25. vyhnout se vystavení dřeně: **avoid exposure of the pulp**
26. zadní zub (třenový či stolička): **a posterior tooth (premolar or molar)**
27. zářivý povrch: **shiny surface**
28. zásady konstrukce kavity: **principles of cavity design**

English–Czech Dictionary

A

abbreviation /əˌbriː.viˈeɪ.ʃən/ zkratka

abdominal /æbˈdɒm.ɪ.nəl/ břišní

abide /əˈbaɪd/ trvat, dodržovat

ability /əˈbɪl.ɪ.ti/ schopnost, dovednost

abnormal /æbˈnɔː.məl/ abnormální

abortion /əˈbɔː.ʃən/ interrupce

above /əˈbʌv/ all /ɔːl/ především

above /əˈbʌv/ nahoře shora (v citaci)

abrasion /əˈbreɪ.ʒən/ obrušování

abrasion /əˈbreɪ.ʒən/ resistance / rɪˈzɪs.tənts/ otěruvzdornost

abscess /ˈæb.ses/ absces

absence /ˈæb.sᵊnts/ absence, nepřítommnost, nedostatek

absent /ˈæb.sənt/ nepřítomný

absolutely /ˌæb.səˈluːt.li/ absolutně, naprosto

absorb /əbˈzɔːb/ pohltit, absorbovat, vstřebat

absorbent /əbˈzɔː.bənt/ pad /pæd/ absorbční tampon

abstain /æbˈsteɪn/ from /frɒm/ zdržovat se (čeho)

abundance /əˈbʌn.dᵊnts/ velké množství

abundant /əˈbʌn.dənt/ početný, hojný

abuse /əˈbjuːs/ zneužívání

abuse /əˈbjuːz/ zneužít

abutment /əˈbʌt.mənt/ vyztužení, podpěra, pilíř zubního můstku, nástavec, sekundární díl

accept /əkˈsept/ akceptovat, přijmout, připustit

acceptable /əkˈsept.ə.bl̩/ přijatelný, vhodný

accepted /əkˈsep.tɪd/ přijatý

access /ˈæk.ses/ přístup, vstup

accessible /əkˈses.ə.bl̩/ dostupný

accident /ˈæk.sɪ.dənt/ nehoda, úraz, havárie

accidentally /ˌæk.sɪˈden.tᵊl.i/ nešťastnou náhodou

accompany /əˈkʌm.pə.ni/ provázet, spojovat

according to /əˈkɔː.dɪŋˌtuː/ podle

account /əˈkaʊnt/ for /fɔːʳ/ odpovídat za, vysvětlit fakt

accumulate /əˈkjuː.mjʊ.leɪt/ hromadit se

accumulation /əˌkjuː.mjʊˈleɪ.ʃən/ nahromadění

accuracy /ˈæk.jʊ.rə.si/ přesnost, správnost věci

accurate /ˈæk.jʊ.rət/ pečlivý, přesný

achievable /əˈtʃiː.və.bl̩/ dosažitelný, proveditelný

achieve /əˈtʃiːv/ dosáhnout, uspět

achiever /əˈtʃiː.vəʳ/ úspěšný člověk

acid /ˈæs.ɪd/ kyselina

acid-etch /ˈæs.ɪd.ˈetʃ/ leptat kyselinou

acidic /'æs.ɪ.dɪk/ acidický, kyselinotvorný, kyselý

acquire /ə'kwaɪəʳ/ získat

acrylic /ə'krɪl.ɪk/ akrylový, pryskyřičný

act /ækt/ působit

action /'æk.ʃən/ akce, postup, působení

active /'æk.tɪv/ účinný, působivý, účinný

actually /'æk.tʃu.ə.li/ vlastně, ve skutečnosti

acupuncture /'æk.jʊ.pʌŋk.tʃəʳ/ akupunktura

acute /ə'kjuːt/ akutní

adapt /ə'dæpt/ přizpůsobit

adapted /ə'dæp.tɪd/ přizpůsobený, upravený

add /æd/ přidat, přimísit, přidávat, doplnit

addition /ə'dɪʃ.ᵊn/ dodatek, přidání

additional /ə'dɪʃ.ən.əl/ dodatečný, další, doplňkový

additive /'æd.ɪ.tɪv/ aditivní, přísada, dodatkový

adequate /'æd.ə.kwət/ adekvátní, odpovídající, přiměřený, dostačující

adequately /'æd.ə.kwət.li/ přiměřeně, dostatečně

adhere /əd'hɪəʳ/ držet na, lepit se na

adherence /əd'hɪə.rənts/ dodržování

adherent /əd'hɪə.rənt/ přilepený

adhesion /əd'hiː.ʒən/ adheze, přilnavost

adhesive /əd'hiː.sɪv/ lepidlo, lepicí páska, přilnavý, ulpívající

adjacent /ə'dʒeɪ.sənt/ přiléhající, sousední, vedlejší, hraničící

adjunct /'ædʒ.ʌŋkt/ doplněk

adjust /ə'dʒʌst/ přizpůsobit, nastavit přístroj, upravit

adjustment /ə'dʒʌst.mənt/ nastavení, přizpůsobování, seřizování

administer /əd'mɪn.ɪ.stəʳ/ podávat lék

administrative /əd'mɪn.ɪ.strə.tɪv/ administrativní

admission /əd'mɪʃ.ən/ přijetí

admit /əd'mɪt/ přijmout, připustit

adopted /ə'dɒp.tɪd/ přijatý

adrenal /ə'driː.nəl/ týkající se nadledviny

adrenaline /ə'dren.əl.ɪn/ adrenalin, epinefrin

adult /'æd.ʌlt/ dospělý člověk

advanced /əd'vɑːntst/ pokročilý

advantage /əd'vɑːn.tɪdʒ/ výhoda

adverse /'æd.vɜːs/ **effect** /ɪ'fekt/ nepříznivý účinek

adverse /'æd.vɜːs/ nepříznivý

adversely /'æd.vɜː.sli/ nepříznivě, příčně

advertising /'æd.və.taɪ.zɪŋ/ inzerát

advice /'æd.vɜːs/ rada, oznámení

advisable /əd'vaɪ.zə.bl̩/ vhodný, doporučeníhodný

advise /əd'vaɪ.z/ poradit

advised /əd'vaɪzd/ doporučený

aerobic /eə'rəʊ.bɪk/ aerobní

aesthetically /es'θet.ɪ.kli/ esteticky

aesthetics /es'θet.ɪks/ estetika

aetiological /ˌiː.ti'ɒl.ə.dʒi.kᵊl/ etiologický, podle příčiny

aetiology /ˌiː.ti'ɒl.ə.dʒi/ etiologie, nauka o původu a příčinách

affect /ə'fekt/ ovlivnit, postihnout, působit, ovlivňovat

affected /ə'fek.tɪd/ ovlivněný, napadený, zasažený

afford /ə'fɔːd/ dovolit si, poskytovat, přinášet

afterwards /'ɑːf.tə.wədz/ potom

agent /'eɪ.dʒənt/ agens, činitel, faktor, přísada, prostředek, zprostředkovatel

aggressive /ə'gres.ɪv/ agresivní

aid /eɪd/ pomoc, pomůcka, pomáhat, podpora, zařízení

aide-memoire /eɪd.ˈmem.wɑːr/ mnemotechnická pomůcka

aim /eɪm/ at /ət/ směřovat k

aim /eɪm/ záměr, cíl, zaměřit

air /eəʳ/ passage /ˈpæs.ɪdʒ/ dýchací cesta

air /eəʳ/ turbine /ˈtɜː.baɪn/ vzduchová turbinka

air /eəʳ/ vzduch

airtight /ˈeə.taɪt/ vzduchotěsný, neprodyšný

airway /ˈeə.weɪ/ dýchací cesty

alcoholism /ˈæl.kə.hɒl.ɪ.zəm/ alkoholismus

aldehyde /ˈæl.dɪ.haɪd/ aldehyd

alert /əˈlɜːt/ varovat

alertness /əˈlɜːt.nəs/ bdělost

alginate /æˈldʒɪ.neɪt/ alginát

align /əˈlaɪn/ vyrovnat se, zaměřit

alignment /əˈlaɪn.mənt/ seřazení, uspořádání

alike /əˈlaɪk/ stejnou měrou

allergen /ˈæl.ə.dʒən/alergen

allergic /əˈlɜː.dʒɪk/ alergický, přecitlivělý

allergy /ˈæl.ə.dʒi/ alergie

alloplastic /ˌælə'plæs.tɪk/ aloplastický

alloplasty /ˈæl.ə,plæs.tɪ/ aloplastika, plastika materiálem cizím lidskému tělu (stříbro, zlato, kovy)

allow /əˈlaʊ/ dovolit, dovolovat, poskytnout, poskytovat umožnit

alloy /ˈæl.ɔɪ/ slitina, příměs, směs

alone /əˈləʊn/ samotný

alphanumeric /ˌæl.fə.njuːˈmer.ɪk/ abecedně číselný

alter /ˈɒl.təʳ/ upravit, změnit, změnit se

alternative /ɒlˈtɜː.nə.tɪv/ alternativa, druhá možnost

alternatively /ɒlˈtɜː.nə.tɪv.li/ alternativně, eventuálně, střídavě

although /ɔːlˈðəʊ/ ačkoli

alum /ˈæl.əm/ kamenec, ledek

alumina /əˈluː.mɪ.nə/ kysličník hlinitý

aluminosilicate /ˌæl.juˈmɪn. əˈsɪl.ɪ.kət/ aluminosilikát, hlinito-křemičitan

alveolar /ˌæl.viˈəʊ.ləʳ/bone /bəʊn/ dásňová kost

alveolar /ˌæl.viˈəʊ.ləʳ/ dásňový

alveolectomy /ˌale.viəˈlek.tə.mi/ alveolektomie, excise alveolárního výběžku čelisti

amalgam /əˈmæl.gəm/ amalgám

Ambu /æmbjʊ/ bag /bæg/ ambu vak

ameloblastoma /æˌme.lə.blæsˈtəʊ.mə/ ameloblastom, tumor dolní čelisti, vzniklý ze sklovinových buněk

amend /əˈmend/ zlepšit, pozměnit

amongst /əˈmʌŋst/ mezi

amount /əˈmaʊnt/ množství

ampicillin /əmˈpəs.ɪ.lɪn/ ampicilin

amplification /ˌæm.plɪ.fɪˈkeɪ.ʃən/ zesílení

amputate /ˈæm.pjʊ.teɪt/ amputovat

amputation /ˌæm.pjʊˈteɪ.ʃən/ amputace, odstranění

anaemia /əˈniː.mi.ə/ chudokrevnost

anaerobic /ˌæn.əˈrəʊ.bɪk/ anaerobní

anaesthesia /ˌæn.əsˈθiː.zi.ə/ anestezie, znecitlivění

anaesthetic /ˌæn.əsˈθet.ɪk/ působící znecitlivění, anestetikum

analgesia /ˌæn.əl.ˈdʒiː.zi.ə/ analgézie, snížená vnímavost bolesti

analgesic /ˌæn.əlˈdʒiː.zɪk/ analgetikum

analysis /əˈnæl.ə.sɪs/ analýza

anaphylactic /ˌæn.ə.fɪˈlæk.tɪk/ shock /ʃɒk/ anafylaktický šok

337

anchorage /ˈæŋ.kər.ɪdʒ/ ukotvení, úchyt

anesthetise /əˈniːs.θə.taɪz/ dát narkózu, umrtvit

angina /æn͵dʒaɪ.nə/ angína

angina pectoris / æn͵dʒaɪ.nəˈpek.tə.rɪs/ angina pectoris

angle /ˈæŋ.gl̩/ úhel, roh

angled /ˈæŋ.gl̩d/ šikmý

angulation /͵æŋ.gjʊˈleɪ.ʃən/ úhel

animal /ˈæn.ɪ.məl/ živočich

annoying /əˈnɔɪ.ɪŋ/ nepříjemný, otravný

annual /ˈæn.ju.əl/ každoroční, roční

anomaly /əˈnɒm.ə.li/ anomálie, odchylka

anorexia /æn.ə͵rek.si.ə/ chorobné nechutenství

anterior /ænˈtɪə.ri.əʳ/ přední

anteriorly /ænˈtɪə.ri.əʳ.li/ zepředu

anti- /æn.ti-/ proti

antihistamine /æn.ti.ˈhɪs.tə.miːn/ protihistaminový prostředek

antibiotics /͵æn.ti.baɪˈɒt.ɪk/ antibiotika

anticipate /ænˈtɪs.ɪ.peɪt/ anticipovat, očekávat

anticoagulant /͵æn.ti.kəʊˈæg.jʊ.lənt/ antikoagulans, látka bránící srážení krve

anticonvulsant /͵æn.ti.kənˈvʌl.sºnt/ antikonvulzívum, protikřečový

antidote /ˈæn.ti.dəʊt/ protilátka

antifungal /͵æn.ti.ˈfʌŋ.gəl/ proti houbám, fungicidní, protiplísňový

anti-inflammatory /͵æn. ti.ɪnˈflæm.ə.tri/ protizánětlivý

antiplatelet /æn.ti.ˈpleɪt.lət/ proti srážení krve

antiretroviral /æn.ti͵ret.rəʊˈvaɪə.rəl/ proti-retrovirový

antiseptic /͵æn.tiˈsep.tɪk/ antiseptický, dezinfekční prostředek

antiviral /͵æn.tiˈvaɪ.rºl/ protivirový prostředek

antral /æn.trəl/ antrální, týkající se dutiny

antrum /ˈæn.trəm/ (pl. antra) antrum, dutina, předsíň

anxiety /æŋˈzaɪ.ə.ti/ pocit úzkosti, úzkost

anxiolytic /͵ænks.ɪ.aɪəl.ɪ.tɪk/ anxiolytikum, lék proti úzkosti

anxious /ˈæŋk.ʃəs/ úzkostný

any /ˈen.i/ libovolný

apex /ˈeɪ.peks/ (pl. apices) vrchol, hrot, vrcholový bod, špička

aphthous /ˈæf.θəs/ aftózní

apical /ˈeɪ.pɪ.kəl/ apikální, ležící v okolí hrotu, vrcholový, hrotový

apicectomy /æ.pɪˈsek.tə.mɪ/ apikektomie, resekce kořenového hrotu

apparatus /͵æp.əˈreɪ.təs/ ústrojí, přístroj

appear /əˈpɪəʳ/ objevit se, zdát se

appearance /əˈpɪə.rənʦ/ vzhled, objevení se, zevnějšek

appetite /ˈæp.ɪ.taɪt/ chuť k jídlu

appliance /əˈplaɪ.ənʦ/ zařízení, přístroj, aparát, spotřebič, obklad

application /͵æp.lɪˈkeɪ.ʃən/ aplikace, užití, použití, léčebný prostředek, přiložení (obkladu)

applicator /ˈæp.lɪ.keɪ.təʳ/ aplikátor, štětec

applied /əˈplaɪd/ aplikovaný, použitý, přiložený

apply /əˈplaɪ/ aplikovat

appointment /əˈpɔɪnt.mənt/ schůzka, sjednané vyšetření, setkání

appointment /əˈpɔɪnt.mənt/ jmenování, úmluva

apposition /ˌæ.pə'zɪʃ.ᵊn/ přiložení,
vzájemné dotýkání

appreciate /ə'priː.ʃi.eɪt/ ocenit

appreciation /əˌpriː.ʃi'eɪ.ʃən/ ocenění,
pochvala, zhodnocení

apprehensive /ˌæp.rɪ'hent.sɪv/
uvědomující si, mající obavy

approach /ə'prəʊtʃ/ přístup, blížit se,
cesta, kontakt

appropriate /ə'prəʊ.pri.ət/ přiměřený,
náležitý, vhodný

approximately /ə'prɒk.sɪ.mət.li/
přibližně, zhruba

arch /ɑːtʃ/ oblouk, klenout

archwire /ɑːtʃ.waɪəʳ/ drátěný oblouk

argue /'ɑːg.juː/ for /fɔːr/ obhajovat

arise /ə'raɪz/ nastat, vyskytnout se,
vystoupit, být důsledkem, vzniknout

arm /ɑːm/ ruka, rukáv, opěradlo

armament /'ɑː.mə.mənt/ armáda,
zbrojní

around /ə'raʊnd/ okolo, přibližně

arrange /ə'reɪndʒ/ zařídit

arrangement /ə'reɪndʒ.mənt/
opatření, uspořádání

arrest /ə'rest/ zástava, zachycení

arrhythmia /æ'riθ.mi.ə/ arytmie

arrhythmic /æ'rɪθ.mɪk/ arytmický

arrive /ə'raɪv/ přijet, dosáhnout

artefact /'ɑː.tɪ.fækt/ artefakt, výtvor

arterial /ɑː'tɪə.ri.əl/ tepenný

arthritis /ɑː'θraɪ.tɪs/ artritida, zánět
kloubů

articulated /ɑː'tɪk.jʊ.leɪ.tɪd/
kloubový, spojený

articulating /ɑː'tɪk.jʊ.leɪ.tɪŋ/ paper /
'peɪ.pəʳ/ artikulační papír

artificial/ˌɑː.tɪ'fɪʃ.ᵊl/ umělý

artificially /ˌɑː.tɪ'fɪʃ.ᵊl.i/ uměle

as /əz/ well /wel/ as /əz/ právě tak jako

ascend /ə'send/ stoupat, nastoupit
(přen.), dostat se

aspect /'æs.pekt/ hledisko, pohled,
poloha, vzhled

aspirate /'æs.pɪ.reɪt/ nasávat

aspirate /'æs.pɪ.rət/ nasátí

aspiration /ˌæs.pɪ'reɪ.ʃən/ vdech,
odsávání (nečistot)

aspirator /ˌæs.pɪ'reɪ.təʳ/ odsavač slin,
krve

aspirin /'æs.pɪ.rɪn/ aspirin

assess /ə'ses/ zhodnotit, určit

assessment /ə'ses.mənt/ stanovení,
posouzení, určení

assign /ə'saɪn/ přiřadit, stanovit

assist /ə'sɪst/ asistovat, pomáhat

assistance /ə'sɪs.tənt s/ asistence,
pomoc, podpora

associate /ə'səʊ.si.eɪt/ asociovat,
spojovat, spolupracovník

associated /ə'səʊ.si.eɪ.tɪd/ spojený
(přidružený)

assume /ə'sjuːm/ předpokládat,
domnívat se, přijmout

asthma /'æs.mə/ astma, dušnost

asystole /ə.sɪs.təli/ asystola

at /ət/ a /ə/ rate /reɪt/ rychlostí

at /ət/ hand /hænd/ k dispozici, po
ruce

at /ət/ once /wʌnt s/ ihned

at /ət/ the same /seɪm/ time /taɪm/
současně

ataxia /ə'tæk.sɪ.ə/ ataxie, ztráta
kontroly volních pohybů

atraumatic /'eɪ.trɔː'mæt.ɪk/
nezraňující

atropine /æt.rəp.ɪn/ atropin

atropine /æt.rəp.ɪn/ sulphate /sʌl.
feɪt/ atropinsíran

attach /ə'tætʃ/ připojit

attached /ə'tætʃt/ spojený, připojený

attachment /ə'tætʃ.mənt/ attachment,
připojení, připevnění, upevnění,
spoj, vazivo

339

attack /əˈtæk/ útok, záchvat postihnout (nemocí apod.)

attain /əˈteɪn/ dosáhnout, docílit

attempt /əˈtemp t/ pokus, pokoušet se, pokusit se, snažit

attend /əˈtend/ navštívit, navštěvovat, ošetřovat (nemocné), mít službu

attendance /əˈten.dənt s/ návštěvnost

attendance /əˈten.dənt s/ **record** /ˈrek. ɔːd/ záznam o návštěvách

attention /əˈten.t ʃən/ pozornost, ošetření, výstraha, pozor!

attention /əˈten.t ʃən/ **span** /spæn/ rozsah pozornosti

attitude /ˈæt.ɪ.tjuːd/ postoj

attraction /əˈtræk.ʃən/ přitažlivost

attrition /əˈtrɪʃ.ən/ otírání

audible /ˈɔː.dɪ.bl̩/ slyšitelný

audio /ˈɔː.di.əʊ/ **tape** /teɪp/ magnetofonová páska

aura /ˈɔː.rə/ předzvěst

auricular /ɔːˈrɪ.kjʊ.ləʳ/ ušní, boltcovitý

autoantibody /ˌɔː.təʊ ˈæn.ti.bɒd.i/ vlastní protilátka

autoclave /ˈɔː.təʊ.kleɪv/ autokláv, tlakový hrnec, autoklávovaný

autoimmune /ˌɔː.təʊ.ɪˈmjuːn/ autoimunní

auxiliary /ɔːɡˈzɪl.i.ər.i/ pomocné zařízení, příslušenství

availability /əˌveɪ.ləˈbɪl.ɪ.ti/ dostupnost, vhodnost, vybavenost

available /əˈveɪ.lə.bl̩/ dostupný, dosažitelný, k dispozici, vhodný

average /ˈæv.ər.ɪdʒ/ průměrný

avoid /əˈvɔɪd/ vyhnout se, vyhýbat se, uchránit se, vyvarovat se

avoidance /əˈvɔɪ.dənt s/ vyvarování se

avulsion /æˈval.ʃən/ avulse, odtržení, vytržení

award /əˈwɔːd/ přisoudit

aware /əˈweəʳ/ být si vědom

awareness /əˈweə.nəs/ informovanost, uvědomění, připravenost

away /əˈweɪ/ **from** /frɒm/ pryč od

away /əˈweɪ/ pryč, daleko

awkward /ˈɔː.kwəd/ špatně přístupný, nešikovný

axillary /æˈksɪl.ər.i/ axilární, podpažní

axis /ˈæk.sɪs/ osa

B

babysitter /ˈbeɪ.bi.sɪt.əʳ/ pečovatelka (k dítěti)

back /bæk/ zadní část, zpět, záda, opěradlo

background /ˈbæk.graʊnd/ zázemí, pozadí

backwards /ˈbæk.wədz/ směrem dozadu

bacterial /bækˈtɪə.ri.əl/ bakteriální

bactericidal /bækˌtɪə.ri.saɪdl/ baktericidní, zabíjející bakterie

bacteriologist /bækˌtɪə.riˈɒl.ə.dʒɪst/ bakteriolog

bacteriostatic /bækˌtɪə.ri.əˈstæt.ɪk/ bakteriostatický, bránící množení

Bacteroides /ˌbæk.tɪəˈrɒɪ.diːz/ druh střevních bacilů

badge /bædʒ/ odznak

bag /bæg/ taška, pytel, sáček

balance /ˈbæl.ənt s/ rovnováha

ball-ended /bɔːl.en.dɪd/ kulatě zakončený, zakončený kuličkou

band /bænd/ obroučka, proužek, spojit páska, kroužek

bar /bɑːʳ/ tyčinka

barbed /bɑːbd/ **broach** /brəʊtʃ/ pulpextraktor

barbed /bɑːbd/ opatřený ostny, opatřený ozubcem, ostnatý

bare /beəʳ/ obnažený

barrier /'bær.i.ə^r/ bariéra, zábrana, překážka

basal /'beɪ.sl/ cell /sel/ bazální, základní buňka

base /beɪs/ základ, základna, opěrný bod, podklad

based /beɪst/ on /ɒn/ založený na

baseplate /beɪs.pleɪt/ bazální deska

basic /'beɪ.sɪk/ základní

basis /'beɪ.sɪs/ báze, základ, podstata

batch /bætʃ/ dávka

battery /'bæt.ər.i/ baterie

beaked /biːkt/ zobákovitý

bearing /'beə.rɪŋ/ nosný, ložisko, opěrný

beat /biːt/ bít

beating /'biː.tɪŋ/ tlukot

become /bɪ'kʌm/ better /'bet.ər/ zlepšit se

become /bɪ'kʌm/ stát se

become /bɪ'kʌm/ worse /wɜːs/ zhoršit

bedding /'bed.ɪŋ/ podklad, navrstvení

bee /biː/ včela, včelí

beforehand /bɪ'fɔː.hænd/ předem

behaviour /bɪ'heɪ.vjər/ chování, jednání, způsob práce, reakce

behavioural /bɪ'heɪ.vjə.rəl/ týkající se chování

behind /bɪ'haɪnd/ za, vzadu

below /bɪ'ləʊ/ níže, dolů

bend /bend/ ohnout se

beneath /bɪ'niːθ/ pod, vespod

beneficial /ˌben.ɪ'fɪʃ.əl/ prospěšný

benefit /'ben.ɪ.fɪt/ prospěch, pomoc, příspěvek, užitek, výhoda

benign /bɪ'naɪn/ nezhoubný

benzodiazepine /ben.'zəʊ. daɪ.æ.sə,paɪn/ benzodiazepin

between /bɪ'twiːn/ mezi

beverage /'bev.ər.ɪdʒ/ nápoj

beware /bɪ'weə^r/ dát si pozor, varovat se

beyond /bɪ'jɒnd/ za, dále než

bib /bɪb/ náprsenka zástěry, náprsenka, bryndáček

bin /bɪn/ koš (na odpadky), popelnice

bind /baɪnd/ down /daʊn/ svazovat

biocompatible /ˌbaɪ.əʊ.kəm'pæt.ɪ.b^{ə}l/ biokompatibilní, biologicky slučitelný

biofeedback /baɪ.əʊ.'fiːd.bæk/ biologická zpětná vazba

biopsy /'baɪ.ɒp.si/ biopsie

birth /bɜːθ/ narození

biscuit /'bɪs.kɪt/ sušenka

bite /baɪt/ kousat, kousnutí, stisková linie

bite /baɪt/ pack /pæk/ skusový tampon

bite /baɪt/ plane /pleɪn/ nákusná deska

bite /baɪt/ skus

bitewing /baɪt.wɪŋ/ bitewing

biting /'baɪ.tɪŋ/ kousání, kousající

bitten /'bɪt.ən/ kousnutý

bladder /'blæd.ə^r/ měchýř

blade /bleɪd/ čepel

blanch /blɑːntʃ/ zblednout

bland /blænd/ jemný, nedráždivý

bleach /bliːtʃ/ bělit, vybělit

bleaching /bliːtʃ.ɪŋ/ bělení, bělicí

bleeding /'bliː.dɪŋ/ krvácení, krvácející

blind /blaɪnd/ spot /spɒt/ slepé místo na sítnici; bolavé místo (přen.)

blindness /'blaɪnd.nəs/ slepota

blistering /'blɪs.tər.ɪŋ/ vytvoření puchýřů

bloating /'bləʊ.tɪŋ/ nadmutí břicha

block /blɒk/ blokovat

blockage /'blɒk.ɪdʒ/ blokáda, ucpání

blood /blʌd/ pressure /'preʃ.ər/ krevní tlak

blood /blʌd/ clot /klɒt/ krevní sraženina

blood /blʌd/ **clotting** /klɒt.ɪŋ/ srážení krve

blood /blʌd/ **count** /kaʊnt/ krevní obraz

blood /blʌd/ **disorder** /dɪˈsɔː.dəʳ/ krevní porucha

blood /blʌd/ **test** /test/ krevní test

bloodstream /ˈblʌd.striːm/ krevní řečiště

blow /bləʊ/ **air** /eəʳ/ vhánět vzduch

blow /bləʊ/ foukat

blow /bləʊ/ úder, rána

blown /bləʊn/ **dry** /draɪ/ vyfoukat, vysušit

blur /blɜːr/ znejasnit

blurred /blɜːd/ rozmazaný

body /ˈbɒd.i/ **cavity** /ˈkæv.ɪ.ti/ tělní dutina

body /ˈbɒd.i/ **fluid** /ˈfluː.ɪd/ tělní tekutina

body /ˈbɒd.i/ tělo, těleso

body /ˈbɒd.i/ **weight** /weɪt/ tělesná váha

bond /bɒnd/ lepit, spojit, spojovat, vazba (chemická ap.), tmelit

bonding /ˈbɒnd.ɪŋ/ **agent** /ˈeɪ.dʒənt/ pojivo, tmel, lepidlo

bonding /ˈbɒnd.ɪŋ/ spojení lepidlem, vázání, slučování,

bone /bəʊn/ kost

border /bɔː.dəʳ/ hrana, hranice, okraj, rámeček, lemovat

borderline /bɔː.dəʳ.laɪn/ hraniční, sporný

bore /bɔːr/ kalibr, vrtání, vývrt

borne /bɔː.ʳn/ nesený

both /bəʊθ/ oba

bottle /ˈbɒt.l/ **brush** /brʌʃ/ malý mezizubní kartáček

bout /baʊt/ záchvat, perioda

bowels /ˈbaʊ.əlz/ vnitřnosti

bowl /bəʊl/ miska, kalíšek

brachial /breɪk.ɪ.əl/ brachiální, pažní

bracket /ˈbræk.ɪt/ ortodontický zámek, podpěra, spojit svorkou

bradycardia /ˌbræd.ɪ.ˈkɑː.di.ə/ bradykardie, zpomalená srdeční činnost

bradykinesia /ˌbræ.di.ki̇ˈniːzɪ.ə/ bradykineze, extrémní zpomalení pohybu

braided /breɪd.ɪd/ **silk** /sɪlk/ opředené hedvábí

brain /breɪn/ mozek, rozum

branch /brɑːntʃ/ rozvětvení

break /breɪk/ přerušení, přestávka, zlámat, porušit

break down /ˈbreɪk.daʊn/ rozbít

breakage /ˈbreɪ.kɪdʒ/ rozbití, zlom

breast /brest/ hruď, prsa

breastfeeding /ˈbrest.fiː.d.ɪŋ/ kojení

breath /breθ/ dech, vdechnutí

breathing /ˈbriː.ðɪŋ/ dýchání

breathless /ˈbreθ.ləs/ bez dechu, udýchaný

bridge /brɪdʒ/ zubní můstek

bridgework /brɪdʒ.wəːk/ zhotovení můstku

briefly /ˈbriː.fli/ krátce

bring /brɪŋ/ **about** /əˈbaʊt/ způsobit

bristle /brɪs.l/ štětina

brittle /ˈbrɪt.l/ křehký

broach /brəʊtʃ/ bodec, kořenová jehla, sonda, čep

broad /brɔːd/ široký, obsáhlý

broken /brəʊ.kᵊn/ rozbitý, prasklý, zlomený

bronchial /ˈbrɒŋ.ki.əl/ průduškový

bronchitis /brɒŋˈkaɪ.tɪs/ bronchitida, zánět průdušek

bronchospasm /ˈbrɒŋ.kə.spæz.ᵊm/ bronchospasmus, křeč průdušek

bronchus /ˈbrɒŋ.kəs/ průduška

brow /braʊ/ obočí, čelo

bruised /bruːzd/ zhmožděný

bruising /ˈbruː.zɪŋ/ podlitina, odřeniny

brush /brʌʃ/ kartáček, vyčistit si kartáčkem

brushing /brʌʃ.ɪŋ/ čistění

bruxism /bruːk.sɪ.zəm/ bruxismus, skřípání zuby

bubble /ˈbʌb.l̩/ bublinka

bucca /bʌk.ə/ (pl. buccae /bʌk.siː/) tvář

buccal /bʌk.l/ bukální, tvářový, lícní

buccolingual /ˌbʌk.əˈlɪŋ.gwᵊl/ bukolingvální, týkající se tváří a jazyka

build /ˌbɪld/ up /ʌp/ výstavba, zvyšování

bulimia /bʊˌlɪm.i.ə/ chorobná chuť k jídlu

bundle /ˈbʌn.dl̩/ svazek

bung /bʌŋ/ čep, zátka

bur /bɜːr/ vrtáček, fréza

burnisher /ˈbɜː.nɪʃ.əʳ/ leštič, leštítko, hladítko, cpátko

burst /bɜːst/ protrhnout

butterfly /ˈbʌt.ə.flaɪ/ motýlek, škrticí klapka

button /ˈbʌt.ᵊn/ tlačítko

by /baɪ/ hand /hænd/ ručně, za ruku

C

cake /keɪk/ koláč, dort

calcium /ˈkæl.si.əm/ vápník

calcium hydroxide /ˌkæl.si.əm. haɪˈdrɒk.saɪd/ hydroxid vápenatý

calculate /ˈkæl.kjʊ.leɪt/ počítat, zamýšlet

call /kɔːl/ for /fɔːr/ vyžadovat, požadovat

campaign /kæmˈpeɪn/ kampaň

canal /kəˈnæl/ kanálek

cancellation /ˌkænt.səlˈeɪ.ʃən/ zrušení

cancer /ˈkænt.səʳ/ rakovina

cancerphobia /ˈkænt.səʳˈfəʊ.bi.ə/ chorobný strach z rakoviny

candidiasis /ˌkæn.diˈdaɪ.ə.sɪs/ kandidóza

candidosis /ˈkæn.dɪ.dəʊ.sɪs/ kandidóza, infekce způsobená některými druhy Candidy

canine /ˈkeɪ.naɪn/ zub špičák

canister /ˈkæn.ɪ.stəʳ/ kanystr

cannula /ˈkæn.jʊ.lə/ (pl. cannulae) kanyla, dutá jehla, trubička

cantilever /ˈkæn.ti.liː.vəʳ/ bridge / brɪdʒ/ samonosný můstek

cantilever /ˈkæn.ti.liː.vəʳ/ samonosný

capsule /ˈkæp.sjuːl/ váček, pouzdro (anat.)

carbide /ˈkɑː.baɪd/ karbid, tvrdý kov

carbonated /ˈkɑː.bən.eɪ.tɪd/ perlivý, sycený, s bublinkami

carboxylate /kɑːˈbɒk.sɪl.eɪt/ karboxylát

carcinoma /ˌkɑː.sɪˈnəʊ.mə/ rakovinný nádor

cardiac /ˈkɑː.di.æk/ srdeční

cardiorespiratory / kɑː.di.əʊ.rɪˈspɪr.ə.tri/ arrest / əˈrest/ zástava srdeční a dechová

cardiovascular / ˌkɑː.di.əʊˈvæs.kjʊ.ləʳ/ kardiovaskulární

care /keəʳ/ mít zájem, ošetřovat

care /keəʳ/ péče, dohled, pozornost

careful /ˈkeə.fəl/ pečlivý, opatrný

caries /ˈkeə.riːz/ zubní kaz

caries /ˈkeə.riːz/ rate /reɪt/ kazivost

cariogenic /ˌkeə.ri.əˈdʒen.ɪk/ kazový

cariostatic /ˌkeər.ɪ.əˈstæt.ɪk/ působící zastavení kazu

carious /ˈkeər.ɪ.əs/ kariézní, kazivý, zkažený zub

carotid /kəˌrɒt.ɪd/ karotida

343

carotid /kəˌrɒt.ɪd/ pulse /pʌls/ puls na karotidě

carrier /ˈkær.i.əʳ/ nosič

carrot /ˈkær.ət/ mrkev

carry /ˈkær.i/ away /əˈweɪ/ nést pryč

carry /ˈkær.i/ nést

carry /ˈkær.i/ out /aʊt/ provést (realizovat), vykonat, vykonávat

cartilage /ˈkɑː.tᵊl.ɪdʒ/ chrupavka

cartridge /ˈkɑː.trɪdʒ/ karpule, kapsle, typ balení, kazeta, náplň, zásobník, výměnný zásobník

carve /kɑːv/ vyřezat

carver /ˈkɑː.vəʳ/ modelovací nůž, kráječ, rydlo

cascade /kæsˈkeɪd/ seřazení za sebou, kaskáda

case /keɪs/ případ, důvod, věc

cast /kɑːst/ odlít, odlitek

casting /kɑːst.ɪŋ/ alloy /ˈæl.ɔɪ/ slévárenská slitina

casting /kɑːst.ɪŋ/ odlévání, odlitek

casualty /ˈkæʒ.ju.əl.ti/ oběť, postižený, zraněný

catch /kætʃ/ zachytit

categorise /ˈkæt̬.ə.gə.raɪz/ vytvářet kategorie

catheter /ˈkæθ.ɪ.təʳ/ katétr, cévka

causation /kɔːˈzeɪ.ʃən/ příčina

cause /kɔːz/ být příčinou, vyvolat, přinutit, způsobit, zapříčinit

cause /kɔːz/ příčina, důvod,

caution /ˈkɔː.ʃᵊn/ opatrnost

cavernous /ˈkæv.ən.əs/ porézní, sklípkový

cavity /ˈkæv.ɪ.ti/ dutina, prohloubení, zubní kaz

cease /siːs/ ustat, zastavit se

ceiling /ˈsiː.lɪŋ/ strop

cell /sel/ buňka

celluloid /ˈsel.jʊ.lɔɪd/ celuloid, film, buničina

celluloid /ˈsel.jʊ.lɔɪd/ strip /strɪp/ celuloidová páska

cellulose /ˈsel.jʊ.ləʊs/ celulóza, buničina

cement /sɪˈment/ cement, tmel, pojivo, tmelit

cementation /ˌsiː.menˈteɪ.ʃᵊn/ nacementování, přitmelení, tmelení, zalévání cementem

central /ˈsen.trəl/ ústřední, nejdůležitější

centreline /sen.trə.laɪn/ střednice, osa

cephalometric /ˌse.fəˈlom.ɪt.rɪk/ cefalometrický, měřící lebku

ceramics /sɪˈræm.ɪks/ keramický materiál

cerebral palsy /ˌser.ə.brəlˈpɔːl.zi/ mozková obrna

cerebrovascular /ˌser.ɪ.brəˈvæs.kjʊ.ləʳ/ accident /ˈæk.sɪ.dᵊnt/ mozková cévní příhoda

cervical /səˈvaɪ.kəl/ cervikální, krčkový

cervical /səˈvaɪ.kəl/ collar /ˈkɒl.əʳ/ krční límec

chain /tʃeɪn/ řetízek

chair /tʃeəʳ/ křeslo

chairside /tʃeəʳ.saɪd/ u křesla, vedle křesla

chalky /ˈtʃɔː.ki/ křídovitý

chamber /ˈtʃeɪm.bəʳ/ vyhloubit

chance /tʃɑːnts/ šance, možnost

change /tʃeɪndʒ/ změna

character /ˈkær.ɪk.təʳ/ charakter, vlastnosti

charge /tʃɑːdʒ/ účtovat si

chart /tʃɑːt/ sestavovat diagramy

check /tʃek/ kontrolovat, zkontrolovat, kontrola

check-up /tʃek. ʌp/ kontrola

cheek /tʃiːk/ tvář

chemical /ˈkem.ɪ.kᵊl/ chemická látka

344

chest /tʃest/ compression / kəmˈpreʃ.ⁿn/ stlačení hrudníku

chest /tʃest/ hrudník, prsní

chew /tʃuː/ the cud /kʌd/ přežvykovat

chew /tʃuː/ žvýkat, rozmělnit

chewing /tʃuː.ɪŋ/ gum /gʌm/ žvýkačka

chickenpox /ˈtʃɪk.ɪn.pɒks/ plané neštovice, varicella

chin /tʃɪn/ brada

chisel /ˈtʃɪz.ⁿl/ dláto, sekáč

chlorhexidine /ˌklɒː.hek.sɪˈdiːn/ chlorhexidin

choclear /kɒk.lɪ.ə/ kochleární, hlemýžďovitý

choice /tʃɔɪs/ volba, výběr, sortiment

choke /tʃəʊk/ dusit se, přestat dýchat

choose /tʃuːz/ vybrat si

chosen /ˈtʃəʊ.zⁿn/ (inf. choose) vybraný

chrome /krəʊm/ chrom

chromium /ˈkrəʊ.mi.əm/ chrom, chromový

chronic /ˈkrɒn.ɪk/ chronický, vleklý, trvalý

circle /ˈsɜː.kl̩/ kruh

circulation /ˌsɜː.kjʊˈleɪ.ʃⁿn/ cirkulace, oběh

circumoral /ˈsɜː.kəm.ˈɔː.rəl/ okolo úst

circumstance /ˈsɜː.kəm.stɑːnts/ okolnost, poměry

citrus /ˈsɪt.rəs/ citrus

claim /kleɪm/ žádost

clamminess /ˈklæm.ɪ.nəs/ vlhká lepkavost

clammy /ˈklæm.i/ chladný a lepkavý, vlhce lepkavý

clamp /klæmp/ upnout, výztuha, svorka

clasp /klɑːsp/ spona, háček, opatřit sponou, připnout

classification /ˌklæs.ɪ.fɪˈkeɪ.ʃⁿn/ klasifikace, třídění

clean /kliːn/ čistit

cleaning /ˈkliː.nɪŋ/ čištění, čistící

cleanser /ˈklen.zəʳ/ čisticí prostředek

clear /klɪəʳ/ čistý, jasný

clear /klɪəʳ/ off /ɒf/ očistit, vyprázdnit

clear /klɪəʳ/ away /əˈweɪ/ odstranit

clearing /ˈklɪə.rɪŋ/ odstranění

clearly /ˈklɪə.li/ jasně

clench /klentʃ/ sevřít, zatnout, pevně uchopit

click /klɪk/ kliknutí, klapnutí

cline /klaɪn/ klín

clinical /ˈklɪn.ɪ.kⁿl/ klinický

clinician /klɪˈnɪʃ.ən/ klinický lékař

clip /klɪp/ sepnout (spínátkem), štípat

clip /klɪp/ svorka, ruční nůžky

clonic /klɒn.ik/ klonický, škubavý

close /kləʊz/ blízko, blízký

closely /ˈkləʊ.sli/ těsně

clot /klɒt/ sraženina

clothing /ˈkləʊ.ðɪŋ/ oděv, oblečení

cluster /ˈklʌs.təʳ/ shluk, hrozen, nahromadit se

coagulation /kəʊˈæg.jʊ.leɪ.ʃⁿn/ koagulace, srážení

coated /ˈkəʊ.tɪd/ pokrytý, povlečený, potažený

cobalt /ˈkəʊ.bɒlt/ kobalt

code /kəʊd/ kód

codeine /ˈkəʊ.diːn/ kodein

coeliac disease /ˈsiː.li.æk.dɪˌziːz/ celiakie, břišní onemocnění

cold /kəʊld/ chlad, studený, nachlazení

cold /kəʊld/ sore /sɔːʳ/ opar

cold-cure /kəʊld.kjʊəʳ/ tuhnout za studena

colitis /kəʊˈlaɪ.təs/ zánět tlustého střeva

collapse /kəˈlæps/ kolaps, zhroucení, zhroutit se

collect /kəˈlekt/ hromadit se

colloid /kɒl.ɒ.id/ koloid, druh roztoku homogenní, želatinový, rosolovitý

colon /ˈkəʊ.lɒn/ tlusté střevo

combine /kəmˈbaɪn/ kombinovat, spojit

comfort /ˈkʌm.fət/ pohodlí, uklidnění

comfortable /ˈkʌmp.fə.tə.bl̩/ pohodlný

comfortably /ˈkʌmf.tə.bli/ pohodlně

command /kəˈmɑːnd/ příkaz, nařídit, ovládat

commence /kəˈments/ otevřít, začínat, zahájit

commensal /ˈkɒm.əns.ᵊl/ symbiont

comminuted /ˈkɒ.mɪˈnjuː.tɪd/ fracture /ˈfræk.t ʃəʳ/ roztříštěná zlomenina

common /ˈkɒm.ən/ běžný, častý, obvyklý, společný

communicate /kəˈmjuː.nɪ.keɪt/ komunikovat

communication /kə.mjuː.nɪˈkeɪ.ʃᵊn/ spojení

community /kəˈmjuː.nə.ti/ komunita, společnost

compact /kəmˈpækt/ pevný, hustý

compactor /kəmˈpæk.təʳ/ lis, zhutňovač

compatible /kəmˈpæt.ɪ.bl̩/ slučitelný, zaměnitelný

compensate /ˈkɒm.pən.seɪt/ vyrovnat, vynahradit, vyvážit

competently /ˈkɒm.pɪ.tənt.li/ schopně

complaint /kəmˈpleɪnt/ stížnost, potíž

complementary /ˌkɒm.plɪˈmen.tər.i/ pomocný, doplňující

complete /kəmˈpliːt/ dokončený, hotový, úplný

complete /kəmˈpliːt/ doplnit, dokončit, skončit

completely /kəmˈpliːt.li/ úplně, zcela

completion /kəmˈpliː.ʃən/ dokončení, dohotovení, ukončení

complex /ˈkɒm.pleks/ komplex, složitý

complexion /kəmˈplek.ʃᵊn/ pleť, pokožka

compliance /kəmˈplaɪ.ənts/ shoda, souhlas, spolupráce, dodržení

complicate /ˈkɒm.plɪ.keɪt/ komplikovat

complicated /ˈkɒm.plɪ.keɪ.tɪd/ složitý

complication /ˌkɒm.plɪˈkeɪ.ʃᵊn/ komplikace, obtíž

comply /kəmˈplaɪ/ with /wɪð/ dodržet (co), vyhovovat

component /kəmˈpəʊ.nənt/ složka

composed /kəmˈpəʊzd/ složený

composite /ˈkɒm.pə.zɪt/ kompozitní výplňový materiál

composition /ˌkɒm.pəˈzɪʃ.ən/ složení

compound /ˈkɒm.paʊnd/ fracture / ˈfræk.t ʃəʳ/ otevřená zlomenina

compound /ˈkɒm.paʊnd/ sloučenina, směs

comprehensive /ˌkɒm.prɪˈhent.sɪv/ komplexní, obsáhlý

compress /kəmˈpres/ působit tlakem, stlačit

compression /kəmˈpreʃ.ən/ komprese, stisk, stlačení, zhuštění

comprise /kəmˈpraɪz/ zahrnovat, obsahovat

compromise /ˈkɒm.prə.maɪz/ oslabit, vydat v nebezpečí

compulsive /kəmˈpʌl.sɪv/ nutkavý (psych.)

computer /kəmˈpjuː.təʳ/ počítačový

computer /kəmˈpjuː.təʳ/ tomography /təˈmɒ.grə.fɪ/ počítačová tomografie

concentration /ˌkɒnt.sənˈtreɪ.ʃᵊn/ hustota, koncentrace, soustřeďování concept /ˈkɒn.sept/ návrh (koncept), představa, způsob, provedení

concern /kənˈsɜːn/ týkat se, zájem, znepokojení

concurrent /kənˈkʌr.ᵊnt/ souběžný

concussion /kənˈkʌʃ.ən/ otřes, pohmoždění

condenser /kənˈden.səʳ/ chladič

condition /kənˈdɪʃ.ən/ stav, kondice, podmínka, podmiňovat, poměry, okolnost

conditioned /kənˈdɪʃ.ənd/ podmíněný, upravený, určený

conditioner /kənˈdɪʃ.ᵊn.ᵊr/ kondicionér

conduct /kənˈdʌkt/ vést, řídit

conduction /kənˈdʌk.ʃən/ vedení, přenos, vodivost

conductivity /ˌkɒn.dʌkˈtɪv.ɪ.ti/ vodivost

condyle /ˌkɒn.dɑɪl/ kondyl, kloubní hrbol

confidence /ˈkɒn.fɪ.dənts/ důvěra, spolehnutí

confidently /ˈkɒn.fɪ.dənt.li/ jistě

confused /kənˈfjuːzd/ zmatený, nejasný

confusing /kənˈfjuː.zɪŋ/ matoucí

congenital /kənˈdʒen.ɪ.tᵊl/ vrozený

congested /kənˈdʒes.tɪd/ překrvený

conjunctiva /ˌkɒn.dʒʌŋkˈtaɪ.və/ oční spojivka

connected /kəˈnek.tɪd/ připojený, spojený

connection /kəˈnek.ʃən/ spojení

connective tissue /kəˌnek.tɪvˈtɪʃ.uː/ pojivová tkáň

conscious /ˈkɒn.tʃəs/ při vědomí, uvědomělý

consciousness /ˈkɒn.tʃə.snəs/ vědomí

consent /kənˈsent/ souhlas, shoda

consequence /ˈkɒnt.sɪ.kwənts/ následek, závažnost, závěr

consequently /ˈkɒnt.sɪ.kwənt.li/ následně

conservation /ˌkɒnt.səˈveɪ.ʃᵊn/ ochrana, zachování, uchování, udržování

consider /kənˈsɪd.əʳ/ uvážit, zvážit, vzít do úvahy

considerable /kənˈsɪd.ər.ə.bḷ/ značný

consideration /kənˌsɪd.əˈreɪ.ʃən/ úvaha

considered /kənˈsɪd.əd/ zvažován

consistency /kənˈsɪs.tᵊnt.si/ konzistence, hutnost, hustota, shoda, důslednost

constant /ˈkɒnt.stᵊnt/ stálý

constipation /ˌkɒnt.stɪˈpeɪ.ʃən/ zácpa

constituent /kənˈstɪt.ju.ənt/ prvek (složka, člen, součást)

constitute /ˈkɒn.stɪ.tjuːt/ vytvářet

constrain /kənˈstreɪn/ omezení, omezovat, škrtit

constrict /kənˈstrɪkt/ stáhnout, stisknout

construct /kənˈstrʌkt/ postavit, vybudovat, vytvořit, sestavit

construction /kənˈstrʌk.ʃən/ konstrukce

consume /kənˈsjuːm/ konzumovat, sníst, zkonzumovat, spotřebovat

consumption /kənˈsʌmp.ʃən/ spotřeba, strávení, opotřebování (člověka), zničení

contagious /kənˈteɪ.dʒəs/ nakažlivý

contain /kənˈteɪn/ obsahovat, pojmout, skládat se, zaujímat

container /kənˈteɪ.nəʳ/ obal, schránka

content /ˈkɒn.tent/ obsah, objem, kapacita

content /ˈkɒn.tent/ spokojený, ochoten

context /ˈkɒn.tekst/ souvislost

continence /ˈkɒn.tɪ.nənt/ schopnost udržet moč

continually /kənˈtɪn.ju.ə.li/
nepřetržitě, ustavičně, neustále

continue /kənˈtɪn.juː/ pokračovat,
vytrvat

continuity /ˌkɒn.tɪˈnjuː.ɪ.ti/
kontinuita, nepřetržitost, souvislost,
neprůchodnost

continuous /kənˈtɪn.ju.əs/ nepřetržitý,
plynulý, neustálý, pravidelný,
souvislý, spojený

contraceptive /ˌkɒn.trəˈsep.tɪv/
antikoncepce

contract /ˈkɒn.trækt/ uzavřít smlouvu,
chytit (nemoc), smrštit se

contraction /kənˈtræk.ʃən/ kontrakce,
stažení, stah, smrštění, zmenšení

contraindicate /ˌkɒn.trə.ˈɪn.dɪ.keɪt/
kontraindikovat

contraindication /ˈkɒn.trə.ˌɪnd.ɪ.ˈkeɪ.ʃən/ kontraindikace

contribute /kənˈtrɪb.juːt/ přispívat

control /kənˈtrəʊl/ kontrola,
kontrolovat, řídit, dohlížet na

convenience /kənˈviː.ni.ənts/ výhoda,
vhodnost, příležitost (vhodná)

convention /kənˈvenʧ.ʃən/ pravidlo

conventional /kənˈvenʧ.ʃən.əl/
konvenční, tradiční

convert /kənˈvɜːt/ přeměnit

cooker /ˈkʊk.əʳ/ sporák

cool /kuːl/ **down** /daʊn/ ochladit

cool /kuːl/ chladný, klidný

coolant /ˈkuː.lənt/ chladivo,
ochlazovací prostředek

cooled /kuːld/ chlazený, zchlazený

cooling /ˈkuː.lɪŋ/ ochlazení

cooperation /kəʊˌɒp. əˈreɪ.ʃən/
spolupráce

cooperative /kəʊˈɒp.əˈr.ə.tɪv/
spolupracující

coordination /kəʊˌɔː.dɪˈneɪ.ʃən/
koordinace, uvedení v soulad

cope /kəʊp/ zvládat, zvládnout, stačit

copious /ˈkəʊ.pi.əs/ hojný, bohatý

copper /ˈkɒp.əʳ/ měď

copy /ˈkɒp.i/ kopie

cord /kɔːd/ šňůra, lanko

core /kɔːʳ/ hlavní, nitro, střed

corner /ˈkɔː.nəʳ/ cíp, růžek, roh, kout,
úhel

correct /kəˈrekt/ správný, přesný

correction /kəˈrek.ʃən/ oprava

corrective /kəˈrek.tɪv/ nápravný,
opravný

correctly /kəˈrekʧ.li/ správně, přesně

correlation /ˌkɒr.əˈleɪ.ʃən/ korelace,
vztah

corrode /kəˈrəʊd/ rezavět

corrosion /kəˈrəʊ.ʒ°n/ rozežírání,
leptání

corrosive /kəˈrəʊ.sɪv/ žíravina

corticosteroid /ˈkɔː.tɪkɒˈster.ɔɪd/
kortikosteroid

cost /kɒst/ finanční náklady

cost-effective /kɒst.ɪˈfek.tɪv/ cenově
přístupný

costly /ˈkɒsʧ.li/ nákladný, drahý

cotton /ˈkɒt.°n/ **wool** /wʊl/ **roll** /rəʊl/
svitek vaty

cotton /ˈkɒt.°n/ **wool** /wʊl/ vata

cough /kɒf/ kašel

counselling /ˈkaʊnʧ.səl.ɪŋ/
poradenství

count /kaʊnt/ počet, spočítat

couple /ˈkʌp.l̩/ dvojice, spojený,
připojit

course /kɔːs/ průběh, kúra
(léčebná),postup

cover /ˈkʌv.əʳ/ pokrýt, kryt, zakrýt, skrýt

coverage /ˈkʌv.°r.ɪdʒ/ pokrytí, rozsah,
šíře záběru

covered /kʌv.əd/ pokrytý

covering /ˈkʌv.ər.ɪŋ/ pokrytí, překrytí,
obložení

CPR /ˌsiː.piːˈɑːˈ/ cardiopulmonary / ˌkɑː.di.əˈpʌl.mə.nə.ri/ resuscitation /rɪˌsʌs.ɪˈteɪ.ʃᵊn/ kardiopulmonární resuscitace

cranial /ˈkreɪ.ni.əl/ lebeční

cranial /ˈkreɪ.ni.əl/ **nerve** /nɜːv/ lebeční nerv

craniomandibular/ˈkreɪ.ni.ə.mæn.ˈdɪ.bjʊ.ləˈ/ kraniomandibulární, týkající se lebky a dolní čelisti

craving /ˈkreɪ.vɪŋ/ touha, bažení

cream /kriːm/ krém, pasta

creamy /ˈkriː.mi/ bělavý, krémový

create /kriˈeɪt/ vytvořit

creep /kriːp/ roztahovat se, tečení

creosote /ˈkriː.ə.səʊt/ kreozot (chem.)

crevice /ˈkrev.ɪs/ prasklina, škvíra, štěrbina, trhlina (úzká)

crevicular /ˈkreˈv.ɪ.kjʊ.ləˈ/ štěrbinový

crib /krɪb/ kotevní spona

cricothyroid /ˌkraɪ.kəˈθaɪə.rɔɪd/ krikotyreoidní, týkající se spoje chrupavky prstencové a štítné

criterion /kraɪˈtɪə.ri.ən/ (pl. criteria) měřítko

critical /ˈkrɪt.ɪ.kᵊl/ kritický, velmi důležitý, rozhodující

crossbite /krɒs.baɪt/ zkřížený skus

cross-infection /krɒs.ɪnˈfek.ʃᵊn/ šíření infekce

cross-section/ˌkrɒsˈsek.ʃᵊn/ příčný řez, průřez

crowding /kraʊd.ɪŋ/ městnání

crown /kraʊn/ korunka (zubu)

crucial /ˈkruː.ʃᵊl/ klíčový, rozhodující, velmi důležitý

crush /krʌʃ/ rozdrtit

crushing /ˈkrʌʃ.ɪŋ/ drtivý, zdrcující

crust /krʌst/ kůra, strup, povlak, usazenina

cryosurgery /kraɪ.əˈsɜːdʒər.i/ kryochirurgie, schlazení tkání pod minus 20 stupňů

crystallisation /ˌkrɪs.təl.aɪˈzeɪ.ʃᵊn/ tvoření krystalů

cuff /kʌf/ opatřit manžetou

cure /kjʊəˈ/ léčba, kúra (léčebná), vyléčit se

cure /kjʊəˈ/ vytvrdit

curettage /ˌkjʊəˈret.ɪdʒ/ kyretáž, výškrab

curette /kjʊəˈret/ kyreta

curing /kjʊəˈ.ɪŋ/ **lamp** /læmp/ polymerační lampa

curing /kjʊər.ɪŋ/ ošetřování, vytvrzení (lepidla, plastu)

current /ˈkʌr.ᵊnt/ aktuální, současný

currently /ˈkʌr.ənt.li/ aktuálně, v současné době

curvature /ˈkɜː.və.tʃəˈ/ zakřivení

curved /kɜːvd/ zakřivený, obloukový

cusp /kʌsp/ vrcholek, hrbolek

cut /kʌt/ řezat, stříhat, říznutí

cutter /ˈkʌt.əˈ/ dláto, fréza

cutting /ˈkʌt.ɪŋ/ řezací

cyanosis /ˈsʌɪəˈnəʊ.sɪs/ cyanóza, promodrání, zmodrání kůže a sliznic

cycle /ˈsaɪ.kl̩/ cyklus

cylinder /ˈsɪl.ɪn.dəˈ/ tlaková láhev, válec

cyst /sɪst/ cysta, váček

cystic /ˌsɪs.tɪk/ cystický

cystic fibrosis /ˌsɪs.tɪk.faɪˈbrəʊ.sɪs/ cystická fibróza, fibrotické onemocnění slinivky

cystitis /sɪˈstaɪ.tɪs/ cystitida, zánět močového měchýře

cytotoxic /saɪ.təˈtɒk.sɪk/ cytotoxický, škodlivý pro buňky

D

damage /ˈdæm.ɪdʒ/ poškození, zničení

danger /ˈdeɪn.dʒəʳ/ nebezpečí

dangerous /ˈdeɪn.dʒºr.əs/ nebezpečný

daydreaming /ˈdeɪ.driːm/ snění

dead /ded/ odumřelý

deafness /ˈdef.nəs/ hluchota

deal /dɪəl/ část, hodně

deal /dɪəl/ with /wɪð/ jednat, zacházet, týkat se

death /deθ/ smrt, zánik

debilitate /dɪˈbɪl.ɪ.teɪt/ oslabit

debond /dɪ.ˈbɒnd/ zeslabit spojení

debridement /dɪˈbriːd.mənt/ excise kavity, odstranění nekrotické tkáně

debris /ˈdeb.riː/, /ˈdeɪ.briː/ úlomky, pozůstatky, poškozená tkáň, zbytky, nečistota

decade /ˈdek.eɪd/ dekáda, desetiletí, desítka

decay /dɪˈkeɪ/ kaz

deciduous /dɪˈsɪd.ju.əs/ teeth /tiːθ/ dočasný, mléčný chrup, vypadavý

decision /dɪˈsɪʒ.ən/ making /ˈmeɪ. kɪŋ/ rozhodování

decision /dɪˈsɪʒ.ən/ rozhodnutí, nález

declare /dɪˈkleəʳ/ prohlašovat

decrease /dɪˈkriːs/ snížení, snížit se, být na ústupu

deep /diːp/ hluboký, hlubina, ponořený

deep-seated /diːp.ˈsiː.tɪd/ hluboce uložený, mající hluboké kořeny

defective /dɪˈfek.tɪv/ vadný, porušený

defibrillator /ˌdiːˈfɪb.rɪ.leɪ.tər/ defibrilátor

deficiency /dɪˈfɪʃ.ənt.si/ nedostatek

deficient /dɪˈfɪʃ.ənt/ deficitní, nedostatečný

deficit /ˈdef.ɪ.sɪt/ deficit, nedostatek

defined /dɪˈfaɪnd/ definovaný

definitive /dɪˈfɪn.ɪ.tɪv/ definitivní

deform /dɪˈfɔːm/ deformovat, změnit tvar

deformity /dɪˈfɔː.mɪ.ti/ deformita, znetvoření

degeneration /dɪˌdʒen.əˈreɪ.ʃən/ degenerace, rozklad

degradable /dɪˈgreɪ.də.bl̩/ rozložitelný, odbouratelný

degree /dɪˈgriː/ stupeň

dehydration /ˌdiː.haɪˈdreɪ.ʃən/ odvodnění, vysychání

delay /dɪˈleɪ/ zdržet, zpoždění, odkládat

delete /dɪˈliːt/ vymazat, vynechat

delicate /ˈdel.ɪ.kət/ jemný

deliver /dɪˈlɪv.əʳ/ dodávat

delusion /dɪˈluː.ʒən/ halucinace, klam

demand /dɪˈmɑːnd/ poptávka

demanding /dɪˈmɑːn.dɪŋ/ náročný

demonstrate /ˈdem.ən.streɪt/ předvádět, vyložit (názorně), ukázat, dokázat

demyelination /dɪˈmaɪ.ə.li.naɪˈzeɪ.ʃən/ demyelinizace, zničení myelinu

density /ˈdent.sɪ.ti/ denzita, objemová hmotnost, hutnost

dental /ˈden.tºl/ history /ˈhɪs.tər.i/ dentální anamnéza

dental /ˈden.tºl/ zubní

dentate /den.teɪt/ ozubený, zubatý, vroubkovaný

dentigerous /denˈtɪ.dʒə.rəs/ obsahující zub

dentine /ˈden.tiːn/ dentin, zubovina

dentist /ˈden.tɪst/ zubní lékař

dentistry /ˈden.tɪ.stri/ zubní lékařství

dentition /denˈtɪʃ.ən/ dentice, chrup

denture /ˈden.tʃə/ base /beɪs/ základna protézy

denture /ˈden.tʃə/ zubní náhrada

depend /dɪˈpend/ záviset, záležet na

dependant /dɪ'pen.dᵊnt/ závislá osoba, rodinný příslušník

dependence /dɪ'pen.dᵊnts/ závislost, vztah

dependent /dɪ'pen.dənt/ on /ɒn/ závislý

deposit /dɪ'pɒz.ɪt/ uložit

depressed /dɪ'prest/ skleslý, stlačený, snížený

depression /dɪ'preʃ.ən/ deprese, potlačení, sklíčenost

depth /depθ/ hloubka, tloušťka

derivative /dɪ'rɪv.ə.tɪv/ derivát, odvozenina

dermatitis /ˌdɜː.mə'taɪ.təs/ dermatitida, zánět kůže

dermatology /ˌdɜː.mə'tɒl.ə.dʒi/ dermatologie, kožní lékařství

describe /dɪ'skraɪb/ popsat

description /dɪ'skrɪp.ʃən/ popis

design /dɪ'zaɪn/ návrh, nákres, schéma

desirable /dɪ'zaɪə.rə.bl̩/ vhodné, žádoucí

desire /dɪ'zaɪəʳ/ přát si, přání

desired /dɪ'zaɪəd/ požadovaný

despise /dɪ'spaɪz/ ignorovat, opovrhovat

despite /dɪ'spaɪt/ navzdory

destruction /dɪ'strʌk.ʃən/ ničení, zkáza, rozložení, zničení, zánik

destructive /dɪ'strʌk.tɪv/ destruktivní, zhoubný, ničící, rušivý

detect /dɪ'tekt/ zjistit, objevit, určit

detection /dɪ'tek.ʃən/ objevení, odhalení, vypátrání

detector /dɪ'tek.təʳ/ detekční přístroj, snímač, čidlo

deteriorate /dɪ'tɪə.ri.ə.reɪt/ kazit se, chátrat, zhoršit

deterioration /dɪˌtɪə.ri.ə'reɪ.ʃən/ deteriorizace, zhoršení, chátrání, porucha

determination /dɪˌtɜː.mɪ'neɪ.ʃᵊn/ určení

determine /dɪ'tɜː.mɪn/ určit, vymezit, rozhodnout, stanovit

detersive /dɪ'tɜːʳ.sɪv/ čisticí

detract /dɪ'trækt/ odvést pozornost

detriment /'det.rɪ.mənt/ neprospěch, poškození

devastating /'dev.ə.steɪ.tɪŋ/ zničující

develop /dɪ'vel.əp/ projevit, projevit se, objevit se, rozvinout se, vypěstovat v sobě (nemoc), vyvinout se

develop /dɪ'vel.əp/ radiograph / reɪ.di.ə.grɑːf/ vyvolat rentgenový snímek

development /dɪ'vel.əp.mənt/ rozvoj

developmental /dɪˌvel.əp'men.tᵊl/ vývojový

deviation /ˌdiː.vi'eɪ.ʃən/ odchylka

device /dɪ'vaɪs/ zařízení, prostředek, vybavení, záměr

dexterity /dek'ster.ə.ti/ obratnost, zručnost

diabetes /ˌdaɪə'biː.tiːz/ úplavice cukrová, cukrovka

diagnosis /ˌdaɪ.əg'nəʊ.sɪs/ diagnóza, rozpoznání (choroby), určení, popsání

dial /'daɪ.əl/ vytočit (telefonní číslo)

diameter /daɪ'æm.ɪ.təʳ/ průměr (kružnice)

diamond /'daɪə.mənd/ bur /bɜːʳ/ diamantový brousek

diamond /'daɪə.mənd/ diamant

diarrhoea /ˌdaɪ.ə'riː.ə/ diarea (průjem)

diastema /ˌdaɪ.əs'tiːm.ə/ diastéma, mezera mezi středními řezáky

diastolic /ˌdaɪ.ə'stɒ.lɪk/ diastolický

diathesis /ˌdaɪ'æ.θiː.sɪs/ diatéza, dispozice

diazepam /ˌdaɪ'æz.ə.pəm/ diazepam, sedativum, valium

dietary /ˈdaɪ.ə.tər.i/ dietní

dietetic /ˌdaɪə.teˈtɪk/ dietetický, dietní

differ /ˈdɪf.ᵊr/ lišit se, neshodovat se, nesouhlasit

difference /ˈdɪf.ər.ənt s/ rozdílnost

differentiation /ˌdɪf.ər.en.t ʃiˈeɪ.ʃən/ rozlišování, rozdílnost

difficulty /ˈdɪf.ɪ.kəl.ti/ obtíž

diffuse /dɪˈfjuːs/ rozptýlený, neohraničený, rozšířit se, pronikat

dig /dɪg/ vrtat, dloubat

digital /ˈdɪdʒ.ɪ.tᵊl/ digitální

dignity /ˈdɪg.nɪ.ti/ důstojnost

dilate /daɪˈleɪt/ rozšiřovat

dimension /ˌdaɪˈmen.t ʃᵊn/ rozměr

dimensional /daɪ.ment.ʃən.ᵊl/ objemový rozměrový

diminish /dɪˈmɪn.ɪʃ/ zmenšit se, slábnout

dip /dɪp/ sklánět se

direct /daɪˈrekt/ dohlížet, nasměrovat, zamířit, řídit

direct /daɪˈrekt/ přímý

direction /daɪˈrek.ʃᵊn/ směr, vedení

dirt /dɜːt/ špína

dirty /ˈdɜː.ti/ špinavý

disadvantage /ˌdɪs.ədˈvɑːn.tɪdʒ/ nevýhoda, nedostatek

disastrous /dɪˈzɑː.strəs/ katastrofální

disc /dɪsk/ kotouč

discard /dɪˈskɑːd/ vyřadit, vyřazení

discharge /dɪsˈtʃɑːdʒ/ výtok

disclose /dɪˈskləʊz/ odhalit, prozradit

discoloration /dɪˌskʌl.əˈreɪ.ʃən/ změna barvy zubů

discomfort /dɪˈskʌmp.fət/ nepohoda, nepohodlí, nevolnost, obtěžovat

discourage /dɪˈskʌr.ɪdʒ/ odradit

discrepancy /dɪˈskrep.ᵊnt.si/ nepoměrnost, odchylka

discrete /dɪˈskriːt/ diskrétní, jednotlivý, oddělený, samostatný

discriminate /dɪˈskrɪm.ɪ.neɪt/ rozlišovat

disease /dɪˈziːz/ nemoc, onemocnění

disinfect /ˌdɪs.ɪnˈfekt/ dezinfikovat

disinfectant /ˌdɪs.ɪnˈfek.tᵊnt/ dezinfekční prostředek

dislocation /ˌdɪs.ləʊ ˈkeɪ.ʃən/ posunutí

dislodge /dɪˈslɒdʒ/ přemístit, pohybovat se, vypudit, vyplavit, vyjmout, vytlačit

disorder /dɪˈsɔː.dəʳ/ porucha (zdraví)

disorganization /dɪˌsɔː.gə.naɪˈzeɪ.ʃᵊn/ rozpad, rozklad, nepořádek

disorientated /dɪˈsɔː.ri.ən.tɪd/ dezorientovaný

dispense /dɪˈspent s/ rozdělit, připravovat léky

displaced /dɪˈspleɪst/ **fracture** /ˈfræk.t ʃəʳ/ dislokovaná zlomenina

displaced /dɪˈspleɪst/ odstraněný, posunutý

displacement /dɪˈspleɪs.mənt/ posunutí, chybné postavení zubu, vytlačení

disposable /dɪˈspəʊ.zə.bḷ/ k dispozici, sloužící, na jedno použití

dispose /dɪˈspəʊz/ **of** /əv/ naložit s, zbavit se, uspořádat, použít, likvidovat, vyhodit

disrupt /dɪsˈrʌpt/ přerušit

disruption /dɪsˈrʌp.ʃən/ přerušení, porucha, protržení

dissatisfaction /dɪsˌsæt.ɪsˈfæk.ʃᵊn/ nespokojenost

dissect /daɪˈsekt/ rozřezat, pitvat

dissection /daɪˈsek.ʃᵊn/ oddělování tkání

dissipate /ˈdɪs.ɪ.peɪt/ rozptýlit se

dissolve /dɪˈzɒlv/ rozpustit, zmizet, odstranit

distal /dɪˈstəl/ distální, vzdálený, zadní (zuby)

distance /'dɪs.tənts/ vzdálenost

distant /'dɪs.tənt/ vzdálený

distillation /ˌdɪs.tɪ'leɪ.ʃən/ destilace, překapávání

distinguish /dɪ'stɪŋ.gwɪʃ/ rozlišovat

distortion /dɪ'stɔː.ʃ°n/ zkřivení, zkroucení

distraction /dɪ'stræk.ʃən/ rozptýlení, rozrušení, napravení zlomeniny tahem

distress /dɪ'stres/ tíseň, stav ohrožení

disturb /dɪ'stɜːb/ rušit, porušit, působit poruchy, vyrušovat

disturbance /dɪ'stɜː.bənts/ nesprávnost funkce, porušení, rozrušení

diving /'daɪ.vɪŋ/ potápění

division /dɪ'vɪʒ.°n/ dělení

dizziness /'dɪz.ɪ.nəs/ závrať, mrákotný stav

docket /'dɒk.ɪt/ stvrzenka, nálepka

domestic /də'mes.tɪk/ domácí, používaný v domácnosti

doppler /'dɒp.ləʳ/ dopler

dormant /'dɔː.mənt/ dormantní, spící, skrytý, latentní (možnosti)

dose /dəʊs/ dávka (zpravidla léku), dávkovat

double /'dʌb.l̩/ dvojitý, dvojnásobný

Down's syndrome /'daʊnz.sɪn.drəʊm/ Downova choroba

drainage /'dreɪ.nɪdʒ/ odčerpání

dressing /'dres.ɪŋ/ obvaz, desinfekční vložka, úprava

dried /draɪd/ vysušený, zaschlý

drift /drɪft/ rozšiřovat, vybočit

drill /drɪl/ vrták, vrtačka, vrtat, vyvrtat

drink /drɪŋk/ pít

droop /druːp/ sklesnout

drop /drɒp/ kapka

drop /drɒp/ klesnout

drowning /'draʊn.ɪŋ/ tonutí

drowsiness /'draʊ.zɪ.nəs/ ospalost, mátožnost

drug /drʌg/ lék

dry /draɪ/ socket /'sɒk.ɪt/ suché zubní lůžko

dry /draɪ/ out /aʊt/ vyschnout, vysušit se, vysychat

dry /draɪ/ suchý, sušit

dryness /draɪ.nəs/ suchost

dual /'djuː.əl/ dvojitý, obousměrný

duct /dʌkt/ kanálek, trubice

ductility /dʌk'tɪl.ɪ.ti/ kujnost, tažnost, poddajnost

due /djuː/ to /tʊ/ kvůli, následkem, v důsledku, díky

dull /dʌl/ tupý

dullness /'dʌl.nəs/ tupost (přen.)

duodenal /ˌdjuː.əʊ'diː.nəl/ duodenální, dvanáctníkový

duration /djʊə'reɪ.ʃən/ trvání

duty /'djuː.ti/ povinnost

dye /daɪ/ barvivo

dying /'daɪ.ɪŋ/ hynoucí

dysaesthesia /dɪs.æs.'θiː.sɪ.ə/ dysestézie, porucha citlivosti

dysmenorrhoea /ˌdɪs.me.nə'riː.ə/ dysmenorea, bolestivá menstruace

dysphagia /dɪ'sfeɪ.dʒiə/ dysfagie, porucha polykání

dysplasia /dis'pleɪ.zɪə/ dysplazie, porucha vývoje nebo růstu

dyspnoea /dɪs.pniː.ə/ dyspnoe, dušnost

dystrophy /dɪs.trə.fi/ dystrofie

dysuria /dɪs.'juː.ə.ri.ə/ dysurie, obtíž při močení

E

early /'ɜː.li/ časný, počáteční

ease /iːz/ off /ɒf/ odstranit, uvolnit

eat /iːt/ jíst

ECG /ˌiː.siː'dʒiː/ electrocardiogram /ɪˌlek.trə'kɑː.di.ə.græm/ elektrokardiogram (EKG)

edentate /ə'den.teɪt/ bezzubý

edentulous /əˈden.tju.ləs/ bez zubů, bezzubý

edentulousness /əˈden.tju.ləs.nəs/ bezzubost

edge /edʒ/ okraj, hrana, hrot

education /ˌed.juˈkeɪ.ʃᵊn/ instruktáž, školení, vzdělání

effect /ɪˈfekt/ účinek, výsledek

effective /ɪˈfek.tɪv/ efektivní (skutečný), účinný (vysoce)

effectively /ɪˈfek.tɪv.li/ efektivně, účinně

effectiveness /ɪˈfek.tɪv.nəs/ účinnost, působení

efficiently /ɪˈfɪʃ.ᵊnt.li/ efektivně, účinně

either /ˈaɪ.ðəʳ/ buď

either /ˈaɪ.ðəʳ/ or /ɔːʳ/ buď anebo, buď jeden nebo druhý

ejector /ɪˈdʒek.təʳ/ ejektor, sací pumpa

elastic /ɪˈlæs.tɪk/ elastický, pružný, pružná tkanina, guma

elastomer /ɪˈlæs.tə.məʳ/ elastomer, pružný kaučuk, gumovitý polymer

elastomeric /ɪˈlæs.təˈmer.ɪk/ elastomerní

elderly /ˈel.dəl.i/ stárnoucí, postarší, vyššího věku

electrical /ɪˈlek.trɪ.kᵊl/ current /ˈkʌr.ᵊnt/ elektrický proud

electrical /ɪˈlek.trɪ.kᵊl/ failure/ˈfeɪ.ljəʳ/ porucha elektřiny

electricity /ɪˌlekˈtrɪs.ɪ.ti/ supply /səˈplaɪ/ zásobování elektřinou

electrocution /ɪˌlek.trəˈkjuː.ʃən/ úraz, smrt způsobená elektřinou

electronic /ɪˌlekˈtrɒn.ɪk/ elektronický

electrotherapy /ɪˌlek.trəʊˈθer.ə.pi/ elektroléčba

elevate /ˈel.ɪ.veɪt/ zvednout

elevation /ˌel.ɪˈveɪ.ʃᵊn/ vyvýšenina, pahrbek

elevator /ˈel.ɪ.veɪ.təʳ/ zdvihák, elevátor, zvedač, páka, zdviž

elicit /ɪˈlɪs.ɪt/ vyžadovat, vyvolat (reakci), získat, dosáhnout

elimination /ɪˌlɪm.ɪˈneɪ.ʃᵊn/ vyloučení, vyřazení

embarrassment /ɪmˈbær.ə.smənt/ rozpaky, nedostatek (vada), potíže

emerge /ɪˈmɜːdʒ/ objevit se (náhle), vyjít najevo

emergency /ɪˈmɜː.dʒənʧ.si/ kit /kɪt/ souprava první pomoci

emergency /ɪˈmɜː.dʒənt.si/ naléhavá nutnost, pohotovost

emission /ɪˈmɪʃ.ᵊn/ vysílání, vyzařování

emit /ɪˈmɪt/ vydávat, vysílat

emotional /ɪˈməʊ.ʃᵊn.ᵊl/ vzrušivý, citový, dojemný

emphasize /ˈemp.fə.saɪz/ zdůraznit

emphysema /ˌemp.fəˈsiː.mə/ emfyzém, rozšíření tkání plynem nebo vzduchem

employed /ɪmˈplɔɪd/ použitý

emulsion /ɪˈmʌl.ʃᵊn/ emulze, emulzní

enable /ɪˈneɪ.bl̩/ umožnit, dát možnost, učinit schopným, umožňovat, uzpůsobit

enamel /ɪˈnæm.ᵊl/ sklovina (zubní)

encircle /ɪnˈsɜː.kl̩/ obemknout, obklopit, obejít kolem

enclose /ɪnˈkləʊz/ uzavřít

encourage /ɪnˈkʌr.ɪdʒ/ povzbudit, povzbuzovat, dodat odvahu, doporučovat

encouragement /ɪnˈkʌr.ɪdʒ.mənt/ povzbuzení, dodání odvahy

ending /ˈen.dɪŋ/ zakončení

endocarditis /ˌen.də̩ˈkɑː.dai.tis/ endokarditida, zánět srdeční nitroblány

endocrine /ˈen.də.krɑ ɪn/ endokrinní, s vnitřním vyměšováním

endodontics /ˌen.dəˈdɒn.tɪks/ endodoncie, prevence a léčení zubní dřeně, nauka o onemocnění zubní dřeně a kořenového kanálku

energy /ˈen.ə.dʒi/ energie, schopnost

engage /ɪnˈgeɪdʒ/ obsadit, zaměstnávat, zapadat, zajistit

engine /ˈen.dʒɪn/ stroj

enhance /ɪnˈhɑːnt s/ zlepšit kvalitu, zvětšit

enlarge /ɪnˈlɑːdʒ/ zvětšit, rozšířit se, vzmáhat se

enough /ɪˈnʌf/ dostatečně

ensuing /ɪnˈsjuː.ɪŋ/ následující, nastávající, vyplývající

ensure /ɪnˈʃɔːʳ/ zajistit, zabezpečit, postarat se

entirety /ɪnˈtaɪə.rɪ.ti/ celistvost

entrance /ˈen.trənt s/ přístup

entry /ˈen.tri/ vstup, záznam, údaj

enucleate /ɪˈnjuː.kli.əɪt/ enukleovat, odstranit celý orgán

environment /ɪnˈvaɪə.rən.mənt/ prostředí

environmental /ɪnˌvaɪə.rənˈmen.tʲl/ vnější, týkající se okolí, životního prostředí

environs /ɪnˈvaɪə.rənz/ prostředí

epilepsy /ˈep.ɪ.lep.si/ epilepsie

epinephrine /ˌep.ɪ.ˈnef.riːn/ epinefrin, adrenalin

episode /ˈep.ɪ.səʊd/ příhoda, záchvat, vedlejší děj

epistaxis /ˌe.pɪ.ˈstæk.sɪs/ epistaxe, krvácení z nosu

epithelial /e.pɪˈθiː.li.əl/ epitelový, výstelkový

epithelium /e.pɪˈθiː.li.əm/ epitel, výstelka

epulis /eˈpjuː.lɪs/ (pl. epulides / eˈpjuː.lɪ.diːz/)epulis, nádorek dásně v okolí zubního krčku

equipment /ɪˈkwɪp.mənt/ vybavení, zařízení

equipped /ɪˈkwɪpt/ vybavený

erosion /ɪˈrəʊ.ʒən/ odírání, mechanické opotřebení

erratic /ɪˈræt.ɪk/ nestálý, neurčitý, bludný

erupt /ɪˈrʌpt/ prořezávat se (zuby)

eruption /ɪˈrʌp.ʃən/ prořezání

erythromycin /əˌrɪθ.rəˈmaɪ.sɪn/ erytromycin

escape /ɪˈskeɪp/ uniknutí, otvor, výlevka

escort /ɪˈskɔːt/ doprovodit, doprovázet, odvést

essential /ɪˈsen.t ʃəl/ základní, podstatná věc, důležitý, hlavní, podstatný, nepostradatelný, nezbytný, výtažkový, základní

essentially /ɪˈsen.t ʃˑl.i/ v podstatě, nezbytně, zásadně

establish /ɪˈstæb.lɪʃ/ ustanovit, zavést, uvést do chodu, zřídit, zabezpečit

etch /etʃ/ leptat, vyrýt

etchant /etʃ.ˑnt/ leptadlo

etching /ˈetʃ.ɪŋ/ leptání

eugenol /juːˈdʒen.ɒl/ eugenol

even /ˈiː.vˑn/ stejný

event /ɪˈvent/ jev, eventualita, událost, případ, výsledek

eventually /ɪˈven.tju.əl.i/ nakonec

evidence /ˈev.ɪ.dˑnt s/ důkaz (očividný), dokázat, jistota

evident /ˈev.ɪ.dˑnt/ zjevný

exacerbate /ɪgˈzæs.ə.beɪt/ zhoršit, přitížit

exacting /ɪgˈzæk.tɪŋ/ náročný

exactly /ɪgˈzækt.li/ přesně, úplně, doslovně

exaggerate /ɪgˈzædʒ.ə.reɪt/ přehánět, zveličovat

examination /ɪgˌzæm.ɪˈneɪ.ʃ°n/ prohlídka, vyšetření

examine /ɪgˈzæm.ɪn/ vyšetřovat, vyšetřit, prohlídka

excavator /ˈek.skə.veɪ.təʳ/ exkavátor

exceed /ɪkˈsiːd/ převládat, přesahovat (míru)

excellent /ˈek.səl.ənt/ vynikající

except /ɪkˈsept/ kromě, vyjmout

exception /ɪkˈsep.ʃ°n/ výjimka

excess /ekˈses/ nadbytek, nadměrný

excessive /ekˈses.ɪv/ nadměrný, nepřiměřený

excessively /ekˈses.ɪv.li/ nadměrně, nepřiměřeně

exchange /ɪksˈtʃeɪndʒ/ výměna, vyměnit si (vzájemně)

excise /ekˈsaɪz/ odstranit, vyříznout

excision /ekˈsɪʒ.°n/ excize, vyříznutí

exclude /ɪkˈskluːd/ vyloučit

exclusive /ɪkˈskluː.sɪv/ vylučující

excrete /ɪkˈskriːt/ vylučovat

excursion /ɪkˈskɜː.ʃ°n/ odchýlení, odbočení

excuse /ɪkˈskjuːs/ omluva, výmluva

exercise /ˈek.sə.saɪz/ cvičení, používání

exert /ɪgˈzɜːt/ použít., snažit se, vynaložit úsilí, vyvolávat

exertion /ɪgˈzɜː.ʃ°n/ úsilí, vypětí

exhausted /ɪgˈzɔː.stɪd/ vyčerpaný

exhaustive /ɪgˈzɔː.stɪv/ kompletní, důkladný

exhibit /ɪgˈzɪb.ɪt/ ukázka, projevit

expand /ɪkˈspænd/ rozpínat se, šířit se, rozšířit, rozšířit se, zvětšit

expansion /ɪkˈspæn.tʃ°n/ expanze, rozšíření

expect /ɪkˈspekt/ očekávat

expectant /ɪkˈspek.t°nt/ **mother** / ˈmʌð.ər/ nastávající matka

expected /ɪkˈspek.tɪd/ očekávaný

expense /ɪkˈspents/ výdaje, náklady

experience /ɪkˈspɪə.ri.°nts/ prožívat, ucítit

experience /ɪkˈspɪə.ri.°nts/ zkušenost, prožitek, zkušenost, praxe

explanation /ˌek.spləˈneɪ.ʃ°n/ vysvětlení

expose /ɪkˈspəʊz/ odkrýt, uvolnit

exposed /ɪkˈspəʊzd/ vystavený

exposure /ɪkˈspəʊ.ʒəʳ/ obnažení, vystavení

expression /ɪkˈspreʃ.ən/ výraz tváře, vyjádření, vytlačení

expressive /ɪkˈspres.ɪv/ výrazový

extend /ɪkˈstend/ rozprostírat se

extended /ɪkˈsten.dɪd/ v extenzi, natažený, rozšířený

extension /ɪkˈsten.tʃən/ natažení, rozšíření

extensive /ɪkˈsten.tsɪv/ rozsáhlý

extent /ɪkˈstent/ rozsah, objem

external /ɪkˈstɜː.nəl/ vnější

externally /ɪkˈstɜː.nə.li/ zevně

extirpation /ˌek.stɜːˈpeɪ.ʃ°n/ extirpace, totální vynětí nervu

extra-articular /ˈek.strə.ˈaː.tɪ.kjʊ.ləʳ/ mimo-kloubní

extract /ɪkˈstrækt/ extrahovat, vytáhnout, vytrhnout

extraction /ɪkˈstræk.ʃən/ extrakce, vytržení

extraoral /ˌek.strəˈɔː.rəl/ mimo ústa

extreme /ɪkˈstriːm/ mimořádný

extremely /ɪkˈstriːm.li/ extrémně

extremity /ɪkˈstrem.ɪ.ti/ končetina

extrusion /ɪkˈstruː.ʒ°n/ extruze, vysunutí, vystrčení, vypuzení

exudate /eks.juːdeɪt/ exsudát, zánětlivá tekutina, výpotek

eye /aɪ/ oko
eyelid /'aɪ.lɪd/ oční víčko
eyesight /'aɪ.saɪt/ zrak

F

face /feɪs/ obličej, čelit (čemu)
facial /'feɪ.ʃᵊl/ faciální, obličejový,
lícní
facial /'feɪ.ʃᵊl/ flushing /flʌʃ.ɪŋ/ nával
horka v obličeji
facial /'feɪ.ʃᵊl/ obličejový
facilitate /fə'sɪl.ɪ.teɪt/ usnadnit
facility /fə'sɪl.ɪ.ti/ zařízení, vybavení
facing /'feɪ.sɪŋ/ fazeta
fail /feɪl/ selhat, chybit, zanedbat
failure /'feɪ.ljəʳ/ chyba, selhání,
porucha, nedostatek
faint /feɪnt/ omdlít, mdloba
fainting /feɪnt.ɪŋ/ mdloba
fall /fɔːl/ asleep /ə'sliːp/ usnout
fall /fɔːl/ back /bæk/ ustoupit,
stáhnout se (zpět)
fall /fɔːl/ into /'ɪn.tuː/ spadat do
fall /fɔːl/ pád, padat, padnout, spadnout
far /fɑːʳ/ daleko
fascial /fæ.ʃɪ.əl/ povázkový, týkající se
povázky
fast /fɑːst/ hladovět
fast /fɑːst/ rychlý
fasting /fɑːst.ɪŋ/ hladovění
fat /fæt/ tuk, tloušťka
fatal /'feɪ.tᵊl/ fatální, smrtelný
fatality /fə'tæl.ə.ti/ smrtelný úraz
fatigue /fə'tiːg/ slabost, schvácenost,
únava (též materiálu), vyčerpání
fault /fɒlt/ vada, chyba
favour /'feɪ.vəʳ/ prospěch, pozornost
fear /fɪəʳ/ obava, strach
fearful /'fɪə.fᵊl/ bojácný
feature /'fiː.tʃəʳ/ rys, znak,
charakteristická vlastnost,
charakteristický rys

feel /fiːl/ cítit, hmatat, pocítit, procítit
feeling /'fiː.lɪŋ/ pocit, hmat, mínění,
nálada
female /'fiː.meɪl/ ženský, žena, pro
ženy
femur /'fiː.məʳ/ femur, stehenní kost
fermentation /ˌfɜː.men'teɪ.ʃᵊn/
fermentace, kvašení
ferromagnetic /ˌfer.ə.mæg'net.ɪk/
feromagnetický
fever /'fiː.vəʳ/ horečka
few /fjuː/ málo
fibre /'faɪ.bəʳ/ vlákno
fibre optic /'faɪ.bəʳ.'ɒp.tɪk/ optické
vlákno
fibrillation /ˌfaɪ.brɪ'leɪ.ʃᵊn/ fibrilace
fibrin /'fɪ.brɪn/ fibrin (biol.)
fiddle /'fɪd.l̩/ pohrávat si nervózně
fight /faɪt/ bojovat, rvačka
fighting /'faɪ.tɪŋ/ rvačka
filament /'fɪl.ə.mənt/ vlákno
file /faɪl/ pilníček, pilník
fill /fɪl/ vyplnit
filler /'fɪl.əʳ/ náplň, vložka, plnič,
plnící nástroj, plnivo
filling /'fɪl.ɪŋ/ material /mə'tɪə.ri.əl/
materiál na výplně
filling /'fɪl.ɪŋ/ výplň, plnění
filter /'fɪl.təʳ/ infiltrovat
final /'faɪ.nᵊl/ konečný, finální
fine /faɪn/ jemný, ryzí, ušlechtilý
finger /'fɪŋ.gəʳ/ prst na ruce, ohmatat
finish /'fɪn.ɪʃ/ skončit, dokončit,
dokončení, závěr
fire /faɪəʳ/ oheň
firm /fɜːm/ pevný
firmly /'fɜːm.li/ pevně
first-aid /'fɜːst.eɪd/ kit /kɪt/
lékárnička první pomoci
fishing /'fɪʃ.ɪŋ/ line /laɪn/ vlasec
fissure /'fɪʃ.əʳ/ sealant /'siː.lənt/
pečetidlo na praskliny

357

fissure /'fɪʃ.əʳ/ fisura, prasklina, rýha

fistula /'fɪs.tjʊ.lə/ fistula, píštěl

fit /fɪt/ and well /wel/ v dobrém zdravotním stavu

fit /fɪt/ hodit se, vhodný, padnout (oděv), upevnit, upravit

fit /fɪt/ v kondici

fit /fɪt/ záchvat, nával

fitting /'fɪt.ɪŋ/ montování, úprava, instalace

fitting /'fɪt.ɪŋ/ přiléhající, příhodný

fixation /fɪk'seɪ.ʃᵊn/ fixace, upevnění

fixed /fɪkst/ bridge /brɪdʒ/ pevný můstek

fixed /fɪkst/ fixovaný, pevný, nepohyblivý, stálý, upevněný

fizzy /'fɪz.i/ pop /pɒp/ šumivý nápoj (šampaňské apod.)

flail /fleɪl/ ochromený, klinkající se

flame /fleɪm/ plamen

flange /flændʒ/ výčnělek, křídlo

flap /flæp/ chlopeň, lalok, kousek volně visící kůže

flat /flæt/ plochý, rovný

flatulence /'flæt.jʊ.lənts/ flatulence, plynatost

flavour /'fleɪ.vəʳ/ příchuť

fleck /flek/ skvrnka, tečka

flexible /'flek.sɪ.bl̩/ flexibilní, pružný

flexion /flek.ʃᵊn/ ohýbání

floor /flɔːʳ/ dno

floss /flɒs/ hedvábí, hedvábná voskovaná nit

flow /fləʊ/ proud (vzduchu), tok, prýštit (krev)

flow /fləʊ/ tok, výtok

fluid /'fluː.ɪd/ tekutina

fluoridation /ˌflʊə.rɪ'deɪ.ʃən/ fluoridace

fluoride /'flʊə.raɪd/ fluorid, s fluoridem

fluorosis /ˌflʊə.'rəʊ.sɪs/ fluoróza

flush /flʌʃ/ přítok, proud (vody), vypláchnout

flush /flʌʃ/ zrudnout

foil /fɔɪl/ folie

folate /fəʊ.leɪt/ folát, sůl kyseliny listové

follicular /fə'lɪk.jʊ.ləʳ/ folikulární (anat.), váčkový

follow /'fɒl.əʊ/ instruction / ɪn'strʌk.ʃᵊn/ plnit pokyn

follow /'fɒl.əʊ/ následovat

following /'fɒl.əʊ.ɪŋ/ následující

food /fuːd/ jídlo, potrava, potravina

for /fɔːʳ/ the sake /seɪk/ kvůli, v zájmu

foramen /fə'reɪ.mən/ (pl. foramina) otvor, průchod

force /fɔːs/ síla, účinnost, nutit, vyvíjet tlak

forceful /'fɔːs.fᵊl/ mocný, prudký

forceps /'fɔː.seps/ lékařské kleště, pinzeta, nůžky, svorka

forcibly /'fɔː.sɪ.bli/ násilně

forehead /'fɒr.ɪd/, /'fɔː.hed/ čelo

foreign /'fɒr.ən/ body /'bɒd.i/ cizí tělísko

form /fɔːm/ forma, formulář, podoba, tvar, utvářet

formation /fɔː'meɪ.ʃən/ formace, tvoření, utváření, sestava, nástup, vznik

former /'fɔː.məʳ/ the latter /'læt.əʳ/ první - druhý

former /'fɔː.məʳ/ tvarovač

forth /fɔːθ/ dopředu, dále

fortunately /'fɔː.tʃᵊn.ət.li/ naštěstí

forward /'fɔː.wəd/ přední, posunout dopředu

forwards /'fɔː.wədz/ kupředu (směřující), směrem dopředu

fossa /fɒs.ə/ jamka

fracture /'fræk.tʃᵊr/ fraktura, zlomenina

fragile /ˈfrædʒ.aɪl/ křehký

fragment /ˈfræg.mənt/ část, úlomek

frame /freɪm/ rámeček

free /friː/ volný, zbavený

freeway /ˈfriː.weɪ/ komunikace, volný prostor

freezing /ˈfriː.zɪŋ/ zmrazování

frenectomy /frɪˈnɒ.tə.mi/ frenotomie, protětí uzdičky

frenum /friː.nəm/ frenum, uzdička

frequency /ˈfriː.kwənt.si/ časté opakování, četnost (výskytu jevu v čase)

frequent /ˈfriː.kwənt/ častý

frequently /ˈfriː.kwənt.li/ často, mnohdy, opakovaně

fresh /freʃ/ čerstvý

friction /ˈfrɪk.ʃən/ tření

frontal /ˈfrʌn.təl/ frontální, přední, čelní

full /fʊl/ plný, úplný

fully /ˈfʊl.i/ zcela, v hojné míře

function /ˈfʌŋk.ʃən/ činnost, fungování, funkce, fungovat

functional /ˈfʌŋk.ʃən.əl/ funkční, fungující

fungal /ˈfʌŋ.gəl/ houbový, plísňový

fungus /ˈfʌŋ.gəs/ (pl. fungi) houba, plíseň

furcation /fɜːˈkeɪ.ʃən/ furkace, rozvětvení

further /ˈfɜː.ðəʳ/ dále, další, vzdálenější, kromě toho

fuse /fjuːz/ roztavit, slít, sloučit se

G

gain /geɪn/ získat

gallium /ˈgæl.ɪ.əm/ gallium, síran galitý

gap /gæp/ mezera, trhlina

gas /gæs/ plyn

gaseous /ˈgeɪ.si.əs/ plynný

gasp /gɑːsp/ těžce dýchat, popadat dech

gastric /ˈgæs.trɪk/ gastrický, žaludeční

gastrointestinal / ˌgæs.trəʊˌɪn.tesˈtaɪ.nəl/ gastrointestinální, týkající se žaludku a střeva

gauge /geɪdʒ/ standardní míra, zkušební přístroj

gauze /gɔːz/ gáza, mul

gelatine /ˈdʒel.ə.tiːn/ želatina

gender /ˈdʒen.dəʳ/ pohlaví

general /ˈdʒen.ər.əl/ anaesthesia / ˌæn.əsˈθiː.zi.ə/ celková anestézie, narkóza

general /ˈdʒen.ər.əl/ hlavní, všeobecný, celkový

generalized /ˈdʒen.ər.ə.laɪzd/ všeobecný, obecný, zobecněný, celkový

generally /ˈdʒen.ə r.əl.i/ obecně, zpravidla

generator /ˈdʒen.ə.reɪ.təʳ/ zdroj, původce

generic /dʒəˈner.ɪk/ všeobecný, druhový (označující druh)

genitourinary /ˌdʒen.ɪ.təʊˈjʊə.rɪn.ri/ genitourinární, močopohlavní

gently /ˈdʒent.li/ jemně, mírně

germ-free /dʒɜːm.friː/ zárodků prostý

gesture /ˈdʒes.tʃəʳ/ gesto, posuněk, ukázat

get /get/ used /juːst/ to /tʊ/ zvyknout si na

gingiva /ˌdʒɪn.dʒaɪ.və/ (pl. gingivae) dáseň

gingival /ˌdʒɪn.dʒɪ.val/ gingivální, dásňový

gingivectomy /ˌdʒɪn.dʒɪˈvekt.ə.mi/ gingivektomie, vynětí dásně nebo její části

gingivitis /ˌdʒɪn.dʒɪˈvaɪ.tɪs/
  gingividita, zánět sliznice dásní

give /ɡɪv/ advice /ədˈvaɪs/ poradit

give /ɡɪv/ dát, podat

gland /ɡlænd/ žláza

glass /ɡlɑːs/ ionomer /ˈaɪ.əˌnɒ.məʳ/
  sklo-ionomer

glass /ɡlɑːs/ sklo, sklenice

glasses /ɡlɑːs.ɪz/ brýle

glenoid /ɡlɪː.nɒɪd/ fossa /fɒs.ə/ jamka
  lopatky pro skloubení v ramenním
  kloubu

glenoid /ɡlɪː.nɒɪd/ glenoidální,
  vyhloubený

glomerulonephritis /ɡlɒˈme.
  ru.ləˌnəfˈraɪ.tɪs/ glomeluronefritida,
  zánět ledvin, spojený se zánětem
  glomerulů

glove /ɡlʌv/ rukavice

glucagon /ɡluː.kəɡ.ən/ glukagon,
  peptidový hormon, tvořený ve
  slinivce břišní

glucose /ˈɡluː.kəʊs/ glukóza, hroznový
  cukr

glyceryl /ˈɡlɪs.ə.rɪl/ trinitrate /
  traɪˈnaɪ.treɪt/ glyceriltrinitrát,
  nitroglycerin

goal /ɡəʊl/ cíl

goitre /ˈɡɔɪ.təʳ/ struma, vole

gold /ɡəʊld/ zlato, zlatý

gonorrhoea /ˌɡɒn.əˈriː.ə/ gonorea,
  kapavka

grade /ɡreɪd/ stupeň

gradual /ˈɡræd.jʊ.əl/, /ˈɡrædʒ.ʊ.əl/
  postupný, pozvolný

graft /ɡrɑːft/ štěp, transplantovat

gram /ɡræm/ negative /ˈneɡ.ə.tɪv/
  gram negativní

gram /ɡræm/ positive /ˈpɒz.ə.tɪv/
  gram pozitivní

grand mal /ˈɡrɑːnd.ˈmæl/ velký
  epileptický záchvat

grasp /ɡrɑːsp/ pevně uchopit, popadat

gravel /ˈɡræv.ᵊl/ štěrk, močové
  kamínky, písek v moči

greatly /ˈɡreɪt.li/ velmi, z velké části

greenstick /ˈɡriːn.stɪk/ fracture /
  ˈfræk.tʃəʳ/ částečná zlomenina kosti

grey /ɡreɪ/ šedivý, šedý

grind /ɡraɪnd/ skřípat

grinding /ˈɡraɪn.dɪŋ/ skřípání

grip /ɡrɪp/ pevně uchopit, uchytit,
  upínadlo

groove /ɡruːv/ rýha, žlábek

grossly /ˈɡrəʊ.sli/ hrubě

growing /ˈɡrəʊ.ɪŋ/ old /əʊld/ stárnutí

growth /ɡrəʊθ/ růst

guarantee /ˌɡær.ᵊnˈtiː/ zaručit

guard /ɡɑːd/ chránit, bránit, ochrana

guide /ɡaɪd/ šablona, příručka

gum /ɡʌm/ dáseň, guma

gumshield /ɡʌm.ʃiːld/ ochrana zubů
  (boxera)

gush /ɡʌʃ/ téci proudem, řinout se

gutta-percha /ˌɡʌt.əˈpɜː.tʃə/ gutaperča

gynaecology /ˌɡaɪ.nəˈkɒl.ə.dʒi/
  gynekologie, ženské lékařství

H

habit /ˈhæb.ɪt/ zvyk, návyk

habitual /həˈbɪtʃ.u.əl/ habituální,
  navyklý, častý, notorický

haematological /ˌhiː.mə.təˈlɒdʒ.ɪ.kəl/
  zabývající se studiem krve a tkání

haemoglobin /ˌhiː.məˈɡləʊ.bɪn/
  hemoglobin

haemophilia /ˌhiː.məˈfɪl.i.ə/ hemofilie,
  dědičná krvácivost

haemophiliac /ˌhiː.məˈfɪl.i.æk/
  hemofilik, jedinec trpící hemofilií

haemoptysis /hiːˈmɒ.ptɪ.sɪs/
  hemoptýza, vykašlávání krve

haemorrhage /ˈhem.ᵊr.ɪdʒ/ krvácení,
  vnitřní krvácení

haemorrhoids /ˈhem.ᵊr.ɔɪdz/
hemeroidy

haemostasis /ˌhiːməˈste.sɪs/
hemostáza, zástava krvácení

halfway /ˌhɑːfˈweɪ/ půl cesty

halitosis /ˌhæl.ɪˈtəʊ.sɪs/ halitóza,
páchnoucí dech

hallucination /həˌluː.sɪˈneɪ.ʃᵊn/
halucinace, přelud

hand /hænd/ předat, podat

handheld /ˌhændˈheld/ ruční (držený v
ruce), přenosný

handle /ˈhæn.dl̩/ ovládat, zacházet

handpiece /hænd.piːs/ držadlo,
rukojeť, násadec, násadec vrtačky

happen /ˈhæp.ᵊn/ stát se

hard /hɑːd/ palate /ˈpæl.ət/ tvrdé
patro

hard /hɑːd/ tvrdý, pevný, nesnadný

hardness /hɑːd.nəs/ odolnost, tvrdost

harm /hɑːm/ poškození, zranění

hazard /ˈhæz.əd/ riziko

head /hed/ hlava, hlavní, směřovat

headache /ˈhed.eɪk/ bolest hlavy

headgear /ˈhed.gɪəʳ/ extraorálné
kotvení, zevní tah

heading /ˈhed.ɪŋ/ záhlaví, hledisko,
přední část

heal /hiːl/ hojit, léčit, léčit se, zahojit
se

healing /ˈhiː.lɪŋ/ hojení, léčivý

health /helθ/ care /keəʳ/ system /ˈsɪs.
təm/ systém zdravotní péče

health /helθ/ zdraví

healthy /ˈhel.θi/ zdravý

hearing /ˈhɪə.rɪŋ/ sluch, schopnost
slyšet

heart /hɑːt/ attack /əˈtæk/ srdeční
záchvat

heart /hɑːt/ massage /ˈmæs.ɑːdʒ/
masáž srdce

heart /hɑːt/ srdce, srdeční

heart /hɑːt/ rate /reɪt/ srdeční frekvence

heartburn /ˈhɑːt.bɜːn/ pálení žáhy

heat /hiːt/ teplo, zahřát, rozžhavit,
způsobený teplem

heater /ˈhiː.təʳ/ zahřívač (přístroj)

heavily /ˈhev.ɪ.li/ silně, velmi

heavy /ˈhev.i/ obtížný

height /haɪt/ výška, úroveň

Heimlich manoeuvre /ˈhaɪm.lɪk.
məˈnuː.vəʳ/ Heimlichův manévr

held /held/ držený

helpful /ˈhelp.fᵊl/ užitečný

hemisection /ˈhem.ɪ.ˈsek.ʃᵊn/
hemisekce, řez v polovině orgánu

hence /henʦ/ odtud, z toho důvodu, a
proto

hepatic /hepˈæt.ɪk/ jaterní

hepatitis /ˌhep.əˈtaɪ.tɪs/ hepatitida,
zánět jater

herald /ˈher.ᵊld/ ohlašovat, hlasatel

hereditary /həˈred.ɪ.tri/ dědičný,
vrozený

hernia /ˈhɜː.ni.ə/ hernie (kýla)

herpes /ˈhɜː.piːz/ herpes, opar

herpetic /hɜːˈpe.tik/ týkající se oparu

hesitancy /ˈhez.ɪ.tᵊnʦ.si/ váhavost,
rozkolísanost

heterogeneous /ˌhet.ər.əˈdʒiː.ni.əs/
heterogenní, různorodý

hiatus /haɪˈeɪ.təs/ mezera, otvor

hide /haɪd/ skrýt

high /haɪ/ pressure /ˈpreʃ.əʳ/ vysoký
tlak, vysokotlaký

high /haɪ/ vysoký

high-frequency /haɪ.ˈfriː.kwənʦ.si/
vysokofrekvenční

high-volume /haɪ.ˈvɒl.juːm/
vysoko-objemový

highlight /ˈhaɪ.laɪt/ zdůraznit

high-speed /ˌhaɪˈspiːd/ handpiece
/hænd.piːs/ vysokoobrátkový
násadec

361

high-speed /ˌhaɪˈspiːd/
vysokorychlostní

hinder /ˈhɪn.dəʳ/ bránit, být překážkou,
zadní

histological /ˌhɪ.stəˈlɒdʒ.ɪ.kᵊl/
histologický, tkáňový

history /ˈhɪs.tᵊr.i/ anamnéza, vývoj
změn

hoe /həʊ/ motyčka

hold /həʊld/ držet

holder /ˈhəʊl.dəʳ/ držadlo

holding /ˈhəʊl.dɪŋ/ držení

hole /həʊl/ dírka

hollow /ˈhɒl.əʊ/ dutý, dutina,
vykotlaný (zub)

home /həʊm/ care /keəʳ/ domácí péče

honest /ˈɒn.ɪst/ poctivý, otevřený,
řádný

hook /hʊk/ háček, ohnout, zahnout

hopeless /ˈhəʊ.pləs/ beznadějný,
bezvýhledný

horizontal /ˌhɒr.ɪˈzɒn.tᵊl/ horizontální,
vodorovný

horizontal /ˌhɒr.ɪˈzɒn.tᵊl/ plane /
pleɪn/ vodorovná plocha

household /ˈhaʊs.həʊld/ domácnost

however /ˌhaʊˈev.əʳ/ avšak

human /ˈhjuː.mən/ člověk, lidský

hurt /hɜːt/ bolet, poranit

hydrochloric acid /ˌhaɪd.rə.klɒr.
ɪkˈæs.ɪd/ kyselina chlorovodíková

hydrocolloid /haɪ.drəʊˈkɒl.ɒid/
hydrokoloid

hydrocortisone /haɪ.drəʊˈkɔː.
tɪ.zəʊn/ hydrocortison

hydrogen /ˈhaɪ.drɪ.dʒən/ vodík

hydrogen/ˈhaɪ.drɪ.dʒən/ peroxide /
pəˈrɒk.saɪd/ peroxid vodíku

hydrophilic /ˌhaɪ.drəˈfɪl.ɪk/ smáčivý

hygiene /ˈhaɪ.dʒiːn/ hygiena,
zdravověda

hygienic /haɪˈdʒiː.nɪk/ hygienický

hygienist /haɪˈdʒiː.nɪst/ hygienic,
hygienista

hyperactivity /haɪ.pəʳ.ækˈtɪv.ɪ.ti/
nadměrná aktivita

hyperglycaemia /ˌhaɪ.pə.glaɪˈsiːmi.ə/
hyperglykémie, zvýšené množství
glukózy v krvi

hyperplasia /ˌhaɪ.pəˈpleɪ.zɪ.ə/
hyperplazie, zbytnění

hypersensitivity /ˈhaɪ.pə.sen.
sɪˈtɪv.ɪ.ti/ hypersensitivita,
nadměrná citlivost

hypertension /ˌhaɪ.pəˈten.tʃᵊn/
hypertenze, zvýšený tlak, vysoký
krevní tlak

hyperthyroidism /
ˌhaɪ.pə.ˈθaɪə.rɔɪdɪ.zᵊm/
hypertyroidismus, zvýšená činnost
štítné žlázy

hypnosis /hɪpˈnəʊ.sɪs/ hypnóza,
zhypnotizování, hypnotický stav

hypnotherapy /ˌhɪp.nəʊ ˈθer.ə.pi/
hypnoterapie, léčení spánkem

hypnotic /hɪpˈnɒt.ɪk/ uspávající, lék
navozující spánek

hypochondria /ˌhaɪ.pəʊ ˈkɒn.dri.ə/
hypochondrie

hypoglycaemia /ˌhaɪ.pəʊ .glaɪˈsiː.
mi.ə/ hypoglykémie

hypotension /ˌhaɪ.pəʊˈten.tʃᵊn/ nízký
tlak

hypothetical /ˌhaɪ.pəˈθet.ɪ.kᵊl/
hypotetický

hypothyroidism /ˌhaɪ.pəʊ.ˈθaɪə.
rɔɪdɪ.zᵊm/ hypotyreóza, snížená
činnost štítné žlázy

hypoxia /haɪˈpɒk.sɪ.ə/ hypoxie,
nedostatečné zásobení krve kyslíkem

I

iatrogenic /aɪˌætrəˈdʒen.ɪk/
iatrogenní, lékařem vyvolaný

ibuprofen /ˌaɪ.bjuːˈprəʊ.fen/
ibuprofen

identify /aɪˈden.tɪ.faɪ/ identifikovat,
určit, ztotožňovat se

idiopathic /ˈɪdiəˈpæθɪk/ idiopatický,
samostatný

ileum /ˈɪl.i.əm/ kyčelník

ill /ɪl/ effect /ɪˈfekt/ škodlivý následek

image /ˈɪm.ɪdʒ/ zobrazení

imaging /ˈɪ'mɪdʒ.ɪŋ/ zobrazování

immediate /ɪˈmiː.di.ət/ okamžitý,
bezprostřední

immediately /ɪˈmiː.di.ət.li/ ihned

immerse /ɪˈmɜːs/ ponořit, ponořit se

immiscibility /ɪˌmɪs.əˈbɪl.ɪ.ti/
nemísivost

immobilization /ɪˌməʊ.bəl.aɪˈzeɪ.ʃən/
znehybnění

immune /ɪˈmjuːn/ imunní, odolný,
bezpečný před něčím

immunocompromised /ɪˈmjuː.
nəˈkɒm.prə.maɪ.zd/ se sníženou
imunitou

immunodeficiency /
ˌɪm.jʊ.nəʊ.dɪˈfɪʃ.ᵊnˈ.si/
imunodeficience, deficit imunity

immunosuppression /ˌɪm.jə.nəʊ.
səˈpreʃ.ᵊn/ imunosuprese, snížení
schopnosti organismu reagovat na
cizí látky

impact /ˈɪm.pækt/ resistance /
rɪˈzɪs.tᵊnˈts/ odolnost proti nárazu

impact /ˈɪm.pækt/ vliv, výsledek,
dopadat, natlačit

impacted /ɪmˈpæk.tɪd/ vpáčený

impaction /ɪmˈpæk.ʃᵊn/ stlačení,
zaklínění

impaired /ɪmˈpeəd/ zhoršený,
poškozený

impalpable /ɪmˈpæl.pə.bļ/
nepalpovatelný, nepostižitelný
(nehmatatelný)

imperative /ɪmˈper.ə.tɪv/ pravidlo,
nevyhnutelný (nutný)

implant /ɪmˈplɑːnt/ implantát

implication /ˌɪm.plɪˈkeɪ.ʃən/ důsledek

importance /ɪmˈpɔː.tᵊnˈts/ důležitost,
význam, závažnost

impossible /ɪmˈpɒs.ɪ.bļ/ nemožný

impression /ɪmˈpreʃ.ᵊn/ otisk

impression /ɪmˈpreʃ.ən/ tray /treɪ/
otiskovací lžíce

improbability /ɪmˌprɒb.əˈbɪl.ɪ.ti/
nepravděpodobnost

improve /ɪmˈpruːv/ zlepšit, zlepšit se,
zdokonalit

impulse /ˈɪm.pʌls/ podnět, náraz

in situ /ˌɪnˈsɪt.juː/ na místě, na
původním místě

in /ɪn/ addition /əˈdɪʃ.ən/ kromě
(čeho), navíc, vedle (navíc)

in /ɪn/ doubt /daʊt/ na pochybách,
nejistý

in /ɪn/ line /laɪn/ v linii, řadový

in /ɪn/ order /ˈɔː.dəʳ/ to /tʊ/ aby mohl,
za účelem

in /ɪn/ turn /tɜːn/ střídavě

in /ɪn/ general /ˈdʒen.ər.əl/ všeobecně

inability /ˌɪn.əˈbɪl.ɪ.ti/ neschopnost,
nemožnost, nezpůsobilost

inaccuracy /ɪnˈæk.jʊ.rə.si/
nepřesnost, chyba

inaccurate /ɪˈnæk.jʊ.rət/ nesprávný,
nepřesný

inadequate /ɪˈnæd.ɪ.kwət/
nepřiměřený, neschopný, chybný,
mentálně opožděný

inadvertent /ˌɪn.ədˈvɜː.tᵊnt/
nepozorný, nedbalý

inadvertently /ˌɪn.ədˈvɜː.tᵊnt.li/
nedopatřením

inappropriate /ˌɪn.əˈprəʊ.pri.ət/
nepatřičný, nevhodný, neúčelný

inattentive /ˌɪn.əˈten.tɪv/ nepozorný

incidence /ˈɪnɾ.sɪ.dənɾs/ dopad, výskyt, rozsah působení

incident /ˈɪnɾ.sɪ.dᵊnt/ nehoda, událost

incisal /ɪnˈsɪ.zᵊl/ edge /edʒ/ řezáková hrana

incisal /ɪnˈsɪ.zᵊl/ řezný

incision /ɪnˈsɪʒ.ᵊn/ incise, naříznutí, vpich, vyříznutí, chirurgické otevření

incisor /ɪnˈsaɪ.zəʳ/ řezák

included /ɪnˈkluː.dɪd/ obsažený, zahrnutý

income /ˈɪn.kʌm/ příjem

incompetent /ɪnˈkɒm.pɪ.tᵊnt/ slabý

incomprehensible /ɪn,kɒm.prɪˈhenɾ.sɪ.bl̩/ nesrozumitelný

incontinence /ɪnˈkɒn.tɪ.nənɾs/ inkontinence, neschopnost udržet moč či stolici

incorporated /ɪnˈkɔː.pᵊr.eɪ.tɪd/ vmíchaný, vpravený, začleněný

incorrect /,ɪn.kərˈºkt/ nesprávný, nevhodný

increase /ɪnˈkriːs/ zvýšit, zvětšování

index /ˈɪn.deks/ (pl. indices /ˈɪn.dɪ.siːz/) index, ukazatel, seznam

indicate /ˈɪn.dɪ.keɪt/ indikovat, označit, ukazovat, signalizovat

indication /,ɪn.dɪˈkeɪ.ʃᵊn/ indikace, údaj, označení

indicator /ˈɪn.dɪ.keɪ.təʳ/ ukazatel

indigestion /,ɪn.dɪ.dʒes.tʃᵊn/ porucha trávení, zažívací potíže

indirect /,ɪn.dɑɪˈrekt/ nepřímý, vedlejší

individual /,ɪn.dɪˈvɪd.ju.əl/ jednotlivec

induce /ɪnˈdjuːs/ navodit

induced /ɪn.djuːst/ indukovaný, přivozený

ineffective /,ɪn.ɪˈfek.tɪv/ neúčinný

inevitably /ɪˈnev.ɪ.tə.bli/ nevyhnutelně

infancy /ˈɪn.fənɾ.si/ dětství, počátek

infection /ɪnˈfek.ʃᵊn/ nákaza, nakažlivost, infekční nemoc

infectious /ɪnˈfek.ʃəs/ nakažlivý, přenosný

inferior /ɪnˈfɪə.ri.əʳ/ spodní

infiltration /,ɪn.fɪlˈtreɪ.ʃᵊn/ infiltrace, pronikání, prosakování

inflammation /,ɪn.fləˈmeɪ.ʃᵊn/ zápal, zánět

inflammatory /ɪnˈflæm.ə.tər.i/ zánětlivý

influence /ˈɪn.flu.ənɾs/ vliv, ovlivnit, ovlivňovat, působit

infusion /ɪnˈfjuː.ʒᵊn/ infuze, nalévání, nálev

ingestion /ɪnˈdʒes.tʃᵊn/ přijímání potravy

inhalation /,ɪn.ɦ əˈleɪ.ʃᵊn/ inhalace, vdechování

inhale /ɪnˈheɪl/ vdechnout, inhalovat (vdechovat)

inhaler /ɪnˈheɪ.ləʳ/ inhalátor

inherent /ɪnˈher.ᵊnt/ inherentní, vnitřní

inhibit /ɪnˈhɪb.ɪt/ inhibovat, bránit (překážet), zakázat, zpomalovat

initial /ɪˈnɪʃ.ᵊl/ původní, výchozí

initially /ɪˈnɪʃ.ᵊl.i/ zpočátku, nejprve

initiate /ɪˈnɪʃ.i.eɪt/ iniciovat, spustit, zahájit, uvést

injection /ɪnˈdʒek.ʃᵊn/ injekce

injury /ˈɪn.dʒᵊr.i/ poranění, zranění, poškození

inlay /ˈɪn.leɪ/ inlej, litá výplň

inner /ˈɪn.əʳ/ vnitřní

input /ˈɪn.pʊt/ přísun, vstup

inquiry /ɪnˈkwaɪə.ri/ dotaz, vyšetřování

insert /ɪnˈsɜːt/ vložit, vsunout, vložka, příloha

insertion /ɪnˈsɜː.ʃᵊn/ vložení, zasazení, aplikace (vložka)

inside /ɪnˈsaɪd/ uvnitř

insomnia /ɪnˈsɒm.ni.ə/ insomnie, nespavost

instead /ɪnˈsted/ of /əv/ namísto

instruction /ɪnˈstrʌk.ʃᵊn/ pokyn, návod, směrnice

instrument /ˈɪn.strə.mənt/ nástroj

instrumentation /ˌɪn.strə.menˈteɪ.ʃᵊn/ vybavení nástroji

insufficient /ˌɪn.səˈfɪʃ.ənt/ nedostatečný

insulin /ˈɪn.sjʊ.lɪn/ inzulín

insurance /ɪnˈʃɔː.rənts/ pojištění, pojistka

intact /ɪnˈtækt/ nedotčený, neporušený

intake /ˈɪn.teɪk/ příjem

integral /ˈɪn.tɪ.grəl/ nedílný

integrate /ˈɪn.tɪ.greɪt/ začlenit, tvořit nedílný celek, doplnit

intended /ɪnˈten.dɪd/ zamýšlený, plánovaný

intensity /ɪnˈtent.sɪ.ti/ intenzita, síla, hustota

interact /ˌɪn.təˈrækt/ reagovat vzájemně, vzájemně na sebe působit

interaction /ˌɪn.təˈræk.ʃᵊn/ spolupůsobení, vzájemná součinnost

intercuspal /ˌɪn.təˈkʌsp.ᵊl/ mezi hrboly, hroty

interfacial /ˌɪn.təˈfeɪ.ʃᵊl/ meziplošný

interfere /ˌɪn.təˈfɪəʳ/ zasahovat, ovlivnit

interference /ˌɪn.təˈfɪə.rᵊnts/ překážení, porucha, rušivé ovlivňování

intermediate /ˌɪn.təˈmiː.di.ət/ střední, prostřední

intermittent /ˌɪn.təˈmɪt.ənt/ občasný, přerušovaný, nestálý, vracející se

internal /ɪnˈtɜː.nəl/ vnitřní, interní

interproximal /ˌɪn.təˈprɒk.sɪ.mᵊl/ aproximální, styčný, interproximální

interrupt /ˌɪn.təˈrʌpt/ přerušit, přerušovat

interruption /ˌɪn.təˈrʌp.ʃᵊn/ přerušení, překážka

interspace /ˈɪn.tə.speɪs/ mezera

intervention /ˌɪn.təˈven.ʃᵊn/ intervence, zakročení, zásah

intolerable /ɪnˈtɒl.ər.ə.bl̩/ netolerovatelný, nesnesitelný, nesnášenlivý

intolerance /ɪnˈtɒl.ᵊr.ᵊnʦ/ nesnášenlivost

intoxication /ɪnˌtɒk.sɪˈkeɪ.ʃᵊn/ intoxikace, omámení

intra-abdominal /ˌɪn.trə.æbˈdɒm.ɪ.nəl/ intraabdominální, vnitrobřišní

intraligament /ˌɪn.trə.ˈlɪg.ə.mənt/ do vaziva

intracanal /ˌɪn.trə.kəˈnæl/ uvnitř kanálku

intracoronally /ˌɪn.trəˈkɒr.ᵊn.ᵊl.i/ mezi korunkami

intraoral /ˌɪn.trəˈɔː.rəl/ intraorální, uvnitř úst

intraorally /ˌɪn.trə.ˈɔː.rə.li/ intraorálně

intraosseous /ˌɪn.trəˈɒs.i.əs/ intraoseální, nitrokostní, ležící uvnitř kosti

intravenous /ˌɪn.trəˈviː.nəs/ intravenózní, nitrožilní

intravenously /ˌɪn.trəˈviː.nə.sli/ intravenózně, do žil

introduction /ˌɪn.trəˈdʌk.ʃᵊn/ úvod, zavedení

intrusion /ɪnˈtruː.ʒᵊn/ intruse, pronikání, vstup, vnikání, vtlačení

intubation /ˌɪŋ.tjʊˈbeɪ.ʃᵊn/ intubace, zavedení rourky do průdušnice

invariably /ɪnˈveə.ri.ə.bli/ trvale, pravidelně

invasion /ɪnˈveɪ.ʒᵊn/ invaze, napadení

invasive /ɪnˈveɪ.sɪv/ invazivní, agresivní, napadající

inventory /ˈɪn.vᵊn.tri/ inventář (věcí)

investigation /ɪnˌves.tɪˈgeɪ.ʃᵊn/ vyšetření, vyšetřování

investment /ɪnˈvesʈ.mənt/ formovací hmota

involve /ɪnˈvɒlv/ obsahovat, postihnout, postihovat, zahrnovat. Vyžadovat, znamenat

involvement /ɪnˈvɒlv.mənt/ zapojení, postižení, komplikace

ion /ˈaɪ.ɒn/ iont

iron /aɪən/ železo

ironmongery /ˈaɪənˌmʌŋ.gər.i/ práce se železem

irradiation /ɪˌreɪ.diˈeɪ.ʃᵊn/ iradiace, ozáření, osvětlení

irregular /ɪˈreg.jə.ləʳ/ nepravidelný

irregularity /ɪˌreg.jəˈlær.ə.ti/ nepravidelnost

irreversible /ˌɪr.ɪˈvɜː.sɪ.bl̩/ nevratný, nezvratný, nevyléčitelný

irrigate /ˈɪr.ɪ.geɪt/ zavlažovat

irrigation /ˌɪr.ɪˈgeɪ.ʃᵊn/ nálev, výplach, zavlažení, zavlažování

irrigation /ˌɪr.ɪˈgeɪ.ʃᵊn/ syringe / sɪˈrɪndʒ/ stříkačka pro výplach

irritable /ˈɪr.ɪ.tə.bl̩/ podrážděný, přecitlivělý

irritant /ˈɪr.ɪ.tᵊnt/ dráždidlo, dráždící, dráždivý

irritate /ˈɪr.ɪ.teɪt/ dráždit

irritation /ˌɪr.ɪˈteɪ.ʃᵊn/ dráždění

ischaemic /ɪsˈkiː.mɪk/ ischemický, nedokrvený

isolate /ˈaɪ.sə.leɪt/ odloučit, izilovat

isolation /ˌaɪ.sᵊl.eɪ.ʃᵊn/ izolace, oddělování, osamocení

isometric /aɪ.səʊˈmet.rɪk/ izometrický, mající stejné rozměry

isotonic /aɪ.səʊˈtɒn.ɪk/ izotonický, se stejným osmotickým tlakem

itchiness /ˈɪtʃ.ɪ.nəs/ svědění

itching /ˈɪtʃ.ɪŋ/ svědění, svědivý

item /ˈaɪ.təm/ položka, jednotlivost

IV /ˌaɪˈviː/, **intravenous** /ˌɪn.trəˈviː. nəs/ intravenózní, nitrožilní

J

jaundice /ˈdʒɔː.n.dɪs/ žloutenka

jaw /dʒɔː/ čelist, dáseň

jerk /dʒɜːk/ trhnout, škubnutí, tik

jet /dʒet/ proud vody, stříkat

jewellery /ˈdʒuː.ᵊl.ri/ šperky

joint /dʒɔɪnt/ kloub, spojení, místo připojení

K

keen /kiːn/ nadšený

keep /kiːp/ ponechat, udržovat

key /kiː/ klíč

keyhole /ˈkiː.həʊl/ klíčová dírka

kidney /ˈkɪd.ni/ ledvina

kit /kɪt/ výbava, sada nástrojů

knife /naɪf/ nůž

knock /nɒk/ uhodit

knot /nɒt/ klička, uzel

knowledge /ˈnɒl.ɪdʒ/ znalost, vědomost

L

LA local /ˈləʊ.kəl/ **anaesthesia** /ˌæn. əsˈθiː.zi.ə/ místní anestezie

label /ˈleɪ.bᵊl/ nálepka, označení

labia /leɪ.bɪə/ rty

labial /ˈleɪ.bi.əl/ labiální, retní, retný

laceration /ˌlæs.ᵊrˈeɪ.ʃᵊn/ lacerace, tržná rána

lack /læk/ **of** /əv/ nedostatek

lack /læk/ postrádat, nedostatek

lacrimation /læk.rɪˈmeɪ.ʃᵊn/ slzení

Lactobacillus /ˈlæk.tʊ.bəˈsɪl.əs/ laktobacil, střevní mikroorganismus, vytvářející kyselinu mléčnou

lancinate /ˈlaːn.sɪ.nəɪt/ řezat

large /lɑːdʒ/ **intestine** /ɪnˈtes.tɪn/ tlusté střevo

laser /ˈleɪ.zəʳ/ laserový

lassitude /ˈlæs.ɪ.tjuːd/ malátnost, únava

latch /lætʃ/ západka, zaklapnout

later /ˈleɪ.təʳ/ později, pozdější

lateral /ˈlæt.rᵊl/ laterální, postranní, vedlejší, příčný

lay /leɪ/ **out** /aʊt/ vyložit, dimenzovat

lay /leɪ/ položit

layer /ˈleɪ.əʳ/ vrstva, úroveň, poloha

leaflet /ˈliː.flət/ leták (propagační), prospekt

leakage /ˈliː.kɪdʒ/ netěsnost, vytékání, unikání, propouštění

learning /ˈlɜː.nɪŋ/ **disability** /ˌdɪs.əˈbɪl.ɪ.ti/ porucha učení

least /liːst/ nejnižší

leg /leg/ noha, nohavice

leisure /ˈleʒ.əʳ/ volný čas

length /leŋk θ/ délka, trvání

lengthen /ˈleŋk.θən/ prodloužit

lesion /ˈliː.ʒᵊn/ léze, zranění, poranění, poškození, porucha, postižené místo

less /les/ **than** /ðən/ méně než

lethargy /ˈləθ.ə.dʒɪ/ letargie, strnulost, netečnost

leukaemia /luːˈkiː.mi.ə/ leukémie

leukoplakia /ˌluːkə.ˈpleɪ.kɪə/ leukoplakie, bělavé skvrny na sliznici

level /ˈlev.ᵊl/ hladina, úroveň, stupeň, vrstva, stejná rovina

licence /ˈlaɪ.sᵊnts/ oprávnění, povolení

lichen /ˈlaɪ.kən/ **planus** /pleɪ.nəs/ lišej

lie /laɪ/ ležet

lifesaver /ˈlaɪfˌseɪ.vəʳ/ životní záchrana

lifestyle /ˈlaɪf.staɪl/ životní styl

life-threatening /ˈlaɪf.θret.ᵊn.ɪŋ/ život ohrožující

lift /lɪft/ nadzvednout, zvednout, zvednutí

ligament /ˈlɪg.ə.mənt/ ligament, vaz, vazivo

ligature /ˈlɪg.ə.tʃəʳ/ ligatura, podvázání

light /laɪt/ lehký

light /laɪt/ světlo, osvětlit, světlý

light-cured /laɪt.kjʊəʳ.d/ světlem tuhnoucí, tvrzený světlem

light-headed /ˌlaɪtˈhed.ɪd/ mající závrať, zmámený

likelihood /ˈlaɪ.kli.hʊd/ pravděpodobnost, možnost

likely /ˈlaɪ.kli/ pravděpodobný, pravděpodobně

limb /lɪm/ končetina

limit /ˈlɪm.ɪt/ limit, omezit, vymezit, krajní hranice, hranice (omezení)

limitation /ˌlɪm.ɪˈteɪ.ʃᵊn/ limitace, omezení, nedostatek, vada

limited /ˈlɪm.ɪ.tɪd/ omezený

line /laɪn/ lemovat

lined /laɪnd/ vyztužený, obložený

lined /laɪnd/ **with** /wɪð/ lemovaný

liner /ˈlaɪ.nəʳ/ podložka, vložka, izolační materiál

lingual /ˈlɪŋ.gwᵊl/ jazykový

lining /ˈlaɪ.nɪŋ/ obložení, výstelka, vložka, výplněk

linked /lɪŋkt/ **to** /tʊ/ spojený s

lip /lɪp/ **competence** /ˈkʊm.pɪ.tənts/ celistvost rtu

lip /lɪp/ ret

lipoma /lɪˈp.əʊ.mə/ lipom, nezhoubný tukový nádor

liposarcoma /ˌlɪp.ə.sɑːˈkəʊ.mə/ liposarkom, zhoubný nádor z tukové tkáně liquid /ˈlɪk.wɪd/ kapalina, kapalný, tekutina, tekutý, průzračný

listen /ˈlɪs.ᵊn/ poslouchat, sledovat, poslech

literally /ˈlɪt.ᵊr.ᵊl.i/ doslova

liver /ˈlɪv.əʳ/ játra

living /ˈlɪv.ɪŋ/ životní, žijící, živý

load /ləʊd/ náplň, naplnit, plnit, zatížení, zatížit

load-carrying /ləʊd.kær.i.ɪŋ/ nesoucí váhu

local /ˈləʊ.kəl/ anaesthetic /ˌæn.əsˈθet.ɪk/ místní anestetikum

local /ˈləʊ.kᵊl/ místní

localise /ˈləʊ.kᵊl.aɪz/ omezit na jedno místo

locally /ˈləʊ.kəl.i/ lokálně, místně

locate /ləʊˈkeɪt/ zjistit polohu (místo), vyhledat

locator /ləʊˈkeɪ.təʳ/ vyhledávač, lokátor

location /ləʊˈkeɪ.ʃən/ lokace, umístění, poloha

lock /lɒk/ zámek, zamknout, uzavřít, zavřít

locking /lɒk.ɪŋ/ uzavírání, blokování

locomotor /ˌləʊ.kəˈməʊ.təʳ/ lokomotorický, pohybový

lodge /lɒdʒ/ ukládat, usazovat

long-acting /lɒŋ.ˈæk.tɪŋ/ dlouhodobě působící

long-term /ˌlɒŋˈtɜːm/ dlouhodobý

look /lʊk/ dívat se, podívat se, vyhledat, brát v úvahu, vypadat, vzhled

look /lʊk/ for /fɔːʳ/ pátrat po

loose /luːs/ uvolnit, uvolněný, viklající se

loose-fitting /ˌluːsˈfɪt.ɪŋ/ volný

loosen /ˈluː.sᵊn/ povolit, uvolnit, rozvázat, rozviklat, vyviklat

loss /lɒs/ of /əv/ consciousness /ˈkɒn.tʃə.snəs/ ztráta vědomí

loss /lɒs/ ztráta, úbytek

lost /lɒst/ ztracený

low /ləʊ/ nízký

lower /ˈləʊ.əʳ/ spodní

low-volume /ləʊ.ˈvɒl.juːm/ nízko-objemový

lump /lʌmp/ boule (na těle), opuchlina

lung /lʌŋ/ plíce (jedna)

luting /luːt.ɪŋ/ upevnění, upnutí, sevření, přitmelení, tmel, utěsňování

lying (inf. lie) /ˈlaɪ.ɪŋ/ ležící

lymph /lɪmp f/ lymfa, míza

lymph /lɪmp f/ node /nəʊd/ lymfatická uzlina

lymphadenopathy /lɪmpˌfædɪˈnɒp.ə.θɪ/ lymfadenopatie, nepřesně určené onemocnění mízních uzlin

lymphatic /lɪmpˈfæt.ɪk/ lymfatický

lymphoma /lɪmpˈfəʊ.mə/ lymfom, maligní tumor lymfatické tkáně

M

machinery /məˈʃiː.nə.ri/ strojové vybavení

magnetic /mægˈnet.ɪk/ field /fiːld/ magnetické pole

magnetic /mægˈnet.ɪk/ magnetický

magnetic /mægˈnet.ɪk/ resonance /ˈrez.ᵊn.ənts/ imaging /ɪˈmɪdʒ.ɪŋ/ zobrazování magnetickou rezonancí

main /meɪn/ hlavní, silný

mains-operated /meɪnz.ˈɒp.ər.eɪt.ɪd/ ručně ovládaný

maintain /meɪnˈteɪn/ podporovat, pokračovat, udržet, udržovat, uchovat, zachovat, živit se

maintain /meɪnˈteɪn/ the airway /ˈeə.weɪ/ udržovat, podporovat dýchací cesty

maintain /meɪnˈteɪn/ **life** /laɪf/ uchovat při životě

maintenance /ˈmeɪn.tɪ.nənt s/ udržování

major /ˈmeɪ.dʒəʳ/ velký, důležitý, významnější, závažný, převážný

major /ˈmeɪ.dʒəʳ/ **vessel** /ˈves.ᵊl/ velká céva

majority /məˈdʒɒr.ə.ti/ většina

malaise /mælˈeɪz/ nevolnost, malátnost

male /meɪl/ muž, mužský

malformed /ˌmælˈfɔːmd/ chybně vytvořený

malignant /məˈlɪg.nənt/ maligní, škodlivý, zhoubný, zákeřný

malnutrition /ˌmæl.njuːˈtrɪ.ʃən/ nesprávná výživa, podvýživa

malocclusion/ˌmæl.əˈkluː.ʒᵊn/ chybný skus

malposition /ˌmæl.pəˈzɪʃ.ᵊn/ chybná poloha, špatné úmístění

manage /ˈmæn.ɪdʒ/ zvládnout, řídit

management /ˈmæn.ɪdʒ.mənt/ péče, ošetření, léčba, snaha o zvládnutí, ovládání, řízení, vedení, ředitelství, zvládnutí

mandible /ˈmæn.dɪ.bᵊl/ mandibula, dolní čelist

mandibular /mænˈdɪ.bjʊ.ləʳ/ mandibulární

mandrel /ˈmæn.drəl/ vřeteno, trn, jádro

manifestation /ˌmæn.ɪ.fesˈteɪ.ʃən/ manifestace, projev, objevení

manipulation /məˌnɪp.jʊˈleɪ.ʃᵊn/ manipulace, obsluha, zpracování

manner /ˈmæn.əʳ/ způsob, chování, metoda

manual /ˈmæn.ju.əl/ ruční (konaný rukama), příručka, rukojeť

manufacture /ˌmæn.jʊˈfæk.t ʃəʳ/ tvořit, zpracovat

margin /ˈmɑː.dʒɪn/ okraj, pokraj, lem, lemovat

marginal /ˈmɑː.dʒɪ.nəl/ okrajový, mezní, krajní

marital /ˈmær.ɪ.tᵊl/ **circumstance** /ˈsɜː.kəm.stɑːnt s/ manželská situace

marked /mɑːkt/ označený, značný

markedly /ˈmɑː.kɪd.li/ značně, zjevně, nápadně

marrow /ˈmær.əʊ/ kostní dřeň

mask /mɑːsk/ maska, zakrýt

mass /mæs/ hmota, masa

massive /ˈmæs.ɪv/ masivní

master /ˈmɑː.stəʳ/ hlavní, originální

masticate /ˈmæs.tɪ.keɪt/ žvýkat

mastication /ˌmæs.tɪˈkeɪ.ʃᵊn/ mastikace, žvýkání

masticatory /ˌmæs.tɪˈkeɪ.tᵊr.i/ žvýkací

matched /mætʃt/ vyrovnaný, sesazený

material /məˈtɪə.ri.əl/ materiál

matrix /ˈmeɪ.trɪks/ forma, matice, matrice, základní hmota

matrix /ˈmeɪ.trɪks/ **band** /bænd/ matriční páska, otiskovací kroužek

mattress /ˈmæt.rəs/ podložka

maturity /məˈtjʊə.rɪ.ti/ zralost, vyspělost

maxilla /mæˈksɪ.lə/ maxilla, horní čelist

maxillary /mæˈksɪ.lᵊr.i/ čelistní

maxillofacial /ˌmæk.sɪ.ləˈfeɪ.ʃᵊl/ maxilofaciální, týkající se horní čelisti a tváře

meal /mɪəl/ jídlo (denní)

meantime /ˈmiːn.taɪm/ mezitím

measurable /ˈmeʒ.ər.ə.bl̩/ měřitelný

measure /ˈmeʒ.əʳ/ měřit, opatření

measurement /ˈmeʒ.ə.mənt/ měření, velikost, opatření

mechanical /məˈkæn.ɪ.kᵊl/ mechanický, bezděčný

medical /ˈmed.ɪ.kᵊl/ history /ˈhɪs.tər.i/ lékařská anamnéza

medical /ˈmed.ɪ.kəl/ lékařský

medicated /ˈmed.ɪ.keɪ.tɪd/ léčebný

medication /ˌmed.ɪˈkeɪ.ʃᵊn/ léčba, lék, léky, léčení

medicine/ˈmed.ɪ.sən/ lék

medium /ˈmiː.di.əm/ medium, přenašeč, střed, prostřední

menopause /ˈmen.ə.pɔːz/ menopauza, klimakterium

menorrhagia /ˌmen.əˈreɪ.dʒɪ.ə/ menoragie, silné menstruační krvácení

menstrual /ˈmen.strəl/ menstruační

menstruation /ˌmen.struˈeɪ.ʃᵊn/ menstruace

mental /ˈmen.tl/ duševní, psychický

mentally /ˈmen.tᵊl.i/ duševně, psychicky

merciless /ˈmɜː.sɪ.ləs/ nelítostný

mercury /ˈmɜː.kjʊ.ri/ rtuť

merely /mɪə.li/ pouze

mesial /miː.zjəl/ střední

mesiodens /ˌmiː.zɪəˈdenz/ přespočetný zub, ve střední čáře horní čelisti

message /ˈmes.ɪdʒ/ sdělení, zpráva

metabolise /məˈtæb.ᵊl.aɪz/ metabolizovat

metal /ˈmet.ᵊl/ kov, kovový, vylít kovem, potáhnout kovem

metastasis /metˈæs.tə.sɪs/ pl. **metastases** metastáza

metastatic /ˌmet.əˈstæ.tɪk/ metastatický, týkající se metastázy

micro- /maɪ.krəʊ -/ mikro-

microbe /ˈmaɪ.krəʊb/ microb, bakterie

microbiology /ˌmaɪ.krəʊ.baɪˈɒl.ə.dʒi/ mikrobiologie

microorganism / maɪ.krəʊ.ˈɔː.gən.ɪ.zᵊm/ mikroorganismus

microscopic /ˌmaɪ.krəˈskɒp.ɪk/ mikroskopický

micturition /ˌmɪkt.juəˈrɪʃ.ᵊn/ močení

middle /ˈmɪd.l̩/ finger /ˈfɪŋ.gəʳ/ prostředníček

midline /ˈmɪd.laɪn/ střednice

migraine /ˈmiː.greɪn/, /ˈmaɪ/ migréna, silná bolest hlavy

migrainous /maɪ.grə.nəs/ migrénový, týkající se migrény

migrate /maɪˈgreɪt/ posunovat se

mild /maɪld/ mírný, klidný, slabý

mimic /ˈmɪm.ɪk/ napodobit

mind /maɪnd/ mysl, vadit, paměť

minimise /ˈmɪn.ɪ.maɪz/ minimalizovat, zmenšit

minor /ˈmaɪ.nəʳ/ malý, menší

minutely /maɪˈnjuːt.li/ nepatrně

mirror /ˈmɪr.əʳ/ zrcadlo, zrcátko, odrážet se

miscarriage /ˈmɪs.kær.ɪdʒ/ potrat, umělé přerušení těhotenství

miscellaneous /ˌmɪs.əlˈeɪ.ni.əs/ rozmanitý

misdiagnosis /mɪs.daɪ.əgˈnəʊ.sɪs/ chybná diagnóza

miss /mɪs/ zmeškat

missing /ˈmɪs.ɪŋ/ teeth /tiːθ/ chybějící zuby

missing /ˈmɪs.ɪŋ/ chybějící, nepřítomný

mix /mɪks/ míchat

mixed /mɪkst/ smíchaný

mixture /ˈmɪks.tʃəʳ/ směs, příměs

mobile /ˈməʊ.baɪl/ mobilní, pohyblivý

mobilisation /ˌməʊ.bɪ.laɪˈzeɪ.ʃᵊn/ uvolnění

mobility /məʊˈbɪl.ɪ.ti/ pohyblivost

model /ˈmɒd.ᵊl/ model, vzor

modelling /ˈmɒd.əl.ɪŋ/ modelový, modelování

moderate /ˈmɒd.ər.ət/ mírný, zmírňovat

modification /ˌmɒd.ɪ.fɪˈkeɪ.ʃᵊn/ modifikace, obměna, přizpůsobení

modify /ˈmɒd.ɪ.faɪ/ modifikovat, přizpůsobit upravit, uzpůsobit

modulus /ˈmɒd.jə.ləs/ modul

moist /mɔɪst/ mokrý, vlhký (vzduch)

moisture /ˈmɔɪs.tʃᵊr/ vlhkost

molar /ˈməʊ.lᵊr/ stolička

monitor /ˈmɒn.ɪ.tər/ monitorovat, sledovat

monomer /mɒn.ə.məʳ/ monomer

mood /muːd/ nálada, kondice

motion /ˈməʊ.ʃᵊn/ pohyb

motivate /ˈməʊ.tɪ.veɪt/ motivovat

motor /ˈməʊ.tər/ **response** /rɪˈspɒnt s/ pohybová reakce

mould /məʊld/ forma, formovat, modelovat, tvar

moulding /məʊld.ɪŋ/ tváření, výlisek

mouth /maʊθ/ **seal** /siːl/ uzavření, obemknutí úst

mouthful /ˈmaʊθ.fʊl/ plná ústa

mouthpiece /ˈmaʊθ.piːs/ náustek

mouth-to-mouth /maʊθ/ z úst do úst

mouthwash /ˈmaʊθ.wɒʃ/ ústní voda, kloktadlo, výplach úst, ústní voda

movable /ˈmuː.və.bl̩/ pohyblivý

movement /ˈmuː.v.mənt/ pohyb, pohybový, postup

movement /ˈmuː.v.mənt/ vyprázdnění střev

mucoperiosteum /ˈmjuː.kəˌper.ɪˈɒs.ti.əm/ mukoperiost, okostice mající mukózní povrch

mucosa /mjuːˈkəʊ.sə/ sliznice

mucosal /ˌmjuːˈkəʊ.sl/ mukózní, slizniční

mucous membrane /ˌmjuː.kəsˈmem.breɪn/ sliznice

multiple /ˈmʌl.tɪ.pl̩/ mnohačetný

multiple /ˈmʌl.tɪ.pl̩/ **sclerosis** /skləˈrəʊ.sɪs/ multiplex, roztroušená skleróza

multiply /ˈmʌl.tɪ.plaɪ/ násobit, rozmnožovat se, vícenásobný

multipurpose /ˌmʌl.tɪˈpɜː.pəs/ víceúčelový

murmur /ˈmɜː.məʳ/ šelest, šeptat

muscle /ˈmʌs.l̩/ sval, svalový

muscular /ˈmʌs.kjʊ.lᵊr/ svalový

musculature /ˈmʌs.kjʊ.lə.tʃəʳ/ svalstvo

musculoskeletal /ˈmʌs.kjʊ.ləˈskel.ɪ.tᵊl/ muskuloskeletální, skládající se ze svalů a kostí

mutant /ˈmjuː.tənt/ mutant, měnící se

myalgia /mʌlˈæl.dʒɪ.ə/ myalgie, svalová bolest

mycoplasma /maɪ.kəˈplæz.mə/ mykoplazma

myocardial /ˌmaɪ.əˈkɑː.diəl/ **infarction** /inˈfɑː.kʃᵊn/ infarkt myokardu

N

nail /neɪl/ nehet

nail /neɪl/ **varnish** /ˈvɑː.nɪʃ/ lak na nehty

name /neɪm/ jmenovat se

nappy /ˈnæp.i/ plenka

narrow /ˈnær.əʊ/ úzký, zužovat se

nasal /ˈneɪ.zəl/ **cavity** /ˈkæv.ɪ.ti/ nosní dutina

nasal /ˈneɪ.zəl/ nosní

natural /ˈnætʃ.ᵊr.ᵊl/ přirozený, přírodní

naturally /ˈnætʃ.ᵊr.ᵊl.i/ přirozeně

nature /ˈneɪ.tʃəʳ/ povaha, přirozená vlastnost, charakter nausea /ˈnɔː.zi.ə/ nausea, nevolnost, pocit nevolnosti, nucení ke zvracení

nauseous /ˈnɔː.zi.əs/ působící zvedání žaludku

nearby /ˌnɪəˈbaɪ/ blízký, sousední

necessary /ˈnes.ə.ser.i/ nutný

necessitate /nəˈses.ɪ.teɪt/ nutně vyžadovat

necessity /nəˈses.ɪ.ti/ nutnost

neck /nek/ krk, hrdlo, límec

need /niːd/ potřeba

needle /ˈniː.dl̩/ holder /ˈhəʊl.dəʳ/ držátko jehel

needle /ˈniː.dl̩/ jehla, sešívat, vpichovat, očkovat

needle /ˈniː.dl̩/ stick /stɪk/ bodnutí jehlou

negative/ˈneg.ə.tɪv/ negativní

neglect /nɪˈglekt/ zanedbat

neither /ˈnaɪ.ðəʳ/ aniž (a také ne), žádný (z obou)

neoplastic /ˈniːəˈplæs.tɪk/ neoplastický, nově vytvořený

nerve /nɜːv/ block /blɒk/ nervový blok

nerve /nɜːv/ nerv

nerve /nɜːv/ trunk /trʌŋk/ nervový kmen

nervousness /ˈnɜː.və.snəs/ nervozita, nervóza

neuralgia /njʊəˈræl.dʒə/ neuralgie, ostrá nervová bolest

neurological /ˌnjʊə.rəˈlɒdʒ.ɪ.kʰl/ neurologický

neuroma /ˌnjʊəˈrəʊ.mə/ neurom, druh nádoru tvořený z nervových buněk

neuromuscular /ˌnjʊəˈrə.mæsk.jʊ.ləʳ/ neuromuskulární, nervosvalový

neuron /ˈnjʊə.rɒn/ neuron, nervová buňka

neuropathy /ˌnjʊəˈrɒ.pə.θi/ neuropatie, onemocnění nervů

neurosis /njʊəˈrəʊ.sɪs/ (pl. neuroses) neuróza

neurovascular /ˌnjʊə.rəʊˈvæs.kjʊ.ləʳ/ neurovaskulární

nibble /ˈnɪb.l̩/ oštipovat

nickel-chromium /ˈnɪk.ᵊl.krəʊ.mi.əm/ steel /stiːl/ niklochromová ocel

nitrous oxide /ˌnaɪ.trəsˈɒk.saɪd/ kysličník dusný, rajský plyn

nocturia /nɒkˈtjʊ.ə.rɪ.ə/ nokturie, noční močení

nodal /ˈnəʊ.dᵊl/ uzlový

node /nəʊd/ uzel, uzlina, otok

noise /nɔɪz/ hluk, zvuk, poruchy

nominate /ˈnɒm.ɪ.neɪt/ jmenovat, navrhnout

non-/nɒn-/ ne (záporná předpona)

nonadhesive /ˌnɒn.ədˈhiː.sɪv/ nepřilnavý

none /nʌn/ žádný

nonstaining /nɒn.ˈsteɪn.ɪŋ/ nešpinící

nonsurgical /nɒnˈsɜː.dʒɪ.kᵊl/ nechirurgický

nonverbal /ˌnɒnˈvɜː.bᵊl/ neverbální, mimoslovní

nonvital /nɒn.ˈvaɪ.tᵊl/ devitalizovaný

notation /nəʊˈteɪ.ʃᵊn/ záznam, označovací soustava

note /nəʊt/ poznámka

notice /ˈnəʊ.tɪs/ zaznamenat

nozzle /ˈnɒz.l̩/ tryska, hubička, licí koncovka

numb /nʌm/ necitlivý

number /ˈnʌm.bəʳ/ počet

numbness /ˈnʌm.nəs/ znecitlivění

numeric /njuːˈmer.ɪk/ číselný

numerous /ˈnjuː.mə.rəs/ početný

nurse /nɜːs/ kojit

nurse /nɜːs/ zdravotní sestra, ošetřovatelka

nursing /ˈnɜː.sɪŋ/ bottle /ˈbɒt.l̩/ dětská lahvička ke krmení nursing /ˈnɜː.sɪŋ/ ošetřování

nut /nʌt/ oříšek

nutrition /njuːˈtrɪʃ.ən/ výživa

nutritional /njuːˈtrɪʃ.ən.əl/ nutriční, výživový

O

obdurate /ˈɒb.djʊ.rət/ zacpat, utěsnit

obesity /əʊˈbiː.sɪ.ti/ obezita, otylost

obey /əʊˈbeɪ/ command /kəˈmɑːnd/ být poslušný příkazu

object /ˈɒb.dʒɪkt/ předmět

objective /əbˈdʒek.tɪv/ cíl

obscure /əbˈskjʊər/ zakrýt, zastírat

observation /ˌɒb.zəˈveɪ.ʃən/ pozorování, dodržování

observe /əbˈzɜːv/ sledovat

obstacle /ˈɒb.stɪ.kḷ/ překážka

obstetric /ɒbˈstet.rɪk/ porodnický, spojený s porodem

obstruction /əbˈstrʌk.ʃən/ překážka, ucpání

obstructive /əbˈstrʌk.tɪv/ obstruktivní, ucpávající

obtain /əbˈteɪn/ získat, dostat (obdržet)

obturate /ˈɒb.tjʊə.reɪt/ ucpat

obturation /ˌɒb.tjʊ.əˈreɪ.ʃən/ utěsnění, uzavření, ucpání

obvious /ˈɒb.vi.əs/ zjevný, zřejmý, samozřejmý, nápadný

obviously/ˈɒb.vi.ə.sli/ zřejmě, evidentně, zjevně

occlude /əˈkluːd/, /ɒkˈluːd/ uzavřít

occlusal /ɒklʊː.zl/ okluzní, skusový

occlusion /əˈklʊː.ʒən/ skus, okluze, závtor

occult /ˈɒk.ʌlt/ skrytý

occupation /ˌɒk.jʊˈpeɪ.ʃən/ zaměstnání, povolání, obsazení

occupational /ˌɒk.jʊˈpeɪ.ʃən.əl/ pracovní

occur /əˈkɜːr/objevit se, nastat, přihodit se, napadnout (přijít na mysl), vyskytovat se

occurrence /əˈkʌr.ənts/ výskyt, případ, událost

ocular /ˈɒk.jʊ.lər/ oční, zrakový, očividný

odontalgia /ˌəʊ.dɒnˈtæl.dʒɪə/ bolest zubů

odontoblast /əʊˈdɒn.tə.blaːst/ odontoblast, buňka dentinu tvořící zubovinu

oedema /ɪˈdiː.mə/ edém, otok

oesophageal /ɪːˌsɒf.əˈdʒɪ.əl/ jícnový

oesophagitis /ˌiːsɒ.fəˈdʒaɪ.tɪs/ ezofagitida, zánět jícnu

oestrogen /ˈiː.strəʊ.dʒən/ estrogen, ženský pohlavní hormon

offending /əˈfen.dɪŋ/ obtížný, zraňující

ointment /ˈɔɪnt.mənt/ mazání, mast

olfactory /ɒlˈfæk.tər.i/ čichový

on /ɒn/ occasion /əˈkeɪ.ʒən/ v případě nutnosti

on /ɒn/ the part /pɑːt/ na straně (koho)

on /ɒn/ waking /ˈweɪ.kɪŋ/ při probuzení

once /wʌnts/ jednou, jakmile jednou, svého času

oncologist /ɒŋˈkɒl.ə.dʒɪst/ onkolog

onlay /ˈɒn.leɪ/ onlej, štěp aplikovaný na povrch tkáně

onlooker /ˈɒn.lʊk.ər/ přihlížející

onset /ˈɒn.set/ nástup, příchod (počátek, začátek

onwards /ˈɒn.wədz/ dále

opacity /əʊˈpæs.ə.ti/ neprůhlednost, temnost, matnost

opening /ˈəʊ.pən.ɪŋ/ otevření

operate /ˈɒp.ər.eɪt/ operovat, řídit, fungovat, obsluhovat (stroj ap.), působit (o léku ap.)

operative /ˈɒp.ªr.ə.tɪv/ operační, operativní

operculum /əˈpɜːk.jʊ.ləm/ operculum, příklopka, víčko

opiate /ˈəʊ.pi.ət/ opiát, narkotický lék

opioid /əʊ.ˈpiː.ɒɪd/ opiát

opposed /əˈpəʊzd/ protikladný

opposing /əˈpəʊ.zɪŋ/ protichůdný, čelící

option /ˈɒp.ʃən/ volba

oral /ˈɔː.rəl/ orální, ústní

orally /ˈɔː.rə.li/ ústně

orbital /ˈɔː.bɪ.tªl/ orbitální, očnicový

order /ˈɔː.dəʳ/ pořadí, postup, objednávka

ordered /ˈɔː.dəd/ napravovaný

ordinary /ˈɔː.dɪ.nə.ri/ obyčejný, obvyklý, běžný

orientated /ˌɔː.ri.ənˈteɪ.tɪd/ orientovaný

origin /ˈɒr.ɪ.dʒɪn/ původ, počátek

originate /əˈrɪdʒ.ɪ.neɪt/ začínat

oroantral /ˌəʊ.rəʊˈæn.trəl/ oroantrální, týkající se úst a vedlejších nosních dutin

orofacial /ˌəʊ.rəˈfeɪ.ʃªl/ orofaciální, týkající se úst a obličeje

oropharyngeal /ˌəʊ.rəˈfær.ɪ.ŋˈdʒɪ.əl/ orofaryngeální, týkající se úst a hltanu

orthodontics /ˌɔː.θəʊ ˈdɒn.tɪks/ ortodoncie, úprava skusu

orthognathic /ˌɔː.θəʊ.ˈnæː.θɪk/ ortognátní, správný skus

orthograde /ɔːˈθəʊ .greɪd/ ortográdní

orthopantomograph /ˌɔː.r.θoʊ ˈpæn.təʊ.mə.grɑːf/ panoramatický snímek

osseointegration /ɒs.i.ə,ɪn.tɪˈgreɪ.ʃªn/ vhojení do kosti

osteitis /ˌɒs.ti ˈaɪ.tɪs/ osteitida, zánět kosti

osteoarthritis /ˌɒs.ti.əʊ.ɑːˈθraɪ.tɪs/ osteoartritida, zánět kostních kloubů

osteoporosis /ˌɒs.ti.əʊ.pəˈrəʊ.sɪs/ osteoporóza, prořídnutí kostí

osteosarcoma /ˌɒs.tɪ.ə.sɑːˈkəʊ.mə/ osteosarkom, maligní kostní nádor

osteotomy /ˌɒs.tiˈɒ.tə.mi/ osteotomie, protětí kosti

otherwise /ˈʌð.ə.waɪz/ jinak, nebo, z jiného hlediska

out /aʊt/ of /əv/ bez

outcome /ˈaʊt.kʌm/ výsledek, závěr

outline /ˈaʊt.laɪn/ kontura, náčrt, náčrtek, obrys přehled, vytyčit, zakreslit

outpatient /ˈaʊt.peɪ.ʃªnt/ ambulantní pacient

outside /ˌaʊtˈsaɪd/ vně

over /ˈəʊ.vəʳ/ dosage /ˈdəʊ.sɪdʒ/ předávkování

over /ˈəʊ.vəʳ/ nad, přes, příliš, u konce, pokrytí celku

over /ˈəʊ.vəʳ/ the counter /ˈkaʊn.təʳ/ přes pult, bez receptu lékaře

overall /ˌəʊ.vəˈrɔːl/ celkový, všude, dohromady

overbite /ˌəʊ.və.baɪt/ překus (vertikální)

overdentures /ˈəʊ.və.ˈden.tʃəz/ hybridní protézy

overeruption /ˈəʊ.və.ɪˈrʌp.ʃªn/ supraokluze

overhang /ˌəʊ.vəˈhæŋ/ přečnívat, odstávat, viset přes

overjet /ˈəʊ.və.dʒet/ předkus (horizontální)

overlay /ˌəʊ.vəˈleɪ/ potažení, překrytí, překrýt (vrstvou)

overload /ˈəʊ.və.ləʊd/ přetížení, přílišný náklad, zahltit, zahlcení

overly /ˈəʊ.vªl.i/ moc, příliš

overlying /ˌəʊ.vªlˈaɪ.ɪŋ/ ležící nad

overnight /ˌəʊ.vəˈnaɪt/ přes noc (též přen.)

overreaction /ˌəʊ.və.riˈæk.ʃ°n/ nadměrná reakce

overspill /ˈəʊ.və.spɪl/ přelití, přebytek

oxide /ˈɒk.saɪd/ layer /ˈleɪ.əʳ/ oxidová vrstva

oxidise /ˈɒk.sɪ.daɪz/ oxidovat, okysličovat

oximeter /ˌɒk.sɪ.miː.təʳ/ oximetr

oxygen /ˈɒk.sɪ.dʒən/ delivery /dɪˈlɪv.ər.i/ podávání kyslíku

oxygen /ˈɒk.sɪ.dʒən/ kyslík

oxygenation /ˌɒk.sɪ.dʒəˈneɪ.ʃ°n/ oxygenace, okysličení

P

pacemaker /ˈpeɪsˌmeɪ.kəʳ/ srdeční stimulátor

pacifier/ ˈpæs.ɪ.faɪ.əʳ/ dudlík, uklidňovací prostředek

pack /pæk/ balíček, balit, cpát, tampon, tamponovat, ucpávat vatou, ucpávka

package /ˈpæk.ɪdʒ/ balení, zabalit

pad /pæd/ čtverec, čtvereček, polštář, polštářek, podložit (vatou), těsnit, blok (na psaní)

pain /peɪn/ bolest, námaha, trápit

painful /ˈpeɪn.f°l/ bolestivý

painkiller /ˈpeɪnˌkɪl.əʳ/ lék proti bolesti

painlessly /ˈpeɪn.lə.sli/ bezbolestně

pair /peəʳ/ of /əv/ pár, jedny

palatal /pæ.lə.tl/ bar /bɑːʳ/ patrový třmen

palatal /pæ.lə.tl/ patrový, předopatrový

pale /peɪl/ bledý

palliative /ˈpæl.i.ə.tɪv/ paliativní, utišující

pallor /ˈpæl.əʳ/ bledost, zsinalost

palm /pɑːm/ dlaň

palpate /ˈpæl.peɪt/ prohmatávat

palpitations /ˌpæl.pɪˈteɪ.ʃ°nz/ palpitace, bušení srdce

panacea /ˌpæn.əˈsiː.ə/ všelék (univerzální lék)

pancarditis /ˌpæn.kɑːˈdaɪ.tɪs/ pankarditida, zánět všech vrstev srdeční stěny

pancreas /ˈpæŋ.kri.əs/ pankreas, slinivka břišní

pancreatic /ˌpæŋ.kriˈæt.ɪk/ pankreatický, slinivkový

panic /ˈpæn.ɪk/ panický strach, zděšení

panoramic /ˌpæn.ərˈæm.ɪk/ celkový, panoramatický

paper /ˈpeɪ.pəʳ/ point /pɔɪnt/ papírový čípek

papilla /pəˈpɪl.ə/ (pl. papillae) bradavka, papila

papilloma /ˌpæp.ɪ.ˈləʊ.mə/ papilom, nezhoubný epitelový nádor

paracetamol /ˌpær.əˈsiː.tə.mɒl/ paracetamol

parachlorphenol /pær.əˌklɒrˈfɪː.nɒl/ parachlorfenol

parachute /ˈpær.ə.ʃuːt/ padákový

paraesthesia /ˌpær.əsˈθiː.sɪ.ə/ parestezie, změněná citlivost

parafunction /ˌpær.əˈfʌnk.ʃ°n/ parafunkce, poškozená funkce

parallel /ˈpær.ə.lel/ souběžný, shodný

paramedic /ˌpær.əˈmed.ɪk/ zdravotník, záchranář

paramount /ˈpær.ə.maʊnt/ nejdůležitější, hlavní, velice důležitý

parathyroid gland /ˌpær.əˈθaɪə.rɔɪdˌglænd/ příštitná žláza

parental /pəˈren.t°l/ rodičovský

parotid /pəˈrɒt.ɪd/ gland /glænd/ příušní žláza

part /pɑːt/ část, součást

partial /ˈpɑː.ʃªl/ částečný, dílčí, neúplný

partial /ˈpɑː.ʃªl/ dentures /ˈden.tʃəz/ částečné protézy

partially /ˈpɑː.ʃªl.i/ částečně

particle /ˈpɑː.tɪ.kl̩/ částečka, zrnko

particular /pəˈtɪk.jʊ.ləʳ/ podrobnost, konkrétní, specifický (určitý), jednotlivý, přesný, zvláštní

particularly /pəˈtɪk.jʊ.lə.li/ obzvláště

pass /pɑːs/ podat, projít, překonat

pass /pɑːs/ through /θruː/ procházet

passive /ˈpæs.ɪv/ pasivní

past /pɑːst/ poslední, minulý, za, přes

paste /peɪst/ keramická směs, pasta, lepidlo, lepit, přilepit

paste /peɪst/ zinkoxid-eugenolová pasta

patent /ˈpeɪ.tənt/ průchodný

path /pɑːθ/ cesta

pathogenesis /ˌpæθəˈdʒen.ɪ.sɪs/ patogeneze, vznik a vývoj onemocnění

pathological /ˌpæθ.əˈlɒdʒ.ɪ.kªl/ patologický, chorobný

pathology /pəˈθɒl.ə.dʒi/ patologie (obor), stav způsobující onemocnění, patologie, choroba

patient /ˈpeɪ.ʃªnt/ pacient

pattern /ˈpæt.ən/ vzor, model

payment /ˈpeɪ.mənt/ platba

pear-shaped /ˈpeə.ʃeɪpt/ ve tvaru hrušky

pea-sized /piː.saɪzd/ velikosti hrášku

peel /piːl/ oškrabat

peer /pɪəʳ/ vrstevník

peg-shaped /peg.ʃeɪpt/ čípkovitý

pellicle /pel.ɪ.kl̩/ povlak

pelvis /ˈpel.vɪs/ pánev

penetrate /ˈpen.ɪ.treɪt/ proniknout

penicillin /ˌpen.əˈsɪl.ɪn/ penicilin

perceive /pəˈsiːv/ vnímat, uvědomit si, pochopit

percentage /pəˈsen.tɪdʒ/ procento

percussion /pəˈkʌʃ.ªn/ poklep

perforated /ˈpɜː.fªr.eɪ.tɪd/ proražený

perforation /ˌpɜː.fªrˈeɪ.ʃªn/ proniknutí, propíchnutí

perform /pəˈfɔːm/ provést, předvést, fungovat, vykonat

periapical /per.ɪˈeɪ.pɪk.l/ periapikální, v okolí hrotu kořene

pericoronitis /ˌper.ɪ.kɒr.əˈnaɪ.tɪs/ perikoronitida, zánět kolem zubní korunky

perinatal /ˌper.ɪˈneɪ.tl/ kolem porodu, do 10 dní po porodu

period /ˈpɪə.ri.əd/ doba, období

periodontal /ˌper.ɪ.əˈdɒn.tl/ periodontální

periodontitis /ˌper.ɪ.əˈdɒn.ˈtaɪ.tɪs/ periodontitida, zánět závěsného aparátu

periodontium /ˌper.ɪ.əˈdɒn.ʃiəm/ periodoncium, parodont

periodontology /ˌper.ɪ.ədɒnˈtɒl.ə.dʒɪ/ periodontologie, odvětví specializující se na léčení tkáně kolem zubů

perioral /ˌper.ɪ.ˈɔː.rəl/ umístěný kolem úst

periosteal /ˌper.ɪˈɒs.ti.əl/ elevator / ˈel.ɪ.veɪ.təʳ/ raspatorium

periosteal /ˌper.ɪˈɒs.ti.əl/ periosteální, okostiční

periosteum /ˌper.ɪˈɒs.ti.əm/ periost, okostice

permanent /ˈpɜː.mə.nənt/ stálý, trvalý, nepřetržitý

permanently /ˈpɜː.mə.nənt.li/ stále

permeability /ˌpɜː.mi.əˈbɪl.ɪ.ti/ permeabilita, propustnost

permit /pə'mɪt/ dovolit, dovolovat, tolerovat, připustit

perpetuate /pə'petʃ.u.eɪt/ zachovat na věky

persevere /ˌpɜː.sɪ'vɪər/ vytrvat

persistent /pə'sɪs.tənt/ dlouhotrvající, neustálý, stálý, neústupný, ustavičný

personality /ˌpɜː.sən'æl.ə.ti/ **disorder** /dɪ'sɔː.dər/ porucha osobnosti

personnel /ˌpɜː.sən'el/ personál

petit mal /ˌpə'tiː'mæl/ malý epileptický záchvat

petroleum /pə'trəʊ.li.əm/ ropa, nafta

pharmacy /'fɑː.mə.si/ farmacie, lékárna, lékárnický, lékárnička

pharynx /'fær.ɪŋks/ farynx, hltan

phase /feɪz/ fáze, etapa

phenomenon /fə'nɒm.ɪ.nən/ fenomén (úkaz, jev, div), vlastnost

philosophy /fɪ'lɒs.ə.fi/ filosofie, strategie

phlebitis /flɪ'baɪ.tɪs/ flebitida, zánět žil

phobic /'fəʊ.bɪk/ panický, týkající se fobie, ustrašený

phosphate /'fɒs.feɪt/ fosfát, fosforečnan

phosphor /'fɒs.fər/ luminofor

phosphoric /fɒs'fɒr.ɪk/ **acid** /'æs.ɪd/ kyselina fosforečná

photo /'fəʊ.təʊ/ foto

photostimulable /'fəʊ.təʊ.'stɪm.jʊ.lə.bl̩/ reagující na světlo

physical /'fɪz.ɪ.kəl/ fyzikální

physically /'fɪz.ɪ.kli/ fyzicky

physician /fɪ'zɪʃ.ən/ ošetřující lékař, lékařský

pick /pɪk/ **up** /ʌp/ zvednout

pickled /'pɪk.l̩d/ **food** /fuːd/ potraviny nakládané do kyselého nálevu

piece /piːs/ kousek, kus

pier /pɪər/ pilíř, pilířový zub

pierce /pɪəs/ probodnout, prorazit

piercing /'pɪə.sɪŋ/ ostrý (pronikavý), bodavý, propichování těla kroužky

pigmentation /ˌpɪg.mən'teɪ.ʃən/ zbarvení

pillow /'pɪl.əʊ/ polštář, položit na polštář

pin /pɪn/ kolík, čípek, špendlík, svorka, připevnit, přišpendlit

pink /pɪŋk/ růžová barva, růžový

pins /pɪnz/ **and needles** /'niː.dlz̩/ brnění (mravenčení)

pit /pɪt/ jamka

pituitary gland /pɪ'tjuː.ɪ.tər.iˌglænd/ hypofýza, podvěsek mozkový

place /pleɪs/ umístit, prostor

placement /'pleɪs.mənt/ kladení, poloha, umístění, uspořádání

plain /pleɪn/ rovina, jednoduchý, jasný (zřetelný)

plane /pleɪn/ plocha (rovina)

planning /'plæn.ɪŋ/ plánování

plaque /plɑːk/ plak, zubní kámen

plasma /'plæz.mə/ plazma

plaster /'plɑː.stər/ náplast

plastic /'plæs.tɪk/ pružná hmota, plast, plastový, plastický

plasticiser /'plæs.tɪ.saɪz.ər/ změkčovadlo

plate /pleɪt/ destička, plát (deska), patro (umělého chrupu)

platelet /'pleɪt.lət/ destička, krevní destička

pledget /pledʒ.ɪt/ tampon z vaty

pleuritic /pluə.rət.ɪk/ nemocný zánětem pohrudnice

pliable /'plaɪ.ə.bl̩/ ohebný, pružný, plastický

pliers /'plaɪ.əz/ kleště, klíšťky, pinzeta

plugger /plʌg.ər/ zátka, cpátko

pocket /'pɒk.ɪt/ kapsa, chobot, váček

377

point /pɔɪnt/ bod, hrot, špička, pracovní konec nástroje

poisonous /ˈpɔɪ.zᵊn.əs/ jedovatý, škodlivý

poisonous /ˈpɔɪ.zᵊn.əs/ **vapour** / ˈveɪ.pəʳ/ jedovatý výpar

poke /pəʊk/ šťourat se, strkat, dloubnout, rýpat

polish /ˈpɒl.ɪʃ/ leštit

polishing /ˈpɒl.ɪʃ.ɪŋ/ **disc** /dɪsk/ leštící kotouč

polypharmacy /pɒl.ɪ.ˈfɑː.mə.si/ užívání více léků, nadměrné užívání léčiv

polyacrylate /pɒl.i.æˈkrɪ.leɪt/ polyakrylan, polyakrylát

polyacrylic /ˈpɒl.i.əˈkrɪl.ɪk/ **acid** / ˈæs.ɪd/ kyselina polyakrylová

polyarthropathy /ˌpɒl.ɪ.ɑːˈθrəp.ə.θi/ současný zánět několika kloubů

polycarboxylate / pɒl.i.kɑːˈbɒk.sɪl.eɪt/ polykarboxylát

polymer /ˈpɒl.ɪ.mər/ polymer

polyuria /ˌpɒl.ɪ.ˈjʊə.rɪə/ polyurie, nadměrné močení

pontic /ˌpɒnt.ɪk/ umělý zub umístěný na můstku

pooling /puː.lɪŋ/ sdílení, shromažďující

poor /pɔːʳ/ chybný, špatný, slabý

population /ˌpɒp.jʊˈleɪ.ʃᵊn/ populace, obyvatelstvo

porcelain /ˈpɔː.səl.ɪn/ porcelán (jemný)

pore /pɔːʳ/ pór

porous /ˈpɔː.rəs/ **porézní,** propustný

portable /ˈpɔː.tə.bl̩/ přenosný, příruční

portion /ˈpɔː.ʃən/ část, podíl

position /pəˈzɪʃ.ən/ místo, poloha, postavení, umístit

positive /ˈpɒz.ə.tɪv/ pozitivní, kladný, jasný, nesporný, prokázaný

post /pəʊst/ čep, sloupek, podpěra, stojan

post /pəʊst/ **crown** /kraʊn/ čepová korunka

poster /ˈpəʊ.stəʳ/ plakát

posterior /pɒsˈtɪə.ri.əʳ/ pozdější, zadní, zadní část

postictal /ˈpəʊstˈɪkt.ᵊl/ následně po prodělaném záchvatu

postmenopausal /pəʊstˌmen.ə.ˈpɔː. zᵊl/ po menopauze

postoperation /pəʊstˌɒp.ᵊrˈeɪ.ʃᵊn/ **(post-op)** pooperačně

postoperative /ˌpəʊstˈɒp.ᵊr.ə.tɪv/ pooperační

postural /ˈpɒs.tjʊ.ə.rəl/ posturální, postojový

posture /ˈpɒs.tʃəʳ/ pozice, postoj

pot /pɒt/ kelímek

potent /ˈpəʊ.tᵊnt/ silně účinný

potential /pəʊˈten.tʃᵊl/ potenciál, potenciální, možnost, možný

potentially /pəʊˈten.tʃᵊl.i/ potenciálně

potentiate /pəʊˈten.tʃi.eɪt/ znásobit, umocnit

powder /ˈpaʊ.dəʳ/ prášek, pudr, posypat, rozemlít, rozdrtit na prášek

powdered /ˈpaʊ.dəd/ **glass** /glɑːs/ práškové sklo

power /paʊəʳ/ **cut** /kʌt/ výpadek elektřiny

practice /ˈpræk.tɪs/ trénink, cvičení, procvičovat, klientela, pracovní technika

practitioner /prækˈtɪʃ.ᵊn.ᵊr/ praktický lékař, odborník

praise /preɪz/ chválit, pochvala

precede /prɪˈsiːd/ předcházet, předstihnout

preceding /prɪˈsiː.dɪŋ/ předcházející, předešlý

precious /ˈpreʃ.əs/ drahý, vzácný

precipitant /prɪˌsɪp.ɪ.ˈtənt/ překotný, spěšný, srážecí činidlo

precipitate /prɪˈsɪp.ɪ.teɪt/ urychlovat

precipitation /prɪˌsɪp.ɪˈteɪ.ʃᵊn/ precipitace, urychlení, srážení, vylučování

precise /prɪˈsaɪs/ přesný

precision /prɪˈsɪʒ.ᵊn/ attachment / əˈtætʃ.mənt/ přesné upevnění

preclude /prɪˈkluːd/ zabránit

predict /prɪˈdɪkt/ předpovídat, tvrdit

predictable /prɪˈdɪk.tə.bl̩/ předvídatelný

predispose /ˌpriː.dɪˈspəʊz/ predisponovat, učinit náchylným

predisposition /ˌpriː.dɪ.spəˈzɪʃ.ᵊn/ predispozice, náchylnost, předpoklad, sklon

predominantly /prɪˈdɒm.ɪ.nənt.li/ převážně, hlavně

prefabricated /ˌpriːˈfæb.rɪ.keɪ.tɪd/ stavebnicový, předmontovaný

prefer /prɪˈfɜːʳ/ preferovat, dávat přednost

preferable /ˈpref.ᵊr.ə.bl̩/ vhodnější, lepší

preference /ˈpref.ᵊr.ᵊnts/ přednost (priorita), volba, větší záliba

pregnancy /ˈpreg.nənt.si/ těhotenství

pregnant /ˈpreg.nənt/ gravidní (těhotná)

premalignant ˌpre.məˈlig.nənt/ před rakovinný

premature /ˈprem.ə.tʃəʳ/ předčasný, raný

premenstrual /ˌpriːˈmen.strəl/ syndrome /ˈsɪn.drəʊ m/ předmenstruační syndrom

premolar /ˌpriːˈməʊ.ləʳ/ třenový zub

prenatal /ˌpriːˈneɪ.tl̩/ prenatální, předporodní

preoperative /ˌpriːˈɒp.ᵊr.ə.tɪv/ předoperační

preparation /ˌprep.ᵊrˈeɪ.ʃᵊn/ preparace, příprava, přípravek, úprava

preparedness /prɪˈpeəd.nəs/ pohotovost (připravenost)

prescribe /prɪˈskraɪb/ předepsat, předepisovat, naordinovat

prescription /prɪˈskrɪp.ʃᵊn/ lékařský předpis

presence /ˈprez.ᵊnts/ přítomnost (osoby, věci ap.), zevnějšek

present /ˈprez.ᵊnt/ přítomný

present /prɪˈz.ent/ představit se, nabídnout

preservation /ˌprez.əˈveɪ.ʃᵊn/ uchování

pressed /prest/ stlačený

pressure /ˈpreʃ.əʳ/ tlak, stisk, napětí

prevalence /ˈprev.ᵊl.ənts/ prevalence, převládání, převaha, častý výskyt

prevalent /ˈprev.ᵊl.ənt/ obvyklý, převládající

prevent /prɪˈvent/ předejít, zajistit prevenci, zabránit čemu

prevention /prɪˈvent.ʃᵊn/ prevence, ochrana, zabránění

preventive /prɪˈven.tɪv/ preventivní, ochranný, předběžný, ochranné opatření

previous /ˈpriː.vi.əs/ dosavadní, před, předešlý, předchozí, překotný

price /praɪs/ cena

prickle /ˈprɪk.l̩/ osten, bodání, brnění, svrbění

primary /ˈpraɪ.mə.ri/ primární, první, prvotní, základní, začáteční

prime /praɪm/ prvotní, hlavní

principally /ˈprɪntʃ.sɪ.pli/ hlavně

principle /ˈprɪnt.sɪ.pl̩/ princip, metoda, postup, zásada, základní pravidlo

printout /ˈprɪnt.aʊt/ výtisk, výpis

prior /praɪəʳ/ **to** /tʊ/ před, dříve než

priority /praɪˈɒr.ɪ.ti/ prvenství, přednost, důležitá věc

prise /praɪz/ páčit

prism /ˈprɪz.ᵊm/ prizma, hranol

probe /prəʊb/ sonda, zubařská sonda, zkoumat sondou

probing /ˈprəʊ.bɪŋ/ sondáž

problem /ˈprɒb.ləm/ problém

procedure /prəˈsiː.dʒəʳ/ procedura (postup), průběh

proceed /prəʊˈsiːd/ postupovat, probíhat, provést

process /ˈprəʊ.ses/ proces, postup, průběh

processed /ˈprəʊ.sest/ zpracovaný

procline /prəʊˈklaɪn/ naklonit dopředu

prodromal /prɒ.drə.ml/ prodromální, předzvěstný

produce /prəˈdjuːs/ vytvářet, vytvořit, product, produkovat

product /ˈprɒd.ʌkt/ produkt

production /prəˈdʌk.ʃᵊn/ produkce, tvorba

professional /prəˈfeʃ.ᵊn.ᵊl/ profesionál, odborník

profound /prəˈfaʊnd/ hluboký (důkladný)

prognosis /prɒgˈnəʊ.sɪs/ **(pl. prognoses)** prognóza, předpověď

progress /prəˈgres/ postupovat, vyvíjet se

progress /ˈprəʊ.gres/ pokrok, postup

progression /prəˈgreʃ.ᵊn/ pokrok, postup, průběh

progressive /prəˈgres.ɪv/ progresivní, postupující, postupný

projection /prəˈdʒek.ʃᵊn/ výběžek, výstupek

proliferate /prəˈlɪf.ᵊr.eɪt/ bujet

prolong /prəˈlɒŋ/ prodloužit

prolonged /prəˈlɒŋd/ dlouhodobý, dlouhotrvající, prodloužený

prominent /ˈprɒm.ɪ.nənt/ vyčnívající

promote /prəˈməʊt/ propagovat, napomáhat, podporovat

promptly /ˈprɒmp t.li/ promptně, okamžitě, rychle

prone /prəʊn/ náchylný, šikmý, ležící na břiše

pronounce /prəˈnaʊnts/ vyslovovat

prop /prɒp/ podpěra

property /ˈprɒp.ə.ti/ kvalita, vlastnost, charakteristika

prophylactic /ˌprɒf.ɪˈlæk.tɪk/ profylaktický, preventivní

prophylaxis /ˌprɒf.ɪˈlæk.sɪs/ profylaxe, prevence

proportional /prəˈpɔː.ʃᵊn.ᵊl/ poměrný, přiměřený

propose /prəˈpəʊz/ navrhnout, nabídnout

proprietary /prəˈpraɪə.tri/ patentovaný

prospective /prəˈspek.tɪv/ předpokládaný, případný

prosthesis /ˈprɒs.θiː.sɪs/ **(pl. prostheses)** protetika, protéza, náhrada

prosthodontics /ˌprɒs.θəˈdɒnt.ɪks/ protetická stomatologie, protézy, specializace na zubní náhrady

protect /prəˈtekt/ chránit, ochrana, ochranný, bezpečnostní

protein /ˈprəʊ.tiːn/ protein, bílkovina

proton /ˈprəʊ.tɒn/ proton

prove /pruːv/ dokázat

provide /prəˈvaɪd/ poskytnout, připravit, poskytovat

provision /prəˈvɪʒ.ᵊn/ poskytnutí,
poskytování, zajištění (zabezpečení)
provisional /prəˈvɪʒ.ᵊn.ᵊl/ provizorní,
dočasný, prozatímní
provoke /prəˈvəʊk/ vyvolat
proximal /prɒˈk.sɪ.məl/ proximální,
bližší trupu, hlavě, středu
proximity /prɒkˈsɪm.ɪ.ti/ blízkost,
těsná blízkost
pseudonym /ˈsuː.də.nɪm/ pseudonym
psoriasis /səˈraɪə.sɪs/ psoriáza,
lupénka
psychiatric /ˌsaɪ.kiˈæt.rɪk/
psychiatrický, duševní
psychogenic /ˈsaɪ.kəˌdʒə.nɪk/
psychogenní, mentálního původu
psychological /ˌsaɪ.kᵊlˈɒdʒ.ɪ.kᵊl/
psychologický, duševní
psychosis /saɪˈkəʊ.sɪs/ psychóza,
porucha myšlení a jednání s
následným rozpadem osobnosti
psychosomatic /ˌsaɪ.kəʊ.səˈmæt.ɪk/
psychosomatický, týkající se vztahu
těla a mysli
ptosis /ˈtəu.sɪs/ ptóza, sklesnutí orgánu
pull /pʊl/ out /aʊt/ vytáhnout
pull /pʊl/ táhnout, trhat (i s kořenem),
zmítat
pulmonary /ˈpʊl.mə.nə.ri/
pulmonární, plicní
pulp /pʌlp/ dřeň, dužnina, vláknina
pulpal /pʌlp.ᵊl/ dřeňový
pulpectomy /pʌlˈpek.tə.mɪ/
pulpektomie, chirurg. vynětí dřeně
pulpitis /pʌlˈaɪ.tɪs/ pulpitida, zánět
zubní dřeně
pulse /pʌls/ impulz, puls
punch /pʌntʃ/ úder, propíchnout,
vytváření malých děr do tkáně
puncture /ˈpʌŋk.tʃəʳ/ punkce, vpich,
otvor
pure /pjʊəʳ/ čistý, pouhý

purple /ˈpɜː.pl̩/ fialový
purpose /ˈpɜː.pəs/ účel, záměr, mít v
úmyslu
pus /pʌs/ hnis
push /pʊʃ/ tlačit, pohánět
put /pʊt/ umístit (kam)
putty /ˈpʌt.i/ tmel (sklenářský), stmelit
pyelonephritis /ˌpaɪ.ə.lə.neˈfraɪ.tɪs/
pyelonefritida, současný zánět
ledvinné pánvičky a ledviny

Q

quadhelix /kwɒdˈhiː.lɪks/ čtvercová
šroubovice
qualitative /ˈkwɒl.ɪ.tə.tɪv/
kvalitativní, jakostní
quantitative /ˈkwɒn.tɪ.tə.tɪv/
kvantitativní (mnohostní)
quantity /ˈkwɒn.tɪ.ti/ množství
quartz /ˈkwɔːts/ krystal, křemen,
křemenný
questionnaire /ˌkwes.tʃəˈneəʳ/
dotazník

R

radial /ˈreɪ.di.əl/ radiální
radiate /ˈreɪ.di.eɪt/ vyzařovat
radiation /ˌreɪ.diˈeɪ.ʃᵊn/ radiace,
ozařovací, emise, záření, vyzařování
radicular /ræˈdɪk.jʊ.ləʳ/ kořenový
radio /ˈreɪ.di.əʊ/ rádio-
radiograph /reɪ.di.ə.grɑːf/
rentgenovat, rentgenový snímek
radiographic /ˌreɪ.diˈɒg.rə.fik/
rentgenový
radiography /ˌreɪ.diˈɒg.rə.fi/
radiografie
radio-opaque /ˈreɪ.di.əʊ.əʊˈpeɪk/
radiopakní, nepropustný,
nepropustný pro záření
radiotherapy /ˌreɪ.di.əʊˈθer.ə.pi/
radioterapie, léčba ozařováním

radius /ˈreɪ.di.əs/ radius, kost vřetenní, okruh, poloměr

raise /reɪz/ vytáhnout, zvýšit, zvýšení, zvednout, zřídit

rake /reɪk/ shrnovač

rampant /ˈræm.pᵊnt/ útočný, nekontrolovatelný

ramus /reɪ.məs/ rameno, větev

random /ˈræn.dəm/ namátkou

range /reɪndʒ/ rozsah, řada, rozmezí, roztřídit, seřadit

rapid /ˈræp.ɪd/ rychlý, prudký

rapidly /ˈræp.ɪd.li/ rychle

rare /reəʳ/ vzácný, zřídka

rarely /ˈreə.li/ zřídka

rat /ræt/ krysa

rate /reɪt/ poměr, rychlost

rather /ˈrɑː.ðəʳ/ **than** /ðən/ spíše než

rating /ˈreɪ.tɪŋ/ ohodnocení

ratio /ˈreɪ.ʃi.əʊ/ podíl, vzájemný poměr, vztah

reach /riːtʃ/ dosah, dosáhnout, rozpětí

reactionary /riˈæk.ʃᵊn.ᵊr.i/ reakční

reactivate /riˈæk.tɪ.veɪt/ reaktivovat, znovu aktivovat, oživit

readily /ˈred.ɪ.li/ pohotově, ihned

realise /ˈrɪə.laɪz/ uvědomit si, uvědomovat si, chápat

realm /relm/ doména, oblast

reamer /ˈriː.məʳ/ výstružník, rozšiřovač

reason /ˈriː.zᵊn/ důvod

reassess /ˌriː.əˈses/ přehodnotit

reassurance /ˌriː.əˈʃɔː.rənts/ opětovné ujištění, uklidnění, uklidňování, útěcha

reassure /ˌriː.əˈʃɔːʳ/ uklidňovat

reassuring /ˌriː.əˈʃɔː.rɪŋ/ uklidňování

recall /rɪˈkɔːl/ opětné pozvání pacienta, znovu zavolat, vzpomenout, přivést k vědomí

receive /rɪˈsiːv/ dostat, přijímat, obdržet, získat

recent /ˈriː.sᵊnt/ současný, poslední (nedávný)

receptionist /rɪˈsep.ʃᵊn.ɪst/ recepční, sestra (u příjmu pacientů)

receptor /rɪˈsep.təʳ/ příjemce, čidlo

recession /rɪˈseʃ.ᵊn/ odstoupení, ústup

reclining /rɪˈklaɪ.nɪŋ/ **chair** /tʃeəʳ/ sklápěcí křeslo

recognise /ˈrek.əg.naɪz/ rozpoznat, připustit, uznat

recognizable /ˈrek.əg.naɪ.zə.bl̩/ rozeznatelný, poznatelný

recommend /ˌrek.əˈmend/ doporučit

recommended /ˌrek.əˈmen.dɪd/ doporučený

record /ˈrek.ɔːd/ záznam

record /rɪˈkɔːd/ zaznamenat

recourse /rɪˈkɔːs/ pomoc, východisko, přístup

recover /rɪˈkʌv.ər/ objevit

recovery /rɪˈkʌv.ᵊr.i/ **position** /pəˈzɪʃ.ᵊn/ zotavovací poloha, stabilizovaná poloha

recovery /rɪˈkʌv.ᵊr.i/ zotavení, uzdravení

recurrence /rɪˈkʌr.ᵊnts/ rekurence, návrat, opětovný výskyt

recurrent /rɪˈkʌr.ᵊnt/ opakující se, recidivující

reduce /rɪˈdjuːs/ snížit, napravit, přemoct

reduction /rɪˈdʌk.ʃᵊn/ omezení, snížení, zmenšení, zmírnění, srovnání kosti, redukce

re-evaluate /riː.ɪˈvæl.ju.eɪt/ přehodnotit

refer /rɪˈfɜːr/ týkat se, odvolávat se, vztahovat se, poukázat, uvést, uvádět

reflect /rɪˈflekt/ odrážet (světlo), reflektovat, uvažovat, vyjadřovat, zrcadlit (se)

reflex /ˈriː.fleks/ reflex, výraz, odraz, přemítání

reflux /ˈriː.flʌks/ reflux, zpětné proudění

regain /rɪˈgeɪn/ znovu získat

regarding /rɪˈgɑː.dɪŋ/ týkající se, s ohledem na

regimen /ˈredʒ.ɪ.mən/ režim, životospráva

region /ˈriː.dʒ°n/ oblast (též správní), část, rozsah

regional /ˈriː.dʒ°n.°l/ týkající se dané oblasti, ohraničený

regionally /ˈriː.dʒ°n.°l.i/ regionálně

registration /ˌredʒ.ɪˈstreɪ.ʃ°n/ registrace, zápis, zaznamenávání

regular /ˈreg.jʊ.lə^r/ pravidelný

regularly /ˈreg.jʊ.lə.li/ pravidelně

regurgitation /rɪˌgɜː.dʒɪˈteɪ.ʃ°n/ opakované zvracení

rehabilitation /ˌriː.hə.bɪl.ɪˈteɪ.ʃ°n/ rehabilitace

reimplantation /ˌriːɪm.plɑːnˈteɪ.ʃ°n/ reimplantace, nahrazení odejmuté časti

reinforce /ˌriː.ɪnˈfɔːs/ posílit, vyztužit, zesílit, zpevnit

reinsert /riː.ɪnˈsɜːt/ znovu vložit

relapse /rɪˈlæps/ recidiva, úpadek, dostat recidivu

related /rɪˈleɪ.tɪd/ mající vztah, vztahující se k, spojený

relation /rɪˈleɪ.ʃ°n/ poměr (vztah)

relationship /rɪˈleɪ.ʃ°n.ʃɪp/ souvislost (vztah), příbuzenství, příbuznost, vzájemný poměr

relative /ˈrel.ə.tɪv/ poměrný, nikoli absolutní, příbuzný

relaxation /ˌriː.lækˈseɪ.ʃ°n/ uvolnění

relaxed /rɪˈlækst/ uvolněný, relaxovaný

release /rɪˈliːs/ uvolnit, pustit, spustit

relevant /ˈrel.ə.v°nt/ relevantní, příslušný

reliable /rɪˈlaɪə.bļ/ spolehlivý

relief /rɪˈliːf/ úleva

relieve /rɪˈliːv/ **pain** /peɪn/ ulevit bolesti

relieve /rɪˈliːv/ ulehčit, ulevit, vykrýt, zmírnit, zmírňovat

reline /riːˈlaɪn/ obložit, vyměnit obložení, podložit vnitřní stranu protézy

relining /riːˈlaɪn.ɪŋ/ obnova vnitřní strany protézy

reluctant /rɪˈlʌk.t°nt/ neochotný, váhavý

rely /rɪˈlaɪ/ **on** /ɒn/ spoléhat se na

remain /rɪˈmeɪn/ zbývat, zůstat, vytrvat

remainder /rɪˈmeɪn.də^r/ zbytek

remaining /rɪˈmeɪ.nɪŋ/ zbývající, zůstávající

remission /rɪˈmɪʃ.°n/ remise, dočasné vymizení projevů nemoci, úleva

remodel /ˌriːˈmɒd.əl/ modelovat znovu, přestavit, přemodelovat

removable /rɪˈmuː.və.bļ/ odstranitelný, pohyblivý, snímatelný, vyjímatelný

removal /rɪˈmuː.v°l/ vyjmutí, odstranění, přesun

remove /rɪˈmuːv/ odstranit, vyjmout

renal /ˈriː.n°l/ renální, ledvinový

render /ˈren.də^r/ poskytovat

renowned /rɪˈnaʊnd/ renomovaný, chvalně známý

repair /rɪˈpeə^r/ opravit, oprava

repeat /rɪˈpiːt/ opakovat, opakovaný, zažít znovu

repeated /rɪˈpiː.tɪd/ opakovaný, častý

repeatedly /rɪˈpiː.tɪd.li/ opakovaně

repetitive /rɪˈpet.ə.tɪv/ opakovaný, opakující se

replace /rɪˈpleɪs/ dát zpět, nahradit

replacement /rɪˈpleɪs.mənt/ náhrada, nahrazení, protéza, nové umístění, výměna (vadné součásti), vrácení, znovudosazení

replica /ˈrep.lɪ.kə/ replika, duplikát

replication /ˌrep.lɪˈkeɪ.ʃ°n/ replikace, reprodukce stejným způsobem

report /rɪˈpɔːt/ hlásit, ohlásit, oznámit, podat zprávu, udělat zápis

reposition /rɪ.pəˈzɪʃ.ən/ přemístit

reposition /rɪ.pəˈzɪʃ.ən/ repozice, nové upevnění, opětné přiložení

request /rɪˈkwest/ požadavek, žádost, požádání, prosba, žádat

require /rɪˈkwaɪəʳ/ nutně potřebovat, požádat, požadovat, chtít, být zapotřebí, vyžadovat

requirement /rɪˈkwaɪə.mənt/ požadavek, potřeba

rescue /ˈres.kjuː/ záchrana, záchranný, zachránit

rescuer /ˈres.kjuː.əʳ/ zachránce, záchranář, záchranný přístroj

residual /rɪˈzɪd.ju.əl/ zbytkový, zbývající, zbytek

resin /ˈrez.ɪn/ pryskyřice

resin /ˈrez.ɪn/ **composite** /ˈkɒm.pə.zɪt/ kompozitní pryskyřice

resin-bonded /ˈrez.ɪn.bɒnd.ɪd/ pojený pryskyřicí

resist /rɪˈzɪst/ odolat, odolávat, vydržet

resistance /rɪˈzɪs.t°nts/ odolnost, stálost, vzdor, odpor, pevnost

resonance /ˈrez.°n.ənts/ rezonance

resorb /rɪˈzɔːb/ vstřebat se

resorption /rɪˈsɔːp.ʃ°n/ chřadnutí

resorption /rɪˈsɔːp.ʃən/ rozpuštění, vstřebání

respectively /rɪˈspek.tɪv.li/ co se každého týče

respiratory /rɪˈspɪr.ə.tri/ **rate** /reɪt/ rytmus dýchání

respiratory /rɪˈspɪr.ə.tri/ respirační, dýchací

respiratory rɪˈspɪr.ə.tri/ **arrest** / əˈrest/ zástava dechu

respond /rɪˈspɒnd/ reagovat (odpovídat)

response /rɪˈspɒnts/ reakce

responsibility /rɪˌspɒnt.sɪˈbɪl.ɪ.ti/ zodpovědnost, spolehlivost

responsible /rɪˈspɒnt.sɪ.bl̩/ odpovědný, významný, rozvážný

responsiveness /rɪˈspɒnt.sɪv.nəs/ schopnost reagovat na podněty, vnímavost

rest /rest/ zbytek

resting /ˈrest.ɪŋ/ klidový

restoration /ˌres.t°rˈeɪ.ʃ°n/ obnovení, zotavení, uzdravení, obnova, oprava, náhrada, výplň, vyplnění

restorative /rɪˈstɒr.ə.tɪv/ obnovený, opravený, konzervační, posilňující, obnovující

restore /rɪˈstɔːʳ/ obnovit, opravit, navrátit do původního stavu, rekonstruovat, uzdravit

restraint /rɪˈstreɪnt/ omezování, bránění

restrict /rɪˈstrɪkt/ omezit

restricted /rɪˈstrɪk.tɪd/ omezený

restrictive /rɪˈstrɪk.tɪv/ omezující

result /rɪˈzʌlt/ být následkem, mít za následek

resultant /rɪˈzʌl.t°nt/ z toho vyplývající (výsledný)

resuscitation /rɪˌsʌs.ɪˈteɪ.ʃ°n/ resuscitace, křísení, oživení

retain /rɪˈteɪn/ ponechat, zachytit, zadržet, zachovat

retained /rɪˈteɪnd/ ponechaný, zadržený

retainer /rɪˈteɪ.nəʳ/ napínač, držák, retenční přístroj, úchytka

retch /retʃ/ říhat, mít mimovolní pocit na zvracení

retention /rɪˈten.tʃən/ paměť

retention /rɪˈten.tʃən/ retence (zubů), upevnění, zadržení, uchování

retention /rɪˈten.tʃən/ nahromadění, zácpa

retentive /rɪˈten.tɪv/ retenční, nepropouštějící, zadržující

retract /rɪˈtrækt/ odtáhnout, stáhnout, stáhnout zpět

retraction /rɪˈtræk.ʃən/ stahování, smršťování

retractor /rɪˈtræk.təʳ/ retraktor, hák na rány, háček, držák

retrieve /rɪˈtriːv/ vrátit, získat zpět

retrocline /ˌret.rəʊ ˈklaɪn/ naklonit dozadu

retrograde /ˈret.rəʊ.greɪd/ retrográdní, obrácený, odvrácený, zpětný

retrosternal /ˌret.rəˈstɔː.nᵊl/ retrosternální, umístěný za hrudní kostí

retruded /rɪˈtruː.dɪd/ ustouplý zpět

retry /ˌriːˈtraɪ/ nový pokus, zkoušet znova

return /rɪˈtɜːn/ návrat

reuse /ˌriːˈjuːz/ znovu použít, opakované použití

reveal /rɪˈviːl/ odhalit

reverse /rɪˈvɜːs/ obrácený

reversible /rɪˈvɜː.sᵊ.bl̩/ reverzibilní, vratný

review /rɪˈvjuː/ překontrolování, přehled, prohlédnout opět, zhodnotit, konfrontovat

revise /rɪˈvaɪz/ zopakovat

revive /rɪˈvaɪv/ oživit

revolution /ˌrev.əˈluː.ʃən/ otáčka

reward /rɪˈwɔːd/ odměna

rheumatic /ruːˈmæt.ɪk/ **fever** /ˈfiː.vəʳ/ revmatická horečka

rheumatoid arthritis /ˌruː.mə.tɔɪd. ɑːˈθraɪ.tɪs/ kloubní revmatismus

rhinorrhoea /ˌraɪ.nəˈriː.ə/ rinorea, vodnatý výtok z nosu

rib /rɪb/ **cage** /keɪdʒ/ hrudní koš

ridge /rɪdʒ/ okraj, lišta, rýha, hřeben, vyvýšenina, okraj

right-angle /raɪt.ˈæŋ.gl̩/ pravý úhel

rigid /ˈrɪdʒ.ɪd/ rigidní, pevný, neohebný, tuhý, strnulý

rigidity /rɪˈdʒɪd.ɪ.ti/ strnulost, tuhost, tvrdost, ztuhlost

rim /rɪm/ lem, hrana, okraj, obroučka

ring /rɪŋ/ prsten

ring /rɪŋ/ zvonit

rinse /rɪnts/ vypláchnout, propláchnout, proprat

rise /raɪz/ vzestup, zdvihat se (stoupat)

risk /rɪsk/ riziko

rodent /ˈrəʊ.dᵊnt/ **ulcer** /ˈʌl.səʳ/ hlodavý vřed

roll /rəʊl/ svitek

rongeur /rɒːnˈʒeəʳ/ štípací kleště

root /ruːt/ **apex** /ˈeɪ.peks/ hrot kořene

root /ruːt/ **canal** /kəˈnæl/ kořenový kanálek

root /ruːt/ **face** /feɪs/ kořenová fréza

root /ruːt/ kořen

root /ruːt/ **planing** /pleɪn.ɪŋ/ vyhlazení stěn kořene

rose /rəʊz/ růže

rose-head /rəʊz.hed/ **bur** /bɜːr/ vrtáček ve tvaru špičatého poupětě

rotary /ˈrəʊ.tᵊr.i/ otočný, otáčivý, rotační

rotation /rəʊ ˈteɪ.ʃən/ rotace, otočení

roughen /ˈrʌf.ᵊn/ zdrsnit

round /raʊnd/ **bur** /bɜːr/ kulatý vrtáček

rounded /ˈraʊn.dɪd/ zakulacený

rounder /ˈraʊn.dəʳ/ zaoblovací nástroj

rouse /raʊz/ vzbudit

route /ruːt/ cesta

routine /ruːˈtiːn/ rutina, běžná praxe, pravidelný postup, obvyklý, rutinní

routinely /ruːˈtiːn.li/ rutinně, běžně

rub /rʌb/ dřít, drhnout

rubber /ˈrʌb.əʳ/ dam /dæm/ gumová blána

rubber /ˈrʌb.əʳ/ guma

ruler /ˈruː.ləʳ/ měřítko, pravítko

run /rʌn/ under /ˈʌn.dəʳ/ cold /kəʊld/ tap /tæp/ nechat pod studenou tekoucí vodou

runny /ˈrʌn.i/ tekutý

rupture /ˈrʌp.tʃəʳ/ ruptura, protržení, zlomení, kýla, výhřez

S

sachet /ˈsæʃ.eɪ/ sáček

saddle /ˈsæd.l̩/ sedlo

safe /seɪf/ bezpečný, důvěryhodný

safely /ˈseɪ.fli/ bezpečně

safety /ˈseɪf.ti/ bezpečnostní

safety /ˈseɪf.ti/ glasses /glɑː.sɪz/ bezpečnostní brýle, ochranné brýle

saline /ˈseɪ.laɪn/ fyziologický roztok

saliva /səˈlaɪ.və/ ejector /ɪːˈdʒekt.əʳ/ ejektor, vývěva, odsavač slin

saliva /səˈlaɪ.və/ sliny

salivary /səˈlaɪ.vᵊr.i/ gland /glænd/ slinná žláza

salt /sɒlt/ sůl

saltwater /sɒlt.ˈwɔː.təʳ/ slaná voda

same /seɪm/ tentýž, stejný

sample /ˈsɑːm.pl̩/ vzorek

sand /sænd/ písek

sandbag /ˈsænd.bæg/ pytel písku na ochranu

sandblast /ˈsænd.blɑːst/ pískovat

sarcoma /sɑːˈkəʊ.mə/ sarkom, zhoubný nádor pojivových tkání

satisfactory /ˌsæt.ɪsˈfæk.tᵊr.i/ uspokojivý, splňující všechny podmínky

satisfied /ˈsæt.ɪs.faɪd/ spokojený

saturation /ˌsæt.jʊˈreɪ.ʃᵊn/ saturace (nasycení)

save /seɪv/ zachránit

scald /skɔːld/ opařenina

scale /skeɪl/ škála (stupnice), váha (na vážení)

scale /skeɪl/ zubní kámen, odstranit zubní kámen

scaler /skeɪl.əʳ/ škrabka

scalloped /ˈskɒl.əpd/ vroubkovaný, zoubkovaný

scalpel /ˈskæl.pᵊl/ blade /bleɪd/ čepelka skalpelu

scalpel /ˈskæl.pᵊl/ skalpel

scan /skæn/ skenovat, postupně snímat (po řádcích)

scar /skɑːʳ/ jizva

scenario /sɪˈnɑː.ri.əʊ/ scénář, postup

schedule /ˈʃed.juːl/ rozvrh, naplánovat, tabulka, cedule

scheme /skiːm/ nákres, plán, projekt, program

scissors /ˈsɪz.əz/ nůžky, kleštičky

sclera /ˈsklɪə.rə/ skléra, oční bělmo

scope /skəʊp/ rozsah

scrape /skreɪp/ oškrabat, škrabat

screening /ˈskriː.nɪŋ/ podrobné prohlížení

screw /skruː/ spirála, šroubek, šroubovat

scrub /skrʌb/ drhnout (kartáčem), vydrhnout

seal /siːl/ off /ɒf/ zablokovat, zatarasit

seal /siːl/ plomba, uzávěr, utěsnění, uzavřít těsně, zaplombovat

sealant /ˈsiː.lənt/ pečetidlo, tmel,
těsnicí materiál

sealed /siːld/ utěsněný, hermeticky
uzavřený, zaplombovaný

sealer /ˈsiː.ləʳ/ pečetidlo, prostředek
pro utěsnění

search /sɜːtʃ/ for /fɔːʳ/ hledat

seat /siːt/ dosedací plocha, sedadlo,
dosedat, umístit, usadit

secondary /ˈsek.ən.dri/ sekundární
(druhotný), závislý-porucha

section /ˈsek.ʃ°n/ část, úsek, průřez,
odříznutí, pitva

sectioning /ˈsek.ʃ°n.ɪŋ/ provádění řezů

sedate /sɪˈdeɪt/ zklidnit

sedation /sɪˈdeɪ.ʃ°n/ uklidňující lék,
utišení

sedative /ˈsed.ə.tɪv/ sedativum,
uklidňující prostředek, uklidňující,
bolesti utišující lék

seek /siːk/ vyhledávat, požadovat,
pátrat

seep /siːp/ prosakovat

segment /ˈseg.mənt/ úsek, segment

seizure /ˈsiː.ʒəʳ/ uchopení, záchvat
(nemoci), záchvatový

selection /sɪˈlek.ʃ°n/ výběr, volba

selective /sɪˈlek.tɪv/ výběrový

self-/self/ sebe-, sobě

self-esteem /ˌself.ɪˈstiːm/ sebe-ocenění

self-healing /self.ˈhiː.lɪŋ/
samoregenerační

self-inflicted /ˌself.ɪnˈflɪk.tɪd/
sebeporanění, sebepoškození

self-limiting /self.ˈlɪm.ɪ.tɪŋ/ spontánně
mizející

semi-/sem.i-/ polo-

semifluid /sem.i.ˈfluː.ɪd/ polotekutý

semipermanent /sem.i.ˈpɜː.mə.nənt/
semipermanentní, polotrvalý

sensation /senˈseɪ.ʃ°n/ pocit, cit, dojem,
vjem, vnímání, smyslové vnímání

sensibility /ˌsent.sɪˈbɪl.ɪ.ti/ citlivost

sensitive /ˈsent.sɪ.tɪv/ citlivý (na
něco), vnímavý, choulostivý

sensitivity /ˌsent.sɪˈtɪv.ɪ.ti/ senzitivita,
citlivost, vnímavost

sensor /ˈsent.səʳ/ snímač

sensory /ˈsent.s°r.i/ disability /
ˌdɪs.əˈbɪl.ɪ.ti/ smyslové postižení

sensory /ˈsent.s°r.i/ smyslový

separate /ˈsep.°r.aɪt/ oddělit,
oddělovat, odtrhnout

separate /ˈsep.°r.ət/ oddělený

sequence /ˈsiː.kwənts/ následnost,
pořadí, postup

series /ˈsɪə.riːz/ sada, sled, skupina

serious /ˈsɪə.ri.əs/ opravdový (vážný)

seriousness /ˈsɪə.ri.ə.snəs/ vážnost,
závažnost, nebezpečnost

seropositive /ˌsɪ.ə.rəˈpɒz.ə.tɪv/
séropozitivní, obsahující sérové
protilátky

set /set/ nastavit, sestavit, upravit,
vsadit, zasadit

set /set/ out /aʊt/ stanovit, vytyčovat,
vyložit (na prodej)

set /set/ sada (souprava), stanovený

set /set/ umístění, tuhnutí

set /set/ určit, stanovit

setback /ˈset.bæk/ zhoršení situace,
zhoršení zdravotního stavu,
neúspěch

setting /ˈset.ɪŋ/ time /taɪm/ doba
tuhnutí

setting /ˈset.ɪŋ/ tuhnutí, nasazení,
nastavení, seřízení

severe /sɪˈvɪəʳ/ těžký, vážný, prudký
(bolest ap.), závažný

severity /sɪˈver.ɪ.ti/ krutost, vážnost,
útrapy, potíže

sexual /ˈsek.sjʊəl/ characteristic /
ˌkær.ɪk.təˈrɪs.tɪk/ pohlavní znak

sexually /ˈsek.sjʊə.li/ pohlavně

shade /ʃeɪd/ odstín

shake /ʃeɪk/ třást, otřes (otřesení), potřesení (též hlavou)

shape /ʃeɪp/ tvar, formovat, tvarovat

shaped /ʃeɪpt/ ve tvaru, tvarovaný, zformovaný

sharp /ʃɑːp/ ostrý, ostrý předmět, prudký (nápor), ostrý (dobře řezající)

sharpness /ˈʃɑːp.nəs/ ostrost

shatter /ˈʃæt.əʳ/ roztříštit se

shattered /ˈʃæt.əd/ zničený, rozpadlý, rozdrcený

shaving /ˈʃeɪ.vɪŋ/ holení

shears /ʃɪəz/ kleště, nůžky (velké)

sheet /ʃiːt/ arch, tenká deska, výkaz

shelf life /ʃelf.laɪf/ záruční doba

shell /ʃel/ skořápka

shield /ʃiːld/ ochrana (přen.), ochranný štít

shifting /ˈʃɪf.tɪŋ/ přesouvání, posunování, přeřaďování

shine /ʃaɪn/ zářit, lesknout se

shiny /ˈʃaɪ.ni/ lesklý, jasný

shooting /ˈʃuː.tɪŋ/ vystřelující

shorten /ˈʃɔː.tⁿn/ zkrátit

shoulder /ˈʃəʊl.dəʳ/ blade /bleɪd/ lopatka (rameno)

shout /ʃaʊt/ volat, křičet

shouting /ˈʃaʊ.tɪŋ/ zvolání, zavolání, křik

shrink /ʃrɪŋk/ srážet se, smršťovat

shrinkage /ˈʃrɪŋ.kɪdʒ/ smrštění, srážení, ztráta na objemu

sialadenitis /ˈsaɪəlˌædəˈnʌɪ.tis/ sialoadenitida, zánět slinné žlázy

sialosis /ˌsaɪəˈləʊ.sɪs/ salivace, slinění

sibling /ˈsɪb.lɪŋ/ vrstevník, sourozenec

sickle /ˈsɪk.l̩/ srpek

sickness /ˈsɪk.nəs/ nevolnost

side /saɪd/ effect /ɪˈfekt/ vedlejší účinek

side /saɪd/ strana, vedlejší

sideropenia /ˌsɪd.ə.rəˈpiː.nɪ.ə/ sideropenie, nedostatek železa v krvi

sideways /ˈsaɪd.weɪz/ stranou

sigh /saɪ/ vzdychat, naříkat

sight /saɪt/ pohled, podívaná, uvidět

sign /saɪn/ znak, příznak, znamení, podpis

signature /ˈsɪg.nɪ.tʃəʳ/ podpis, podepsání

significance /sɪgˈnɪf.ɪ.kənts/ význam, hodnota

significant /sɪgˈnɪf.ɪ.kənt/ důležitý, význačný, významný

significantly /sɪgˈnɪf.ɪ.kənt.li/ významně, závažně

silicone /ˈsɪl.ɪ.kəʊn/ silikon

similar /ˈsɪm.ɪ.lər/ podobný

similarly /ˈsɪm.ɪ.lə.li/ podobně

simple /ˈsɪm.pl̩/ fracture /ˈfræk.tʃəʳ/ zavřená zlomenina

simple /ˈsɪm.pl̩/ jednoduchý, prostý

singing /ˈsɪŋ.ɪŋ/ zpívání

single /ˈsɪŋ.gl̩/ jediný, jednotlivý, samostatný

single-stage /ˈsɪŋ.gl̩.steɪdʒ/ jednostupňový

singly /ˈsɪŋ.gli/ po jednom, jednotlivě

sink /sɪŋk/ dřez

sinus /ˈsaɪ.nəs/ dutina

site /saɪt/ místo, poloha, umístění, být umístěn

situs /saɪ.təs/ místo, poloha

size /saɪz/ velikost

skeletal /ˈskel.ɪ.tⁿl/ kosterní

skeletal /ˈskel.ɪ.tⁿl/ pattern /ˈpæt.ən/ kosterní typ

skeleton /ˈskel.ɪ.tⁿn/ kostra

skill /skɪl/ dovednost, schopnost, dovednost

skin /skɪn/ kůže (pokožka), pokrýt se kůží (zahojit se)

skull /skʌl/ lebka

slab /slæb/ destička

slap /slæp/ plácnout, plesknutí

sleep /sliːp/ loss /lɒs/ nespavost

slice /slaɪs/ seškrábnout, krájet na plátky

slide /slaɪd/ sklouznout, sjet

slight /slaɪt/ nepatrný, mírný, tenký, lehký

slightly /ˈslaɪt.li/ mírně, trochu, slabě

slip /slɪp/ prokluzovat, sklouznout, upadnout

slope /sləʊp/ sklánět se, naklonění

sloth /sləʊθ/ loudavost, nemotornost

slow /sləʊ/ down /daʊn/ zpomalovat

slow /sləʊ/ pomalý, zvolna, zpomalit

slow-speed /sləʊ.spiːd/ pomalý

slump /slʌmp/ pokles, propadnout, sesunout

slurred /slɜːʳd/ nezřetelný

smear /smɪəʳ/ nepatrné množství, skvrna, šmouha, namazat

smell /smel/ čich, cítit (čichem), být cítit

smile /smaɪl/ usmívat se

smoking /ˈsməʊ.kɪŋ/ kouření

smooth /smuːð/ jemný, hladký, vyhladit

snack /snæk/ lehké jídlo, přesnídávka

snack /snæk/ svačit, pojídat malá jídla

snore /snɔːʳ/ chrápat

snuff /snʌf/ šňupat (tabák), čichat, nadýchnutí nosem

soak /səʊk/ up /ʌp/ nasakovat, vstřebat, vsáknout se

soaked /səʊkt/ prosáknutý

social /ˈsəʊ.ʃəl/ history /ˈhɪs.tər.i/ sociální anamnéza

socialise /ˈsəʊ.ʃəl.aɪz/ socializovat, stýkat se (společensky)

socket /ˈsɒk.ɪt/ jamka, dutina, ložisko, zubní lůžko, zásuvka, zdířka

sodium /ˈsəʊ.di.əm/ hypochlorite / haɪ.pəʊˈklɔː.raɪt/ chlornan sodný

soft /sɒft/ tissue /ˈtɪʃ.uː/, /ˈtɪs.juː/ měkká tkáň

soften /ˈsɒf.ən/ změkčit, sejmout

solid /ˈsɒl.ɪd/ pevný, tuhá hmota

solubility /ˌsɒl.jʊˈbɪl.ɪ.ti/ rozpustnost, tavitelnost

solution /səˈluː.ʃən/ řešení, roztok, rozpuštění

soon /suːn/ dříve, brzy

sore /sɔːʳ/ bolavý

soreness /ˈsɔː.nəs/ bolestivost

sound /saʊnd/ pořádný, seriózní, zdravý

sound /saʊnd/ sonda

sound /saʊnd/ zvuk, znít

source /sɔːs/ zdroj

space /speɪs/ maintainer /meɪnˈteɪn.əʳ/ mezerník

space /speɪs/ prostor, prázdné místo, volný prostor, mezera, vzdálenost

span /spæn/ šíře, rozpětí, oblouk

spark /spɑːk/ erosion /ɪˈrəʊ.ʒən/ elektrojiskrové obrábění

spasm /ˈspæz.əm/ křeč

spatula /ˈspæt.jʊ.lə/ lopatička, třecí lopatka, špachtle, stěrka

spatulation /ˌspæt.jəˈleɪ.ʃən/ míchání, tření

speaking /ˈspiː.kɪŋ/ mluvení

specialised /ˈspeʃ.əl.aɪzd/ specializovaný

species /ˈspiː.ʃiːz/ druhy

specimen /ˈspes.ə.mɪn/ zkušební vzorek

speck /spek/ zrníčko

speckled /ˈspek.l̩d/ skvrnitý (flíčky)

spectacles /ˈspek.tɪ.kl̩z/ brýle (dioptrické)

speech /spiːtʃ/ řeč

speed /spiːd/ rychlost

sphenopalatine /ˌsfiːn.əˈpæl.ə.taɪn/ sfenopalatální, týkající se kosti klínové a patrové sphygmomanometer / sfɪg.məʊ.mænˈɒm.ɪ.təʳ/ sfygmomanometr, tlakoměr

spicule /ˈspɪk.juːl/ úlomek, štěpina

spicy /ˈspaɪ.si/ kořeněný

spillage /ˈspɪl.ɪdʒ/ rozlité (rozsypané) množství

spina bifida /ˌspaɪ.nəˈbɪf.ɪ.də/ zadní rozštěp páteře, obratle

spine /spaɪn/ páteř

spiral /ˈspaɪə.rᵊl/ spirálovitý

spiral /ˈspaɪə.rᵊl/ točit se

spit /spɪt/ plivat, odplivnout, vyplivnout

splint /splɪnt/ dlaha, klínek, štěpina

split /splɪt/ rozštěpit, roztrhnout

spontaneous /spɒnˈteɪ.ni.əs/ spontánní, samovolný

spontaneously /spɒnˈteɪ.ni.ə.sli/ spontánně, samovolně

spoon /spuːn/ excavator / ˈek.skə.veɪ.təʳ/ exkavační lžička

spoon /spuːn/ lžíce, lopatka

spot /spɒt/ tečka, skvrna, kapka

spotted /ˈspɒt.ɪd/ spatřený

spray /spreɪ/ rozprašovat, rozšířit, šíření

spreader /spred.əʳ/ cpátko pro kořenové kanálky

spring /sprɪŋ/ pero, pružina

spring /sprɪŋ/ tryskat, pramen

spun /spʌn/ roztočen, vtlačen

spurt /spɜːt/ tryskat, vytrysknout

sputum /ˈspjuː.təm/ sputum, výměšek dýchacího ústrojí

squamous /skweɪ.məs/ cell /sel/ plochá (dlaždicová) buňka

square /skweəʳ/ čtverec

squash /skwɒʃ/ rozmačkat, kašovitá hmota

squeeze /skwiːz/ mačkat, protlačit, stisknout, stlačit, vymačkat

stabbing /ˈstæb.ɪŋ/ bodnutí, očkovat vpichem, cukavý

stability /stəˈbɪl.ɪ.ti/ stabilita

stabilization /ˌsteɪ.bɪ.lɑ ɪˈzeɪ.ʃᵊn/ stabilizace (ustálení)

stable /ˈsteɪ.bḷ/ stabilní, stálý

staff /stɑːf/ zaměstnanci, vybavit personálem

stage /steɪdʒ/ etapa, stupeň, stádium (období)

staging /ˈsteɪ.dʒɪŋ/ představení, rozdělování do stupňů

stagnation /stægˈneɪ.ʃᵊn/ stagnace, váznutí, hniloba

stain /steɪn/ kaz, vada

stainless /ˌsteɪn.ləs/ nerezavící

stainless steel /ˌsteɪn.ləsˈstiːl/ nerezavějící ocel

standard /ˈstæn.dəd/ norma, pravidlo (určitý poměr), úroveň

stare /steəʳ/ zírat

starved /stɑːvd/ hladový

state /steɪt/ prohlásit

state /steɪt/ status, stav, skupenství, okolnosti

status /ˈsteɪ.təs/ status (stav), životní úroveň, společenské postavení

steadily /ˈsted.ɪ.li/ neustále, pevně

steady /ˈsted.i/ trvalý, pevný

steam /stiːm/ pára

steatorrhoea /ˌstɪ.ə.təˈriː.ə/ steatorea, tuková stolice

steel /stiːl/ ocel

step /step/ krok

sterile /ˈster.aɪl/ sterilní

sterilise /ˈster.ɪ.laɪz/ sterilizovat

steriliser /ˈster.ᵊl.aɪz.əʳ/ sterilizační zařízení

sternum /ˈstɜː.nəm/ sternum, hrudní kost

steroid /ˈste.rɔɪd/, /ˈstɪər.ɔɪd/ steroid, organická látka, např. hormony pohlavní nebo kůry nadledvin

stethoscope /ˈsteθ.ə.skəʊp/ stetoskop, fonendoskop

stick /stɪk/ přilepit

stick /stɪk/ tyčinka

sticker /ˈstɪk.əʳ/ štítek, cedulka

stickiness /ˈstɪk.ɪ.nəs/ soudržnost, lepivost

sticking plaster /ˈstɪk.ɪŋ ˌplɑː.stəʳ/ lepicí náplast

sticky /ˈstɪk.i/ lepkavý

stiff /stɪf/ tuhý

stiffly /ˈstɪf.li/ ztuha

stiffness /ˈstɪf.nəs/ strnulost, ztuhnutí

stimulant /ˈstɪm.jʊ.lənt/ povzbuzující prostředek

stimulate /ˈstɪm.jʊ.leɪt/ stimulovat, podněcovat

stimulation /ˌstɪm.jʊˈleɪ.ʃ°n/ podnět, povzbuzení, podráždění (svalů, nervů)

stimulus /ˈstɪm.jʊ.ləs/ (pl. stimuli) podnět

stippled /ˈstɪp.l̩d/ dolíčkovaný, tečkovaný

stippling /ˈstɪp.lɪŋ/ tečkování, dolíčkování

stitch /stɪtʃ/ **cutter** /kʌt.əʳ/ nůžky na stehy

stomatitis /ˌstəʊ.məˈtaɪ.tɪs/ stomatitida, zánět sliznice ústní dutiny

stone /stəʊn/ kámen

stool /stuːl/ sedačka

stool /stuːl/ stolice (vyprazdňování střev)

store /stɔːʳ/ skladovat, uložit, zásoba, materiál

straight /streɪt/ přímo, přímý, rovný

straight-bladed /streɪt.bleɪd.ɪd/ s rovnou čepelí

strain /streɪn/ napětí, napnout, usilovat, námaha

streak /striːk/ tvořit proužky, pruhovat, čmouha

stream /striːm/ běh, chod, příval, dělit, plynout

strength /streŋθ/ síla (moc), stabilita, silná stránka, houževnatost, mez pevnosti

Streptococcus /ˌstrep.təˈkɒk.əs/ (pl. streptococci) streptokok

stress /stres/ namáhat, tlačit, zdůraznit

stress /stres/ stres, nepohoda, tlak, stlačení, napětí, namáhání

string /strɪŋ/ provázek, zde: pramének

strip /strɪp/ pásek, proužek, plátek

stroke /strəʊk/ mrtvice

stroke /strəʊk/ pohladit

stroke /strəʊk/ úder, bití (pulsu), rána

strong /strɒŋ/ silný (mocný), silně

structural /ˈstrʌk.tʃ°r.°l/ strukturální

stuck /stʌk/ přilepen

study /ˈstʌd.i/ rozbor, studijní

subject /ˈsʌb.dʒekt/ předmět

subjective /ˈsʌb.dʒek.tɪv/ subjektivní (osobní)

sublining /sʌb.ˈlaɪ.nɪŋ/ podložení

subluxation /ˌsʌb.lʌkˈseɪ.ʃ°n/ subluxace, neúplné vykloubení

submit /səbˈmɪt/ předložit

subperiosteal /sʌbˌper.ɪˈɒs.ti.əl/ subperiostální, ležící pod okosticí

subsequent /ˈsʌb.sɪ.kwənt/ pozdější, následující

subsequently /ˈsʌb.sɪ.kwənt.li/ následovně, postupně, později

substance /ˈsʌb.st°nɪs/ látka

substitute /ˈsʌb.stɪ.tjuːt/ nahradit, zastupovat, náhražka

success /səkˈses/ úspěch

suck /sʌk/ cucat, sát

suction /ˈsʌk.ʃən/ odsávání, nasávání (vzduchu)

suction /ˈsʌk.ʃən/ **tip** /tɪp/ sací špička

sudden /ˈsʌd.ən/ náhlý

suffer /ˈsʌf.əʳ/ **from** /frɒm/ trpět něčím

suffer /ˈsʌf.əʳ/ trpět, utrpět, být poškozen

sufferer /ˈsʌf.ᵊr.ᵊr/ trpící

sufficient /səˈfɪʃ.ᵊnt/ dostatečný, přiměřený

sufficiently /səˈfɪʃ.ᵊnt.li/ dostatečně

sugar /ˈʃʊg.əʳ/ cukr

suggestion /səˈdʒes.tʃᵊn/ sugesce (vnuknutí)

suicidal /ˌsuː.ɪˈsaɪ.dᵊl/ **idea** /aɪˈdɪə/ sebevražedná myšlenka

suitable /ˈsjuː.tə.bl̩/ vhodný, přiměřený

suited /ˈsjuː.tɪd/ **to** /tʊ/ vhodný k

sulcus /sʌl.kəs/ **(pl: sulci)** rýha, sulkus

sulphate /ˈsʌl.feɪt/ sulfát, síran, kyselina sírová

summon /ˈsʌm.ən/ zavolat, přivolat

sunlight /ˈsʌn.laɪt/ sluneční světlo

super /ˈsuː.pəʳ/ extra, výborný

superb /suːˈpɜːb/ znamenitý

superficial /ˌsuː.pəˈfɪʃ.ᵊl/ povrchový

supernumerary /ˌsuː.pəˈnjuː.mᵊr.ᵊr.i/ nadpočetný

supervise /ˈsuː.pə.vaɪz/ dohlížet

supine /ˈsuː.paɪn/ ležící naznak, ležící tváří vzhůru, klidný

supplement /ˈsʌp.lɪ.mənt/ doplněk

supply /səˈplaɪ/ dodávat, dodání, zásobovat, zásoba

support /səˈpɔːt/ podpora, podpírat

supportive /səˈpɔː.tɪv/ **surgery** /ˈsɜː.dʒᵊr.i/ podpůrný chirurgický zákrok

surface /ˈsɜː.fɪs/ povrch, plocha, hladina, stěna, opracovat povrch

surgeon /ˈsɜː.dʒᵊn/ praktický lékař, chirurg

surgery /ˈsɜː.dʒᵊr.i/ chirurgie, chirurgický zákrok, operace

surgery /ˈsɜː.dʒᵊr.i/ ordinace, ošetřovna

surgical /ˈsɜː.dʒɪ.kᵊl/ chirurgický, pooperační

surgical /ˈsɜː.dʒɪ.kᵊl/ **site** /saɪt/ operační místo

surgically /ˈsɜː.dʒɪ.kli/ chirurgicky

surpass /səˈpɑːs/ překonat

surround /səˈraʊnd/ obklopit, okraj

surrounding /səˈraʊn.dɪŋ/ obklopující, okolní, sousední, sousední tkáň

surroundings /səˈraʊn.dɪŋz/ okolí

susceptibility /səˌsep.tɪˈbɪl.ɪ.ti/ susceptibilita, náchylnost, citlivost, vnímavost

susceptible /səˈsep.tɪ.bl̩/ náchylný k

suspected /səˈspek.tɪd/ suspektní, podezřelý, předpokládaný

suspicion /səˈspɪʃ.ᵊn/ podezření

sustain /səˈsteɪn/ utrpět

sustained /səˈsteɪnd/ utrpěný, vytrvalý

suture /ˈsuː.tʃəʳ/ **end** /end/ koneček stehů

suture /ˈsuː.tʃəʳ/ **needle** /ˈniː.dl̩/ šicí jehla s vláknem

suture /ˈsuː.tʃəʳ/ **removal** /rɪˈmuː.vᵊl/ odstranění stehů

suture /ˈsuː.tʃəʳ/ sutura, šev, steh, sešití rány

swab /swɒb/ vata na špejli, vysušit tamponem

swallow /ˈswɒl.əʊ/ polykat, pozřít, hlt

sweat /swet/ potit se, pot

sweaty /ˈswet.i/ propocený, opocený

sweep /swiːp/ odstranit, vymést

sweetener /ˈswiː.t.nəʳ/ umělé sladidlo

sweets /swiːts/ sladkosti

swelling /ˈswel.ɪŋ/ otok, edém, nádor, boule

swill /swɪl/ **out** /aʊt/ spláchnout, vymýt

swing /swɪŋ/ rozkývat, houpat

swollen /ˈswəʊ.lən/ oteklý, zduřený

sympathetic /ˌsɪm.pəˈθet.ɪk/ sympatický, účastný (soucitný)

symptom /ˈsɪmp.təm/ symptom

syndrome /ˈsɪn.drəʊ m/ syndrom, příznak

synergistic /ˌsɪn.əːˈdʒi.stik/ synergistický, souhlasně působící

syphilis /ˈsɪf.ɪ.lɪs/ syfilis (příjice)

syringe /sɪˈrɪndʒ/ injekční stříkačka, vstříknout, injekční

system /ˈsɪs.təm/ systém

systemic /sɪˈstem.ɪk/ systemický, systémový

systolic /sɪs.tʊl.ɪk/ systolický

T

tablet /ˈtæb.lət/ tabletka

tactile /ˈtæk.taɪl/ taktilní, dotekový

tailored /ˈteɪ.ləd/ upravený na míru

take /teɪk/ **account** /əˈkaʊnt/ **of** /əv/ počítat s (čím), přihlížet (k)

take /teɪk/ brát

take /teɪk/ **care** /keəʳ/ dávat pozor, pečovat

take /teɪk/ **into** /ˈɪn.tuː/ **account** /əˈkaʊnt/ vzít v úvahu

take /teɪk/ **precedence** /ˈpres.ɪ.dⁿnts/ mít přednost

take /teɪk/ **pulse** /pʌls/ měřit puls

take /teɪk/ **time** /taɪm/ dát si na čas, využít času

take /teɪk/ **up** /ʌp/ zvednout, nabrat, nasát, upevnit

take /teɪk/ vzít, brát

take /teɪk/ **over**/ˈəʊ.vəʳ/ převzetí, přijmout

talk /tɔːk/ hovor, mluvit

tangential /tænˈdʒen.tʃⁿl/ tangenciální, tečný

tape /teɪp/ proužek, stužka

tapered /ˈteɪ.pəʳ/ zužující se, zahrocený, kuželový

target /ˈtɑː.gɪt/ cíl, terč, zamířit, plán

taste /teɪst/ chuť, chutnat, záliba

tasting /teɪ.stɪŋ/ chutnající

tattoo /təˈtuː/, /tætˈuː/ tetovat

tear /teəʳ/ **resistance** /rɪˈzɪs.tⁿnts/ pevnost proti natržení

tear /teəʳ/ roztrhnout, trhat, trhlina

tear /tɪəʳ/ slza

tease /tiːz/ škádlit

technical /ˈtek.nɪ.kⁿl/ technický

technician /tekˈnɪʃ.ⁿn/ technik

technique /tekˈniːk/ pracovní postup, metoda

teenager /ˈtiːnˌeɪ.dʒəʳ/ -náctiletý

temperature /ˈtem.prə.tʃəʳ/ teplota

temporal /ˈtem.pər.əl/ temporální, skráňový (na spáncích), přechodný

temporary /ˈtem.pⁿr.ⁿr.i/ dočasný, prozatímní

temporisation /tem.pə.raɪˈzeɪ.ʃⁿn/ vyčkávání

temporomandibular /ˌtem.pər.ə.mænˈdɪ.bjʊ.ləʳ/ **joint** /dʒɔɪnt/ kloub spánkový a dolní čelisti

tend /tend/ **to** /tʊ/ mít sklon, inklinovat

tendency /ˈten.dⁿnt.si/ tendence

tenderness /ˈten.də.nəs/ bolestivost, citlivost (na dotek)

tensile /ˈten.saɪl/ tažný (síla)

tension /ˈtent.ʃⁿn/ napětí, tenze, napínání (tahem), tlak

terminal /ˈtɜː.mɪ.nəl/ koncový, termínový, mezní, konečný, smrtelný

tertiary /ˈtɜː.ʃⁿr.i/ terciálně, v třetí řadě

tetanus /ˈtet.ⁿn.əs/ tetanus

texture /ˈteks.tʃəʳ/ struktura, tkáň, vazba

theoretically /θɪəˈret.ɪ.kli/ teoreticky

therapeutic /ˌθer.əˈpjuː.tɪk/ terapeutický (léčebný), lék

therapist /ˈθer.ə.pɪst/ terapeut

therapy /ˈθer.ə.pi/ terapie, léčba

thereby /ˌðeəˈbaɪ/ čímž, a tím

therefore /ˈðeə.fɔːʳ/ proto tedy, tudíž, z toho důvodu

thermal /ˈθɜː.məl/ **expansion** /ɪkˈspæn.tʃ°n/ tepelná rozpínavost

thermal /ˈθɜː.məl/ termální, tepelný

thin /θɪn/ nepatrný, tenký, řídký, zeslabit

third /θɜːd/ **molar** /ˈməʊ.ləʳ/ zub moudrosti

third /θɜːd/ třetina

thorough /ˈθʌr.ə/ dokonalý, důkladný, úplný

thoroughly /ˈθʌr.ə.li/ řádně, důkladně

thought /θɔːt/ myšlenka

thread /θred/ niť

threaded /θred.ɪd/ navlečený, niťový, se závitem

threader /θred.əʳ/ závitnice

thready /θred.i/ **pulse** /pʌls/ nitkovitý tep

threshold /ˈθreʃ.h əʊld/ práh, mez citlivosti

thrive /θraɪv/ prospívat (dobře růst), dařit se

throat /θrəʊt/ hrdlo

throb /θrɒb/ tepat, tep

thrombus /θrɒm.bəs/ thrombus, sraženina

through and through /θruː/ skrz naskrz

throughout /θruːˈaʊt/ celkový, od počátku do konce, docela, úplně (veskrze), všude v

thrush /θrʌʃ/ moučnivka

thrust /θrʌst/ úder, probodnout, cpát

thumb /θʌm/ palec na ruce

thus /ðʌs/ takto, tudíž

thyroid gland /ˈθaɪə.rɔɪdˌglænd/ štítná žláza

tidy /ˈtaɪ.di/ uklidit

tie /taɪ/ svázat, zavázat

tight /taɪt/ pevný, těsný

tighten /ˈtaɪ.t°n/ utažený, napjatý

tilt /tɪlt/ nachýlit, naklonit, vyklonit, sklon

time /taɪm/ doba

time /taɪm/ **off** /ɒf/ **work** /wɜːk/ volno z práce

time /taɪm/ **related** /rɪˈleɪ.tɪd/ vztahující se k času

time-consuming /ˈtaɪm.kənˌsjuː.mɪŋ/ časově náročný

tin /tɪn/ cín

tingle /ˈtɪŋ.gl̩/ zvonit (v uších), brnět (v těle), tetelit se (chvět se)

tingling /ˌtɪŋ.lɪŋ/ mravenčení

tinnitus /ˈtɪn.ɪ.təs/ tinitus, hučení v uších

tiny /ˈtaɪ.ni/ tenounký (nepatrný)

tip /tɪp/ hrot, špička, zahrocení, naklonit, sklopit

tiring /ˈtaɪə.rɪŋ/ únavný, vyčerpávající

tissue /ˈtɪʃ.uː/, /ˈtɪs.juː/ papírový kapesník, tkáň

titanium /tɪˈteɪ.ni.əm/ titan

to /tʊ/ **hand** /hænd/ v dosahu, k ruce

toddler /ˈtɒd.ləʳ/ batole

toe /təʊ/ prst (na noze)

toffee /ˈtɒf.i/ karamelový bonbón

together /təˈgeð.əʳ/ proti sobě, pohromadě

toilet /ˈtɔɪ.lət/ toaleta, čistění

tolerance /ˈtɒl.°r.°nt s/ tolerance (dovolená úchylka), snášenlivost, odolnost

tolerate /ˈtɒl.°r.eɪt/ tolerovat

tomography /təˈmɒg.rə.fi/ tomografie

tongue /tʌŋ/ jazyk, špice

tonic /'tɒn.ɪk/ phase /feɪz/ tonický, napjatý

tooth /tuːθ/ extraction /ɪk'stræk.ʃən/ vytrhnutí zubu

tooth /tuːθ/ wear /weəʳ/ opotřebení zubů

toothed /tuːθt/ ozubený

top /tɒp/ navršit, navýšit

topical /'tɒp.ɪ.kᵊl/ místní, aktuální (soudobý)

torrential /təˈren.tʃᵊl/ řinoucí se, proudící

totally /'təʊ.tᵊl.i/ úplně

touch /tʌtʃ/ dotek, hmat, dotýkat se

tough /tʌf/ tuhý

tourniquet /'tʊə.nɪ.keɪ/ škrtidlo

towards /təˈwɔːdz/ směrem k

towel /taʊəl/ ručník, utěrka

toy /tɔɪ/ hračka

trace /treɪs/ stopa

trachea /trəˈkiː.ə/ trachea, průdušnice

tract /trækt/ trakt

traction /'træk.ʃᵊn/ trakce, náprava tahem

traditionally /trəˈdɪʃ.ᵊn.ᵊl.i/ tradičně

trained /treɪnd/ vyškolený

tranquilliser /'træŋ.kwɪ.laɪ.zəʳ/ uklidňující prostředek

transducer /trænz'djuː.səʳ/ snímač, čidlo

transfer /'træns.fɜːʳ/ převoz, přenést

transformation /ˌtræns.fəˈmeɪ.ʃᵊn/ transformace (přeměna), přechod

transillumination /ˌtræn.zɪ'luː.mɪ'neɪ.ʃᵊn/ prosvícení

translate /træns'leɪt/ chápat, vysvětlit

translucence /trænz'luː.sənt s/ průsvitnost

transmission /trænz'mɪʃ.ᵊn/ transmise (převod), zaslání, odevzdání

transmit /trænz'mɪt/ přenášet, rozšířit

transplant /træn'splɑːnt/ transplantovat, transplantace, transplantovaný orgán

transplantation /ˌtræn.splɑːn'teɪ.ʃᵊn/ transplantace

transport /'træn.spɔːt/ transport, převoz

trap /træp/ zachycovat

trauma /'trɔː.mə/, /'traʊ-/ trauma, úraz

traumatic /trɔː'mæt.ɪk/, /traʊ-/ traumatický, úrazový

traumatise /'trɔː.mə.taɪz/ traumatizovat, poranit

tray /treɪ/ otiskovací lžíce, miska, destička, tác, tácek

treatment /'triːt.mənt/ léčba, ošetření, zacházení (s), léčebný postup, pohoštění

treatment /'triːt.mənt/ modality /mə'dæl.ə.ti/ varianta léčby

tremor /'trem.əʳ/ třes, chvění, strach

trial /traɪəl/ zkouška, pokus

trigeminal /'traɪ'dʒem.ɪ.nᵊl/ nerve /nɜːv/ trojklaný nerv

trigeminal /'traɪ'dʒem.ɪ.nᵊl/ trigeminální, trojklaný

trigger /'trɪg.əʳ/ spustit, začít, spustit (náhle uvolnit), spouštěč

trim /trɪm/ odstřihnout, oříznout, vyčistit, úprava

trimmer /'trɪm.əʳ/ nůž, ořezávačka

trimming /'trɪm.ɪŋ/ upravování

triple /'trɪp.ļ/ trojitý

trismus /trɪz.məs/ trizmus, křeč žvýkacího svalstva

trochlear /trə.kli.ə/ horní sval oční

troubled /'trʌb.ļ d/ problémový

troublesome /'trʌb.ļ.sᵊm/ obtížný, komplikující situaci, otravný (nepříjemný)

try /traɪ/ pokusit se, vyzkoušet, zkusit, zkoušet, zkouška

tuberculosis /tjuːˌbɜːˈkjʊˈləʊ.sɪs/ tuberkulóza

tuberosity /ˈtjuː.bəˈrɒs.ə.ti/ hrbol na kosti, drsnatina

tubular /ˈtjuː.bjʊ.ləʳ/ tubulární, trubicovitý

tubule /ˈtjuː.bjuːl/ tubulus, kanálek

tufted /ˈtʌf.tɪd/ chomáčkovitý

tumour /ˈtjuː.məʳ/ tumor, nádor

tungsten /ˈtʌŋ.stən/ wolfram

tunnel /ˈtʌn.ᵊl/ tunel, nálevka, trychtýř, chodba

turbine /ˈtɜː.baɪn/ turbína

tweezers /ˈtwiː.zəz/ pinzeta

twice /twaɪs/ dvakrát

U

ulcer /ˈʌl.səʳ/ vřed, nádor

ulceration /ˌʌl.sᵊrˈeɪ.ʃᵊn/ ulcerace, tvoření vředů, vředovitost

ulcerative /ˈʌl.sər.ə.tɪv/ colitis / kəʊˈlaɪ.təs/ ulcerativní kolitida (zánět tlustého střeva)

ulcerative /ˈʌl.sᵊr.ə.tɪv/ vředový

ultimate /ˈʌl.tɪ.mət/ základní, konečný

ultimately /ˈʌl.tɪ.mət.li/ nakonec, skutečně

ultrasonic /ˌʌl.trəˈsɒn.ɪk/ ultrazvukový

ultrasonography /ˌʌl.trəˈsɒn.ˈnɒg.rə.fi/ nauka o ultrazvuku

ultrasound /ˈʌl.trə.saʊnd/ ultrazvukový, sonogram

ultraviolet /ˌʌl.trəˈvaɪə.lət/ ultrafialový (UV)

unacceptable /ˌʌn.əkˈsep.tə.bl̩/ nepřijatelný

unaccompanied /ˌʌn.əˈkʌm.pᵊn.id/ samotný, nedoprovázený

unaffected /ˌʌn.əˈfek.tɪd/ nedotčený, neovlivněný

unaided /ˌʌnˈeɪ.dɪd/ bez pomoci

unattended /ˌʌn.əˈten.dɪd/ bez pomoci

unavoidable /ˌʌn.əˈvɔɪ.də.bl̩/ nevyhnutelný

uncertainty /ʌnˈsɜː.tᵊn.ti/ nejistota, nespolehlivost

uncomfortable /ʌnˈkʌmp f. tə.bl̩/ diskomfortní, nepříjemný, nepohodlný

uncommon /ʌnˈkɒm.ən/ neobvyklý, neobyčejný

unconscious /ʌnˈkɒn.tʃəs/ bezvědomý

unconsciousness /ʌnˈkɒn.tʃə.snəs/ bezvědomí, mdloby

uncontrollably /ˌʌn.kənˈtrəʊ.lə.bli/ nekontrolovatelně

uncoordinated /ˌʌn.kəʊˈɔː.dɪn.eɪ.tɪd/ nekoordinovaný, nesladěný

undercut /ˌʌn.dəˈkʌt/ podebrat, spodní zářez, odkrojit spodní část, podříznout, vrub, zářez

undergo /ˌʌn.dəˈgəʊ/ podstoupit, snášet, přestát

underlying/ˌʌn.dəˈlaɪ.ɪŋ/ ležící pod, vespod ležící, základní

underneath /ˌʌn.dəˈniːθ/ pod

understand /ˌʌn.dəˈstænd/ pochopit

understandable /ˌʌn.dəˈstæn.də.bl̩/ pochopitelný

understanding /ˌʌn.dəˈstæn.dɪŋ/ pochopení (porozumění), rozum (inteligence), dohoda (vzájemná)

undertake /ˌʌn.dəˈteɪk/ podniknout, provést, ujmout se

undiagnosed /ˌʌnˈdaɪ.əg.nəʊzd/ nediagnostikovaný

undo /ʌnˈduː/ rozvázat

unerupted /ˌʌn.ɪrˈʌp.tᵊd/ neprořezaný

unevenness /ʌnˈiː.vᵊn.nəs/ nerovnost, nepravidelnost

uneventful /ˌʌn.ɪˈvent.fᵊl/ bez událostí

unexpected /ˌʌn.ɪkˈspek.tɪd/
neočekávaný

unfavourable /ʌnˈfeɪ.vᵊr.ə.bl̩/
nepříznivý

unfit /ʌnˈfɪt/ neschopný (čeho),
nezpůsobilý

unfocused /ʌn.ˈfəʊ.kəst/ nezaostřený

unhindered /ˌʌnˈhɪn.dəd/ nenarazivší
na překážku

unilateral /ˌjuː.nɪˈlæt.ᵊr.ᵊl/
unilaterální, pouze na jedné straně

unintended /ˌʌn.ɪnˈten.dɪd/
neúmyslný, nezamýšlený

unit /ˈjuː.nɪt/ jednotka, celek

unknown /ʌnˈnəʊn/ neznámý

unless /ənˈles/ pokud ne

unlikely /ʌnˈlaɪ.kli/ nepravděpodobný

unnatural /ʌnˈnætʃ.ᵊr.ᵊl/ nepřirozený

unnecessary /ʌnˈnes.ə.ser.i/ zbytečný
(nepodstatný)

unpolished /ʌnˈpɒl.ɪʃt/ nevyleštěný

unpredictable /ˌʌn.prɪˈdɪk.tə.bl̩/
nepředvídatelný, neočekávaný

unrecordable /ˌʌn.rɪˈkɔːd.ə.bl̩/
nezaznamenatelný

unresponsive /ˌʌn.rɪˈspɒnt.sɪv/ bez
reakce

unsightly /ʌnˈsaɪt.li/ nevzhledný

unstable /ʌnˈsteɪ.bl̩/ nepevný,
pohyblivý, nestabilní, proměnlivý,
nestálý

unsuccessful /ˌʌn.səkˈses.fᵊl/
neúspěšný, nepodařený (nezdařilý)

unsupported /ˌʌn.səˈpɔː.tɪd/ bez
podpory

unsusceptible /ˌʌn.səˈsep.tɪ.bl̩/
necitlivý, nevnímavý

unused /ʌnˈjuːzd/ nepoužitý

unusual /ʌnˈjuː.ʒu.əl/ pozoruhodný
(neobvyklý), mimořádný

unwanted /ʌnˈwɒn.tɪd/ nežádoucí

unwell /ʌnˈwel/ nedobře

unwillingness /ʌnˈwɪl.ɪŋ.nəs/
neochota

up /ʌp/ **to** /tʊ/ až do, do výše

update /ʌpˈdeɪt/ aktualizovat

upper /ˈʌp.əʳ/ horní, vrchní

upright /ˈʌp.raɪt/ **position** /pəˈzɪʃ.ᵊn/
vzpřímená poloha

upright /ˈʌp.raɪt/ vzpřímený

upwards /ˈʌp.wədz/ nahoru

uraemia /jʊəˈriː.mi.ə/ uremie,
chronické selhání činnosti ledvin

urea /jʊᵊˈriː.ə/ močovina

urgency /ˈɜː.dʒᵊnt.si/ nutná potřeba,
nutnost (naléhavost)

urgent /ˈɜː.dʒᵊnt/ nutný (naléhavý)

urine /ˈjʊə.rɪn/ moč, močový

use /juːs/ použití, užití, užívání,
funkce, praxe

use /juːz/ použít

useful /ˈjuːs.fᵊl/ užitečný

user /ˈjuː.zᵊr/ uživatel

uterine /ˈjuː.tᵊr.aɪn/ děložní

utilise /ˈjuː.tɪ.laɪz/ využít

V

vacant /ˈveɪ.kᵊnt/ prázdný

valid /ˈvæl.ɪd/ platný, oprávněný

validate /ˈvæl.ɪ.deɪt/ uznat platnost,
schválit

valuable /ˈvæl.jʊ.bl̩/ cenný, hodnotný

value /ˈvæl.juː/ cena, hodnota,
význam, ocenit, ohodnotit

valve /vælv/ chlopeň

vanity /ˈvæn.ɪ.ti/ marnivost

vapocoolant /ˈveɪ.pə.ˈkuː.lənt/
chladicí prostředek s použitím
odpařování

vapour /ˈveɪ.pəʳ/ výpary

variable /ˈveə.ri.ə.bl̩/ variabilní
(proměnlivý), nestálý, kolísavý

variant /ˈveə.ri.ənt/ variantní, lišící se,
proměnný

variation /ˌveə.riˈeɪ.ʃ°n/ odchylka, změna, různost

varicella /ˌvæ.rɪˈsel.ə/ varicella, plané neštovice

varicose vein /ˌvær.ɪ.kəʊ sˈveɪn/ varikózní žíla (křečová)

variety /vəˈraɪə.ti/ varianta, druh, odrůda, rozmanitost, mnohotvárnost

varnish /ˈvɑː.nɪʃ/ lak, lesk, nalakovat

vascular /ˈvæs.kjʊ.ləʳ/ vaskulární, cévní

vasculitis /ˌvæs.kjʊˈlaɪ.tɪs/ vaskulitida, zánět cév

vasoconstrictor /ˌveɪz.ə.kənˈstrɪkt.əʳ/ vazokonstrikční látka, vyvolávající smrštění cévy

vasodilatation /ˌveɪ.zə.daɪˈlə.teɪ.ʃ°n/ vazodilatace, rozšíření cév

vast /vɑːst/ rozsáhlý

vehicle /ˈviː.ɪ.kl̩/ dopravní prostředek

veneer /vəˈnɪəʳ/ dýha, fazeta, tenká vrstva, nátěr, obložení

venous /ˈviː.nəs/ žilní

ventilation /ˌven.tɪˈleɪ.ʃ°n/ vdech

verbal /ˈvɜː.bəl/ slovní

vertebra /ˈvɜː.tɪ.brə/ obratel, páteř

vertical /ˈvɜː.tɪ.k°l/ vertikální, kolmý

vertigo /ˈvɜː.tɪ.gəʊ/ závrať

vesicle /ˈvesɪkl/ váček, dutina, puchýřek

vesiculobullous /ve.ˈsɪ.kju.lə.buːləʊs/ týkající se puchýřků a velkých puchýřů

vessel /ˈves.°l/ céva, prázdná nádoba

via /vaɪə/, /ˈviː.ə/ skrz, pomocí (čeho)

vibrate /vaɪˈbreɪt/ vibrovat (kmitat), chvět se

vicinity /vɪˈsɪn.ɪ.ti/ těsná blízkost

view /vjuː/ pohled, dívat se

viral /ˈvaɪə.r°l/ virový

visibility /ˌvɪz.ɪˈbɪl.ɪ.ti/ viditelnost

visible /ˈvɪz.ɪ.bl̩/ viditelný

vision /ˈvɪʒ.°n/ vidění, zrak (pohled), zorný

visual /ˈvɪʒ.u.əl/ zrakový

visualisation /ˌvɪʒ.u.°l.aɪˈzeɪ.ʃ°n/ znázornění (vizuální)

visualise /ˈvɪʒ.u.°l.aɪz/ vyšetřit zrakem

vitality /vaɪˈtæl.ɪ.ti/ životnost

vitamin /ˈvɪt.ə.mɪn/ vitamin, vitaminový

voice /vɔɪs/ hlas, hlasový, vyjádřit (názor, mínění)

volume /ˈvɒl.juːm/ objem

vomit /ˈvɒm.ɪt/ zvracet, zvracení

vouch /vaʊtʃ/ **for** /fɔːʳ/ zaručit

vulnerability /ˌvʌl.nər.əˈbɪl.ɪ.ti/ zranitelnost, náchylnost

W

waken /ˈweɪ.kən/ probouzet se, procitnout (probudit se), budit se

wall /wɑːl/ stěna

ward /wɔːd/ **off** /ɒf/ uchránit

warm /wɔːm/ nahřát

warn /wɔːn/ varovat

warning /ˈwɔː.nɪŋ/ upozornění

wash /wɒʃ/ mýt, promýt, prát

washout /ˈwɒʃ.aʊt/ pohroma

waste /weɪst/ odpad

wasting /weɪst.ɪŋ/ zhoubný, ničivý, plýtvání

watch /wɒtʃ/ sledovat (zrakem), hlídat, dávat pozor

water /ˈwɔː.təʳ/ **syringe** /sɪˈrɪndʒ/ vodní stříkačka

waterproof /ˈwɔː.tə.pruːf/ nepromokavý

wave /weɪv/ vlna

wax /wæks/ vosk

waxed /wækst/ voskovaný

weak /wiːk/ slabý, křehký, nedostatečný

weakness /ˈwiːk.nəs/ slabá stránka, slabá odolnost, vada

wear /weə^r/ mít na sobě, obléknout, nosit na sobě, oblékat si

wear /weə^r/ **off** /ɒf/ mizet (ztrácet se), opotřebovat se

wear /weə^r/ opotřebování

wear /weə^r/ **resistance** /rɪˈzɪs.t^ənt s/ otěruvzdornost

wearer /weə.rə^r/ nositel, kdo nosí

wedge /wedʒ/ klín, klínek, vklínit, vtlačit, zaklínit

weekly /ˈwiː.kli/ týdně

weight /weɪt/ **loss** /lɒs/ úbytek váhy

weight /weɪt/ váha

weight /weɪt/ **bearing** /ˈbeə.rɪŋ/ nesoucí váhu

welcoming /ˈwel.kəm.ɪŋ/ přívětivý

well /wel/ správně (dobře)

well timed /ˌwelˈtaɪmd/ dobře načasovaný

well-being /ˌwelˈbiː.ɪŋ/ blaho, prospěch, dobré zdraví

wet /wet/ mokrý, vlhký, namočit (navlhčit)

whatever /wɒtˈev.ə^r/ kterýkoliv

whatsoever /ˌwɒt.səʊˈev.ə^r/ vůbec

wheeze /wiːz/ sípat

whereas /weəˈræz/ zatímco, kdežto, naopak

whereby /weəˈbaɪ/ čímž (pomocí něhož)

wherever /weəˈrev.ə^r/ kdekoli

whether /ˈweð.ə^r/ jestli

whichever /wɪˈtʃev.ə^r/ kterýkoli (z určitého počtu)

while /waɪl/ zatímco

whilst /waɪlst/ zatímco, kdežto, když

whiten /ˈwaɪ.t^ən/ bělit

whole /həʊl/ celý, celistvý

wide /waɪd/ široký

widely /ˈwaɪd.li/ široce

widen /ˈwaɪ.d^ən/ rozšířit

width /wɪtθ/ šíře, vůle

wind /wɪnd/ **instrument** /ˈɪn.strə.mənt/ dechový nástroj

wipe /waɪp/ utřít, otřít

wire /waɪə^r/ drát

withdrawal /wɪðˈdrɔː.^əl/ stažení (ústup), odnětí, vysazení

withdrawn /wɪðˈdrɔːn/ stáhnutý

withstand /wɪðˈstænd/ odolávat, snést, vydržet

womb /wuːm/ děloha

wooden /ˈwʊd.^ən/ dřevěný

work /wɜːk/ fungovat

worker /ˈwɜː.kə^r/ dělník, pracovník

working /ˈwɜː.kɪŋ/ pracovní

worldwide /wɜːld.waɪd/ světový, celosvětově

worn /wɔːn/ opotřebovaný

worse /wɜːs/ horší

worsen /ˈwɜː.sən/ zhoršit, zhoršit se, poškodit, pokazit se

worsening /ˈwɜː.sən.ɪŋ/ zhoršující se

worth /wɜːθ/ mít cenu, za něco stát

wound /wuːnd/ rána

wrapped /ræpt/ zabalený

wrapping /ˈræp.ɪŋ/ zabalení

wrist /rɪst/ zápěstí

write /raɪt/ **up** /ʌp/ dokončit (dopsat)

written /ˈrɪt.^ən/ psaný

wrought /rɔːt/ **alloy** /ˈæl.ɔɪ/ tvářecí slitina, kujná slitina

X

xerostomia /ˈzɪə.rəˈstəʊ.mɪə/ xerostomie, suchost úst

Y

yawn /jɔːn/ zívat

yawning /ˈjɔː.nɪŋ/ zívání

youngster /ˈjʌŋk.stə^r/ výrostek

Z

zinc /zɪŋk/ oxide /oxide/ˈɒk.saɪd/ zinková běloba

zinc /zɪŋk/ oxide /ˈɒk.saɪd/ /eugenol /juːˈdʒen.ɒl/ zinkoxid-eugenolová pasta

zinc /zɪŋk/ phosphate /ˈfɒs.feɪt/ cement /sɪˈment/ zink-fosfátový cement

zinc /zɪŋk/ phosphate /ˈfɒs.feɪt/ fosforečnan zinečnatý

zinc /zɪŋk/ zinek

zone /zəʊn/ zóna, oblast

zygomatic /zʌɪˈgəʊ.mə.tɪk/ lícní

Czech–English Dictionary

A

abecedně číselný alphanumeric /ˌæl.fə.njuːˈmer.ɪk/

abnormální abnormal /æbˈnɔː.məl/

absolutně, naprosto absolutely /ˌæb.səˈluːt.li/

absorbční tampon absorbent /əbˈzɔː.bənt/ pad /pæd/

absorbovat, pohltit, vstřebat absorb /əbˈzɔːb/

acidický, kyselinotvorný, kyselinový, kyselý acidic /ˈæs.ɪ.dɪk/

adekvátní, přiměřený, dostačující adequate /ˈæd.ə.kwət/

adhezivní materiál, lepidlo, lepicí páska adhesive /ədˈhiː.sɪv/

aditivní, přísada, dodatkový additive /ˈæd.ɪ.tɪv/

administrativní administrative /ədˈmɪn.ɪ.strə.tɪv/

aerobní aerobic /eəˈrəʊ.bɪk/

agresivní aggressive /əˈgres.ɪv/

akceptovat, přijmout, připustit accept /əkˈsept/

akrylový, pryskyřičný acrylic /əˈkrɪl.ɪk/

aktuálně, v současné době currently /ˈkʌr.ənt.li/

aktuální (soudobý) topical /ˈtɒp.ɪ.kəl/

akupunktura acupuncture /ˈæk.jʊ.pʌŋk.tʃəʳ/

akutní, naléhavý acute /əˈkjuːt/

alergický, přecitlivělý allergic /əˈlɜː.dʒɪk/

alergie allergy /ˈæl.ə.dʒi/

alkoholismus alcoholism /ˈæl.kə.hɒl.ɪ.zəm/

allergen allergen /ˈæl.ə.dʒən/

aloplastický alloplastic /ˌæləˈplæs.tɪk/

aloplastika, plastika materiálem cizím lidskému tělu (stříbro, zlato, kovy) alloplasty /ˈæl.ə.plæs.tɪ/

alternativa, druhá možnost, náhrada, náhradní, jiná možnost alternative /ɒlˈtɜː.nə.tɪv/

aluminosilikát, hlinito-křemičitan aluminosilicate /ˌæl.jʊˈmɪn.əˈsɪl.ɪ.kət/

alveolektomie, excise alveolárního výběžku čelisti alveolectomy /ˌale.viəˈlek.tə.mi/

alveolus, hřbet, hřeben, lišta, okraj, rýha, val, výběžek, vyvýšenina ridge /rɪdʒ/

amalgám amalgam /əˈmæl.gəm/

ambu vak Ambu bag /æm.bjʊ.bæg/

ambulantní pacient outpatient /ˈaʊt.peɪ.ʃənt/

ameloblastom, tumor dolní čelisti, vzniklý ze sklovinových buněk ameloblastoma /æˌme.lə.blæsˈtəʊ.mə/

ampicilin ampicillin /əmˈpəs.ɪ.lɪn/

amputace, odstranění amputation /
,æm.pjʊˈteɪ.ʃən/

amputovat amputate /ˈæm.pjʊ.teɪt/

anafylaktický šok anaphylactic /
,æn.ə.fɪˈlæk.tɪk/ shock /ʃɒk/

analgetikum analgesic /,æn.əlˈdʒiː.zɪk/

analgézie, snížená vnímavost bolesti
analgesia /,æn.əl.ˈdʒiː.zi.ə/

analýza, rozbor analysis /əˈnæl.ə.sɪs/

anestezie, znecitlivění anaesthesia /
,æn.əsˈθiː.zi.ə/

anomálie, odchylka anomaly /
əˈnɒm.ə.li/

antibiotika antibiotics /,æn.ti.baɪˈɒt.ɪk/

anticipovat, očekávat anticipate /
ænˈtɪs.ɪ.peɪt/

antikoagulans, látka bránící srážení
krve anticoagulant /
,æn.ti.kəʊˈæg.jʊ.lənt/

antikoncepce contraceptive /
,kɒn.trəˈsep.tɪv/

antikonvulzívum, protikřečový
anticonvulsant /,æn.ti.kənˈvʌl.sᵊnt/

antiseptický, dezinfekční prostředek
antiseptic /,æn.tiˈsep.tɪk/

antrální, týkající se dutiny antral /
æn.trəl/

antrum, dutina, předsíň antrum /
ˈæn.trəm/ (pl. antra)

anxiolytikum anxiolytic /
,æŋksˈ.aɪəl.ɪ.tɪk/

aparát, přístroj, nástroj, pomůcka,
zařízení, spotřebič, obklad
appliance /əˈplaɪ.ənt s/

apikektomie, resekce kořenového
hrotu apicectomy /æ.pɪˈsek.tə.mɪ/

aplikace (vložka), vložení, zasazení
insertion /ɪnˈsɜː.ʃən/

aplikace, použití, léčebný prostředek,
přiložení (obkladu) application /
,æp.lɪˈkeɪ.ʃən/

aplikátor, štětec applicator /
ˈæp.lɪ.keɪ.təʳ/

aplikovaný, použitý, přiložený
applied /əˈplaɪd/

aplikovat, používat, týkat se apply /
əˈplaɪ/

aproximální, mezizubní, styčný
interproximal /,ɪn.təˈ.prɒk.sɪm.l/

areál, prostor, provozovna premises /
ˈprem.ɪ.sɪz/

arch, fólie, kus, list, tenká deska,
výkaz sheet /ʃiːt/

armáda, zbrojní armament /
ˈɑː.mə.mənt/

artefakt, výtvor artefact /ˈɑː.tɪ.fækt/

articulátor articulator /ɑːˈtɪk.jʊ.lət.əʳ/

artikulační papír articulating /
ɑːˈtɪk.jʊ.leɪ.tɪŋ/ paper /ˈpeɪ.pəʳ/

artritida, zánět kloubů arthritis /
ɑːˈθraɪ.tɪs/

arytmický arrhythmic /æˈrɪθ.mɪk/

arytmie arrhythmia /æˈrɪθ.mɪ.ə/

asistence, podpora, pomoc assistance
/əˈsɪs.tənt s/

asistovat, pomáhat assist /əˈsɪst/

asociovat, spojovat, spojit, přidružit
associate /əˈsəʊ.si.eɪt/

aspirate /ˈæs.pɪ.reɪt/ nasávat

aspirin aspirin /ˈæs.pɪ.rɪn/

astma, dušnost asthma /ˈæs.mə/

ataxie, ztráta kontroly volních
pohybů ataxia /əˈtæk.sɪ.ə/

atropine atropine /æt.rəp.ɪn/

atropinsíran atropine /æt.rəp.ɪn/
sulphate /sʌl.feɪt/

autoimunní autoimmune /
,ɔː.təʊ.ɪˈmjuːn/

autorita (pravomoc) authority /
ɔːˈθɒr.ɪ.ti/

avšak however /,haʊˈev.əʳ/

axilární, podpažní axillary /æˈksɪl.ᵊr.i/

až do, do výše up /ʌp/ to /tʊ/

B

baktericidní, zabíjející bakterie
bactericidal /bæk͵tɪə.ri.saɪdl/

bakterie, mikrob, mikroorganismus
microorganism /
maɪ.krəʊ.ˈɔː.gən.ɪ.zᵊm/

bakteriolog bacteriologist /
bæk͵tɪə.ri.ˈɒl.ə.dʒɪst/

balení, balíček, tampon, ucpávka
pack /pæk/

balit, cpát, tamponovat, ucpávat
vatou pack /pæk/

bariéra, zábrana, překážka barrier /
ˈbær.i.əʳ/

baterie battery /ˈbæt.ər.i/

batole toddler /ˈtɒd.ləʳ/

bazální deska baseplate /beɪs.pleɪt/

bazální, základní buňka basal /
ˈbeɪ.sl/ cell /sel/

bdělost alertness /əˈlɜːt.nəs/

běh, chod, příval stream /striːm/

během, uvnitř, v rozmezí within /
wɪˈðɪn/

bělavý, krémový creamy /ˈkriː.mi/

bělení, bělicí bleaching /bliːtʃ.ɪŋ/

bělit whiten /ˈwaɪ.tᵊn/

benzodiazepin benzodiazepine /
ben.ˈzəʊ.daɪ.æ.sə͵paɪn/

bez dechu, udýchaný breathless /
ˈbreθ.ləs/

bez pomoci unaided /͵ʌnˈeɪ.dɪd/,
unattended /͵ʌn.əˈten.dɪd/

bez reakce unresponsive /
͵ʌn.rɪˈspɒnt.sɪv/

bez zubů, bezzubý edentulous /
əˈden.tju.ləs/

bezbolestně painlessly /ˈpeɪn.lə.sli/

beznadějný, bezvýhledný hopeless /
ˈhəʊ.pləs/

bezpečnostní zařízení safety /ˈseɪf.ti/
device /dɪˈvaɪs/

bezpečný, důvěryhodný safe /seɪf/

bezprostřední, okamžitý immediate /
ɪˈmiː.di.ət/

bezvědomí, mdloby unconsciousness /
ʌnˈkɒn.t ʃə.snəs/

bezvědomý unconscious /ʌnˈkɒn.t ʃəs/

bezzubost edentulousness /əˈden.tju.
ləs.nəs/

bezzubý edentate /əˈden.teɪt/

biokompatibilní, biologicky
slučitelný biocompatible /
͵baɪ.əʊ.kəmˈpæt.ɪ.bᵊl/

biologická zpětná vazba biofeedback /
baɪ.əʊ.ˈfiːd.bæk/

biopsie biopsy /ˈbaɪ.ɒp.si/

bít beat /biːt/

blaho, dobré zdraví, prospěch
well-being /͵welˈbiː.ɪŋ/

bledost, zsinalost pallor /ˈpæl.əʳ/

bledý pale /peɪl/

blízkost, těsná blízkost proximity /
prɒkˈsɪm.ɪ.ti/

blízký, sousední nearby /͵nɪəˈbaɪ/

blokáda, ucpání blockage /ˈblɒk.ɪdʒ/

blokovat, zatarasit block /blɒk/

bodání, brnění, osten, píchat, svrbění
prickle /ˈprɪk.ḷ/

bodavý, ostrý (pronikavý),
propichování těla kroužky piercing
/ˈpɪə.sɪŋ/

bodec, jehla, kořenová jehla, sonda,
čep broach /brəʊtʃ/

bodnout, píchnout prick /prɪk/

bodnutí, cukavý, očkovat vpichem
stabbing /ˈstæb.ɪŋ/

bodnutí, píchnutí jehlou needlestick͵ /
ˈniː.dḷ stɪk/

bojácný, strašný fearful /ˈfɪə.fᵊl/

bojovat proti combat /kəmˈbæt/

bolavý sore /sɔːr/

bolest hlavy headache /ˈhed.eɪk/

bolest zubů odontalgia /
͵əʊ.dɒnˈtæl.dʒɪə/

bolest, námaha, trápit pain /peɪn/

bolestivost soreness /'sɔː.nəs/

bolestivost, citlivost (na dotek) tenderness /'ten.də.nəs/

bolet, poranit hurt /hɜːt/

boule (na těle), bulka, opuchlina lump /lʌmp/

brada chin /tʃɪn/, mentum /men.təm/

bradykardie, zpomalená srdeční činnost bradycardia / ˌbræd.ɪ.ˈkɑː.di.ə/

bradykineze, extrémní zpomalení pohybu bradykinesia /ˌbræ. di.ki'niːzɪ.ə/

brachiální, pažní brachial /breɪk.ɪ.əl/

brát v úvahu, dívat se, pátrat, podívat se, vyhledat look /lʊk/

brát, pojit se, ujmout se take /teɪk/

brnění (mravenčení) pins /pɪns/ and needles /'niː.dl̩z/

brnět (v těle), tetelit se (chvět se), zvonit (v uších) tingle /'tɪŋ.gl̩/

bronchitida, zánět průdušek bronchitis /brɒŋ'kaɪ.tɪs/

bronchospasmus, křeč průdušek bronchospasm /'brɒŋ.kə.spæz.əm/

bruxismus, skřípání zuby bruxism / brʊːk.sɪ.zəm/

brýle (dioptrické) spectacles / 'spek.tɪ.kl̩ z/

brýle glasses /glɑːs.ɪz/

bublinka bubble /'bʌb.l̩/

buď either /'aɪ.ðəʳ/

bujet proliferate /prə'lɪf.əʳ.eɪt/

bukální, tvářový, lícní buccal /bʌk.l/

bukolingvální, týkající se tváří a jazyka buccolingual / ˌbʌk.ə.'lɪŋ.gwəl/

být následkem, mít za následek, výsledek result /rɪ'zʌlt/

být poslušný příkazu obey /əʊ 'beɪ/ command /kə'mɑːnd/

být umístěn, místo, poloha, umístění site /saɪt/

být zapotřebí, chtít, nutně potřebovat require /rɪ'kwaɪəʳ/

C

cákanec, skvrna splash /splæʃ/

cefalometrický, měřící lebku cephalometric /ˌse.fə'lom.ɪt.rɪk/

celek, jednotka, přístroj unit /'juː.nɪt/

celiakie, břišní onemocnění coeliac disease /'siː.li.æk.dɪˌziːz/

celistvost entirety /ɪn'taɪə.rɪ.ti/

celistvost rtu lip /lɪp/ competence / 'kɒm.pɪ.tənt s/

celková anestezie, narkóza general / 'dʒen.ᵊr.ᵊl/ anaesthesia / ˌæn.əs'θiː.zi.ə/

celkový, panoramatický panoramic / ˌpæn.ər'æm.ɪk/

celuloid, film, buničina celluloid / 'sel.jʊ.lɔɪd/

celuloidová páska celluloid / 'sel.jʊ.lɔɪd/ strip /strɪp/

celulóza, buničina cellulose / 'sel.jʊ.ləʊs/

celý, celistvý whole /həʊl/

cement, tmel, pojivo, stmelit cement / sɪ'ment/

cena price /praɪs/

cena, hodnota, ocenit, ohodnotit, význam value /'væl.juː/

cenný, hodnotný valuable /'væl.jʊ.bl̩/

cenově přístupný cost-effective / kɒst.ɪ'fek.tɪv/

cervikální, krčkový cervical /sə'vaɪ.kəl/

cesta path /pɑːθ/, route /ruːt/

cíl goal /gəʊl/, objective /əb'dʒek.tɪv/

cíl, plán, terč, zamířit target /'tɑː.gɪt/

cín tin /tɪn/

cíp, roh, růžek, kout, úhel corner / 'kɔː.nəʳ/

cirkulace, oběh circulation /ˌsɜːkjʊˈleɪ.ʃᵊn/

cit, dojem, pocit, smyslové vnímání, vjem sensation /senˈseɪ.ʃᵊn/

cítit feel /fiːl/

citron lemon /ˈlem.ən/

cizí tělísko foreign /ˈfɒr.ən/ body /ˈbɒd.i/

co se každého týče, podle pořadí (uvedeného) respectively /rɪˈspek.tɪv.li/

cpát, probodnout, úder thrust /θrʌst/

cpátko pro kořenové kanálky spreader /ˈspred.əʳ/

cpátko, zátka plugger /plʌg.əʳ/

cucat, nasát, sát suck /sʌk/

cukr sugar /ˈʃʊg.əʳ/

cyanóza, zmodrání kůže a sliznic cyanosis /ˈsʌɪəˈnəʊ.sɪs/

cyklus cycle /ˈsaɪ.kl̩/

cystická fibróza, fibrotické onemocnění slinivky cystic fibrosis /ˌsɪs.tɪk.faɪˈbrəʊ.sɪs/

cystický cystic /ˌsɪs.tɪk/

cystitida, zánět močového měchýře cystitis /sɪˈstaɪ.tɪs/

cytotoxický, škodlivý pro buňky cytotoxic /saɪ.təˈtɒk.sɪk/

Č

časný, počáteční, ranný early /ˈɜː.li/

časově náročný time-consuming /ˈtaɪm.kənˌsjuː.mɪŋ/

část, hodně, podíl deal /dɪəl/

část, oblast (též správní), rozsah region /ˈriː.dʒᵊn/

část, součást part /pɑːt/

část, úlomek fragment /ˈfræg.mənt/

část, úsek section /ˈsek.ʃᵊn/

částečka, částice, zrnko particle /ˈpɑː.tɪ.kl̩/

částečná zlomenina kosti greenstick /ˈgriːn.stɪk/ fracture /ˈfræk.tʃᵊr/

částečně partially /ˈpɑː.ʃᵊl.i/

částečné protézy partial /ˈpɑː.ʃᵊl/ dentures /ˈden.tʃəz/

částečný, dílčí, neúplný partial /ˈpɑː.ʃᵊl/

častý frequent /ˈfriː.kwənt/

častý, opakovaný repeated /rɪˈpiː.tɪd/

čelistní maxillary /mæˈksɪ.lᵊr.i/

čep, podpěra, sloupek, stojan post /pəʊst/

čep, zátka bung /bʌŋ/

čepelka skalpelu scalpel /ˈskæl.pᵊl/ blade /bleɪd/

čepová korunka post /pəʊst/ crown /kraʊn/

černý kašel, pertussis pertussis /pəˈtʌs.ɪs/

čerstvý fresh /freʃ/

červenat, rudnout, zrudnout flush /flʌʃ/

čidlo, příjemce receptor /rɪˈsep.təʳ/

čich, být cítit, cítit (čichem) smell /smel/

čichat, nadýchnutí nosem, šňupat (tabák) snuff /snʌf/

čichový olfactory /ɒlˈfæk.tᵊr.i/

čímž (pomocí něhož) whereby /weəˈbaɪ/

čímž, a tím thereby /ˌðeəˈbaɪ/

čípek, kolík, připevnit, přišpendlit, svorka, špendlík pin /pɪn/

čípkovitý peg-shaped /peg.ʃeɪpt/

číselný numeric /njuːˈmer.ɪk/

čisticí detersive /dɪˈtɜːˑr.sɪv/

čisticí prostředek cleanser /ˈklen.zəʳ/

čistit clean /kliːn/

čistý, jasný, zřetelný, průhledný clear /klɪəʳ/

čistý, pouhý pure /pjʊəʳ/

čištěný, rafinovaný (zušlechtěný)
refined /rɪˈfaɪnd/
člověk, lidský human /ˈhjuː.mən/
čmouha, pruhovat, tvořit proužky
streak /striːk/
čtvercová šroubovice quadhelix /
kwɒdˈhiː.lɪks/
čtverec square /skweəʳ/
čtvrtina kruhu (kvadrant) quadrant /
ˈkwɒd.rənt/

D

dále onwards /ˈɒn.wədz/
daleko far /fɑːʳ/
dařit se, prospívat (dobře růst) thrive
/θraɪv/
dásňová kost alveolar /ˌæl.viˈəʊ.ləʳ/
bone /bəʊn/
dát náplast, hojivý obvaz, náplast
plaster /ˈplɑː.stəʳ/
dát narkózu, umrtvit anesthetise /
əˈniːs.θə.taɪz/
dát si na čas, využít čas take /teɪk/
time /taɪm/
dát si pozor, varovat se beware /
bɪˈweəʳ/
dát signál (signalizovat), popud
signal /ˈsɪg.nəl/
dát zpět, nahradit, vyměnit, znovu
umístit replace /rɪˈpleɪs/
dát, podat give /gɪv/
dávat pozor, hlídat, sledovat
(zrakem) watch /wɒtʃ/
dávka batch /bætʃ/
defibrilátor defibrillator /
ˌdiːˈfɪb.rɪ.leɪ.tər /
deficit, nedostatek deficit /ˈdef.ɪ.sɪt/
deficitní, nedostatečný deficient /
dɪˈfɪʃ.ənt/
definitivní, konečný, nesporný
definite /ˈdef.ɪ.nət/

deformita, znetvoření deformity /
dɪˈfɔː.mɪ.ti/
deformovat, změnit tvar deform /
dɪˈfɔːm/
degenerace, rozklad degeneration /
dɪˌdʒen.əˈreɪ.ʃən/
dehet tar /tɑːʳ/
dech, vdechnutí breath /breθ/
dechový nástroj wind /wɪnd/
instrument /ˈɪn.strə.mənt/
dekáda, desetiletí, desítka decade /
ˈdek.eɪd/
delegovat delegate /ˈdel.ɪ.geɪt/
dělit, plynout stream /striːm/
dělník, pracovník worker /ˈwɜː.kəʳ/
děloha womb /wuːm/
děložní uterine /ˈjuː.tər.aɪn/
demyelinizace, zničení myelinu
demyelination /
dɪˈmaɪ.ə.li.naɪˈzeɪ.ʃən/
dentální anamnéza dental /ˈden.tᵊl/
history /ˈhɪs.tər.i/
dentice, chrup dentition /denˈtɪʃ.ən/
denzita, objemová hmotnost, hutnost
density /ˈdent.sɪ.ti/
deprese, sklíčenost, potlačení
depression /dɪˈpreʃ.ən/
derivát, odvozenina derivative /
dɪˈrɪv.ə.tɪv/
dermatitida, zánět kůže dermatitis /
ˌdɜː.məˈtaɪ.təs/
dermatologie, kožní lékařství
dermatology /ˌdɜː.məˈtɒl.ə.dʒi/
deska, destička, plát, patro (umělého
chrupu) plate /pleɪt/
destička slab /slæb/
destička, krevní destička platelet /
ˈpleɪt.lət/
destička, miska, lžíce, otiskovací
lžíce, podnos, tác, tácek tray /treɪ/
destilace, překapávání distillation /
ˌdɪs.tɪˈleɪ.ʃən/

destruktivní, zhoubný, ničící, rušivý destructive /dɪˈstrʌk.tɪv/

deteriorizace, zhoršení, chátrání, poškození, porucha deterioration / dɪˌtɪə.ri.əˈreɪ.ʃən/

dětinský babyish /ˈbeɪ.bi.ɪʃ/

dětská lahvička na krmení nursing / ˈnɜː.sɪŋ/ bottle /ˈbɒt.l̩/

devitalizovaný nonvital /nɒn.ˈvaɪ.tᵊl/

dezinfekční prostředek disinfectant / ˌdɪs.ɪnˈfek.tᵊnt/

dezinfikovat disinfect /ˌdɪs.ɪnˈfekt/

dezorientovaný disorientated / dɪˈsɔː.ri.ən.tɪd/

diagnóza, rozpoznání choroby, určení, popsání diagnosis / ˌdaɪ.əgˈnəʊ.sɪs/

diamant diamond /ˈdaɪə.mənd/

diamantový brousek diamond / ˈdaɪə.mənd/ bur /bɜːʳ/

diarea (průjem) diarrhoea /ˌdaɪ.əˈriː.ə/

diastolický diastolic /ˌdaɪ.əˈstɒ.lɪk/

diatéza, dispozice diathesis / ˌdaɪˈæ.θiː.sɪs/

diazepam, sedativum, hovor. valium diazepam /ˌdaɪˈæz.ə.pəm/

dietetický, dietní dietetic /ˌdaɪə.teˈtɪk/

digitální digital /ˈdɪdʒ.ɪ.tᵊl/

dimenzovat, vyložit, vystavit lay /leɪ/ out /aʊt/

diskomfortní, nepohodlný, nepříjemný uncomfortable / ʌnˈkʌmp f.tə.bl̩ /

diskrétní, jednotlivý, oddělený, samostatný discrete /dɪˈskriːt/

dislokovaná zlomenina displaced / dɪˈspleɪst/ fracture /ˈfræk.t ʃəʳ/

dívat se, podívat se (kam), prohlížet, vidět view /vjuː/

dlaha, klínek, štěpina splint /splɪnt/

dlaň palm /pɑːm/

dláto, dlátko, sekáč chisel /ˈtʃɪz.ᵊl/

dláto, fréza cutter /ˈkʌt.əʳ/

dloubnout, rýpat, strkat, šťourat se poke /pəʊk/

dlouhodobě působící long-acting / lɒŋ.ˈæk.tɪŋ/

dlouhodobý long-term /ˌlɒŋˈtɜːm/

dlouhodobý, dlouhotrvající, prodloužený prolonged /prəˈlɒŋd/

dlouhotrvající, neustálý, neústupný, stálý, ustavičný persistent / pəˈsɪs.tᵊnt/

dno floor /flɔːʳ/

doba time /taɪm/

doba tuhnutí setting /ˈset.ɪŋ/ time / taɪm/

doba, období period /ˈpɪə.ri.əd/

dobře načasovaný well timed / ˌwelˈtaɪmd/

docílit score /skɔːʳ/

dočasný, mléčný chrup deciduous / dɪˈsɪd.ju.əs/ teeth /tiːθ/

dočasný, mléčný, vypadavý deciduous /dɪˈsɪd.ju.əs /

dočasný, prozatímní temporary / ˈtem.pᵊr.ᵊr.i/

dodávat deliver /dɪˈlɪv.əʳ/

dodávat, zásobovat supply /səˈplaɪ/

dodržování adherence /ədˈhɪə.rənt s/

dohlížet na oversee /ˌəʊ.vəˈsiː/

dohlížet supervise /ˈsuː.pə.vaɪz/

dohlížet, kontrola, ovladač, ovládací prvek control /kənˈtrəʊl/

dokázaný, vyřízený (urovnaný) settled /ˈset.l̩ d/

dokázat prove /pruːv/

dokonalý, důkladný, naprostý, úplný thorough /ˈθʌr.ə/

dokončit (dopsat) write /raɪt/ up /ʌp/

dolíčkování, tečkování stippling/ ˈstɪp.lɪŋ/

dolíčkovaný, tečkovaný stippled / ˈstɪp.l̩ d/

dolít, doplnit, navršit, navýšit top / tɒp/ up /ʌp/

domácí péče home /həʊm/ care /keəʳ/

domácí, používaný v domácnosti domestic /dəˈmes.tɪk/

doména, oblast realm /relm/

domněnka, hypotéza assumption / əˈsʌmp.ʃən/

dopadat na, natlačit impact / ˈɪm.pækt/

dopler doppler /ˈdɒp.ləʳ/

doporučený advised /ədˈvaɪzd/, recommended /ˌrek.əˈmen.dɪd/

dopravní prostředek vehicle /ˈviː.ɪ.kļ/

doprovázet, provázet, spojovat accompany /əˈkʌm.pə.ni/

dopředu, dále forth /fɔːθ/

dormantní, spící, skrytý, latentní (možnosti), nepoužívaný dormant / ˈdɔː.mənt/

dosáhnout, docílit attain /əˈteɪn/

dosáhnout, uspět achieve /əˈtʃiːv/

dosavadní, před, předešlý, předchozí, překotný previous /ˈpriː.vi.əs/

dosažitelný, proveditelný achievable / əˈtʃiː.və.bļ/

dosedací plocha zubu, zatížení tooth-bearing /tuːθ.beə.rɪŋ/

dosedací plocha, dosedat seat /siːt/

doslova literally /ˈlɪt.ºr.ºl.i/

dospělý člověk adult /ˈæd.ʌlt/

dost, dostatečně enough /ɪˈnʌf/

dostat (obdržet), získat obtain /əbˈteɪn/

dostat, přijímat, získat receive / rɪˈsiːv/

dostupnost, vhodnost, vybavenost availability /əˌveɪ.ləˈbɪl.ɪ.ti/

dostupný accessible /əkˈses.ə.bļ/

dotaz query /ˈkwɪə.ri/ (pl. queries)

dotazník questionnaire /ˌkwes.tʃəˈneəʳ/

dovolit si, poskytovat, přinášet afford /əˈfɔːd/

dovolit, dovolovat, poskytnout, poskytovat, přípustit, povolit, umožnit allow /əˈlaʊ/

dovolit, připustit, tolerovat permit / pəˈmɪt/

Downova choroba Down's syndrome / ˈdaʊnz.sɪn.drəʊm/

drahý, nákladný costly /ˈkɒst.li/

drahý, vzácný precious /ˈpreʃ.əs/

drát wire /waɪəʳ/

drátěný oblouk archwire /ɑːtʃ.waɪəʳ/

dráždění irritation /ˌɪr.ɪˈteɪ.ʃən/

drhnout (kartáčem, vydrhnout scrub /skrʌb/

drtivý, zdrcující crushing /ˈkrʌʃ.ɪŋ/

druh střevních bacilů Bacteroides / ˌbæk.tɪəˈrɒɪ.diːz/

druhový (označující druh), všeobecný generic /dʒəˈner.ɪk/

druhy species /ˈspiː.ʃiːz/

držadlo holder /ˈhəʊl.dəʳ/

držadlo, rukojeť, násadec, násadec vrtačky handpiece /hænd.piːs/

držák, napínač, retenční přístroj, úchytka retainer /rɪˈteɪ.nəʳ/

držátko jehel needle /ˈniː.dļ/ holder / ˈhəʊl.dəʳ/

držení, držící holding /ˈhəʊl.dɪŋ/

držený held /held/

dřeňový pulpal /pʌlp.ºl/

dřevěný wooden /ˈwʊd.ºn/

dříve, brzy soon /suːn/

dříve, předem beforehand / bɪˈfɔː.hænd/

dudlík, uklidňovací prostředek pacifier /ˈpæs.ɪ.faɪ.əʳ/

důkaz (očividný), dokázat, jistota, svědectví evidence /ˈev.ɪ.dºnts/

důkladně, řádně, svědomitě (starostlivě) thoroughly /ˈθʌr.ə.li/

důležitost, význam, závažnost importance /ɪmˈpɔː.tºnts/

důležitý, převážný, velký, větší (velikostí i významem), významnější, závažný major /
'meɪ.dʒəʳ/

důležitý, význačný, významný
significant /sɪg'nɪf.ɪ.kənt/

duodenální, dvanáctníkový duodenal
/ˌdjuː.əʊ'diː.nəl/

dusit se, přestat dýchat choke /tʃəʊk/

důsledek implication /ˌɪm.plɪ'keɪ.ʃən/

důstojnost dignity /'dɪg.nɪ.ti/

duševně, psychicky mentally /
'men.tᵊl.i/

duševní, psychický mental /'men.tl/

dutina sinus /'saɪ.nəs/

**dutina, kavita, prohloubení, zubní
kaz** cavity /'kæv.ɪ.ti/

důvěra, spolehnutí confidence /
'kɒn.fɪ.dənts/

důvěrný confidential /ˌkɒn.fɪ'den.tʃᵊl/

důvod, mít v úmyslu, účel, záměr
purpose /'pɜː.pəs/

důvod, příčina reason /'riː.zᵊn/

dvojice, spojený, připojit couple /
'kʌp.ļ/

dvojitý, dvojnásobný, zdvojnásobit
double /'dʌb.ļ/

dvojitý, obousměrný dual /'djuː.əl/

**dýha, fazeta, nátěr, obložení, tenká
vrstva** veneer /və'nɪəʳ/

dýchací cesta air /eəʳ/ passage /
'pæs.ɪdʒ/

dýchací cesty airway /'eə.weɪ/

dýchání breathing /'briː.ðɪŋ/

dysestézie, porucha citlivosti
dysaesthesia /dɪs.æs.'θiːsɪ.ə/

dysfagie, porucha polykání dysphagia
/dɪ'sfeɪ.dʒiə/

dysmenorea, bolestivá menstruace
dysmenorrhoea /ˌdɪs.me.nə'riː.ə/

dysplazie, porucha vývoje nebo růstu
dysplasia /dis'pleɪ.zɪə/

dyspnoe, dušnost dyspnoea /
dɪs.pniː.ə/

dystrofie dystrophy /dɪs.trə.fi/

dysurie, obtíž při močení dysuria /
dɪs.'ju.ə.ri.ə/

E

edém, otok oedema /ɪ'diː.mə/

efektivně, účinně effectively /
ɪ'fek.tɪv.li/, efficiently /ɪ'fɪʃ.ᵊnt.li/

**efektivní (skutečný), působivý,
účinný (vysoce)** effective /ɪ'fek.tɪv/

ejektor, odsavač slin, vývěva saliva /
sə'laɪ.və/ ejector /ɪː'dʒekt.əʳ/

ejektor, sací pumpa ejector /
ɪ'dʒek.təʳ/

**elastický, pružný, pružná tkanina,
guma** elastic /ɪ'læs.tɪk/

**elastomer, pružný kaučuk, gumovitý
polymer** elastomer /ɪ'læs.tə.məʳ/

elastomerní elastomeric /
ɪ'læs.tə'mer.ɪk/

elektrický proud electrical /
ɪ'lek.trɪ.kᵊl/ current /'kʌr.ᵊnt/

elektrojiskrové obrábění spark /
spɑːk/ erosion /ɪ'rəʊ.ʒᵊn/

elektrokardiogram (EKG) ECG /
ˌiː.siː'dʒiː/ electrocardiogram /
ɪˌlek.trə'kɑː.di.ə.græm/

elektroléčba electrotherapy /
ɪˌlek.trəʊ'θer.ə.pi/

elektronický electronic /ɪˌlek'trɒn.ɪk/

**elevator, zdvihák, zvedač, páka,
zdviž** elevator /'el.ɪ.veɪ.təʳ/

**emfyzém, rozšíření tkání plynem
nebo vzduchem** emphysema /
ˌemp.fə'siː.mə/

**emise, ozařovací, radiace,
vyzařování, záření** radiation /
ˌreɪ.di'eɪ.ʃᵊn/

**endodoncie, nauka o onemocnění
zubní dřeně a kořenového**

kanálku, prevence a léčení zubní dřeně endodontics /ˌen.dəˈdɒn.tɪks/

endokarditida, zánět srdeční nitroblány endocarditis /ˌen.dəˈkɑː.ˈdai.tis/

endokrinní, s vnitřním vyměšováním endocrine /ˈen.də.krɑ ɪn/

energie, schopnost energy /ˈen.ə.dʒi/

enukleovat, odstranit celý orgán enucleate /ɪˈnjuː.kli.əɪt/

epilepsie epilepsy /ˈep.ɪ.lep.si/

epinefrin, adrenalin epinephrine /ˌep.ɪ.ˈnef.riːn/

epistaxe, krvácení z nosu epistaxis /ˌe.pɪ.ˈstæk.sɪs/

epitel, výstelka epithelium /e.pɪˈθiː.li.əm/

epitelový, výstelkový epithelial /e.pɪˈθiː.li.əl/

erytromycin erythromycin /ə.rɪθ.rəˈmaɪ.sɪn/

esteticky aesthetically /esˈθet.ɪ.kli/

estetika aesthetics /esˈθet.ɪks/

estrogen, ženský pohlavní hormon oestrogen /ˈiː.strəʊ .dʒ°n/

etapa (období), stádium, stav, stupeň stage /steɪdʒ/

etapa, fáze phase /feɪz/

etiologický, podle příčiny aetiological /ˌiː.ti.ˈɒl.ə.dʒi.k°l/

etiologie, nauka o původu a příčinách aetiology /ˌiː.ti.ˈɒl.ə.dʒi/

etylchlorid ethyl /eθɪl/ chloride /ˈklɔː.raɪd/

eugenol eugenol /juːˈdʒen.ɒl/

eventuálně, střídavě alternatively /ɒlˈtɜː.nə.tɪv.li/

excise kavity, odstranění nekrotické tkáně, toaleta kavity debridement /dɪˈbriːd.mənt/

excize, vyříznutí excision /ekˈsɪʒ.°n/

exkavační lžička spoon /spuːn/ excavator /ˈek.skə.veɪ.təʳ/

exkavátor excavator /ˈek.skə.veɪ.təʳ/

expanze, rozšíření expansion /ɪkˈspæn.tʃ°n/

exsudát, zánětlivá tekutina, výpotek exudate /eks.juːdeɪt/

extirpace, totální vynětí nervu extirpation /ˌek.stɜːˈpeɪ.ʃ°n/

extra, výborný super /ˈsuː.pəʳ/

extrahovat, vytáhnout, vytrhnout extract /ɪkˈstrækt/

extraorální kotvení, zevní tah headgear /ˈhed.gɪəʳ/

extrémně extremely /ɪkˈstriːm.li/

extruze, vysunutí, vystrčení, vypuzení extrusion /ɪkˈstruː.ʒ°n/

ezofagitida, zánět jícnu oesophagitis /ˌiːsɒ.fəˈdʒaɪ.tɪs/

F

faciální, obličejový, lícní facial /ˈfeɪ.ʃ°l/

farmacie, lékárna, lékárnička, lékárnický pharmacy /ˈfɑː.mə.si/

farynx, hltan pharynx /ˈfær.ɪŋks/

fatální, smrtelný fatal /ˈfeɪ.t°l/

fazeta facing /ˈfeɪ.sɪŋ/

femur, stehenní kost femur /ˈfiː.məʳ/

fenomén (úkaz, jev, div), vlastnost phenomenon /fəˈnɒm.ɪ.nən/

fermentace, kvašení fermentation /ˌfɜː.menˈteɪ.ʃ°n/

feromagnetický ferromagnetic /ˌfer.ə.mægˈnet.ɪk/

fialový purple /ˈpɜː.pl̩/

fibrilace fibrillation /ˌfaɪ.brɪˈleɪ.ʃ°n/

fibrin (biol.) fibrin /ˈfɪ.brɪn/

filosofie, strategie philosophy /fɪˈlɒs.ə.fi/

finální, konečný final /ˈfaɪ.n°l/

fistula, píštěl fistula /ˈfɪs.tjʊ.lə/

fixace, upevnění fixation /fɪk'seɪ.ʃ°n/

fixovaný, upevněný, pevný, nepohyblivý, stálý fixed /fɪkst/

flatulence, plynatost flatulence / 'flæt.jʊ.lən*t* s/

flebitida, zánět žil phlebitis / flɪ'baɪ.tɪs/

flexibilní, pružný flexible /'flek.sɪ.bl̩/

fluoridace fluoridation / ˌflʊə.rɪ'deɪ.ʃən/

folát, sůl kyseliny listové folate / fəʊ.leɪt/

folikulární (anat.), váčkový follicular /fə'lɪk.jʊ.lə^r/

forma, tvar mould /məʊld/

formovat, tvarovat shape /ʃeɪp/

fosforečnan zinečnatý zinc /zɪŋk/ phosphate /'fɒs.feɪt/

foto photo /'fəʊ.təʊ/

fraktura, zlomenina fracture / 'fræk.*t*ʃ°r /

frenotomie, protětí uzdičky frenectomy /frɪ'nɒ.tə.mi/

frontální, přední, čelní frontal / 'frʌn.təl/

fungicidní, proti houbám, protiplísňový antifungal / ˌæn.ti'fʌŋ.gəl/

fungovat work /wɜːk/

fungovat, provést, předvést, vykonat perform /pə'fɔːm/

fungovat, působit (o léku ap.) operate /'ɒp.°r.eɪt/

funkce, použití, praxe, užití, užívání use /juːs/

funkční, fungující functional / 'fʌŋk.ʃ°n.°l/

furkace, rozvětvení furcation / fɜː'keɪ.ʃ°n/

fyzikální physical /'fɪz.ɪ.k°l/

G

gallium, síran galitý gallium / 'gæl.ɪ.əm/

gastrický, žaludeční gastric /'gæs.trɪk/

gastrointestinální, týkající se žaludku a střeva gastrointestinal / ˌgæs.trəʊˌɪn.tes'taɪ.n°l/

genitourinární, močopohlavní genitourinary /ˌdʒen.ɪ.təʊ'jʊə.rɪn.ri/

gesto, posuněk, ukázat gesture / 'dʒes.tʃə^r/

gingivální, dásňový gingival / ˌdʒɪn.dʒɪ.val/

glomeluronefritida, zánět ledvin, spojený se zánětem glomerulů glomerulonephritis / glɒ'me.ru.lə.nəf'raɪ.tɪs/

glukagon, peptidový hormon, tvořený ve slinivce břišní glucagon /gluː.kəg.ən/

glyceriltrinitrát, nitroglycerin glyceryl /'glɪs.ə.rɪl/ trinitrate / traɪ'naɪ.treɪt/

gonorea, kapavka gonorrhoea / ˌgɒn.ə'riː.ə/

gram negativní gram /græm/ negative /'neg.ə.tɪv/

gram pozitivní gram /græm/ positive / 'pɒz.ə.tɪv/

gumová blána rubber /'rʌb.ə^r/ dam / dæm/

gutaperča gutta-percha /ˌgʌt.ə'pɜː.tʃə/

gynekologie, ženské lékařství gynaecology /ˌgaɪ.nə'kɒl.ə.dʒi/

H

habituální, navyklý, častý, notorický habitual /hə'bɪtʃ.u.əl/

háček hook /hʊk/

halucinace, klam delusion /dɪ'luː.ʒən/

halucinace, přelud hallucination / həˌluː.sɪ'neɪ.ʃ°n/

hantýrka (odborná) jargon /
ˈdʒɑː.gən/

Heimlichův manévr Heimlich
manoeuvre /ˈhaɪm.lɪk.mə'nuː.vəʳ/

hemisekce, řez v polovině orgánu
hemisection /ˈhem.ɪ.ˈsek.ʃᵊn/

hemofilie, dědičná krvácivost
haemophilia /ˌhiː.mə'fɪl.i.ə/

hemofilik, jedinec trpící hemofilií
haemophiliac /ˌhiː.mə'fɪl.i.æk/

hemoptýza, vykašlávání krve
haemoptysis /hiː'mɒ.ptɪ.sɪs/

hemoroidy haemorrhoids /
ˈhem.ᵊr.ɔɪdz/

hemostáza, zástava krvácení
haemostasis /ˌhiːmə'ste.sɪs/

hepatitida, zánět jater hepatitis /
ˌhep.ə'taɪ.tɪs/

hernie (kýla) hernia /ˈhɜː.ni.ə/

herpes, opar herpes /ˈhɜː.piːz/

heterogenní, různorodý
heterogeneous /ˌhet.ər.ə'dʒiː.ni.əs/

histologický, tkáňový histological /
ˌhɪ.stə'lɒdʒ.ɪ.kᵊl/

hladce smoothly /ˈsmuː.ð.li/

hladina, plocha, opracovat povrch,
povrch, stěna surface /ˈsɜː.fɪs/

hladina, stejná rovina, stupeň,
úroveň, vrstva level /ˈlev.ᵊl/

hladovění fasting /fɑː.st.ɪŋ/

hladovět fast /fɑːst/

hlas, hlasový, vyjádřit (názor,
mínění) voice /vɔɪs/

hlásit, ohlásit, oznámit, podat
zprávu, udělat zápis report /rɪ'pɔːt/

hlasitý loud /laʊd/

hlavně principally /ˈprɪnt.sɪ.pli/

hlavní, nejdůležitější, nejvyšší, velice
důležitý, vrcholný paramount /
ˈpær.ə.maʊnt/

hlavní, originální master /ˈmɑː.stəʳ/

hlavní, prvotní prime /praɪm/

hlavní, silný main /meɪn/

hlavní, všeobecný, celkový general /
ˈdʒen.ᵊr.ᵊl/

hledat, pátrání po, zjistit search /
sɜːtʃ/ for /fɔːʳ/

hledisko, přední část, záhlaví heading
/ˈhed.ɪŋ/

hlodavý vřed rodent /ˈrəʊ.dᵊnt/ ulcer /
ˈʌl.səʳ/

hluboce uložený, mající hluboké
kořeny deep-seated /diːp.'siː.tɪd/

hluboký (důkladný) profound /
prə'faʊnd/

hluboký, hlubina, ponořený deep /
diːp/

hluchota deafness /ˈdef.nəs/

hluk, porucha, zvuk noise /nɔɪz/

hmatat, cítit, pocítit feel /fiːl/

hmota, masa mass /mæs/

hodit se, vhodný, padnout (oděv) fit /
fɪt/

hodnota, význam significance /
sɪg'nɪf.ɪ.kənt s/

hodnotit, ohodnotit, zhodnotit,
posuzovat, určit assess /ə'ses/

hojný, bohatý copious /ˈkəʊ.pi.əs/

holení shaving /ˈʃeɪ.vɪŋ/

horečka fever /ˈfiː.vəʳ/

horní sval oční trochlear /trə.kli.ə/

horší worse /wɜːs/

houbový, plísňový fungal /ˈfʌŋ.gəl/

houpat, rozkývat swing /swɪŋ/

houževnatost, mez pevnosti strength /
streŋθ/

hovor, mluvit talk /tɔːk/

hračka toy /tɔɪ/

hrana, lem, obroučka, okraj rim /rɪm/

hranice, hrana, okraj, rámeček,
lemovat border /bɔː.dəʳ/

hranice, limit, omezení limit /ˈlɪm.ɪt/

hraniční, sporný borderline /
bɔː.dəʳ.laɪn/

hrbol na kosti, drsnatina tuberosity / ˈtjuː.bəˈrɒs.ə.ti/

hrdina heroe /ˈhɪə.rəʊ/

hromadit se, nahromadit accumulate /əˈkjuː.mjʊ.leɪt/

hrot kořene root /ruːt/ apex /ˈeɪ.peks/

hrot, pracovní konec nástroje, špička point /pɔɪnt/

hrot, špička, zahrocení tip /tɪp/

hrozivý sinister /ˈsɪn.ɪ.stəʳ/

hrubě grossly /ˈgrəʊ.sli/

hruď, prsa breast /brest/

hrudní koš rib /rɪb/ cage /keɪdʒ/

hrudník, prsní chest /tʃest/

hubička, licí koncovka, tryska nozzle /ˈnɒz.l̩/

hybridní protézy overdentures / ˈəʊ.və.ˈden.tʃəz/

hydrocortison hydrocortisone / haɪ.drəʊˈkɔː.tɪ.zəʊn/

hydrokoloid hydrocolloid / haɪ.drəʊˈkɒl.ɒid/

hygiena, zdravověda hygiene / ˈhaɪ.dʒiːn/

hygienický hygienic /haɪˈdʒiː.nɪk/

hygienik hygienist /haɪˈdʒiː.nɪst/

hynoucí, umírající dying /ˈdaɪ.ɪŋ/

hyperglykémie, zvýšené množství glukózy v krvi hyperglycaemia / ˌhaɪ.pə.glaɪˈsiː.mi.ə/

hypersensitivita, přecitlivělost hypersensitivity / ˈhaɪ.pə.ˌsen.sɪˈtɪv.ɪ.ti/

hypertyroidismus, zvýšená činnost štítné žlázy hyperthyroidism / ˌhaɪ.pə.ˈθaɪə.rɔɪdɪ.zᵊm/

hypnoterapie, léčení spánkem hypnotherapy /ˌhɪp.nəʊ ˈθer.ə.pi/

hypofýza, podvěsek mozkový pituitary gland /pɪˈtjuː.ɪ.tᵊr.i,glænd/

hypoglykémie hypoglycaemia / ˌhaɪ.pəʊ .glaɪˈsiː.mi.ə/

hypochondrie hypochondria /ˌhaɪ. pəʊ ˈkɒn.dri.ə/

hypotetický hypothetical /ˌhaɪ. pəˈθet.ɪ.kᵊl/

hypotyreóza, snížená činnost štítné žlázy hypothyroidism /ˌhaɪ.pəʊ. ˈθaɪə.rɔɪdɪ.zᵊm/

CH

chápat, vysvětlit translate /trænsˈleɪt/

charakter, povaha, přirozená vlastnost nature /ˈneɪ.tʃəʳ/

charakter, vlastnosti character / ˈkær.ɪk.təʳ/

charakteristický rys, znak, vlastnost feature /ˈfiː.tʃəʳ/

charakteristika, kvalita, vlastnost property /ˈprɒp.ə.ti/

chirurg, praktický lékař surgeon / ˈsɜː.dʒᵊn/

chirurgický, pooperační surgical / ˈsɜː.dʒɪ.kᵊl/

chlad, studený, nachlazení cold / kəʊld/

chladicí prostředek s použitím odpařování vapocoolant / ˈveɪ.pə.ˈkuː.lənt/

chladič condenser /kənˈden.səʳ/

chladivo, ochlazovací prostředek coolant /ˈkuː.lənt/

chladný, vlhce lepkavý clammy / ˈklæm.i/

chlazený, zchlazený cooled /kuːld/

chlopeň, lalok, kousek volně visící kůže flap /flæp/

chodba, tunel tunnel /ˈtʌn.ᵊl/

chomáčkovitý tufted /ˈtʌf.tɪd/

choroba, patologie (obor), stav způsobující onemocnění pathology /pəˈθɒl.ə.dʒi/

chorobná chuť k jídlu bulimia / bʊˌlɪm.i.ə/

chorobné nechutenství anorexia nervosa /æn.ə‚rek.si.ə.nə'vəʊ.sə/

chorobný strach z rakoviny cancerphobia /'kænt.sə'ˈfəʊ.bi.ə/

chránit, bránit, ochrana guard /gɑːd/

chránit, ochrana protect /prə'tekt/

chrápat snore /snɔːʳ/

chrom chrome /krəʊm/

chrom, chromový chromium /ˈkrəʊ.mi.əm/

chronický, vleklý, trvalý chronic /ˈkrɒn.ɪk/

chřadnutí, rozpuštění, vstřebání resorption /rɪˈsɔːp.ʃən/

chudokrevnost anaemia /əˈniː.mi.ə/

chuť k jídlu appetite /ˈæp.ɪ.taɪt/

chutnající-tasting /-teɪ.stɪŋ/

chválit, pochvala praise /preɪz/

chvění, strach, třes tremor /ˈtrem.əʳ/

chybějící zuby missing /ˈmɪs.ɪŋ/ teeth /tiːθ/

chybějící, nepřítomný missing /ˈmɪs.ɪŋ/

chybná diagnóza misdiagnosis /mɪs‚daɪ.əgˈnəʊ.sɪs/

chybná poloha, špatné úmístění malposition /mæl.pəˈzɪʃ.ən/

chybně vytvořený malformed /‚mælˈfɔːmd/

chybný, malý, slabý, špatný poor /pɔːʳ/

chytlavý, snadno zapamatovatelný catchy /ˈkætʃ.i/

I

iatrogenní, lékařem vyvolaný iatrogenic /aɪ‚ætrəˈdʒen.ɪk/

ibuprofen ibuprofen /‚aɪ.bjuːˈprəʊ.fen/

idiopatický, samostatný idiopathic /ˈɪdiəˈpæθɪk/

ignorovat, opovrhovat despise /dɪˈspaɪz/

ihned at /ət/ once /wʌnts/

ihned, pohotově readily /ˈred.ɪ.li/

implantát implant /ɪmˈplɑːnt/

impulz, puls pulse /pʌls/

imunodeficience, nedostatek imunity immunodeficiency /‚ɪm.jʊ.nəʊ .dɪˈfɪʃ.ⁿt.si/

imunokompromitovaný, se sníženou imunitou immunocompromised /ɪˈmjuː.nə‚kɒm.prə.maɪzd/

imunosuprese, snížení schopnosti organismu reagovat na cizí látky immunosuppression /‚ɪm.jə.nəʊ.səˈpreʃ.ⁿn/

incizální, řezný, řezací, kousací incisal /ɪnˈsɪ.zⁿl/

indikovat, označit, označovat, signalizovat, ukazovat indicate /ˈɪn.dɪ.keɪt/

infiltrovat filter /ˈfɪl.təʳ/

informovaný, bdělý, být si vědom, uvědomovat si aware /əˈweəʳ/

injekční stříkačka, stříkačka, vstříknout syringe /sɪˈrɪndʒ/

inkontinence, neschopnost udržet moč či stolici incontinence /ɪnˈkɒn.tɪ.nənts/

insulin insulin /ˈɪn.sjʊ.lɪn/

interní, vnitřní internal /ɪnˈtɜː.nəl/

interrupce abortion /əˈbɔː.ʃən/

intraorálně, uvnitř úst intraorally /‚ɪn.trə.ˈɔː.rə.li/

intraoseální, ležící uvnitř kosti, nitrokostní intraosseous /‚ɪn.trəˈɒs.i.əs/

intravenózně, do žil intravenously /‚ɪn.trəˈviː.nə.sli/

intravenózní, nitrožilní IV /‚aɪˈviː/, intravenous /‚ɪn.trəˈviː.nəs/

intruse, vnikání, vtlačení intrusion /ɪnˈtruː.ʒⁿn/

intubace, zavedení rourky do průdušnice intubation /ˌɪŋ.tjʊˈbeɪ.ʃᵊn/

invaze, napadení invasion /ɪnˈveɪ.ʒᵊn/

invazivní, agresivní invasive / ɪnˈveɪ.sɪv/

inzerát advertising /ˈæd.və.taɪ.zɪŋ/

iont ion /ˈaɪ.ɒn/

iradiace, osvětlení, ozáření irradiation /ɪˌreɪ.diˈeɪ.ʃᵊn/

ischemický, nedokrvený ischaemic / ɪsˈkɪː.mɪk/

izolace, oddělování, osamocení isolation /ˌaɪ.sᵊl.eɪ.ʃᵊn/

izolační materiál, obal, podložka, vložka liner /ˈlaɪ.nəʳ/

izometrický, mající stejné rozměry isometric /aɪ.səʊ ˈmet.rɪk/

izotonický, se stejným osmotickým tlakem isotonic /aɪ.səʊ ˈtɒn.ɪk/

J

jádro, nitro, střed hlavní core /kɔːʳ/

jádro, trn, vřeteno mandrel / ˈmæn.drəl/

jamka fossa /ˈfɒs.ə/

jamka lopatky pro skloubení v ramenním kloubu glenoid / glɪː.nɒɪd/ fossa /ˈfɒs.ə/

jasný, lesklý shiny /ˈʃaɪ.ni/

jaterní hepatic /hepˈæt.ɪk/

jazylka hyoid /haɪ.oɪd/

jednání (chování), způsob práce, reakce behaviour /bɪˈheɪ.vjər /

jednat, zacházet, týkat se deal /dɪəl/ with /wɪð/

jednoduchý, jasný (zřetelný) plain / pleɪn/

jednoduchý, prostý simple /ˈsɪm.pl̩ /

jednostupňový single-stage / ˈsɪŋ.gl̩.steɪdʒ/

jednotlivě, po jednom singly /ˈsɪŋ.gli/

jednou, jakmile jednou, svého času once /wʌnt s/

jedovatý výpar poisonous /ˈpɔɪ.zᵊn.əs/ vapour /ˈveɪ.pəʳ/

jedovatý, škodlivý, toxický poisonous /ˈpɔɪ.zᵊn.əs/

jemně, mírně gently /ˈdʒent.li/

jemný delicate /ˈdel.ɪ.kət/, gentle / ˈdʒen.tl̩ /

jemný, nedráždivý bland /blænd/

jemný, ryzí, ušlechtilý fine /faɪn/

jestli whether /ˈweð.əʳ/

jev, eventualita, událost, případ, výsledek event /ɪˈvent/

jícnový oesophageal /ɪːˌsɒf.ə.ˈdʒɪ.əl/

jídlo (denní) meal /mɪəl/

jíst eat /iːt/

jistě confidently /ˈkɒn.fɪ.dənt.li/

jizva scar /skɑːʳ/

jmenovaný, určený designated / ˈdez.ɪg.neɪ.tɪd/

jmenovat se name /neɪm/

jmenovat, navrhnout nominate / ˈnɒm.ɪ.neɪt/

K

k dispozici, k jednou použití (pouze) disposable /dɪˈspəʊ.zə.bl̩ /

k dispozici, po ruce at /ət/ hand /hænd/

kalibr, vývrt bore /bɔːr /

kámen stone /stəʊn/

kamenec, ledek alum /ˈæl.əm/

kampaň campaign /kæmˈpeɪn/

kanálek canal /kəˈnæl/

kanálek, trubice duct /dʌkt/

kandidóza, infekce způsobená některými druhy Candidy candidiasis /ˌkæn.di.ˈdaɪ.ə.sɪs/, candidosis /ˈkæn.dɪ.dəʊ.sɪs/

kanyla, dutá jehla, trubička cannula / ˈkæn.jʊ.lə/ (pl. cannulae)

kanystr canister /ˈkæn.ɪ.stəʳ/

kapalina, kapalný, průzračný, tekutina, tekutý liquid /ˈlɪk.wɪd/

kapka, klesnout, upustit drop /drɒp/

kapsa, chobot zubu, váček pocket / ˈpɒk.ɪt/

karamelový bonbón toffee /ˈtɒf.i/

karbid, tvrdý kov carbide /ˈkɑː.baɪd/

karboxylát carboxylate /kɑːˈbɒk.sɪl.eɪt/

kardiovaskulární cardiovascular / ˌkɑː.di.əʊˈvæs.kjʊ.ləʳ/

kariézní, kazivý, zkažený (zub), zasažený kazem carious /ˈkeər.ɪ.əs/

karotida carotid /kəˌrɒt.ɪd/

karta, záznam record /ˈrek.ɔːd/

kaskáda, seřazení za sebou cascade / kæsˈkeɪd/

kašel cough /kɒf/

kašovitá hmota, rozmačkat squash / skwɒʃ/

katastrofální, ničivý disastrous / dɪˈzɑː.strəs/

katétr, cévka catheter /ˈkæθ.ɪ.təʳ/

kaz, vada, zabarvit, zanechat skvrny stain /steɪn/

kazit se, chátrat, zhoršit deteriorate / dɪˈtɪə.ri.ə.reɪt/

kazový, podporující vznik kazu, vyvolávající kaz cariogenic/ˌkeərɪ.əˈdʒen.ɪk/

kdežto, když, zatímco whilst /waɪl.st/

kdežto, zatímco whereas /weəˈræz/

kelímek pot /pɒt/

keramická směs, lepidlo, lepit, pasta, přilepit paste /peɪst/

keramický materiál ceramics / sɪˈræm.ɪks/

kladení, poloha, umístění, uspořádání placement /ˈpleɪs.mənt/

kleště, klíšťky, pinzeta pliers /ˈplaɪ.əz/

kleště, nůžky (velké) shears /ʃɪəz/

klíč key /kiː/

klička, uzel knot /nɒt/

klíčová dírka keyhole /ˈkiː.həʊl/

klidový resting /ˈrest.ɪŋ/

kliknutí, klapnutí click /klɪk/

klín cline /klaɪn/

klín, vklínit, vtlačit, zaklínit wedge / wedʒ/

klonický, škubavý clonic /klɒn.ik/

kloub spánkový a dolní čelisti temporomandibular / ˌtem.pər.ə.mænˈdɪ.bjʊ.ləʳ/ joint / dʒɔɪnt/

kloub, místo připojení, spojení joint / dʒɔɪnt/

kloubní revmatismus, revmatická artritida rheumatoid arthritis / ˌruː.mə.tɔɪd.ɑːˈθraɪ.tɪs/

kloubový, spojený articulated /ɑːˈtɪk.jʊ.leɪ.tɪd/

koagulace, srážení coagulation / kəʊˈæg.jʊ.leɪ.ʃən/

kobalt cobalt /ˈkəʊ.bɒlt/

kód, zásada, kodex, kódovat code / kəʊd/

kodein codeine /ˈkəʊ.diːn/

kódovaný coded /kəʊd.ɪd/

kochleární, hlemýžďovitý choclear / kɒk.lɪ.ə/

kojení breastfeeding /ˈbrestˌfiːd.ɪŋ/

kojit nurse /nɜːs/

koláč, dort cake /keɪk/

kolaps, hroutit se, zhroutit se, zhroucení (přen.) collapse /kəˈlæps/

koloid, druh roztoku, homogenní, želatinový, rosolovitý colloid / kɒl.ɒ.id/

kombinovat, spojit combine / kəmˈbaɪn/

kompletní, důkladný exhaustive / ɪgˈzɔː.stɪv/

komplex, složitý complex /ˈkɒm.pleks/

komplexní, obsáhlý, úplný comprehensive /ˌkɒm.prɪˈhenʃ.sɪv/

komplikace, obtíž complication /
ˌkɒm.plɪˈkeɪ.ʃᵊn/

komplikovat complicate /
ˈkɒm.plɪ.keɪt/

komplikující situaci, obtížný,
otravný (nepříjemný) troublesome
/ˈtrʌb.l̩.sᵊm/

kompozitní pryskyřice resin /ˈrez.ɪn/
composite /ˈkɒm.pə.zɪt/

komprese, stisk, stlačení, zhuštění
compression /kəmˈpreʃ.ən/

komunikace, volný prostor freeway /
ˈfriː.weɪ/

komunikovat communicate /
kəˈmjuː.nɪ.keɪt/

komunita, společnost, veřejnost
community /kəˈmjuː.nə.ti/

končetina extremity /ɪkˈstrem.ɪ.ti/,
limb /lɪm/

kondicionér conditioner /kənˈdɪʃ.ᵊn.ᵊr/

kondyl, kloubní hrbol condyle /
ˌkɒn.dɑɪl/

koneček stehů suture /ˈsuː.tʃəʳ/ end /
end/

konstrukce construction /kənˈstrʌk.ʃən/

kontinuita, nepřetržitost, souvislost,
neprůchodnost continuity /
ˌkɒn.tɪˈnjuː.ɪ.ti/

kontraindikace contraindication /
ˈkɒn.trə.ˌɪnd.ɪ.ˈkeɪ.ʃᵊn/

kontrola check-up /tʃek.ʌp/

kontrola, bilance, prověřit, prověrka
audit /ˈɔː.dɪt/

kontrolovaný, řízený controlled /
kənˈtrəʊld/

kontura, obrys, nárys, náčrtek
outline /ˈaʊt.laɪn/

konvenční, tradiční conventional /
kənˈvent.ʃən.əl/

konzistence, hutnost, hustota, tuhost,
soudržnost consistency /
kənˈsɪs.tᵊnt.si/

konzumovat, sníst, zkonzumovat,
spotřebovat consume /kənˈsjuːm/

koordinace, uvedení v soulad
coordination /kəʊ.ˌɔː.dɪˈneɪ.ʃən/

kopie copy /ˈkɒp.i/

korelace, vztah correlation /
ˌkɒr.əˈleɪ.ʃən/

kortikosteroid corticosteroid /
ˈkɔː.tɪkɒˈster.ɔɪd/

kořeněný spicy /ˈspaɪ.si/

kořenová fréza root /ruːt/ face /feɪs/

kořenový kanálek root /ruːt/ canal /
kəˈnæl/

kost vřetenní radius /ˈreɪ.di.əs/

kosterní typ skeletal /ˈskel.ɪ.tᵊl/ pattern
/ˈpæt.ən/

kostní bony /ˈbəʊ.ni/

kostra skeleton /ˈskel.ɪ.tᵊn/

kotevní spona crib /krɪb/

kotouč disc /dɪsk/

kouření smoking /ˈsməʊ.kɪŋ/

kousání, kousající biting /ˈbaɪ.tɪŋ/

kousek, kus piece /piːs/

kousnutý bitten /ˈbɪt.ən/

krájet na plátky, seškrábnout slice /
slaɪs/

krajní, zoufalý dire /daɪəʳ/

kraniomandibulární, týkající
se lebky a dolní čelisti
craniomandibular /
ˈkreɪ.ni.ə.ˌmæn.ˈdɪ.bjʊ.ləʳ/

krční límec cervical /səˈvaɪ.kəl/ collar
/ˈkɒl.əʳ/

krém, pasta cream /kriːm/

kreozot (chem.) creosote /ˈkriː.ə.səʊt/

kreslit (pastelkou) crayon /ˈkreɪ.ɒn/

krevní obraz blood /blʌd/ count /
kaʊnt/

krevní porucha blood /blʌd/ disorder /
dɪˈsɔː.dəʳ/

krevní sraženina blood /blʌd/ clot /
klɒt/

krevní test blood /blʌd/ test /test/

krevní tlak blood /blʌd/ pressure / ˈpreʃ.ər/

krikotyreoidní, týkající se spoje chrupavky prstencové a štítné cricothyroid /ˌkraɪ.kəˈθaɪə.rɔɪd/

kromě toho, dále, další, vzdálenější further /ˈfɜː.ðəʳ/

kromě, vyjmout except /ɪkˈsept/

kruh circle /ˈsɜː.kl̩/

krutost, náročnost, potíže, útrapy, vážnost severity /sɪˈver.ɪ.ti/

kryochirurgie, schlazení tkání pod minus 20 stupňů cryosurgery / kraɪ.əˈsɜːdʒər.i/

krysa rat /ræt/

krystal, křemen, křemenný quartz / ˈkwɔːts/

kryt, pokrytí cover /ˈkʌv.əʳ/

kryt, příklop, víčko, víko lid /lɪd/

křehký brittle /ˈbrɪt.l̩/, fragile / ˈfrædʒ.aɪl/

křeslo chair /tʃeəʳ/

křídovitý chalky /ˈtʃɔː.ki/

křik, zavolání, zvolání shouting / ˈʃaʊ.tɪŋ/

kterýkoli (z určitého počtu) whichever /wɪˈtʃev.əʳ/

kterýkoliv whatever /wɒtˈev.əʳ/

kujnost, tažnost, poddajnost ductility /dʌkˈtɪl.ɪ.ti/

kulatě zakončený, zakončený kuličkou ball-ended /bɔːl.ˈen.dɪd/

kulatý vrtáček round /raʊnd/ bur / bɜːr /

kůra, strup, povlak, usazenina crust / krʌst/

kuželový, zahrocený, zužující se tapered /ˈteɪ.pəd/

kvalitativní, jakostní qualitative / ˈkwɒl.ɪ.tə.tɪv/

kvantita, množství quantity / ˈkwɒn.tɪ.ti/

kvantitativní (mnohostní) quantitative /ˈkwɒn.tɪ.tə.tɪv/

kvůli, v zájmu for /fɔːʳ/ the sake /seɪk/

kyretáž, výškrab curettage /ˌkjʊəˈret.ɪdʒ/

kyselina polyakrylová polyacrylic / ˈpɒl.i.əˈkrɪl.ɪk/ acid /ˈæs.ɪd/

kysličník dusný, rajský plyn nitrous oxide /ˌnaɪ.trəsˈɒk.saɪd/

kysličník hlinitý alumina /əˈluː.mɪ.nə/

L

lacerace, tržná rána laceration / ˌlæs.ºrˈeɪ.ʃºn/

lak, lesk, nalakovat varnish /ˈvɑː.nɪʃ/

laktobacil, střevní mikroorganismus, vytvářející kyselinu mléčnou Lactobacillus /ˈlæk.tʊ.bəˈsɪl.əs/

laserový laser /ˈleɪ.zəʳ/

laterální, postranní, vedlejší, příčný lateral /ˈlæt.rºl/

lebeční nerv cranial /ˈkreɪ.ni.əl/ nerve /nɜːv/

léčba, lék, medikace medication / ˌmed.ɪˈkeɪ.ʃºn/

léčba, ošetření, péče management / ˈmæn.ɪdʒ.mənt/

léčebný medicated /ˈmed.ɪ.keɪ.tɪd/

léčebný postup, ošetření, pohoštění, zacházení (s) treatment /ˈtriːt.mənt/

léčit, léčit se, hojit, zahojit se heal / hiːl/

ledvina kidney /ˈkɪd.ni/

legrace fun /fʌn/

lehký light /laɪt/

lehký, mírný, nepatrný, tenký slight /slaɪt/

lék drug /drʌg/, medicine /ˈmed.ɪ.sən/

lék proti bolesti painkiller/ˈpeɪn.kɪl.əʳ/

lékárnička první pomoci, příruční lékárnička first-aid /ˈfɜːst.eɪd/ kit / kɪt/

lékařská anamnéza medical / ˈmed.ɪ.kəl/ history /ˈhɪs.tər.i/

lékařský medical /ˈmed.ɪ.kəl/

lekce, ordinace, sezení (porada) session /ˈseʃ.ən/

lemovat, linka (čárka) line /laɪn/

lemující, obložení, vložka, výplněk, výstelka lining /ˈlaɪ.nɪŋ/

lepení, tmelení, spojení, spojení lepidlem, vazba, vázání, slučování, spojování bonding /ˈbɒnd.ɪŋ/

lepicí náplast sticking plaster / ˈstɪk.ɪŋˌplɑː.stər/

lepivost, soudržnost stickiness / ˈstɪk.ɪ.nəs/

lepší, vhodnější preferable / ˈpref.ər.ə.bl̩ /

leptadlo etchant /etʃ.ənt/

lesknout se, zářit shine /ʃaɪn/

lešticí kotouč polishing /ˈpɒl.ɪʃ.ɪŋ/ disc /dɪsk/

leštit polish /ˈpɒl.ɪʃ/

leštítko, hladítko, cpátko burnisher / ˈbɜː.nɪʃ.ər/

letargie, strnulost, netečnost lethargy /ˈleθ.ə.dʒɪ/

leukemie leukaemia /luːˈkiː.mi.ə/

leukoplakie, bělavé skvrny na sliznici leukoplakia /ˌluːkə.ˈpleɪ.kɪə/

léze, poranění, poškození, porucha, postižené místo, zranění lesion / ˈliː.ʒən/

ležící lying (inf. lie) /ˈlaɪ.ɪŋ/

ležící na břiše prone /prəʊn/

ležící naznak, ležící tváří vzhůru, klidný supine /ˈsuː.paɪn/

libovolný any /ˈen.i/

ligament, vaz, vazivo ligament / ˈlɪg.ə.mənt/

ligatura, podvázání ligature / ˈlɪg.ə.tʃər/

limitace, omezení, nedostatek, vada limitation /ˌlɪm.ɪˈteɪ.ʃən/

lipom, nezhoubný tukový nádor lipoma /lɪˈp.əʊ.mə/

liposarkom, zhoubný nádor z tukové tkáně liposarcoma /ˌlɪp.ə.sɑːˈkəʊ.mə/

lis, zhutňovač compactor /kəmˈpæk.tər/

lišej lichen /ˈlaɪ.kən/ planus /pleɪnəs/

lišit se, neshodovat se, nesouhlasit differ /ˈdɪf.ər /

lokace, poloha, umístění location / ləʊ ˈkeɪ.ʃən/

lokálně, místně locally /ˈləʊ.kəl.i/

lokomotorický, pohybový locomotor / ˌləʊ.kəˈməʊ.tər/

lopatička, třecí lopatka, stěrka, špachtle spatula /ˈspæt.jʊ.lə/

lopatka shoulder /ˈʃəʊl.dər/ blade / bleɪd/

loudavost, nemotornost sloth /sləʊθ/

luminofor phosphor /ˈfɒs.fər/

lymfa, míza lymph /lɪmp f/

lymfadenopatie, nepřesně určené onemočnění mízních uzlin lymphadenopathy / lɪmpˌfædɪˈnɒp.ə.θɪ/

lymfatická uzlina lymph /lɪmp f/ node /nəʊd/

lymfatický lymphatic /lɪmp ˈfæt.ɪk/

lymfom, maligní tumor lymfatické tkáně lymphoma /lɪmpˈfəʊ.mə/

lžíce, lopatka spoon /spuːn/

M

mačkat, protlačit, stisknout, stlačit, vymačkat squeeze /skwiːz/

magnetické pole magnetic / mægˈnet.ɪk/ field /fiːld/

magnetofonová páska audio / ˈɔː.di.əʊ/ tape /teɪp/

mající vztah, spojený, vztahující se k related /rɪˈleɪ.tɪd/

mající závrať, zmámený light-headed /ˌlaɪtˈhed.ɪd/

malátnost, únava lassitude / ˈlæs.ɪ.tjuːd/

maligní, škodlivý, zákeřný, zhoubný malignant /məˈlɪg.nənt/

málo few /fjuː/

malování painting /ˈpeɪn.tɪŋ/

malý epileptický záchvat petit mal / ˌpəˈtiːˈmæl/

malý mezizubní kartáček bottle / ˈbɒt.l/ brush /brʌʃ/

malý, menší minor /ˈmaɪ.nəʳ/

manifestace, objevení, projev manifestation /ˌmæn.ɪ.fesˈteɪ.ʃən/

manuál, příručka, ruční (konaný rukama), rukojeť manual / ˈmæn.ju.əl/

manželská situace marital /ˈmær.ɪ.tºl/ circumstance /ˈsɜː.kəm.stɑːnts/

marnivost vanity /ˈvæn.ɪ.ti/

masáž srdce heart /hɑːt/ massage / ˈmæs.ɑːdʒ/

masivní massive /ˈmæs.ɪv/

maska, zakrýt mask /mɑːsk/

mastikace, žvýkání mastication / ˌmæs.tɪˈkeɪ.ʃºn/

materiál material /məˈtɪə.ri.əl/

materiál na výplně filling /ˈfɪl.ɪŋ/ material /məˈtɪə.ri.əl/

matice, matrice, základní hmota matrix /ˈmeɪ.trɪks/

matoucí confusing /kənˈfjuː.zɪŋ/

mátový bonbon mint /mɪnt/

matrice, forma, lůžko, nálitek, pojivo, základní látka matrix / ˈmeɪ.trɪks/

matriční páska, otiskovací kroužek matrix /ˈmeɪ.trɪks/ band /bænd/

maxilofaciální, týkající se horní čelisti a tváře maxillofacial / ˌmæk.sɪ.ləˈfeɪ.ʃºl/

mazání, mast ointment /ˈɔɪnt.mənt/

mdloba fainting /feɪnt.ɪŋ/

měchýř / bladder /ˈblæd.əʳ/

měď copper /ˈkɒp.əʳ/

medium, přenašeč, prostřední, střed medium /ˈmiː.di.əm/

mechanický, bezděčný mechanical / məˈkæn.ɪ.kºl/

méně než less /les/ than /ðən/

menopauza, klimakterium menopause /ˈmen.ə.pɔːz/

menoragie, silné menstruační krvácení menorrhagia / ˌmen.əˈreɪ.dʒɪ.ə/

menstruace menstruation / ˌmen.struˈeɪ.ʃºn/

menstruační menstrual /ˈmen.strəl/

měřit puls take /teɪk/ pulse /pʌls/

měřitelný measurable /ˈmeʒ.ər.ə.bl̩/

měřítko criterion /kraɪˈtɪə.ri.ən/ (pl. criteria)

měřítko, pravítko ruler /ˈruː.ləʳ/

městnání crowding /kraʊd.ɪŋ/

metabolizovat metabolise / məˈtæb.ºl.aɪz/

metastatický, týkající se metastázy metastatic /ˌmet.əˈstæ.tɪk/

metastáza metastasis /metˈæs.tə.sɪs/

metoda, postup, zásada policy / ˈpɒl.ə.si/

metoda, pracovní postup technique / tekˈniːk/

mezera interspace /ˈɪn.tə.speɪs/

mezera, místo, prázdné místo, volný prostor, vzdálenost space /speɪs/

mezera, otvor hiatus /haɪˈeɪ.təs/

mezera, trhlina gap /gæp/

mezerník space /speɪs/ maintainer / meɪnˈteɪn.əʳ/

mezi among /əˈmʌŋ/, amongst / əˈmʌŋst/

mezi dvěma between /bɪˈtwiːn/

mezitím meantime /ˈmiːn.taɪm/

mezní, koncový, konečný, termínový terminal /ˈtɜː.mɪ.nəl/

migréna, silná bolest hlavy migraine / ˈmiː.greɪn/, /ˈmaɪ/

migrénový, týkající se migrény migrainous /maɪ.grə.nəs/

míchání, tření spatulation / ˌspæt.jəˈleɪ.ʃᵊn/

míchat mix /mɪks/

mikro- micro- /maɪ.krəʊ -/

mikrobiologie microbiology / ˌmaɪ.krəʊ.baɪˈɒl.ə.dʒi/

mimo ústa extraoral /ˌek.strəˈɔː.rəl/

mimokloubní extra-articular / ˈek.strə.ˈaːɪ.tɪ.kjʊ.ləʳ/

minulý, poslední, přes, za past /paːst/

mírně, slabě, trochu slightly /ˈslaɪt.li/

mírný, klidný, slabý mild /maɪld/

mírný, zmírňovat moderate /ˈmɒd.ər.ət/

mířit point /pɔɪnt/

miska, kalíšek bowl /bəʊl/

místní anestetikum local /ˈləʊ.kəl/ anaesthetic /ˌæn.əsˈθet.ɪk/

místní anestezie LA local /ˈləʊ.kəl/ anaesthesia /ˌæn.əsˈθiː.zi.ə/

místní pravidlo, norma s místní platností local /ˈləʊ.kᵊl/ rule /ruːl/

místo, poloha situs /saɪ.təs/

místo, postavení, poloha position / pəˈzɪʃ.ᵊn/

mít cenu, za něco stát worth /wɜːθ/

mít na sobě, obléknout wear /weəʳ/

mít námitky proti object /əbˈdʒekt/ to /tʊ/

mít přednost take /teɪk/ precedence / ˈpres.ɪ.dᵊnₜs/

mizet (ztrácet se), opotřebovat se wear /weəʳ/ off /ɒf/

mladší junior /ˈdʒuː.ni.əʳ/

mluvení speaking /spiː.kɪŋ/

mnemotechnická pomůcka aide-memoire /eɪd.ˈmem.waːr/

mnohačetný multiple /ˈmʌl.tɪ.pl̩/

mnohdy, opakovaně frequently / ˈfriː.kwənt.li/

mobilní, pohyblivý mobile /ˈməʊ.baɪl/

moc, příliš overly /ˈəʊ.vᵊl.i/

mocný, prudký forceful /ˈfɔːs.fᵊl/

moč, močový urine /ˈjʊə.rɪn/

močení micturition /ˌmɪkt.juəˈrɪʃ.ᵊn/

močovina urea /jʊᵊˈriː.ə/

model, tvar shape /ʃeɪp/

model, vzor model /ˈmɒd.ᵊl/

modelovací nůž, kráječ, rydlo carver /ˈkaː.vəʳ/

modelování, modelový modelling / ˈmɒd.əl.ɪŋ/

modelovat znovu, přemodelovat, přestavit remodel /ˌriːˈmɒd.əl/

modelovat, formovat mould /məʊld/

modifikace, obměna, přizpůsobení modification /ˌmɒd.ɪ.fɪˈkeɪ.ʃᵊn/

modifikovat, přizpůsobit, upravit, uzpůsobit modify /ˈmɒd.ɪ.faɪ/

modul modulus /ˈmɒd.jə.ləs/

mokrý, namočit (navlhčit), vlhký wet /wet/

mokrý, vlhký (vzduch) moist /mɔɪst/

monitorovat, kontrolovat, sledovat monitor /ˈmɒn.ɪ.təʳ/

monomer monomer /mɒn.ə.məʳ/

montáž, montování, úprava, instalace fitting /ˈfɪt.ɪŋ/

motivovat motivate /ˈməʊ.tɪ.veɪt/

motýlek, škrticí klapka butterfly / ˈbʌt.ə.flaɪ/

mozková cévní příhoda cerebrovascular /ˌser.ɪ.brəˈvæs.kjʊ. ləʳ/ accident /ˈæk.sɪ.dᵊnt/

mozková obrna cerebral palsy /ˌser.ə.brəlˈpɔːl.zi/

možnost volby, volba option /ˈɒp.ʃən/

mrkev carrot /ˈkær.ət/

mrtvice stroke /strəʊk/

mukoperiost, okostice mající mukózní povrch mucoperiosteum /ˈmjuː.kə‚per.ɪˈɒs.ti.əm/

mukózní, slizniční mucosal /ˌmjuːˈkəʊ.sl/

multiplex, roztroušená skleróza multiple /ˈmʌl.tɪ.pl̩/ sclerosis /sklə'rəʊ.sɪs/

muskuloskeletární, skládající se ze svalů a kostí musculoskeletal /ˈmʌs.kjʊ.ləˈskel.ɪ.t°l/

Muslim, mohamedán Moslem /ˈmʊz.lɪm/

mutant, měnící se mutant /ˈmjuː.tənt/

myalgie, svalová bolest myalgia /mʌɪˈæl.dʒɪ.ə/

mykoplazma mycoplasma /maɪ.kəˈplæz.mə/

myšlenka thought /θɔːt/

mýt, prát, promýt, vyprat wash /wɒʃ/

N

na původním místě in situ /ˌɪnˈsɪt.juː/

na straně (koho) on /ɒn/ the part /pɑːt/

nabídnout, navrhovat, navrhnout propose /prəˈpəʊz/

nabídnout, představit se present /prɪˈz.ent/

náboženské vyznání religion /rɪˈlɪdʒ.°n/

nabrat, nasát take /teɪk/ up /ʌp/

nacementování, přitmelení, tmelení, zalévání cementem cementation /ˌsɪː.menˈteɪ.ʃ°n/

náctiletý teenager /ˈtiːn‚eɪ.dʒəʳ/

nadbytek, nadměrný excess /ekˈses/

nadměrná aktivita hyper-activity /haɪ.pəʳˈæk.tɪv.ɪ.ti/

nadměrná reakce overreaction /ˌəʊ.və.riˈæk.ʃ°n/

nadměrně, nepřiměřeně excessively /ekˈses.ɪv.li/

nadmutí břicha bloating /ˈbləʊ.tɪŋ/

nadpočetný, přespočetný supernumerary /ˌsuː.pəˈnjuː.m°r.°r.i/

nadšený keen /kiːn/

nadzvednout, vyzvednout, zdvihnout, zvednout, zvednutí lift /lɪft/

náhoda, případ, událost, výskyt occurrence /əˈkʌr.°n‍t s/

nahoru upwards /ˈʌp.wədz/

náhrada, nahrazení, nahrazování replacement /rɪˈpleɪs.mənt/

náhrada, obnova, obnovení, oprava, výplň restoration /ˌres.t°rˈeɪ.ʃ°n/

nahradit, náhražka, zastupovat substitute /ˈsʌb.stɪ.tjuːt/

nahradit, opravit, úprava repair /rɪˈpeəʳ/

nahromadění accumulation /ə‚kjuː.mjʊˈleɪ.ʃən/

nahřát warm /wɔːm/

nachýlit, naklonit, sklon, vychýlit, vyklonit tilt /tɪlt/

náchylnost, zranitelnost vulnerability /ˌvʌl.n°r.əˈbɪl.ɪ.ti/

náchylný, šikmý prone /prəʊn/

náchylný, zranitelný vulnerable /ˈvʌl.n°r.ə.bl̩/

naklonění, sklánět se slope /sləʊp/

naklonit dopředu procline /prəʊ ˈklaɪn/

naklonit dozadu retrocline /ˌret.rəʊ ˈklaɪn/

naklonit, sklopit tip /tɪp/

nakonec, skutečně ultimately /ˈʌl.tɪ.mət.li/

nákres, plán, projekt, program scheme /skiːm/

nákusná deska bite /baɪt/ plane /pleɪn/

nálada, kondice mood /muːd/

naléhat insist /ɪnˈsɪst/

naléhavá nutnost, pohotovost emergency /ɪˈmɜː.dʒənt.si/

nálepka, označení, označit (štítkem) label /ˈleɪ.bəl/

nálev, výplach, oplach, zavlažení irrigation /ˌɪr.ɪˈgeɪ.ʃən/

nálevka, trychtýř funnel /ˈfʌn.əl/

náležitý, vhodný, odpovídající, patřičný, přiměřený, příslušný appropriate /əˈprəʊ.pri.ət/

namáhat, tlačit, zdůraznit stress / stres/

namátkou random /ˈræn.dəm/

namazat, nepatrné množství, skvrna, šmouha smear /smɪəʳ/

namísto instead /ɪnˈsted/ of /əv/

nános, usazenina, ložisko uložit deposit /dɪˈpɒz.ɪt/

naordinovat, předepisovat, předepsat prescribe /prɪˈskraɪb/

nápadně, zjevně, značně markedly / ˈmɑː.kɪd.li/

napadnout (přijít na mysl) occur / əˈkɜːʳ/

napjatý, utažený tighten /ˈtaɪ.tən/

naplánovat, rozvrh, tabulka (cedule) schedule /ˈʃed.juːl/

náplň, vložka, plnič, plnící nástroj, plnivo filler /ˈfɪl.əʳ/

náplň, zatížení load /ləʊd/

napnout, usilovat strain /streɪn/

nápoj beverage /ˈbev.ər.ɪdʒ/

napomáhat, podporovat, propagovat promote /prəˈməʊt/

napravit, omezit, přemoct, redukovat, snížit, zmenšit reduce / rɪˈdjuːs/

nápravný, opravný corrective / kəˈrek.tɪv/

napravovaný ordered /ˈɔː.dəd/

náprsenka zástěry, bryndáček bib / bɪb/

náročný demanding /dɪˈmɑːn.dɪŋ/, exacting /ɪgˈzæk.tɪŋ/

naříkat, vzdychat sigh /saɪ/

nařízení, pravidlo, předpis regulation /ˌreg.jʊˈleɪ.ʃən/

nasakovat, vstřebat soak /səʊk/ up / ʌp/

nasátí aspirate /ˈæs.pɪ.rət/

nasávání (vzduchu), odsávání suction /ˈsʌk.ʃən/

nasazení, nastavení, seřízení, tuhnutí setting /ˈset.ɪŋ/

násilně forcibly /ˈfɔː.sɪ.bli/

následně po prodělaném záchvatu postictal /ˈpəʊstˈɪkt.əl/

následnost, pořadí, postup, sled sequence /ˈsiː.kwənts/

následovně, postupně, později subsequently /ˈsʌb.sɪ.kwənt.li/

následující following /ˈfɒl.əʊ.ɪŋ/

následující, nastávající, vyplývající ensuing /ɪnˈsjuː.ɪŋ/

násobit, znásobit, vícenásobný multiply /ˈmʌl.tɪ.plaɪ/

nastat, vyskytnout se, vystoupit, být důsledkem, vzniknout arise /əˈraɪz/

nastávající matka expectant /ɪkˈspek.tənt/ mother /ˈmʌð.ər/

nastavení, přizpůsobování, seřizování adjustment /əˈdʒʌst.mənt/

nastavit, seřídit polohu, umístit position /pəˈzɪʃ.ən/

nastavit, sestavit, upravit, vsadit, zasadit set /set/

nástroj instrument /ˈɪn.strə.mənt/

nástroj, prostředek tool /tuːl/

nástup, příchod, začátek onset /ˈɒn.set/

naštěstí fortunately /ˈfɔː.tʃⁿn.ət.li/

natažení, rozšíření extension / ɪkˈsten.t ʃən/

natažený, rozšířený, v extenzi extended /ɪkˈsten.dɪd/

nauka o ultrazvuku ultrasonography / ˌʌl.trəˈsɒn.ˈnɒg.rə.fi/

náustek mouthpiece /ˈmaʊθ.piːs/

nával horka v obličeji facial /ˈfeɪ.ʃəl/ flushing /flʌʃ.ɪŋ/

navlečený, niťový, se závitem threaded /ˈθred.ɪd/

návrat return /rɪˈtɜːn/

návštěvníci, publikum audience / ˈɔː.di.ənt s/

navzdory despite /dɪˈspaɪt/

nazpaměť, jako když bičem mrská by /baɪ/ rote /rəʊt/

nebezpečí danger /ˈdeɪn.dʒəʳ/

nebezpečnost, vážnost, závažnost seriousness /ˈsɪə.ri.ə.snəs/

necitlivý numb /nʌm/

necitlivý, nevnímavý unsusceptible / ˌʌn.səˈsep.tɪ.bļ/

nedbalost negligence /ˈneg.lɪ.dʒⁿnt s/

nediagnostikovaný undiagnosed / ˌʌnˈdaɪ.əg.nəʊzd/

nedílný integral /ˈɪn.tɪ.grəl/

nedobře unwell /ʌnˈwel/

nedodržení, porušení breach /briːtʃ/

nedopatřením inadvertently / ˌɪn.ədˈvɜː.tⁿnt.li/

nedoprovázený, samotný unaccompanied /ˌʌn.əˈkʌm.pⁿn.id/

nedotčený, neovlivněný unaffected / ˌʌn.əˈfek.tɪd/

negativní negative /ˈneg.ə.tɪv/

nehet nail /neɪl/

nehoda, událost, případ incident / ˈɪnt .sɪ.dⁿnt/

nehorázný, očividný blatant /ˈbleɪ.tⁿnt/

nechat pod studenou tekoucí vodou run /rʌn/ under /ˈʌn.dəʳ/ cold /kəʊld/ tap /tæp/

nechirurgický nonsurgical / nɒn.ˈsɜː.dʒɪ.kəl/

nejistota, nespolehlivost uncertainty / ʌnˈsɜː.tⁿn.ti/

nejnižší least /liːst/

nekontrolovatelně uncontrollably / ˌʌn.kənˈtrəʊ.lə.bli/

nekoordinovaný, nesladěný uncoordinated /ˌʌn.kəʊˈɔː.dɪn.eɪ.tɪd/

nelítostný merciless /ˈmɜː.sɪ.ləs/

nemísivost immiscibility /ɪˌmɪs.əˈbɪl.ɪ.ti/

nemocný zánětem pohrudnice pleuritic /pluə.rət.ɪk/

nemožný impossible /ɪmˈpɒs.ɪ.bļ/

nenarazivší na překážku unhindered / ˌʌnˈhɪn.dəd/

neobhajitelný, neomluvitelný indefensible /ˌɪn.dɪˈfent .sɪ.bļ/

neoblomný, neústupný adamant / ˈæd.ə.mənt/

neobvyklý, neobyčejný uncommon / ʌnˈkɒm.ən/

neočekávaný unexpected / ˌʌn.ɪkˈspek.tɪd/

neočekávaný, nepředvídatelný unpredictable /ˌʌn.prɪˈdɪk.tə.bļ/

neochota unwillingness /ʌnˈwɪl.ɪŋ.nəs/

neochotný, váhavý reluctant / rɪˈlʌk.tⁿnt/

neoplastický neoplastic /ˈniːə'plæs.tɪk/

nepalpovatelný, nepostižitelný (nehmatatelný) impalpable / ɪmˈpæl.pə.bļ/

nepatrně minutely /maɪˈnjuːt.li/

nepatrný, řídký, tenký, zeslabit thin / θɪn/

nepevný, nestabilní, nestálý, pohyblivý, proměnlivý unstable / ʌnˈsteɪ.bļ/

nepohoda, nepohodlí, nevolnost, obtěžovat discomfort /dɪˈskʌmp .fət/

nepoměrnost, odchylka discrepancy / dɪˈskrep.ᵊnt .si/

nepoužitý unused /ʌnˈjuːzd/

nepozorný inattentive /ˌɪn.əˈten.tɪv/

nepravděpodobnost improbability / ɪmˌprɒb.əˈbɪl.ɪ.ti/

nepravidelnost irregularity / ɪˌreg.jəˈlær.ə.ti/

nepravidelnost, nerovnost unevenness /ʌnˈiː.vᵊn.nəs/

nepravidelný irregular /ɪˈreg.jə.ləʳ/

nepropustný pro záření, radiopakní radio-opaque /ˈreɪ.di.əʊ.əʊˈpeɪk/

neprořezaný unerupted /ʌn.ɪrˈʌp.tᵊd/

neprospěch, poškození detriment / ˈdet.rɪ.mənt/

neprůhlednost, temnost, matnost opacity /əʊˈpæs.ə.ti/

nepřesnost, chyba, nedostatek inaccuracy /ɪnˈæk.jʊ.rə.si/

nepřetržitě, ustavičně, neustále continually /kənˈtɪn.ju.ə.li/

nepříjemný, otravný annoying / əˈnɔɪ.ɪŋ/

nepřilnavý nonadhesive / ˌnɒn.ədˈhiː.sɪv/

nepřiměřený inappropriate / ˌɪn.əˈprəʊ.pri.ət/

nepříznivě, příčně adversely / ˈæd.vɜː.sli/

nerezavějící, nerezavící stainless / ˌsteɪn.ləs/

nervový blok nerve /nɜːv/ block /blɒk/

nervový kmen nerve /nɜːv/ trunk / trʌŋk/

nervozita, nervóza nervousness / ˈnɜː.və.snəs/

neschopný (čeho), nezpůsobilý unfit / ʌnˈfɪt/

nesoucí váhu load-carrying / ləʊd.kær.i.ɪŋ/, weight /weɪt/ bearing /ˈbeə.rɪŋ/

nespavost sleep /sliːp/ loss /lɒs/

nespokojenost dissatisfaction / dɪsˌsæt.ɪsˈfæk.ʃᵊn/

nesprávná výživa, podvýživa malnutrition /ˌmæl.njuːˈtrɪ.ʃən/

nesprávnost funkce, porušení, rozrušení disturbance / dɪˈstɜː.bənt s/

nesprávný, nepřesný inaccurate / ɪˈnæk.jʊ.rət/

nesprávný, nevhodný incorrect / ˌɪn.kərˈᵊkt/

nést pryč carry /ˈkær.i/ away /əˈweɪ/

nestálý, neurčitý, bludný erratic / ɪˈræt.ɪk/

nešpinící nonstaining /nɒn.ˈsteɪn.ɪŋ/

netěsnost, propouštění, unikání, vytékání leakage /ˈliː.kɪdʒ/

neúčinný ineffective /ˌɪn.ɪˈfek.tɪv/

neúmyslný, nezamýšlený unintended / ˌʌn.ɪnˈten.dɪd/

neuralgie, ostrá nervová bolest neuralgia /njʊəˈræl.dʒə/

neurologický neurological / ˌnjʊə.rəˈlɒdʒ.ɪ.kᵊl/

neurom, druh nádoru tvořený z nervových buněk neuroma / ˌnjʊəˈrəʊ.mə/

neuromuskulární, nervosvalový neuromuscular /ˌnjʊəˈrə.mæsk.jʊ.ləʳ/

neuron, nervová buňka neuron / ˈnjʊə.rɒn/

neuropatie, onemocnění nervů neuropathy /ˌnjʊəˈrɒ.pə.θi/

neurovaskulární neurovascular / ˌnjʊə.rəʊˈvæs.kju.ləʳ/

neuróza neurosis /njʊəˈrəʊ.sɪs/ (pl. neuroses)

neúspěšný, nepodařený (nezdařilý) unsuccessful /ˌʌn.səkˈses.fəl/

neustále, pevně steadily /ˈsted.ɪ.li/

neverbální, mimoslovní nonverbal /ˌnɒnˈvɜː.bəl/

nevolnost sickness /ˈsɪk.nəs/

nevolnost, malátnost malaise /mælˈeɪz/

nevratný irrefutable /ˌɪr.ɪˈfjuː.tə.bl̩/

nevýhoda, nedostatek disadvantage /ˌdɪs.ədˈvɑːn.tɪdʒ/

nevýhodný inconvenient /ˌɪn.kənˈviː.ni.ᵊnt/

nevyleštěný unpolished /ʌnˈpɒl.ɪʃt/

nezákonný illegal /ɪˈliː.gᵊl/

nezaostřený unfocused /ʌn.ˈfəʊ.kəst/

nezaznamenatelný unrecordable /ˌʌn.rɪˈkɔːd.ə.bl̩/

nezbytný, podstatný, důležitý, základní, hlavní, nepostradatelný essential /ɪˈsen.t ʃəl/

nezhoubný benign /bɪˈnaɪn/

neznámý unknown /ʌnˈnəʊn/

nezpůsobilost, invalidita disability /ˌdɪs.əˈbɪl.ɪ.ti/

nezraňující atraumatic /ˈeɪ.trɔːˈmæt.ɪk/

nezřetelný slurred /slɜːʳd/

ničivý, zhoubný wasting /weɪst.ɪŋ/

niklochromová ocel nickel-chromium /ˈnɪk.ᵊl.ˈkrəʊ.mi.əm/ steel /stiːl/

niť thread /θred/

nitkovitý tep thready /θred.i/ pulse /pʌls/

nízko objemový low-volume /ləʊ.ˈvɒl.juːm/

nízký low /ləʊ/

nízký tlak hypotension /ˌhaɪ.pəʊˈten.t ʃᵊn/

noha, nohavice leg /leg/

nokturie, noční močení nocturia /nɒkˈtjʊ.ə.rɪ.ə/

norma, pravidlo (určitý poměr), standard, úroveň standard /ˈstæn.dəd/

nosič, bacilonosič carrier /ˈkær.i.əʳ/

nositel, kdo nosí na sobě weare /weə.rəʳ/

nosní dutina nasal /ˈneɪ.zəl/ cavity /ˈkæv.ɪ.ti/

nosní nasal /ˈneɪ.zəl/

nový pokus, zkoušet znova retry /ˌriːˈtraɪ/

nucení ke zvracení, pocit nevolnosti nausea /ˈnɔː.zi.ə/

nutkavý (psych.) compulsive /kəmˈpʌl.sɪv/

nutná potřeba, nutnost (naléhavost) urgency /ˈɜː.dʒᵊnt .si/

nutně vyžadovat necessitate /nəˈses.ɪ.teɪt/

nutnost necessity /nəˈses.ɪ.ti/

nutný (naléhavý) urgent /ˈɜː.dʒᵊnt/

nutriční, výživový nutritional /njuːˈtrɪʃ.ᵊn.ᵊl/

nůž, ořezávačka trimmer /ˈtrɪm.əʳ/

nůžky na stehy stitch /stɪtʃ/ cutter /kʌt.əʳ/

nůžky, kleštičky scissors /ˈsɪz.əz/

O

oba both /bəʊθ/

obava, strach fear /fɪəʳ/

obava, týkat se, příslušet, zájem, znepokojení concern /kənˈsɜːn/

obecně, zpravidla generally /ˈdʒen.ə r.əl.i/

obemknout, obklopit, obejít kolem encircle /ɪnˈsɜː.kl̩/

oběť, postižený, zraněný casualty /ˈkæʒ.ju.əl.ti/

obezita, otylost obesity /əʊˈbiː.sɪ.ti/

obeznámený, důvěrně známý familiar /fəˈmɪl.i.əʳ/

okraj, pokraj, lem, lemovat margin / ˈmɑː.dʒɪn/

okrajový, krajní, mezní marginal / ˈmɑː.dʒɪ.nəl/

omezení, omezovat, škrtit constrain / kənˈstreɪn/

omezený limited /ˈlɪm.ɪ.tɪd/

omezit na jedno místo localise / ˈləʊ.kəl.aɪz/

omezit, vymezit limit /ˈlɪm.ɪt/

omezování, bránění restraint / rɪˈstreɪnt/

omezující restrictive /rɪˈstrɪk.tɪv/

omluva apology /əˈpɒl.ə.dʒi/

omluva, výmluva excuse /ɪkˈskjuːs/

onkolog oncologist /ɒŋˈkɒl.ə.dʒɪst/

onlej, štěp aplikovaný na povrch tkáně onlay /ˈɒn.leɪ/

opakované použití, znovu použít reuse /ˌriːˈjuːz/

opakované zvracení regurgitation / rɪˌɡɜː.dʒɪˈteɪ.ʃᵊn/

opakující se, opakovaný repetitive / rɪˈpet.ə.tɪv/

opakující se, recidivující recurrent / rɪˈkʌr.ᵊnt /

oparový herpetic /hɜːˈpe.tik/

opatření measure /ˈmeʒ.əʳ/, measurement /ˈmeʒ.ə.mənt/

opatřený ozubcem, opatřený ostny, ostnatý barbed /bɑːbd/

opatřit manžetou cuff /kʌf/

operační místo surgical /ˈsɜː.dʒɪ.kᵊl/ site /saɪt/

operační, operativní operative / ˈɒp.ᵊr.ə.tɪv/

opěrný, nosný, ložisko bearing / ˈbeə.rɪŋ/

operovat, obsluhovat (stroj ap.), řídit operate /ˈɒp.ᵊr.eɪt/

opětné pozvání pacienta, znovu zavolat recall /rɪˈkɔːl/

opětovné ujištění, uklidnění, uklidňování, útěcha reassurance / ˌriː.əˈʃɔː.rənt s/

opiát opioid /əʊˈpiː.ɒɪd/

opiát, narkotický lék opiate /ˈəʊ.pi.ət/

opocený, propocený sweaty /ˈswet.i/

opomenutí omission /əʊˈmɪʃ.ᵊn/

opotřebení zubů tooth /tuːθ/ wear / weəʳ/

opravdový (vážný) serious /ˈsɪə.ri.əs/

oprávnění, povolení, souhlas permission /pəˈmɪʃ.ᵊn/

opředené hedvábí braided /breɪd.ɪd/ silk /sɪlk/

optická vlákna fibre optic / ˈfaɪ.bəʳ.ˈɒp.tɪk/

orální, ústní oral /ˈɔː.rəl/

orbitální, očnicový orbital /ˈɔː.bɪ.tᵊl/

ordinace, ošetřovna surgery / ˈsɜː.dʒᵊr.i/

orientovaný orientated /ˌɔː.ri.ənˈteɪ.tɪd/

oroantrální, týkající se úst a vedlejších nosních dutin oroantral / ˌəʊ.rəʊˈæn.trəl/

orofaciální, týkající se úst a obličeje orofacial /ˌəʊ.rəˈfeɪ.ʃᵊl/

orofaryngeální, týkající se úst a hltanu oropharyngeal / ˌəʊ.rəˈfær.ɪ.ŋˈdʒɪ.əl/

ortodoncie orthodontics / ˌɔː.θəʊ ˈdɒn.tɪks/

ortodontický zámek, sklápěcí polička, podpěra, spojit svorkou bracket /ˈbræk.ɪt/

ortognátní, správný skus orthognathic /ˌɔː.θəʊˈnæː.θɪk/

ortográdní, správně postavený orthograde /ɔːˈθəʊ.greɪd/

ortopantomograf, panoramatický snímek orthopantomograph / ˌɔːr.θoʊˈpæn.təʊ.mə.grɑːf/

oříšek nut /nʌt/

ospalost, mátožnost drowsiness / ˈdraʊ.zɪ.nəs/

osteitida, zánět kosti osteitis / ˌɒs.tiˈaɪ.tɪs/

osteoartritida, zánět kostních kloubů osteoarthritis /ˌɒs.ti.əʊ.ɑːˈθraɪ.tɪs/

osteoporóza, prořídnutí kostí osteoporosis /ˌɒs.ti.əʊ.pəˈrəʊ.sɪs/

osteosarkom, maligní kostní nádor osteosarcoma /ˌɒs.tɪ.ə.sɑːˈkəʊ.mə/

osteotomie, protětí kosti osteotomy / ˌɒs.tiˈɒ.tə.mi/

ostrost sharpness /ˈʃɑːp.nəs/

osvětlit illuminate /ɪˈluː.mɪ.neɪt/

osvobodit, záchrana, záchranný, zachránit rescue /ˈres.kjuː/

ošetřování nursing /ˈnɜː.sɪŋ/

ošetřování, vytvrzení (lepidla, plastu) curing /kjʊər.ɪŋ/

ošetřovat nurse /nɜːs/

ošetřující lékař, lékařský physician / fɪˈzɪʃ.ən/

oškrabat peel /piːl/

oškrabat, škrabat scrape /skreɪp/

oštipovat nibble /ˈnɪb.l̩/

otáčet, uvažovat revolve /rɪˈvɒlv/

otáčka revolution /ˌrev.əˈluː.ʃən/

otěruvzdornost abrasion /əˈbreɪ.ʒən/ resistance /rɪˈzɪs.tənt s/, wear /weəʳ/ resistance /rɪˈzɪs.tᵊnt s/

otevřená zlomenina compound / ˈkɒm.paʊnd/ fracture /ˈfræk.t ʃəʳ/

otevření opening /ˈəʊ.pᵊn.ɪŋ/

otevřít, začínat, zahájit commence / kəˈment s/

otírání attrition /əˈtrɪʃ.ən/

otiskovací lžíce impression / ɪmˈpreʃ.ən/ tray /treɪ/

otočný, otáčivý, rotační rotary / ˈrəʊ.tᵊr.i/

otok, uzel, uzlina node /nəʊd/

otřes, pohmoždění concussion / kənˈkʌʃ.ən/

otvor, punkce, vpich puncture / ˈpʌŋk.tʃəʳ/

ovládání, řízení, snaha o zvládnutí management /ˈmæn.ɪdʒ.mənt/

ovlivnit, zasahovat interfere / ˌɪn.təˈfɪəʳ/

oxidová vrstva oxide /ˈɒk.saɪd/ layer / ˈleɪ.əʳ/

oxidovat, okysličovat oxidise / ˈɒk.sɪ.daɪz/

oximetr oximeter /ˌɒk.sɪ.miː.təʳ/

oxygenace, okysličení oxygenation / ˌɒk.sɪ.dʒəˈneɪ.ʃᵊn/

označit, rozpoznat, určit, identifikovat, ztotožňovat se identify /aɪˈden.tɪ.faɪ/

ozubený toothed /tuːθt/

ozubený, zubatý, vroubkovaný dentate /den.teɪt/

oživit revive /rɪˈvaɪv/

oživit, reaktivovat, znovu aktivovat reactivate /riˈæk.tɪ.veɪt/

P

pacient patient /ˈpeɪ.ʃᵊnt/

páčit prise /praɪz/

padákový parachute /ˈpær.ə.ʃuːt/

padnout, spadat, spadnout, upadnout, pád, padat, poklesnout fall /fɔːl/

palec na ruce thumb /θʌm/

pálení žáhy heartburn /ˈhɑːt.bɜːn/

paliativní, utišující palliative / ˈpæl.i.ə.tɪv/

palpitace, bušení srdce palpitations / ˌpæl.pɪˈteɪ.ʃᵊnz/

paměť, uchování, zadržení, zácpa retention /rɪˈten.t ʃᵊn/

pánev pelvis /ˈpel.vɪs/

panický, týkající se fobie, ustrašený phobic /ˈfəʊ.bɪk/

pankarditida, zánět všech vrstev srdeční stěny pancarditis / ˌpæn.kɑːˈdaɪ.tɪs/

pankreatický, slinivkový pancreatic / ˌpæŋ.kriˈæt.ɪk/

papilla, bradavka papilla /pəˈpɪl.ə/ (pl. papillae)

papilom, nezhoubný epitelový nádor papilloma /ˌpæp.ɪ.ˈləʊ.mə/

papírový čípek paper /ˈpeɪ.pəʳ/ point / pɔɪnt/

papírový kapesník paper /ˈpeɪ.pəʳ/ towel /taʊəl/, tissue /ˈtɪʃ.uː/

pár, jedny pair /peəʳ/ of /əv/

paracetamol paracetamol / ˌpær.əˈsiː.tə.mɒl/

parafunkce, poškozená funkce parafunction /ˌpær.əˈfʌnk.ʃᵊn/

parachlorfenol parachlorphenol / pær.əˌklɒrˈfiː.nɒl/

parestezie, změněná citlivost paraesthesia /ˌpær.əsˈθiː.sɪ.ə/

pásek, plátek, proužek strip /strɪp/

páska, proužek, kroužek, obroučka, spojit band /bænd/

patentovaný, zákonem chráněný proprietary /prəˈpraɪə.tri/

páteř spine /spaɪn/

patogeneze, vznik a vývoj onemocnění pathogenesis / ˌpæθəˈdʒen.ɪ.sɪs/

patologický, chorobný pathological / ˌpæθ.əˈlɒdʒ.ɪ.kᵊl/

pátrat po look /lʊk/ for /fɔːʳ/

patrový třmen palatal /pæ.lə.tl/ bar / bɑːʳ/

patrový, předopatrový palatal /pæ.lə.tl/

pečetění, utěsnění, zaplnění sealing / ˈsiː.lɪŋ/

pečetidlo, prostředek pro utěsnění sealer /ˈsiː.ləʳ/

pečetidlo, těsnicí materiál, tmel sealant /ˈsiː.lənt/

pečlivý, opatrný careful /ˈkeə.fəl/

pečlivý, přesný accurate /ˈæk.jʊ.rət/

pečovatelka (k dítěti) babysitter / ˈbeɪ.biˌsɪt.əʳ/

penicilin penicillin /ˌpen.əˈsɪl.ɪn/

perinatální, kolem porodu, do 10 dní po porodu perinatal /ˌper.ɪˈneɪ.tl/

periodoncium, parodont periodontium /ˌper.ɪ.əˈdɒn.ʃiəm/

periodontitida, zánět závěsného aparátu periodontitis / ˌper.ɪ.əˈdɒn.ˈtaɪ.tɪs/

periodontologie, odvětví specializující se na léčení tkáně kolem zubů periodontology / ˌper.ɪ.ədɒnˈtɒl.ə.dʒɪ/

periost, okostice periosteum / ˌper.ɪˈɒs.ti.əm/

periosteální, okostiční periosteal / ˌper.ɪˈɒs.ti.əl/

perlivý, sycený, s bublinkami carbonated /ˈkɑː.bən.eɪ.tɪd/

permeabilita, propustnost permeability /ˌpɜː.mi.əˈbɪl.ɪ.ti/

pero, pružina spring /sprɪŋ/

peroxid vodíku hydrogen / ˈhaɪ.drɪ.dʒən/ peroxide /pəˈrɒk.saɪd/

personál, zaměstnanci personnel / ˌpɜː.sᵊnˈel/

pevně uchopit, popadat grasp / grɑːsp/

pevně uchopit, uchytit, upínadlo grip /grɪp/

pevný firm /fɜːm/

pevný můstek fixed /fɪkst/ bridge / brɪdʒ/

pevný, hustý compact /kəmˈpækt/

pevný, stabilní, stálý, trvalý, upevněný steady /ˈsted.i/

pevný, těsný tight /taɪt/

pilíř zubního můstku, nástavec, sekundární díl, vyztužení, podpěra abutment /əˈbʌt.mənt/

pilíř, pilířový zub pier /pɪəʳ/

pinzeta tweezers /ˈtwiː.zəz/

písemně in /ɪn/ writing /ˈraɪ.tɪŋ/

pít drink /drɪŋk/

plácnout, plesknutí slap /slæp/

plánování planning /ˈplæn.ɪŋ/

plánovaný, zamýšlený intended / ɪnˈten.dɪd/

plastový, plastický plastic /ˈplæs.tɪk/

platný, oprávněný valid /ˈvæl.ɪd/

plenka nappy /ˈnæp.i/

plivat, odplivnout spit /spɪt/

plná ústa mouthful /ˈmaʊθ.fʊl/

plnit pokyn follow /ˈfɒl.əʊ/ instruction /ɪnˈstrʌk.ʃ°n/

plocha (rovina) plane /pleɪn/

plochý, rovný flat /flæt/

plomba, utěsnění, uzávěr seal /siːl/

plynný gaseous /ˈgeɪ.si.əs/

plynulý, neustálý, pravidelný, souvislý, spojený, nepřetržitý continuous /kənˈtɪn.ju.əs/

plýtvání wasting /weɪst.ɪŋ/

po celém, v celém, úplně (veskrze), všude v throughout /θruːˈaʊt/

po menopauze postmenopausal / pəʊst.ˌmen.ə'pɔː.zəl/

poctivý, otevřený, řádný, upřímný honest /ˈɒn.ɪst/

počet, spočítat count /kaʊnt/

početný numerous /ˈnjuː.mə.rəs/

početný, hojný abundant /əˈbʌn.dənt/

počítačová tomografie computer / kəmˈpjuː.təʳ/ tomography / təˈmɒ.grə.fɪ/

počítačový computer /kəmˈpjuː.təʳ/

počítat s (čím), přihlížet (k) take / teɪk/ account /əˈkaʊnt/ of /əv/

počítat, zamýšlet calculate / ˈkæl.kjʊ.leɪt/

pod- sub- /sʌb/

pod tlakem pressurised /ˈpreʃ.ªr.aɪzd/

pod underneath /ˌʌn.dəˈniːθ/

podání (předvedení) presentation / ˌprez.ªnˈteɪ.ʃ°n/

podávání kyslíku oxygen /ˈɒk.sɪ.dʒən/ delivery /dɪˈlɪv.ər.i/

podávat lék administer /ədˈmɪn.ɪ.stəʳ/

poddásňový subgingival / sʌb.dʒɪn.dʒɪv.ªl/

podezření suspicion /səˈspɪʃ.ªn/

podíl, vzájemný poměr, vztah ratio / ˈreɪ.ʃi.əʊ/

podklad, navrstvení bedding /ˈbed.ɪŋ/

podle toho, adekvátně accordingly / əˈkɔː.dɪŋ.li/

podlitina, odřenina bruising / ˈbruː.zɪŋ/

podložení sublining /sʌb.ˈlaɪ.nɪŋ/

podložit (vatou), těsnit pad /pæd/

podložka mattress /ˈmæt.rəs/

podmíněný, upravený, určený conditioned /kənˈdɪʃ.ənd/

podnět stimulus /ˈstɪm.jʊ.ləs/ (pl. stimuli)

podnět, náraz impulse /ˈɪm.pʌls/

podnět, podráždění (svalů, nervů), povzbuzení stimulation / ˌstɪm.jʊˈleɪ.ʃ°n/

podobně, stejnou měrou alike /əˈlaɪk/

podpěra prop /prɒp/

podpírat, podpora, podporovat support /səˈpɔːt/

podporovat, pokračovat, přidržet, udržet, udržovat, živit se maintain / meɪnˈteɪn/

podpůrný chirurgický zákrok supportive /sə'pɔː.tɪv/ surgery / 'sɜː.dʒᵊr.i/

podrážděný, přecitlivělý irritable / 'ɪr.ɪ.tə.bl̩ /

podrobné prohlížení screening / 'skriː.nɪŋ/

podstatná věc essential /ɪ'sen.tʃəl/

pohánět, strkat, tlačit push /pʊʃ/

pohladit stroke /strəʊk/

pohlaví, rod gender /'dʒen.dəʳ/

pohlavně sexually /'sek.sjʊə.li/

pohlavní znak sexual /'sek.sjʊəl/ characteristic /ˌkær.ɪk.tə'rɪs.tɪk/

pohled, podívaná, uvidět, zrak sight / saɪt/

pohodlí, uklidnění comfort /'kʌm.fət/

pohodlně comfortably /'kʌmf.tə.bli/

pohodlný, klidný, příjemný comfortable /'kʌmp.fə.tə.bl̩ /

pohotovost (připravenost) preparedness /prɪ'peəd.nəs/

pohrávat si nervózně fiddle /'fɪd.l̩ /

pohroma washout /'wɒʃ.aʊt/

pohyb motion /'məʊ.ʃᵊn/

pohyb, pohybový, postup movement / 'muːv.mənt/

pohyblivost mobility /məʊ 'bɪl.ɪ.ti/

pohyblivý movable /'muː.və.bl̩ /

pohybová reakce motor /'məʊ.tər/ response /rɪ'spɒnt s/

pochopení (porozumění), rozum (inteligence), dohoda (vzájemná) understanding /ˌʌn.də'stæn.dɪŋ/

pochopit understand /ˌʌn.də'stænd/

pochopitelný understandable / ˌʌn.də'stæn.də.bl̩ /

pojený pryskyřicí resin-bonded / 'rez.ɪn.bɒnd.ɪd/

pojivo, tmel, lepidlo bonding /'bɒnd. ɪŋ/ agent /'eɪ.dʒənt/

pojivová tkáň connective tissue / kəˌnek.tɪv'tɪʃ.uː/

pokazit se, poškodit, zhoršit se worsen /'wɜː.sᵊn/

poklep percussion /pə'kʌʃ.ᵊn/

pokles, propadnout, sesunout slump / slʌmp/

pokožka, pleť complexion / kəm'plek.ʃᵊn/

pokročilý advanced /əd'vɑːnt st/

pokrok, postup progress /'prəʊ.gres/

pokrytí, rozsah, šíře záběru coverage /'kʌv.ᵊr.ɪdʒ/

pokrytý covered /kʌv.əd/

pokrytý, povlečený, potažený coated / 'kəʊ.tɪd/

pokus, zkouška trial /traɪəl/

pokusit se, zkouška, zkoušet, zkusit, vyzkoušet try /traɪ/

polo- semi- /sem.i-/

poloha, úroveň, vrstva layer /'leɪ.əʳ/

polotekutý semifluid /sem.i.'fluː.ɪd/

polštář, položit na polštář pillow / 'pɪl.əʊ/

polyakrylan, polyakrylát polyacrylate /pɒl.i.æ'krɪ.leɪt/

polykarboxylát polycarboxylate / pɒl.i.kɑː'bɒk.sɪl.eɪt/

polykat, hlt, pozřít, spolknout swallow /'swɒl.əʊ/

polymer polymer /'pɒl.ɪ.mər/

polymerační lampa curing /kjʊər.ɪŋ/ lamp /læmp/

polyurie, nadměrné močení polyuria / ˌpɒl.ɪ.'jʊə.rɪə/

pomalý slow-speed /sləʊ.spiːd/

pomalý, zvolna, zpomalit slow /sləʊ/

pomenopauzální postmenopausal / ˌpəʊst'men.ə'pɔː.zᵊl/

poměr, podíl, rychlost rate /reɪt/

poměrný, přiměřený proportional / prə'pɔː.ʃᵊn.ᵊl/

pomoc, přístup, východisko recourse /rɪˈkɔːs/

pomocné zařízení, příslušenství auxiliary /ɔːgˈzɪl.i.ər.i/

pomocný, doplňující complementary / ˌkɒm.plɪˈmen.tər.i/

ponechaný, zadržený retained / rɪˈteɪnd/

ponechat, udržovat keep /kiːp/

pooperačně postoperation / pəʊst.ˌɒp.ªrˈeɪ.ʃªn/ (post-op)

pooperační postoperative / ˌpəʊstˈɒp.ªr.ə.tɪv/

popis description /dɪˈskrɪp.ʃən/

popsat describe /dɪˈskraɪb/

poptávka, požadavek demand / dɪˈmɑːnd/

populace, obyvatelstvo population / ˌpɒp.juˈleɪ.ʃªn/

pór pore /pɔːʳ/

poradenství counselling / ˈkaʊnʧ.səl.ɪŋ/

poradit advise /ədˈvaɪz/, give /gɪv/ advice /ədˈvaɪs/

porézní, sklípkový cavernous / ˈkæv.ən.əs/

porodnický, spojený s porodem obstetric /ɒbˈstet.rɪk/

porovnání comparison /kəmˈpær.ɪ.sªn/

porucha osobnosti personality / ˌpɜː.sªnˈæl.ə.ti/ disorder /dɪˈsɔː.dəʳ/

porucha sítě, výpadek napájení power /paʊəʳ/ failure /ˈfeɪ.ljəʳ/

porucha učení learning /ˈlɜː.nɪŋ/ disability /ˌdɪs.əˈbɪl.ɪ.ti/

porucha, chyba, opomenutí, zanedbání, selhání failure /ˈfeɪ.ljəʳ/

poskytnutí, zajištění (zabezpečení), zásoby provision /prəˈvɪʒ.ªn/

poslouchat, sledovat, poslech listen / ˈlɪs.ªn/

postavit, vybudovat, vytvořit, sestavit construct /kənˈstrʌkt/

postoj, postavení, názor, poměr attitude /ˈæt.ɪ.tjuːd/

postrádat, nedostatek lack /læk/

postranice (bočnice) strana, vedlejší side /saɪd/

postup (pokrok), průběh progression /prəˈgreʃ.ªn/

postupně snímat (po řádcích), skenovat scan /skæn/

postupovat, probíhat, provést proceed /prəʊˈsiːd/

postupovat, vyvíjet se progress / prəˈgres/

posturální, postojový postural / pɒs.tjʊ.ə.rl/

posunování, přeřaďování, přesouvání shifting /ˈʃɪf.tɪŋ/

posunovat se migrate /maɪˈgreɪt/

posunutí dislocation /ˌdɪs.ləʊˈkeɪ.ʃən/

posunutí, chybné postavení zubu, vytlačení displacement / dɪˈspleɪs.mənt/

posuzovat judge /dʒʌdʒ/

posypat, rozdrtit na prášek, rozemlít powder /ˈpaʊ.dər/

poškodit harm /hɑːm/

pot, potit se sweat /swet/

potápění diving /ˈdaɪ.vɪŋ/

potažení, překrytí, překrýt (vrstvou) overlay /ˌəʊ.vəˈleɪ/

potom afterwards /ˈɑːf.tə.wədz/

potrat, umělé přerušení těhotenství miscarriage /ˈmɪs.kær.ɪdʒ/

potrava feed /fiːd/

potravina foodstuff /ˈfuːd.stʌf/

potraviny nakládané do kyselého nálevu pickled /ˈpɪk.l̩d/ food /fuːd/

potvrdit acknowledge /əkˈnɒl.ɪdʒ/, confirm /kənˈfɜːm/

použít use /juːz/

použít, snažit se, vynaložit úsilí, vyvolávat exert /ɪgˈzɜːt/

použitý employed /ɪmˈplɔɪd/

použitý, odpadní waste /weɪst/

povázkový, týkající se povázky fascial /fæ.ʃɪ.əl/

povinnost, závazek obligation / ˌɒb.lɪˈgeɪ.ʃᵊn/

povlak pellicle /pel.ɪ.kl/

povolený granted /ˈgrɑːn.tɪd/

povolit, rozvázat, rozviklat, uvolnit, vyviklat loosen /ˈluː.sᵊn/

povrchový superficial /ˌsuː.pəˈfɪʃ.ᵊl/

povýšený patronising /ˈpæt.rə.naɪ.zɪŋ/

povzbuzení, dodání odvahy encouragement /ɪnˈkʌr.ɪdʒ.mənt/

později, pozdější later /ˈleɪ.təʳ/

pozdější, zadní část, zadní posterior / pɒsˈtɪə.ri.əʳ/

pozice, postoj posture /ˈpɒs.tʃəʳ/

pozitivní, jasný, kladný, nesporný, prokázaný positive /ˈpɒz.ə.tɪv/

poznatelný, rozeznatelný recognizable /ˈrek.əg.naɪ.zə.bl̩ /

pozornost, ošetření, výstraha, pozor! attention /əˈten.tʃən/

pozorování, dodržování observation / ˌɒb.zəˈveɪ.ʃᵊn/

pozoruhodný (neobvyklý), mimořádný unusual /ʌnˈjuː.ʒu.əl/

požadovaný desired /dɪˈzaɪəd/

požadovat, pátrat, vyhledávat seek / siːk/

požadovat, žádat request /rɪˈkwest/

práce se železem ironmongery / ˈaɪən.mʌŋ.gər.i/

pracovní working /ˈwɜː.kɪŋ/

pracovní, týkající se výkonu zaměstnání occupational /ˌɒk.juˈpeɪ.ʃᵊn.ᵊl/

práh, mez citlivosti threshold / ˈθreʃ.h əʊld/

praktický hands-on /ˈhænd.zɒn/

pramének, provázek string /strɪŋ/

prasklina, škvíra, štěrbina, skulina, trhlina crevice /ˈkrev.ɪs/

práškové sklo powdered /ˈpaʊ.dəd/ glass /glɑːs/

pravděpodobně, pravděpodobný likely /ˈlaɪ.kli/

pravděpodobnost, možnost likelihood /ˈlaɪ.kli.hʊd/

pravdivost truthfulness /ˈtruːθ.fᵊl.nəs/

pravdivý, přesný truthful /ˈtruːθ.fᵊl/

právě tak jako as /əz/ well /wel/ as /əz/

pravidelně regularly /ˈreg.jʊ.lə.li/

pravidlo convention /kənˈvent.ʃən/, imperative /ɪmˈper.ə.tɪv/, rule /ruːl/

právo right /raɪt/

praxe experience /ɪkˈspɪə.ri.ᵊnts/

precipitace, urychlení precipitation / prɪˌsɪp.ɪˈteɪ.ʃᵊn/

predisponovat, učinit náchylným predispose /ˌpriː.dɪˈspəʊz/

predispozice, náchylnost, předpoklad, sklon predisposition / ˌpriː.dɪ.spəˈzɪʃ.ᵊn/

preferovat, dávat přednost prefer / prɪˈfɜːʳ/

prenatální, předporodní prenatal / ˌpriːˈneɪ.tl/

preparace, příprava, přípravek, úprava preparation /ˌprep.ᵊrˈeɪ.ʃᵊn/

prevalence, častý výskyt, převaha převládání prevalence /ˈprev.ᵊl.ənts/

preventivní, ochranné opatření, ochranný, předběžný preventive / prɪˈven.tɪv/

prizma, hranol prism /ˈprɪz.ᵊm/

problém problem /ˈprɒb.ləm/

problémový troubled /ˈtrʌb.l̩ d/

probodnout, prorazit pierce /pɪəs/

procento percentage /pəˈsen.tɪdʒ/

proces, postup, průběh, zpracování, zpracovávat process /ˈprəʊ.ses/

procitnout (probudit se), budit se waken /ˈweɪ.kən/

prodloužit lengthen /ˈleŋk.θən/, prolong /prəˈlɒŋ/

prodromální, předzvěstný prodromal /prɒ.drə.ml/

produkce, tvorba production / prəˈdʌk.ʃⁿn/

produkt product /ˈprɒd.ʌkt/

professionál, odborník, odborný professional /prəˈfeʃ.ⁿn. əl/

profylaktický, preventivní prophylactic /ˌprɒf.ɪˈlæk.tɪk/

prognóza, předpověď prognosis / prɒgˈnəʊ.sɪs/ (pl. prognoses)

progresivní, postupující, postupný progressive /prəˈgres.ɪv/

prohlásit, uvádět state /steɪt/

prohlašovat declare /dɪˈkleəʳ/

prohlídka, vyšetření examination / ɪgˌzæm.ɪˈneɪ.ʃⁿn/

prohmatávat palpate /ˈpæl.peɪt/

prokluzovat, sklouznout, upadnout slip /slɪp/

promptně, okamžitě, rychle promptly /ˈprɒmp t.li/

proniknutí, propíchnutí perforation / ˌpɜː.fⁿrˈeɪ.ʃⁿn/

propláchnout, proprat, vypláchnout rinse /rɪnts/

propustit, vyhodit z práce sack /sæk/

proražený perforated /ˈpɜː.fⁿr.eɪ.tɪd/

prořezání eruption /ɪˈrʌp.ʃən/

prosáknutý soaked /səʊkt/

prospěch, pozornost favour /ˈfeɪ.vəʳ/

prospěšný beneficial /ˌben.ɪˈfɪʃ.əl/

prostředí, okolí environs / ɪnˈvaɪə.rənz/

prostředí, zázemí, pozadí background /ˈbæk.graʊnd/

prostředníček middle /ˈmɪd.l̩/ finger / ˈfɪŋ.gəʳ/

prosvícení transillumination / ˌtræn.zɪˈluː.mɪˈneɪ.ʃⁿn/

protetická stomatologie, protézy, specializace na zubní náhrady prosthodontics /ˌprɒs.θəˈdɒnt.ɪks/

protetika, náhrada, protéza prosthesis /ˈprɒs.θiː.sɪs/ (pl. prostheses)

protéza, přeložení, výměna (vadné součásti) replacement /rɪˈpleɪs.mənt/

proti anti- /æn.ti-/

proti srážení krve antiplatelet / æn.tiˈpleɪt.lət/

protihistaminový prostředek antihistamine /æn.tiˈhɪs.tə.miːn/

protichůdný, čelící opposing / əˈpəʊ.zɪŋ/

protikladný, protilehlý opposed / əˈpəʊzd/

protilátka antidote /ˈæn.ti.dəʊt/

proti-retrovirový antiretroviral / æn.tiˌret.rəʊ ˈvaɪə.rəl/

protivirový prostředek antiviral / ˌæn.tiˈvaɪ.rəl/

protizánětlivý anti-inflammatory / ˌæn.ti.ɪnˈflæm.ə.tri/

protlačovat, tryskat squirt /skwɜːt/

proto, proto tedy, tudíž, z toho důvodu therefore /ˈðeə.fɔːʳ/

proton proton /ˈprəʊ.tɒn/

protrhnout burst /bɜːst/

proud vody, stříkat jet /dʒet/

proudící, řinoucí se torrential / təˈren.tʃⁿl/

provádění řezů sectioning /ˈsek.ʃⁿn.ɪŋ/

proximální, bližší trupu, hlavě, středu proximal /prɒˈk.sɪ.məl/

prozrazení disclosure /dɪˈskləʊ.ʒəʳ/

prožívat, pocítit, ucítit, zakusit, prodělat, zkušenost, prožitek experience /ɪkˈspɪə.ri.ᵊnt s/

prst na noze toe /təʊ/

prst na ruce, ohmatat finger /ˈfɪŋ.gəʳ/

prudký (nápor), ostrý (dobře řezající), ostrý nástroj sharp /ʃɑːp/

průduška bronchus /ˈbrɒŋ.kəs/

průdušnice, trachea windpipe / ˈwɪnd.paɪp/

průchodný patent /ˈpeɪ.tənt/

průměr (kružnice) diameter / daɪˈæm.ɪ.təʳ/

průřez, odříznutí, pitva section / ˈsek.ʃᵊn/

průsvitnost translucence / trænzˈluː.sənt s/

pružná hmota, plast plastic /ˈplæs.tɪk/

prvenství, přednost, důležitá věc priority /praɪˈɒr.ɪ.ti/

první – druhý former /ˈfɔː.məʳ/, the latter /ˈlæt.əʳ/

prvotní, původní, výchozí, začáteční initial /ɪˈnɪʃ.ᵊl/

pryč, daleko, stranou, vzdálený away /əˈweɪ/

přání, přát si, požadovat desire / dɪˈzaɪəʳ/

přebytek, přelití overspill /ˈəʊ.və.spɪl/

před rakovinný premalignant / ˌpre.məˈlig.nənt/

před, dříve než prior /praɪəʳ/ to /tʊ/

předat pass /pɑːs/ on /ɒn/

předat, podat hand /hænd/

předávkování over /ˈəʊ.vəʳ/ dosage / ˈdəʊ.sɪdʒ/

předčasný, raný premature / ˈprem.ə.tʃəʳ/

předejít, zabránit čemu, zajistit prevenci prevent /prɪˈvent/

předešlý, předcházející preceding / prɪˈsiː.dɪŋ/

především above /əˈbʌv/ all /ɔːl/

předcházet, předstihnout precede / prɪˈsiːd/

předkus (horizontální) overjet / ˈəʊ.və.dʒet/

předložit submit /səbˈmɪt/

předmenstruační syndrom premenstrual /priːˈmen.strəl/ syndrome /ˈsɪn.drəʊ m/

předmět object /ˈɒb.dʒɪkt/, subject / ˈsʌb.dʒekt/

předmontovaný, stavebnicový prefabricated /ˌpriːˈfæb.rɪ.keɪ.tɪd/

přední, posunout dopředu forward / ˈfɔː.wəd/

přednost (priorita) preference / ˈpref.ᵊr.ᵊnt s/

předoperační preoperative / priːˈɒp.ᵊr.ə.tɪv/

předpokládaný, případný prospective /prəˈspek.tɪv/

předpovídat, tvrdit predict /prɪˈdɪkt/

představa, návrh (koncept), způsob, provedení, myšlenka concept / ˈkɒn.sept/

představení, rozdělování do stupňů staging /ˈsteɪ.dʒɪŋ/

předvídatelný predictable /prɪˈdɪk.tə.bl̩/

předzvěst aura /ˈɔː.rə/

přehánět, zveličovat exaggerate / ɪgˈzædʒ.ə.reɪt/

přehled, překontrolování review / rɪˈvjuː/

přehodnotit reassess /ˌriː.əˈses/, re-evaluate /riː.ɪˈvæl.ju.eɪt/

přechodný temporal /ˈtem.pər.əl/

překážka obstacle /ˈɒb.stɪ.kl̩/

překládat, obnovovat relay /ˌrɪˈleɪ/, / ˈriː.leɪ/

překonat surpass /səˈpɑːs/

překotný, spěšný, srážecí činidlo precipitant /prɪˌsɪp.ɪ.ˈtənt/

překrvený congested /kənˈdʒes.tɪd/

překus (vertikální) overbite /ˌəʊ.və.baɪt/

přemístit reposition /rɪ.pəˈzɪʃ.ən/

přenést transfer /trænsˈfɜːʳ/

přerušení, porucha, protržení disruption /dɪsˈrʌp.ʃən/

přerušení, přestávka, zlámat, porušit break /breɪk/

přerušit disrupt /dɪsˈrʌpt/

přerušit interrupt /ˌɪn.təˈrʌpt/

přes pult, bez receptu lékaře over /ˈəʊ.vəʳ/ the counter /ˈkaʊn.təʳ/

přes, pomocí (čeho), prostřednictvím, skrz via /vaɪə/, /ˈviː.ə/

přesně strictly /ˈstrɪkt.li/

přesné upevnění precision /prɪˈsɪʒ.ᵊn/ attachment /əˈtætʃ.mənt/

přesně, úplně, doslovně exactly /ɪgˈzækt.li/

přesnídávka, lehké jídlo snack /snæk/

přesný precise /prɪˈsaɪs/

přesto none /nʌn/ the /ðə/ less /les/

převážně, hlavně predominantly /prɪˈdɒm.ɪ.nənt.li/

převzetí, přijmout take /teɪk/ over /ˈəʊ.vəʳ/

převzít, upevnit, zachytit take /teɪk/ up /ʌp/

přežvykovat chew /tʃuː/ the cud /kʌd/

při probuzení on /ɒn/ waking /ˈweɪ.kɪŋ/

při vědomí, uvědomělý, vědomý si čeho conscious /ˈkɒn.tʃəs/

příbuznost, souvislost (vztah), vzájemný poměr relationship /rɪˈleɪ.ʃᵊn.ʃɪp/

příbuzný relative /ˈrel.ə.tɪv/

příčina causation /kɔːˈzeɪ.ʃən/

příčný řez, průřez cross-section /ˌkrɒsˈsek.ʃᵊn/

přidání, dodatek addition /əˈdɪʃ.ᵊn/

přihlížející onlooker /ˈɒnˌlʊk.əʳ/

příhoda, záchvat, vedlejší děj episode /ˈep.ɪ.səʊd/

přichytit se, připojit attach /əˈtætʃ/

přijatý adopted /əˈdɒp.tɪd/

přijet, dosáhnout arrive /əˈraɪv/

přijetí admission /ədˈmɪʃ.ən/

přijmout, připustit, doznávat admit /ədˈmɪt/

příkaz, nařídit, ovládat command /kəˈmɑːnd/

přiléhající, přilehlý, sousední, vedlejší, hraničící adjacent /əˈdʒeɪ.sənt/

přilepený adherent /ədˈhɪə.rənt/

přilepit stick /stɪk/

přilnavost adhesion /ədˈhiː.ʒən/

přilnavý, ulpívající, lepkavý, lepicí, přirostlý adhesive /ədˈhiː.sɪv/

přiložení, vzájemné dotýkání apposition /ˌæ.pəˈzɪʃ.ᵊn/

přiměřeně, dostatečně adequately /ˈæd.ə.kwət.li/

příměs, směs mixture /ˈmɪks.tʃəʳ/

přímo, přímý, rovně, rovný straight /streɪt/

přímý, nasměrovat, zamířit, řídit, dohlížet direct /daɪˈrekt/

případ, důvod, věc case /keɪs/

připojení, připevnění, spoj, vazivo attachment /əˈtætʃ.mənt/

připojený, spojený connected /kəˈnek.tɪd/

připustit, respektovat, rozpoznat, uznat, uznávat recognise /ˈrek.əg.naɪz/

přirozeně naturally /ˈnætʃ.ᵊr.ᵊl.i/

přiřadit, stanovit assign /əˈsaɪn/

přisoudit award /əˈwɔːd/

příspěvek, výhoda, prospěch, pomoc, užitek benefit /ˈben.ɪ.fɪt/

přispívat contribute /kənˈtrɪb.juːt/

přístroj na odsátí, odsavač slin, krve aspirator /ˌæs.pɪˈreɪ.təʳ/

přístup entrance /ˈen.trənt s/

přístup, blížit se, cesta, kontakt approach /əˈprəʊtʃ/

přístupný, vlídný approachable / əˈprəʊ.tʃə.bl̩ /

příštitná žláza parathyroid gland / ˌpær.əˈθaɪə.rɔɪdˌglænd/

přitažlivost attraction /əˈtræk.ʃən/

přitmelení, sevření, upevnění, upnutí, utěsňování, tmel luting / luːt.ɪŋ/

přítok, proud (vody), vypláchnout flush /flʌʃ/

přítomný present /ˈprez.ᵊnt/

příušní žláza parotid /pəˈrɒt.ɪd/ gland /glænd/

přivést k vědomí, vzpomenout recall /rɪˈkɔːl/

přívětivý welcoming /ˈwel.kəm.ɪŋ/

přizpůsobený, upravený adapted / əˈdæp.tɪd/

přizpůsobit adapt /əˈdæpt/

přizpůsobit, nastavit přístroj, upravit adjust /əˈdʒʌst/

psaný written /ˈrɪt.ᵊn/

pseudonym pseudonym /ˈsuː.də.nɪm/

psoriáza, lupénka psoriasis /səˈraɪə.sɪs/

psychiatrický, duševní psychiatric / ˌsaɪ.kiˈæt.rɪk/

psychogenní, mentálního původu psychogenic /ˈsaɪ.kəˌdʒə.nɪk/

psychologický, duševní psychological /ˌsaɪ.kᵊlˈɒdʒ.ɪ.kᵊl/

psychosomatický, týkající se vztahu těla a mysli psychosomatic / ˌsaɪ.kəʊ.səˈmæt.ɪk/

psychóza, porucha myšlení a jednání s následným rozpadem osobnosti psychosis /saɪˈkəʊ.sɪs/

ptóza, sklesnutí orgánu ptosis / təu.sɪs/

půl cesty halfway /ˌhɑːfˈweɪ/

pulpektomie, chirurg. vynětí dřeně pulpectomy /pʌlˈpek.tə.mɪ/

pulpextraktor barbed /bɑːbd/ broach / brəʊtʃ/

pulpitida, zánět zubní dřeně pulpitis / pʌlˈpaɪ.tɪs/

puls na karotidě carotid /kəˌrɒt.ɪd/ pulse /pʌls/

působící zvedání žaludku nauseous / ˈnɔː.zi.əs/

působit tlakem, stlačit compress / kəmˈpres/

pustit, spustit, uvolnit release /rɪˈliːs/

původce, zdroj generator /ˈdʒen.ə.reɪ.təʳ/

pyelonefritida, současný zánět ledvinné pánvičky a ledviny pyelonephritis /ˌpaɪ.ə.lə.neˈfraɪ.tɪs/

pytel písku na ochranu sandbag / ˈsænd.bæg/

R

rada, oznámení, informace, pokyn advice /ˈæd.vɜːs/

radiální radial /ˈreɪ.di.əl/

radiografie radiography / ˌreɪ.diˈɒg.rə.fi/

radioterapie, léčba ozařováním radiotherapy /ˌreɪ.di.əʊˈθer.ə.pi/

radius, okruh, poloměr radius / ˈreɪ.di.əs/

ramadam, devátý měsíc muslimského roku, kdy během dne není dovoleno jíst a pít Ramadan / ˈræm.ə.dæn/

rámeček frame /freɪm/

rameno, větev ramus /reɪ.məs/

rasa race /reɪs/

raspatorium periosteal /ˌper.ɪˈɒs.ti.əl/ elevator /ˈel.ɪ.veɪ.təʳ/

reagovat (odpovídat) respond /rɪˈspɒnd/

reagující na světlo photostimulable /ˈfəʊ.təʊ.ˈstɪm.jʊ.lə.bļ/

reakční reactionary /riˈæk.ʃᵊn.ᵊr.i/

recepční, sestra (u příjmu pacientů) receptionist /rɪˈsep.ʃᵊn.ɪst/

recidiva, dostat recidivu, úpadek relapse /rɪˈlæps/

redukce, omezení, snížení, zmenšení, zmírnění reduction /rɪˈdʌk.ʃᵊn/

reflektovat, odrážet, vyjadřovat, zrcadlit (se) reflect /rɪˈflekt/

reflex, odraz, přemítání, výraz reflex /ˈriː.fleks/

reflux, zpětné proudění reflux /riː.flʌks/

regionálně regionally /ˈriː.dʒᵊn.ᵊl.i/

registrace, zápis, zaznamenávání registration /ˌredʒ.ɪˈstreɪ.ʃᵊn/

rehabilitace rehabilitation /ˌriː.hə.bɪl.ɪˈteɪ.ʃᵊn/

reimplantace, nahrazení odejmuté části reimplantation /ˌriː.ɪm.plɑːnˈteɪ.ʃᵊn/

rekurence, návrat, opětovný výskyt recurrence /rɪˈkʌr.ᵊnt s/

relativní, nikoli absolutní, poměrný relative /ˈrel.ə.tɪv/

relevantní, příslušný relevant /ˈrel.ə.vᵊnt/

remise, dočasné vymizení projevů nemoci, úleva remission /rɪˈmɪʃ.ᵊn/

renální, ledvinový renal /ˈriː.nᵊl/

renomovaný, chvalně známý, vyhlášený, známý renowned /rɪˈnaʊnd/

rentgenový film X-ray /ˈeks.reɪ/ film /fɪlm/

replika, duplikát replica /ˈrep.lɪ.kə/

replikace, reprodukce stejným způsobem replication /ˌrep.lɪˈkeɪ.ʃᵊn/

repozice, nové upevnění, opětné přiložení reposition /rɪ.pəˈzɪʃ.ən/

respirační, dýchací respiratory /rɪˈspɪr.ə.tri/

resuscitace, křísení, oživení resuscitation /rɪˌsʌs.ɪˈteɪ.ʃᵊn/

retence (zubů), nahromadění, upevnění retention /rɪˈten.t ʃᵊn/

retenční, nepropouštějící, zadržující retentive /rɪˈten.tɪv/

retraktor, držák, háček, hák na rány retractor /rɪˈtræk.təʳ/

retrográdní, obrácený, odvrácený, zpětný retrograde /ˈret.rəʊ .greɪd/

retrosternální, umístěný za hrudní kostí retrosternal /ˌret.rəˈstɜː.nᵊl/

reverzibilní, vratný reversible /rɪˈvɜː.sᵊ.bļ/

rigidní, neohebný, pevný, strnulý, tuhý rigid /ˈrɪdʒ.ɪd/

rinorea, vodnatý výtok z nosu rhinorrhoea /ˌraɪ.nəˈri.ə/

rodičovský parental /pəˈren.tᵊl/

rodový původ ancestry /ˈæn.ses.tri/

roentgen X-ray /ˈeks.reɪ/

ropa, nafta petroleum /pəˈtrəʊ.li.əm/

rotace, otočení rotation /rəʊ ˈteɪ.ʃᵊn/

rovnováha balance /ˈbæl.ᵊnt s/

rozbitý, prasklý, zlomený broken /brəʊ.kᵊn/

rozbor, studijní study /ˈstʌd.i/

rozdělit (na části, podíly ap.), rozštěpit, roztrhnout split /splɪt/

rozdělit apportion /əˈpɔː.ʃᵊn/

rozdělit, připravovat léky dispense /dɪˈspent s/

rozdílnost difference /ˈdɪf.ər.ᵊnt s/

rozdrcený, rozpadlý, zničený shattered /ˈʃæt.əd/

rozdrtit crush /krʌʃ/

rozhodnutí, nález decision /dɪˈsɪӡ.ən/

rozhodování decision /dɪˈsɪʒ.ən/ making /ˈmeɪ.kɪŋ/

rozhodující, klíčový, velmi důležitý crucial /ˈkruː.ʃəl/

rozlišování, rozdílnost differentiation / ˌdɪf.ər.en.t ʃiˈeɪ.ʃən/

rozlišovat discriminate / dɪˈskrɪm.ɪ.neɪt/, distinguish / dɪˈstɪŋ.gwɪʃ/

rozložitelný, odbouratelný degradable /dɪˈgreɪ.də.bl̩/

rozmanitý miscellaneous / ˌmɪs.əlˈeɪ.ni.əs/

rozmazaný blurred /blɜːd/

rozměr dimension /ˌdaɪˈmen.t ʃən/, proportion prəˈpɔː.ʃən/

rozmezí, rozsah, roztřídit, řada, seřadit range /reɪndʒ/

rozmnožit, rozmnožovat se multiply / ˈmʌl.tɪ.plaɪ/

rozpad, rozklad, nepořádek disorganization /dɪˌsɔː.gə.naɪˈzeɪ.ʃən/

rozpaky, nedostatek (vada), potíže embarrassment /ɪmˈbær.ə.smənt/

rozpárat se, roztrhnout se rip /rɪp/

rozpínat se, šířit se, rozšířit, rozšířit se, zvětšit expand /ɪkˈspænd/

rozprašovat spray /spreɪ/

rozptýlení, rozrušení, napravení zlomeniny tahem distraction / dɪˈstræk.ʃən/

rozptýlený, neohraničený diffuse / dɪˈfjuːs/

rozptýlit se dissipate /ˈdɪs.ɪ.peɪt/

rozptýlit, rozšířit se, pronikat diffuse /dɪˈfjuːz /

rozpustnost, tavitelnost solubility / ˌsɒl.juˈbɪl.ɪ.ti/

rozrušený, nešťastný distressed / dɪˈstrest/

rozřešit resolve /rɪˈzɒlv/

rozřezat, pitvat dissect /daɪˈsekt/

rozsah pozornosti attention / əˈten.t ʃən/ span /spæn/

rozsah scope /skəʊp/

rozšířit widen /ˈwaɪ.dən/

rozšířit, prostírat se, rozprostírat se, táhnout se extend /ɪkˈstend/

rozšiřovač, výstružník reamer / ˈriː.məʳ/

rozšiřovat dilate /daɪˈleɪt/

rozšiřovat, vybočit drift /drɪft/

roztahovat se, tečení creep /kriːp/

roztavit, slít, sloučit se fuse /fjuːz/

roztočen, vtlačen spun /spʌn/

roztok, rozpuštění solution /səˈluː.ʃən/

roztrhnout, roztrhnout se, trhlina tear /teəʳ/

roztříštěná zlomenina comminuted / ˈkɒ.mɪˈnjuː.tɪd/ fracture /ˈfræk.t ʃəʳ/

roztříštit se shatter /ˈʃæt.əʳ/

rozvázat undo /ʌnˈduː/

rty labia /ˈleɪ.bi.ə/

ručně ovládaný mains-operated / meɪnz.ˈɒp.ər.eɪt.ɪd/

ručně, za ruku by /baɪ/ hand /hænd/

ruční (držený v ruce), přenosný handheld /ˌhændˈheld/

ručník, utěrka towel /taʊəl/

ruka, rukáv, opěradlo arm /ɑːm/

rukavice glove /glʌv/

ruptura, kýla, protržení, výhřez, zlomení rupture /ˈrʌp.tʃəʳ/

rušit, porušit, vyrušovat, působit poruchy disturb /dɪˈstɜːb/

rutinní, běžný routine /ruːˈtiːn/

růže rose /rəʊz/

rýha, sulkus sulcus /sʌl.kəs/ (pl: sulci)

rychlostí at /ət/ a rate /reɪt/

rychlý fast /fɑːst/

rychlý, prudký rapid /ˈræp.ɪd/

rytmus dýchání respiratory / rɪˈspɪr.ə.tri/ rate /reɪt/

Ř

řeč speech /spiːtʃ/

ředitelství, vedení management / ˈmæn.ɪdʒ.mənt/

řešení, vyřešení solution /səˈluː.ʃᵊn/

řezací cutting /ˈkʌt.ɪŋ/

řezáková hrana incisal /ɪnˈsɪ.zᵊl/ edge /edʒ/

řezat lancinate /ˈlaːn.sɪ.nəɪt/

řídit, zvládnout manage /ˈmæn.ɪdʒ/

říhat, mít mimovolní pocit na zvracení retch /retʃ/

řinout se, téci proudem gush /gʌʃ/

S

s rovnou čepelí straight-bladed / streɪt.bleɪd.ɪd/

sací špička suction /ˈsʌk.ʃən/ tip /tɪp/

sáček sachet /ˈsæʃ.eɪ/

sada (souprava), soubor, umístění set /set/

sada, skupina, sled series /ˈsɪə.riːz/

salivace, slinění sialosis /ˌsɑɪəˈləʊ.sɪs/

sami (udělat něco) on /ɒn/ their /ðeər/ own /əʊn/

samonosný cantilever /ˈkæn.ti.liː.vəʳ/

samonosný můstek cantilever / ˈkæn.ti.liː.vəʳ/ bridge /brɪdʒ/

samoregenerační self-healing / self.ˈhiː.lɪŋ/

samotný alone /əˈləʊn/

sandblast /ˈsænd.blɑːst/ pískovat

sarkom, zhoubný nádor pojivových tkání sarcoma /sɑːˈkəʊ.mə/

saturace (nasycení) saturation / ˌsæt.jʊˈreɪ.ʃᵊn/

sdělení, zpráva message /ˈmes.ɪdʒ/

sdílení, shromažďující pooling / puː.lɪŋ/

sebe-ocenění self-esteem /ˌself.ɪˈstiːm/

sebeporanění, sebepoškození self-inflicted /ˌself.ɪnˈflɪk.tɪd/

sebevražedná myšlenka suicidal / ˌsuː.ɪˈsaɪ.dᵊl/ idea /aɪˈdɪə/

sedačka stool /stuːl/

sedadlo, umístit, usadit seat /siːt/

sedativum, bolesti utišující lék, uklidňující prostředek sedative / ˈsed.ə.tɪv/

sedlo saddle /ˈsæd.l̩/

segment, úsek segment /ˈseg.mənt/

sejmout, změkčit soften /ˈsɒf.ᵊn/ důkladný, pevný, tuhá hmota solid /ˈsɒl.ɪd/

semipermanentní, polotrvalý semipermanent /sem.i.ˈpɜː.mə.nənt/

senzitivita, citlivost, vnímavost sensitivity /ˌsent.sɪˈtɪv.ɪ.ti/

sepnout (spínátkem), štípat clip /klɪp/

séropozitivní, obsahující sérové protilátky seropositive / ˌsɪ.ə.rəˈpɒz.ə.tɪv/

seřazení, uspořádání alignment / əˈlaɪn.mənt/

sesazený, vyrovnaný matched /mætʃt/

sevřít, zatnout, pevně uchopit, stisknout clench /klentʃ/

sfygmomanometr, tlakoměr sphygmomanometer / sfɪg.məʊ.mænˈɒm.ɪ.təʳ/

shluk, hrozen, nahromadit se cluster / ˈklʌs.təʳ/

shoda, důslednost consistency / kənˈsɪs.tᵊnt.si/

shoda, souhlas, spolupráce, dodržení compliance /kəmˈplaɪ.ənt s/

shodný, souběžně probíhat, souběžný parallel /ˈpær.ə.lel/

shrnovač rake /reɪk/

schopně competently /ˈkɒm.pɪ.tənt.li/

schopnost reagovat na podněty, vnímavost responsiveness / rɪˈspɒnt .sɪv.nəs/

schopnost udržet moč continence / ˈkɒn.tɪ.nənt/

schopnost, dovednost ability / əˈbɪl.ɪ.ti/

schválit, odsouhlasit approve /əˈpruːv/

sialoadenitida, zánět slinné žlázy sialadenitis /ˈsaɪəlˌædəˈnʌɪ.tis/

sideropenie, nedostatek železa v krvi sideropenia /ˌsɪd.ə.rəˈpiː.nɪ.ə/

síla, účinnost, nutit, vyvíjet tlak force /fɔːs/

silikon silicone /ˈsɪl.ɪ.kəʊn/

silně účinný potent /ˈpəʊ.tᵊnt/

silně, velmi heavily /ˈhev.ɪ.li/

silný (mocný), silně strong /strɒŋ/

sípat wheeze /wiːz/

situace, stav, kondice, podmínka, podmiňovat, poměry, okolnost condition /kənˈdɪʃ.ən/

sjet, sklouznout slide /slaɪd/

skalpel scalpel /ˈskæl.pᵊl/

sklánět se dip /dɪp/

skléra, oční bělmo sclera /ˈsklɪə.rə/

skleslý, stlačený, snížený depressed / dɪˈprest/

sklesnout droop /druːp/

sklo, sklenice glass /glɑːs/

sklo-ionomer glass /glɑːs/ ionomer / ˈaɪ.ə.nɒ.məʳ/

skloněný, šikmý oblique /əʊ ˈbliːk/

skončit, dokončit, dokončení, závěr finish /ˈfɪn.ɪʃ/

skořápka shell /ʃel/

skrytý hidden /hid.ᵊn/, occult /ˈɒk.ʌlt/

skrz naskrz through and through /θruː/

skřípání grinding /ˈgraɪn.dɪŋ/

skřípat grind /graɪnd/

skusový tampon bite /baɪt/ pack /pæk/

skvrna, kaz blemish /ˈblem.ɪʃ/

skvrnitý (flíčky) speckled /ˈspek.l̩ d/

skvrnka, tečka fleck /flek/

slabá odolnost, slabá stránka, vada weakness /ˈwiːk.nəs/

slabost, schvácenost, únava (též materiálu), vyčerpání fatigue / fəˈtiːg/

slabý, křehký, nedostatečný weak / wiːk/

slaná voda saltwater /sɒlt.ˈwɔː.təʳ/

sledovat observe /əbˈzɜːv/

slepé místo na sítnici; bolavé místo (přen.) blind /blaɪnd/ spot /spɒt/

slepota blindness /ˈblaɪnd.nəs/

slévárenská slitina casting /kɑːst.ɪŋ/ alloy /ˈæl.ɔɪ/

slinný salivary /səˈlaɪ.vᵊr.i/

slitina, směs, příměs alloy /ˈæl.ɔɪ/

slovní verbal /ˈvɜː.bəl/

složení composition /ˌkɒm.pəˈzɪʃ.ən/

složitý complicated /ˈkɒm.plɪ.keɪ.tɪd/

slučitelný, zaměnitelný compatible / kəmˈpæt.ɪ.bl̩/

sluch, schopnost slyšet hearing / ˈhɪə.rɪŋ/

služební odznak, odznak, označit odznakem badge /bædʒ/

slyšitelný audible /ˈɔː.dɪ.bl̩ /

slzení lacrimation /læk.rɪˈmeɪ.ʃᵊn/

smáčivý hydrophilic /ˌhaɪ.drəˈfɪl.ɪk/

směrem dopředu, kupředu (směřující) forwards /ˈfɔː.wədz/

směrem dozadu backwards / ˈbæk.wədz/

směřovat k aim /eɪm/ at /ət/

smíchaný mixed /mɪkst/

smrštění, srážení, ztráta objemu shrinkage /ˈʃrɪŋ.kɪdʒ/

smršťovat, srážet se shrink /ʃrɪŋk/

smrt, zánik death /deθ/

smrtelný terminal /ˈtɜː.mɪ.nəl/

smrtelný úraz fatality /fəˈtæl.ə.ti/

smyslové postižení sensory /ˈsent .sᵊr.i/ disability /ˌdɪs.əˈbɪl.ɪ.ti/

smyslový sensory /'sent̬.sᵊr.i/

snaha, úsilí effort /'ef.ət/

snění daydreaming /'deɪ.driːm/

snímač sensor /'sent̬.səʳ/

snímač, čidlo transducer /trænz'djuː.səʳ/

snímač, čidlo, detekční přístroj
  detector /dɪ'tek.təʳ/

snížení, snížit se, být na ústupu
  decrease /dɪ'kriːs/

snížení, úbytek, ztráta loss /lɒs/

socializovat, stýkat se (společensky)
  socialise /'səʊ.ʃᵊl.aɪz/

sociální anamnéza social /'səʊ.ʃᵊl/
  history /'hɪs.tər.i/

sonogram, ultrazvukový ultrasound /
  'ʌl.trə.saʊnd/

souběžný concurrent /kən'kʌr.ᵊnt/

současně at /ət/ the same /seɪm/ time /
  taɪm/

současný contemporaneous /
  kən̩tem.pə'reɪ.ni.əs/

současný zánět několika kloubů
  polyarthropathy /ˌpɒl.ɪ.ɑː'θrəp.ə.θi/

souprava první pomoci emergency /
  ɪ'mɜː.dʒənt̬.si/ kit /kɪt/

sourozenec, vrstevník sibling /
  'sɪb.lɪŋ/

souvislost context /'kɒn.tekst/

spadat do fall /fɔːl/ into /'ɪn.tuː/

spatřený spotted /'spɒt.ɪd/

specializovaný specialised /
  'speʃ.ᵊl.aɪzd/

spirála, spirálovitý, točit se, závitnice
  spiral /'spaɪə.rᵊl/

spirála, šroubek, šroubovat screw /
  skruː/

spláchnout, vymýt swill /swɪl/ out /aʊt/

spodní zářez, vrub, zářez undercut /
  ˌʌn.də'kʌt̬/

spojení communication /
  kə̩mjuː.nɪ'keɪ.ʃᵊn/, connection /
  kə'nek.ʃən/

spojený, připojený attached /ə'tætʃt/

spojit, spojovat, tmelit, lepit, vazba
  (chemická ap.) bond /bɒnd/

spokojený satisfied /'sæt̬.ɪs.faɪd/

spokojený, ochoten content /'kɒn.tent/

společenské postavení, status (stav),
  životní úroveň status /'steɪ.təs/

spolehlivý reliable /rɪ'laɪə.bl̩/

spolupráce cooperation /
  kəʊˌɒp.ᵊr'eɪ.ʃᵊn/

spolupracovník associate /ə'səʊ.si.eɪt/

spolupracující cooperative /
  kəʊ'ɒp.ᵊr.ə.tɪv/

spolužák classmate /'klɑːs.meɪt/

spona, háček, opatřit sponou,
  připnout clasp /klɑːsp/

spontánně mizející self-limiting /
  self.'lɪm.ɪ.tɪŋ/

spontánně, samovolně spontaneously /
  spɒn'teɪ.ni.ə.sli/

spontánní, samovolný spontaneous /
  spɒn'teɪ.ni.əs/

sporák cooker /'kʊk.əʳ/

spotřeba, strávení, opotřebování,
  zničení consumption /kən'sʌmp.ʃən/

spouštěč, spustit (náhle uvolnit),
  začít trigger /'trɪg.əʳ/

správně (dobře) well /wel/

sputum, výměšek dýchacího ústrojí
  sputum /'spjuː.təm/

srážení, vylučování precipitation /
  prɪˌsɪp.ɪ'teɪ.ʃᵊn/

srdce, srdeční heart /hɑːt/

srdeční cardiac /'kɑː.di.æk/

srdeční stimulátor pacemaker /
  'peɪsˌmeɪ.kəʳ/

srovnání kosti reduction /rɪ'dʌk.ʃᵊn/

stabilita stability /stə'bɪl.ɪ.ti/

stabilizace (ustálení) stabilization /
  ˌsteɪ.bɪ.la ɪ'zeɪ.ʃᵊn/

stabilní, stálý stable /'steɪ.bl̩/

stah, smrštění, tažení, zmenšení, stažení, kontrakce contraction / kənˈtræk.ʃən/

stáhnutý withdrawn /wɪðˈdrɔːn/

stahování, smršťování retraction / rɪˈtræk.ʃ°n/

stále permanently /ˈpɜː.mə.nənt.li/

stálý constant /ˈkɒnɪ.st°nt/

standardní míra, zkušební přístroj gauge /geɪdʒ/

stanovení, zhodnocení, posouzení, určení assessment /əˈses.mənt/

stanovený, stanovit, určit set /set/

stanovit, vyložit, vytyčovat set /set/ out /aʊt/

stárnoucí, postarší, vyššího věku elderly /ˈel.dəl.i/

stárnutí growing /ˈgrəʊ.ɪŋ/ old /əʊld/

steatorea, tuková stolice steatorrhoea / ˌstɪ.ə.təˈriː.ə/

stejný, dokonce even /ˈiː.v°n/

stejný, tentýž same /seɪm/

stěna wall /wɑːl/

sterilizační zařízení steriliser / ˈster.°l.aɪz.ə°/

sterilizovat sterilise /ˈster.ɪ.laɪz/

sterilní sterile /ˈster.aɪl/

sternum, hrudní kost sternum / ˈstɜː.nəm/

steroid, organická látka, např. hormon pohlavní nebo kůry nadledvin steroid /ˈste.rɔɪd/, / ˈstɪər.ɔɪd/

stetoskop, fonendoskop stethoscope / ˈsteθ.ə.skəʊp/

stěžovatel complainant /kəmˈpleɪ.nənt/

stlačení hrudníku chest /tʃest/ compression /kəmˈpreʃ.°n/

stlačení, zaklínění impaction / ɪmˈpæk.ʃ°n/

stlačený pressed /prest/

stolice (vyprazdňování střev) stool / stuːl/

stoupat, nastoupit (přen.), dostat se ascend /əˈsend/

stres, napětí, namáhání, nepohoda, stlačení, tlak stress /stres/

strnulost, tuhost, tvrdost, ztuhlost rigidity /rɪˈdʒɪd.ɪ.ti/

strnulost, ztuhnutí stiffness /ˈstɪf.nəs/

stroj engine /ˈen.dʒɪn/

strojové vybavení machinery / məˈʃiː.nə.ri/

strop ceiling /ˈsiː.lɪŋ/

struktura, tkáň, vazba texture / ˈteks.tʃə°/

strukturální structural /ˈstrʌk.tʃ°r.°l/

struma, vole goitre /ˈgɔɪ.tə°/

střednice midline /ˈmɪd.laɪn/

střednice, osa centreline /sen.trə.laɪn/

stříbro silver /ˈsɪl.və°/

stříkačka pro výplach irrigation / ˌɪr.ɪˈgeɪ.ʃ°n/ syringe /sɪˈrɪndʒ/

stříkanec, šplouchat splatter /ˈsplæt.ə°/

stupeň grade /greɪd/

stvrzenka, nálepka docket /ˈdɒk.ɪt/

subjektivní (osobní) subjective / ˈsʌb.dʒek.tɪv/

subluxace, neúplné vykloubení subluxation /ˌsʌb.lʌkˈseɪ.ʃ°n/

subperiostální, ležící pod okosticí subperiosteal /sʌb.per.ɪˈɒs.ti.əl/

sugesce (vnuknutí) suggestion / səˈdʒes.tʃ°n/

suché zubní lůžko dry /draɪ/ socket / ˈsɒk.ɪt/

suchost dryness /draɪ.nəs/

sulfát, kyselina sírová, síran sulphate /ˈsʌl.feɪt/

supraokluze overeruption / ˈəʊ.və.ɪˈrʌp.ʃ°n/

susceptibilita, náchylnost, vnímavost susceptibility /səˌsep.tɪˈbɪl.ɪ.ti/

suspektní, domnělý, očekávaný, podezřelý, předpokládaný suspected /sə'spek.tɪd/

sušenka biscuit /'bɪs.kɪt/

sutura, sešití (stehy), sešití rány, steh, šev suture /'suː.tʃəʳ/

svačit, pojídat malá jídla snack /snæk/

svalový muscular /'mʌs.kjʊ.lᵊr/

svalstvo musculature /'mʌs.kjʊ.lə.tʃəʳ/

svár, spor contention /kən'tent.ʃᵊn/

svázat, zavázat tie /taɪ/

svazovat bind /baɪnd/ down /daʊn/

svědění itchiness /'ɪtʃ.ɪ.nəs/

svědění, svědivý itching /'ɪtʃ.ɪŋ/

světlem tuhnoucí, tvrzený světlem light-cured /laɪt.kjʊəʳ.d /

světlo, světlý, osvětlit light /laɪt/

světový, celosvětově worldwide /w3ːld.waɪd/

svícený shone /ʃɒn/

svitek roll /rəʊl/

svorka, ruční nůžky clip /klɪp/

syfilis (příjice) syphilis /'sɪf.ɪ.lɪs/

symbiont commensal /'kɒm.əns.ᵊl/

sympatický, účastný (soucitný) sympathetic /ˌsɪm.pə'θet.ɪk/

symptom symptom /'sɪmp.təm/

synergistický, souhlasně působící synergistic /ˌsɪn.əː'dʒi.stik/

systém system /'sɪs.təm/

systém zdravotní péče health /helθ/ care /keəʳ/ system /'sɪs.təm/

systolický systolic /sɪs.tɒl.ɪk/

Š

šablona, příručka guide /gaɪd/

šance, možnost chance /tʃɑːnt s/

šedivý, šedý grey /greɪ/

šicí jehla s vláknem suture /'suː.tʃəʳ/ needle /'niː.dl̩ /

šikmý angled /'æŋ.gl̩ d/

široce widely /'waɪd.li/

široký, obsáhlý broad /brɔːd/

šíře, vůle width /wɪtθ/

škádlit tease /tiːz/

škála (stupnice), váha (na vážení) scale /skeɪl/

škodlivý následek ill /ɪl/ effect /ɪ'fekt/

škrtidlo tourniquet /'tʊə.nɪ.keɪ/

škubnutí, tik, trhnout jerk /dʒ3ːk/

šňůra, lanko cord /kɔːd/

špatně informovat misinform /ˌmɪs.ɪn'fɔːm/

špatně přístupný, nešikovný awkward /'ɔː.kwəd/

šperky jewellery /'dʒuː.ᵊl.ri/

špína dirt /d3ːt/

špinavý dirty /'d3ː.ti/

štěp, transplantovat graft /grɑːft/

štěpina, úlomek spicule /'spɪk.juːl/

štěrbinový crevicular /'kre'v.ɪ.kjʊ.ləʳ/

štěrk, močové kamínky, písek v moči gravel /'græv.ᵊl/

štípací kleště rongeur /rɒn'ʒeəʳ/

štítek, cedulka sticker /stɪk.əʳ/

šumivý nápoj (šampaňské apod.) fizzy /'fɪz.i/ pop /pɒp/

T

tabletka tablet /'tæb.lət/

táhnout, trhat (i s kořenem), zmítat pull /pʊl/

taktilní, dotekový tactile /'tæk.taɪl/

tampon z vaty pledget /pledʒ.ɪt/

tangenciální, tečný tangential /tæn'dʒen.tʃᵊl/

taška, pytel, sáček, dávat do pytle bag /bæg/

tažný (síla) tensile /'ten.saɪl/

technický technical /'tek.nɪ.kᵊl/

technik technician /tek'nɪʃ.ᵊn/

tekutý runny /'rʌn.i/

tělesná váha body /'bɒd.i/ weight / weɪt/

tělní dutina body /'bɒd.i/ cavity / 'kæv.ɪ.ti/

tělo, těleso body /'bɒd.i/

temporální, skráňový (na spáncích) temporal /'tem.pər.əl/

temporomandibulární temporomandibular /ˌtem. pər.ə.mæn'dɪ.bjʊ.ləʳ/

tendence tendency /'ten.dənt.si/

tenounký (nepatrný) tiny /'taɪ.ni/

tenze, napětí, napínání (tahem), tlak tension /'tent.ʃªn/

teoreticky theoretically /θɪə'ret.ɪ.kli/

tepat, tep throb /θrɒb/

tepelná rozpínavost thermal /'θɜː.məl/ expansion /ɪk'spæn.tʃªn/

terapeut therapist /'θer.ə.pɪst/

terapeutický (léčebný), lék therapeutic /ˌθer.ə'pjuː.tɪk/

terapie, léčba therapy /'θer.ə.pi/

terciálně, v třetí řadě tertiary / 't3ː.ʃªr.i/

termální, tepelný thermal /'θɜː.məl/

těsná blízkost vicinity /vɪ'sɪn.ɪ.ti/

tetanus tetanus /'tet.ªn.əs/

tetovat tattoo /tə'tuː/, /tæt'uː/

těžce dýchat, popadat dech gasp / gɑːsp/

tinitus, hučení v uších tinnitus / 'tɪn.ɪ.təs/

tíseň, stav ohrožení distress /dɪ'stres/

titan titanium /tɪ'teɪ.ni.əm/

tlukot beating /'biː.tɪŋ/

tmel (sklenářský), stmelit putty / 'pʌt.i/

toaleta, čistění toilet /'tɔɪ.lət/

tok, výtok, proud (vzduchu), prýštit (krev) flow /fləʊ/

tolerance (dovolená úchylka), odolnost, shovívavost, snášenlivost tolerance /'tɒl.ªr.ªnt s/

tolerovat tolerate /'tɒl.ªr.eɪt/

tomografie tomography /tə'mɒg.rə.fi/

tonická fáze, napětí tonic /'tɒn.ɪk/ phase /feɪz/

tonutí drowning /'draʊn.ɪŋ/

totožnost identity /aɪ'den.tɪ.ti/

touha, bažení craving /'kreɪ.vɪŋ/

tradičně traditionally /trə'dɪʃ.ªn.ªl.i/

trakce, náprava tahem traction / 'træk.ʃªn/

transformace (přeměna), přechod transformation /ˌtræns.fə'meɪ.ʃªn/

transmise (převod), odevzdání, přenášení, zaslání transmission / trænz'mɪʃ.ªn/

transplantace transplantation / ˌtræn.splɑːn'teɪ.ʃªn/

transplantace, transplantovat, transplantovaný orgán transplant / træn'splɑːnt/

transport, převoz transport / 'træn.spɔːt/

trauma, úraz trauma /'trɔː.mə/

traumatický, úrazový traumatic / trɔː'mæt.ɪk/, /traʊ-/

trigeminální, trojklaný trigeminal / 'traɪ'dʒem.ɪ.nªl/

trizmus, křeč žvýkacího svalstva trismus /trɪz.məs/

trvání, doba duration /djʊə'reɪ.ʃªn/

trvanlivost, životnost longevity / lɒn'dʒev.ə.ti/

třást, otřes (otřesení), potřesení (též hlavou) shake /ʃeɪk/

tření friction /'frɪk.ʃªn/

třenový zub premolar /ˌpriː'məʊ.ləʳ/

třetina third /θɜːd/

tuberkulóza tuberculosis / tjuːˌbɜː.kjʊ'ləʊ.sɪs/

tubulární, trubicovitý tubular /
'tjuː.bjʊ.lər/

tubulus, kanálek tubule /'tjuː.bjuːl/

tuhnout za studena cold-cure /
kəʊld.kjʊər/

tuhnutí set /set/

tuhý stiff /stɪf/, tough /tʌf/

tuk, tloušťka fat /fæt/

tupost (přen.) dullness /'dʌl.nəs/

tupý dull /dʌl/

tvar, podoba, forma, formulář,
podoba, utvářet form /fɔːm/

tvarovač former /'fɔː.mər/

tvarovaný, ve tvaru, zformovaný
shaped /ʃeɪpt/

tvář bucca /bʌk.ə/ (pl. buccae) /
bʌk.siː/, cheek /tʃiːk/

tvářecí slitina, kujná slitina wrought /
rɔːt/ alloy /'æl.ɔɪ/

tváření, výlisek moulding /məʊld.ɪŋ/

tvoření krystalů crystallisation /
ˌkrɪs.təl.aɪ'zeɪ.ʃᵊn/

tyčinka (vosku apod.) stick /stɪk/

tyčinka bar /bɑːr/

týdně weekly /'wiː.kli/

týkající se chování behavioural /
bɪ'heɪ.vjə.rəl/

týkající se puchýřků a velkých
puchýřů vesiculobullous /
ve.'sɪ.kju.ləˌbuːləʊs/

týkající se, příslušný concerned /
kən's3ːnd/

U

u křesla, vedle křesla chairside /
tʃeər.saɪd/

ublížení, úraz, zranění, škoda,
poškození harm /hɑːm/

úbytek váhy weight /weɪt/ loss /lɒs/

ucpat obturate /'ɒb.tjʊə.reɪt/

účinek, výsledek, provést, způsobit
effect /ɪ'fekt/

účinný, působivý active /'æk.tɪv/

úder, bití (pulsu), rána stroke /strəʊk/

úder, propíchnout, vytváření malých
děr do tkáně punch /pʌntʃ/

úder, rána blow /bləʊ/

uhodit knock /nɒk/

uchopení, záchvat (nemoci),
záchvatový seizure /'siː.ʒər/

uchování, záchrana preservation /
ˌprez.ə'veɪ.ʃᵊn/

uchovat preserve /prɪ'z3ːv/

uchovat při životě maintain /
meɪn'teɪn/ life /laɪf/

uchránit ward /wɔːd/ off /ɒf/

ujistit, uklidnit assure /ə'ʃɔːr/

ukazatele indices /'ɪn.dɪ.siːz/

ukázka, projevit exhibit /ɪg'zɪb.ɪt/

uklidit tidy /'taɪ.di/

uklidnit put /pʊt/ at /ət/ ease /iːz/

uklidňovat reassure /ˌriː.ə'ʃɔːr/

uklidňující lék, utišení sedation /
sɪ'deɪ.ʃᵊn/

uklidňující prostředek tranquilliser /
'træŋ.kwɪ.laɪ.zər/

ukotvení, úchyt anchorage /
'æŋ.kər.ɪdʒ/

ulcerace, vředovitost, tvoření vředů
ulcer /'ʌl.sər/

ulcerativní kolitida (zánět tlustého
střeva) ulcerative /'ʌl.sər.ə.tɪv/
colitis /kəʊ 'laɪ.təs/

ulehčit, ulevit, vykrýt, zmírnit,
zmírňovat relieve /rɪ'liːv/

úlomky, pozůstatky, poškozená tkáň,
zbytky, nečistota debris /'deb.riː/, /
'deɪ.briː/

uložení, uskladnění, zásoba, materiál
storage /'stɔː.rɪdʒ/

ultrafialový (UV) ultraviolet /
ˌʌl.trə'vaɪə.lət/

ultrazvukový ultrasonic /ˌʌl.trə'sɒn.ɪk/

umělé sladidlo sweetener /'swiːt.nər/

umělý zub umístěný na můstku
pontic /ˌpɒnt.ɪk/

umístěný kolem úst perioral /
ˌper.ɪ.ˈɔː.rəl/

umožnit, umožňovat, dát možnost,
učinit schopným, uzpůsobit enable
/ɪˈneɪ.bl̩ /

únavný, vyčerpávající tiring /ˈtaɪə.rɪŋ/

uniknutí, otvor, výlevka escape /
ɪˈskeɪp/

unilaterální, pouze na jedné straně
unilateral /ˌjuː.nɪˈlæt.ᵊr.ᵊl/

úplně totally /ˈtəʊ.tᵊl.i/

upnout, výztuha, svorka clamp /
klæmp/

úprava skusu orthodontic /
ˌɔː.θəʊ ˈdɒn.tɪk/

upravený na míru tailored /ˈteɪ.ləd/

upravit, pozměnit, změnit, změnit se
alter /ˈɒl.təʳ/

upravování trimming /ˈtrɪm.ɪŋ/

úraz, smrt způsobená elektřinou
electrocution /ɪˌlek.trəˈkjuː.ʃən/

určení determination /dɪˌtɜː.mɪˈneɪ.ʃᵊn/

uremie, chronické selhání činnosti
ledvin uraemia /jʊəˈriː.mi.ə/

urovnat spor kompromisem, ústupky
compromise /ˈkɒm.prə.maɪz/

usmívat se smile /smaɪl/

usnadnit facilitate /fəˈsɪl.ɪ.teɪt/

usnout fall /fɔːl/ asleep /əˈsliːp/

uspávající, lék navozující spánek
hypnotic /hɪpˈnɒt.ɪk/

úspěšný člověk achiever /əˈtʃiː.vər/

uspokojivý, splňující všechny
podmínky satisfactory /
ˌsæt.ɪsˈfæk.tᵊr.i/

uspořádat, použít, likvidovat dispose
/dɪˈspəʊz/

ustanovit, zavést, uvést do chodu,
zřídit, zabezpečit establish /
ɪˈstæb.lɪʃ/

ustat, zastavit se cease /siːs/

ústně orally /ˈɔː.rə.li/

ústní voda, kloktadlo, výplach úst
mouthwash /ˈmaʊθ.wɒʃ/

ustoupit, stáhnout se (zpět) fall /fɔːl/
back /bæk/

ustouplý zpět retruded /rɪˈtruː.dɪd/

ústrojí apparatus /ˌæp.əˈreɪ.təs/

ušní, boltcovitý auricular /ɔːˈrɪ.kjʊ.ləʳ/

utěsnění, ucpání, uzavření obturation
/ˌɒb.tjʊ.əˈrəɪ.ʃᵊn/

utíkat, cupitat scurry /ˈskʌr.i/

útočný, nekontrolovatelný rampant /
ˈræm.pᵊnt/

útok, záchvat attack /əˈtæk/

utrpěný, vytrvalý sustained /səˈsteɪnd/

utrpět sustain /səˈsteɪn/

úvaha consideration /kənˌsɪd.əˈreɪ.ʃən/

uvědomění, připravenost,
informovanost awareness /əˈweə.nəs/

uvědomit si, uvědomovat si v chápat
realise /ˈrɪə.laɪz/

uvědomovat si, vědomý si aware /
əˈweəʳ/of /əv/

uvědomující si, mající obavy
apprehensive /ˌæp.rɪˈhent.sɪv/

uvést v omyl mislead /ˌmɪsˈliːd/

uvolnění mobilisation /
ˌməʊ.bɪ.laɪˈzeɪ.ʃᵊn/, relaxation /
ˌriː.lækˈseɪ.ʃᵊn/

uvolněný, relaxovaný relaxed /
rɪˈlækst/

uvolnit ease /iːz/

uvolnit, uvolněný, viklající se, volný
loose /luːs/

uzavírání, blokování locking /lɒk.ɪŋ/

uzavření, obemknutí úst mouth /
maʊθ/ seal /siːl/

uzavřít close /kləʊz/, occlude /
əˈkluːd/, /ɒkˈluːd/

uzavřít smlouvu, chytit (nemoc),
smrštit se contract /ˈkɒn.trækt/

449

uzavřít těsně, zaplombovat seal /siːl/

uzdravení, zotavení recovery /
rɪˈkʌv.ᵊr.i/, restoration /ˌres.tᵊrˈeɪ.ʃᵊn/

uzlový nodal /ˈnəʊ.dᵊl/

uznat platnost, schválit validate /
ˈvæl.ɪ.deɪt/

uznávaný accomplished /əˈkʌm.plɪʃt/,
respected /rɪˈspek.tɪd/

užitečný helpful /ˈhelp.fᵊl/, useful /
ˈjuːs.fᵊl/

užívání více léků, nadměrné užívání
léčiv polypharmacy /
pɒl.ɪ.ˈfɑː.mə.si/

uživatel user /ˈjuː.zᵊr/

V

v dobrém zdravotním stavu fit /fɪt/
and well /wel/

v dosahu, k ruce to /tʊ/ hand /hænd/

v linii, řadový in /ɪn/ line /laɪn/

v plechovce konzervovaná potravina
tinned /tɪnd/

v podstatě, nezbytně, zásadně
essentially /ɪˈsen.tʃᵊl.i/

v případě nutnosti on /ɒn/ occasion /
əˈkeɪ.ʒᵊn/

váček, dutina, puchýřek vesicle /
ˈvesɪkl/

váček, pouzdro (anat.), kapsle,
tabletka capsule /ˈkæp.sjuːl/

vadit mind /maɪnd/

vadný, porušený defective /dɪˈfek.tɪv/

váha weight /weɪt/

váhavost, rozkolísanost hesitancy /
ˈhez.ɪ.tᵊnt.si/

variabilní (proměnlivý), nestálý,
kolísavý variable /ˈveə.ri.ə.bl̩/

varianta léčby treatment /ˈtriːt.mənt/
modality /məˈdæl.ə.ti/

varianta, druh, mnohotvárnost,
odrůda, rozmanitost, výběr
(široký) variety /vəˈraɪə.ti/

variantní, lišící se, proměnný variant /
ˈveə.ri.ənt/

varicella, plané neštovice varicella /
ˌvæ.rɪˈsel.ə/

varikózní žíla (křečová) varicose vein
/ˌvær.ɪ.kəʊ sˈveɪn/

varovat alert /əˈlɜːt/, warn /wɔːn/

vaskulární, cévní vascular /
ˈvæs.kjʊ.ləʳ/

vaskulitida, zánět cév vasculitis /
ˌvæs.kjʊ.ˈlaɪ.tɪs/

vata cotton /ˈkɒt.ᵊn/ wool /wʊl/

vata na špejli, vysušit tamponem
swab /swɒb/

vazodilatace, rozšíření cév
vasodilatation /ˌveɪ.zə.daɪˈlə.teɪ.ʃᵊn/

včela, včelí bee /biː/

vdech, odsávání (nečistot) aspiration /
ˌæs.pɪˈreɪ.ʃən/

vdech, větrání ventilation /
ˌven.tɪˈleɪ.ʃᵊn/

vdechnout inhale /ɪnˈheɪl/

ve tvaru hrušky pear-shaped /ˈpeə.ʃeɪpt/

vedení, přenos, vodivost conduction /
kənˈdʌk.ʃən/

vedlejší účinek side /saɪd/ effect /
ɪˈfekt/

vědomí consciousness /ˈkɒn.tʃə.snəs/

vedoucí (osoba) leader /ˈliː.dəʳ/

velikost size /saɪz/

velikosti hrášku pea-sized /piː.saɪzd/

velká céva major /ˈmeɪ.dʒəʳ/ vessel /
ˈves.ᵊl/

velké množství abundance /
əˈbʌn.dᵊnt s/

velký epileptický záchvat grand mal /
ˈgraːnd.ˈmæl/

velmi, z velké části greatly /ˈgreɪt.li/

věnovat pozornost heed /hiːd/

vertikální, kolmý vertical /ˈvɜː.tɪ.kᵊl/

vést, řídit conduct /kənˈdʌkt/

vhánět vzduch blow /bləʊ/ air /eəʳ/

vhodný k suited /ˈsjuː.tɪd/ to /tʊ/

vhodný, žádoucí desirable / dɪˈzaɪə.rə.bl̩ /

vhojení do kosti osseointegration / ɒs.i.ə͵ɪn.tɪˈgreɪ.ʃən/

vibrovat (kmitat), chvět se vibrate / vaɪˈbreɪt/

víceúčelový multipurpose / ͵mʌl.tɪˈpɜː.pəs/

vidění, zrak (pohled), zorný vision / ˈvɪʒ.ən/

viditelnost visibility /͵vɪz.ɪˈbɪl.ɪ.ti/

vina, dávat vinu blame /bleɪm/

virový viral /ˈvaɪə.rəl/

vitamin, vitaminový vitamin / ˈvɪt.ə.mɪn/

vlasec fishing /ˈfɪʃ.ɪŋ/ line /laɪn/

vlastní protilátka autoantibody / ɔː.təʊ.ˈæn.ti͵bɒd.i/

vlhká lepkavost clamminess / ˈklæm.ɪ.nəs/

vlhkost moisture /ˈmɔɪs.tʃər/

vliv, výsledek impact /ˈɪm.pækt/

vlna wave /weɪv/

vmíchaný, začleněný incorporated / ɪnˈkɔː.pər.eɪ.tɪd/

vně outside /͵aʊtˈsaɪd/

vnější, týkající se okolí, životního prostředí environmental / ɪn͵vaɪə.rən.ˈmen.təl/

vnímat, uvědomit si, pochopit perceive /pəˈsiːv/

vodík hydrogen /ˈhaɪ.drɪ.dʒən/

vodivost conductivity /͵kɒn. dʌkˈtɪv.ɪ.ti/

vodní stříkačka water /ˈwɔː.tər/ syringe /sɪˈrɪndʒ/

vodorovná plocha horizontal / ͵hɒr.ɪˈzɒn.təl/ plane /pleɪn/

volat, křičet shout /ʃaʊt/

volba, větší záliba preference / ˈpref.ər.ənts/

volba, výběr, sortiment choice /tʃɔɪs/

volná chvíle, volný čas leisure /ˈleʒ.ər/

volně, otevřeně freely /ˈfriː.li/

volno z práce time /taɪm/ off /ɒf/ work /wɜːk/

volný loose-fitting /͵luːsˈfɪt.ɪŋ/

vosk wax /wæks/

voskovaný waxed /wækst/

vpáčený impacted /ɪmˈpæk.tɪd/

vrácení, znovudosazení replacement / rɪˈpleɪs.mənt/

vrchol, hrot, vrcholový bod, špička apex /ˈeɪ.peks/ (pl. apices)

vroubkovaný, zoubkovaný scalloped / ˈskɒl.əpd/

vrstevník peer /pɪər/

vrtáček ve tvaru špičatého poupětě rose-head /ˈrəʊz.hed/ bur /bɜːr /

vrták, vrtačka, vrtat, vyvrtat drill / drɪl/

vrtat, dloubat dig /dɪg/

vsáknout se soak /səʊk/

vstup, záznam, údaj entry /ˈen.tri/

všelék (univerzální lék) panacea / ͵pæn.əˈsiː.ə/

vůbec whatsoever /͵wɒt.səʊˈev.ər/

výbava, sada nástrojů kit /kɪt/

vybavený equipped /ɪˈkwɪpt/

výběr, volba selection /sɪˈlek.ʃən/

výběrový selective /sɪˈlek.tɪv/

vybraný chosen /ˈtʃəʊ.zən/ (inf. choose)

vybrat si choose /tʃuːz/

vyčerpaný exhausted /ɪgˈzɔː.stɪd/

vyčkávání temporisation / tem.pə.raɪˈzeɪ.ʃən/

výčnělek, křídlo flange /flændʒ/

vyčnívající prominent /ˈprɒm.ɪ.nənt/

výdaje, finanční náklady cost /kɒst/

vydávat, vysílat, vypouštět (páru, tekutinu) emit /ɪˈmɪt/

451

vyfoukaný, vysušený blown /bləʊn/ dry /draɪ/

vyhledat, zjistit polohu (místo) locate /ləʊ ˈkeɪt/

vyhledávač, lokátor locator / ləʊ ˈkeɪ.təʳ/

výhoda advantage /əd'vɑːn.tɪdʒ/

výhoda, vhodnost, příležitost (vhodná) convenience / kən'viː.ni.ənts/

výjimka exception /ɪk'sep.ʃᵊn/

vykřiknout shout /ʃaʊt/ out /aʊt/

vyloučení, vyřazení elimination / ɪˌlɪm.ɪ'neɪ.ʃᵊn/

vyloučit exclude /ɪk'skluːd/

vylučující exclusive /ɪk'skluː.sɪv/

vymazat, vynechat delete /dɪ'liːt/

vynikající excellent /'ek.səl.ənt/

vynutit coerce /kəʊ'ɜːs/

výpadek elektřiny power /paʊəʳ/cut / kʌt/

vyplivnout spit /spɪt/ out /aʊt/

vyplňování zubu, plomba, výplň, plnění, plnící filling /'fɪl.ɪŋ/

vyprávění narrative /'nær.ə.tɪv/

vyprázdnění střev movement / 'muːv.mənt/

výraz tváře, vyjádření, vytlačení expression /ɪk'spreʃ.ən/

výrazový expressive /ɪk'spres.ɪv/

výrostek youngster /'jʌŋk.stəʳ/

vyrovnat se, zaměřit align /ə'laɪn/

vyrovnat, vynahradit, vyvážit compensate /'kɒm.pən.seɪt/

vyřezat carve /kɑːv/

vyschnout, vysušit, vysušit se, vysychat dry /draɪ/ out /aʊt/

vysílání, vyzařování emission / ɪ'mɪʃ.ᵊn/

vyslovovat pronounce /prə'naʊnts/

vysokofrekvenční (VF) high-frequency /haɪ.'friː.kwənt.si/

vysoko-objemový high-volume / haɪ.'vɒl.juːm/

vysokoobrátkový násadec high-speed /ˌhaɪ'spiːd/ handpiece /hænd.piːs/

vysokorychlostní high-speed / ˌhaɪ'spiːd/

vysoký high /haɪ/

vysoký tlak, vysokotlaký high /haɪ/ pressure /'preʃ.əʳ/

výstavba, zvyšování, vystavět, vytvořit build /ˌbɪld/ up /ʌp/

vystřelující shooting /'ʃuː.tɪŋ/

vysvětlení explanation / ˌek.splə'neɪ.ʃᵊn/

vyšetřit zrakem visualise / 'vɪʒ.u.ᵊl.aɪz/

vyšetřit, prohlídka, vyšetřovat examine /ɪg'zæm.ɪn/

vyšetřovat investigate /ɪn'ves.tɪ.geɪt/

vytáhnout, vytrhnout pull /pʊl/ out / aʊt/

výtažkový essential /ɪ'sen.tʃəl/

výtisk, výpis printout /'prɪnt.aʊt/

vytlačovat express /ɪk'spres/

vytočit (telefonní číslo) dial /'daɪ.əl/

výtok discharge /dɪs'tʃɑːdʒ/

vytrhnutí zubu tooth /tuːθ/ extraction /ɪk'stræk.ʃən/

vytrvat persevere /ˌpɜː.sɪ'vɪəʳ/

vytvářet kategorie categorise / 'kæt.ə.gə.raɪz/

vytvoření puchýřů blistering / 'blɪs.tər.ɪŋ/

vytvořit create /kri'eɪt/

vytvrdit cure /kjʊəʳ/

vytyčit, zakreslit outline /'aʊt.laɪn/

využít utilise /'juː.tɪ.laɪz/

vyvažovat, kompenzovat neutralise / 'njuː.trə.laɪz/

vývojový developmental / dɪˌvel.əp'men.tᵊl/

vyvolat provoke /prə'vəʊk/

vyvolat rentgenový snímek develop /
dɪ'vel.əp/ radiograph /reɪ.di.ə.grɑːf/

vyvolat, přinutit, způsobit, být
příčinou cause /kɔːz/

vyvýšenina, pahrbek elevation /
ˌel.ɪ'veɪ.ʃ ⁿn/

vyzařovat radiate /'reɪ.di.eɪt/

význam meaning /'miː.nɪŋ/

významně, závažně significantly /
sɪg'nɪf.ɪ.kənt.li/

vyžadovat, požadovat call /kɔːl/ for /
fɔːr/

vyžadovat, vyvolat (reakci), získat,
dosáhnout elicit /ɪ'lɪs.ɪt/

výživa nutrition /njuː'trɪʃ.ən/

vzbudit rouse /raʊz/

vzdálenost distance /'dɪs.tənt s/

vzdálený distant /'dɪs.tənt/

vzdělání instruktáž, školení education
/ˌed.jʊ'keɪ.ʃ ⁿn/

vzduch air /eər/

vzduchová turbinka air /eər/ turbine /
't3ː.baɪn/

vzestup, zdvihat se (stoupat) rise /
raɪz/

vzít v úvahu take /teɪk/ into account /
ə'kaʊnt/

vzor, model pattern /'pæt.ən/

vzorek sample /'sɑːm.pl̩ /

vzpřímená poloha upright /'ʌp.raɪt/
position /pə'zɪʃ.ⁿn/

vzpřímený upright /'ʌp.raɪt/

vzrůstat, zvětšit, zvýšit se increase /
ɪn'kriːs/

vzrušivý, citový, dojemný emotional /
ɪ'məʊ.ʃⁿn.ⁿl/

vztahující se k času time /taɪm/
related /rɪ'leɪ.tɪd/

W

wolfram tungsten /'tʌŋ.stən/

Z

z úst do úst mouth-to-mouth /maʊθ/

za, dále než, nad, mimo, za
hranicemi beyond /bi'jɒnd/

za, vzadu behind /bɪ'haɪnd/

zabarvení coloration /ˌkʌl.ə'reɪ.ʃⁿn/

zablokovat, zatarasit seal /siːl/ off /ɒf/

zabývající se studiem krve a tkání
haematological /
ˌhiː.mə.tə'lɒdʒ.ɪ.kəl/

zácpa constipation /ˌkɒnt.stɪ'peɪ.ʃən/

začínat originate /ə'rɪdʒ.ɪ.neɪt/

zadní hinder /'hɪn.dər/

zadní rozštěp páteře, obratle spina
bifida /ˌspaɪ.nə'bɪf.ɪ.də/

zahájit initiate /ɪ'nɪʃ.i.eɪt/

zahrnovat, obsahovat comprise /
kəm'praɪz/

zahřát, rozžhavit heat /hiːt/

zahřívač (přístroj) heater /'hiː.tər/

zacházení, manipulace handling /
'hænd.lɪŋ/

zachovat na věky perpetuate /
pə'petʃ.u.eɪt/

záchranář, zachránce, záchranný
přístroj rescuer /'res.kjuː.ər/

záchvat, nával fit /fɪt/

záchvat, perioda bout /baʊt/

základ, základna, podklad, opěrný
bod base /beɪs/

základna protézy denture /'den.tʃə/
base /beɪs/

základní basic /'beɪ.sɪk/

základní, konečný ultimate /'ʌl.tɪ.mət/

zakončení ending /'en.dɪŋ/

zakrýt, skrýt cover /'kʌv.ər/ up /ʌp/

zakrýt, zastírat obscure /əb'skjʊər/

zakřivený, obloukový curved /kɜːvd/

zakulacený rounded /'raʊn.dɪd/

záležitost, sporná otázka issue /
'ɪʃ.uː/, /'ɪs.juː/

založený na based /beɪst/ on /ɒn/

záměr, cíl, zaměřit aim /eɪm/

zanedbat neglect /nɪˈglekt/

zánět tlustého střeva colitis / kəʊ ˈlaɪ.təs/

zaoblovací nástroj rounder /ˈraʊn.dəʳ/

zapadat, zajistit, obsadit, zaměstnávat engage /ɪnˈgeɪdʒ/

západka, zaklapnout latch /lætʃ/

zápěstí wrist /rɪst/

zapojení, postižení, komplikace involvement /ɪnˈvɒlv.mənt/

zapsat, zaznamenat record /rɪˈkɔːd/

zárodků prostý germ-free /dʒɜːm.friː/

zaručit vouch /vaʊtʃ/ for /fɔːʳ/

záření shining /ˈʃaɪ.nɪŋ/

zařízení, prostředek, vybavení, záměr device /dɪˈvaɪs/

zařízení, vybavení facility /fəˈsɪl.ɪ.ti/

zásobování elektřinou electricity / ɪˌlekˈtrɪs.ɪ.ti/ supply /səˈplaɪ/

zástava srdeční a dechová cardiorespiratory /kɑː.di.əʊ. rɪˈspɪr.ə.tri/ arrest /əˈrest/

zástava, zachycení arrest /əˈrest/

zásuvka, zdířka socket /ˈsɒk.ɪt/

závazný, nutný, nevyhnutelný imperative /ɪmˈper.ə.tɪv/

záviset, záležet na depend /dɪˈpend/

závislá osoba, rodinný příslušník dependant /dɪˈpen.dənt/

závislost, vztah dependence / dɪˈpen.dənts/

závislý na dependent /dɪˈpen.dənt/ on /ɒn/

závitnice threader /θred.əʳ/

zavlažovat irrigate /ˈɪr.ɪ.geɪt/

zavolat, přivolat summon /ˈsʌm.ən/

závrať vertigo /ˈvɜː.tɪ.gəʊ/

závrať, mrákotný stav dizziness / ˈdɪz.ɪ.nəs/

zavřená zlomenina simple /ˈsɪm.pl̩/ fracture /ˈfræk.tʃəʳ/

záznam o návštěvách attendance / əˈten.dənt s/ record /ˈrek.ɔːd/

záznam recording /rɪˈkɔː.dɪŋ/

záznam, označovací soustava notation /nəʊ ˈteɪ.ʃən/

zaznamenat notice /ˈnəʊ.tɪs/

zbarvení pigmentation / ˌpɪg.mənˈteɪ.ʃən/

zbavený, volný free /friː/

zblednout blanch /blɑːnt ʃ/

zbytečný (nepodstatný) unnecessary / ʌnˈnes.ə.ser.i/

zbytek remainder /rɪˈmeɪn.dəʳ/, rest / rest/

zbývající, zůstávající remaining / rɪˈmeɪ.nɪŋ/

zdravotní sestra nurse /nɜːs/

zdravotník, záchranář paramedic / ˌpær.əˈmed.ɪk/

zdržet, zpoždění, odkládat delay / dɪˈleɪ/

zdůraznit emphasize /ˈemp.fə.saɪz/

zdvořilý polite /pəˈlaɪt/

zepředu anteriorly /ænˈtɪə.ri.əʳ.li /

zesílení amplification / ˌæm.plɪ.fɪˈkeɪ.ʃən/

zeslabit spojení debond /dɪˈbɒnd/

zevně externally /ɪkˈstɜː.nə.li/

zhmožděný bruised /bruːzd/

zhoršení situace, zhoršení zdravotního stavu, neúspěch setback /ˈset.bæk/

zhoršený, poškozený impaired / ɪmˈpeəd/

zhoršit se become /bɪˈkʌm/ worse / wɜːs/

zhoršit, přitížit exacerbate / ɪgˈzæs.ə.beɪt/

zhoršující se worsening /ˈwɜː.sən.ɪŋ/

zhotovení můstku bridgework / brɪdʒ.wɜːk/

zhoubný detrimental /ˌdet.rɪˈmen.tᵊl/

zhypnotizování, hypnotický stav hypnosis /hɪp'nəʊ.sɪs/

zinek zinc /zɪŋk/

zink-fosfátový cement zinc /zɪŋk/ phosphate /'fɒs.feɪt/ cement / sɪ'ment/

zinková běloba zinc /zɪŋk/ oxide / 'ɒk.saɪd/

zinkoxid-eugenolová pasta zinc /zɪŋk/ oxide /'ɒk.saɪd/ eugenol /juː'dʒen. ɒl/ paste /peɪst/

zírat stare /steəʳ/

získat zpět, vrátit retrieve /rɪ'triːv/

zívání yawning /'jɔː.nɪŋ/

zívat yawn /jɔːn/

zklidnit sedate /sɪ'deɪt/

zkoumat sondou probe /prəʊb/

zkrátit shorten /'ʃɔː.tᵊn/

zkřivení, zkroucení distortion / dɪ'stɔː.ʃᵊn/

zkřížený skus crossbite /krɒs.baɪt/

zlato, zlatý gold /gəʊld/

zlepšit kvalitu, zvětšit enhance / ɪn'hɑːnts/

zlepšit se become /bɪ'kʌm/ better / 'bet.ər/

zlepšit, pozměnit amend /ə'mend/

zlepšit, zlepšit se, zdokonalit improve /ɪm'pruːv/

zmatek, zmatení confusion / kən'fjuː.ʒᵊn/

zmatený, nejasný confused / kən'fjuːzd/

změkčovadlo plasticiser / 'plæs.tɪ.saɪz.əʳ/

změna change /tʃeɪndʒ/

zmocněnec, zástupce deputy / 'dep.jʊ.ti/

zmrazování freezing /'friː.zɪŋ/

značný considerable /kən'sɪd.ər.ə.bl̩/

znamenitý superb /suː'pɜːb/

znázornění (vizuální) visualisation / ˌvɪʒ.u.ᵊl.aɪ'zeɪ.ʃᵊn/

znecitlivění numbness /'nʌm.nəs/

znehybnění immobilization / ɪˌməʊ.bəl.aɪ'zeɪ.ʃən/

znejasnit blur /blɜːr /

zneužít abuse /ə'bjuːz/

ničující devastating /'dev.ə.steɪ.tɪŋ/

znít, zvuk sound /saʊnd/

znovu vložit reinsert /riː.ɪn's3ːt/

znovu získat regain /rɪ'geɪn/

zobákovitý beaked /biːkt/

zobrazování imaging /ɪ'mɪdʒ.ɪŋ/

zobrazování magnetickou rezonancí magnetic /mæg'net.ɪk/ resonance / 'rez.ᵊn.ənt s/ imaging /ɪ'mɪdʒ.ɪŋ/

zobrazovat depict /dɪ'pɪkt/

zóna, oblast zone /zəʊn/

zopakovat revise /rɪ'vaɪz/

zotavovací poloha, stabilizovaná poloha recovery /rɪ'kʌv.ᵊr.i/ position /pə'zɪʃ.ᵊn/

zpět, záda, zadní část, opěradlo back /bæk/

zpívání singing /'sɪŋ.ɪŋ/

zpracovaný processed /'prəʊ.sest/

způsobit bring /brɪŋ/ about /ə'baʊt/, induce /ɪn'djuːs/

zrakový visual /'vɪʒ.u.əl/

zralost, vyspělost maturity / mə'tjʊə.rɪ.ti/

zrcadlo, zrcátko, odrážet se mirror / 'mɪr.əʳ/

zrníčko speck /spek/

zrušení cancellation /ˌkænt .səl'eɪ.ʃən/

zřejmý (viditelný) visible /'vɪz.ɪ.bl̩/

zřejmý apparent /ə'pær.ᵊnt/

zřídka rarely /'reə.li/

ztracený lost /lɒst/

ztráta vědomí loss /lɒs/ of /əv/ consciousness /'kɒn.t ʃə.snəs/

ztuha stiffly /'stɪf.li/

zubní kaz caries /ˈkeə.riːz/

zubní lékař dentist /ˈden.tɪst/

zubní můstek bridge /brɪdʒ/

zuby moudrosti wisdom /ˈwɪz.dəm/
teeth /tiːθ/

zvážit, rozvážit si, vzít v úvahu
consider /kənˈsɪd.əʳ/

zvednout elevate /ˈel.ɪ.veɪt/, pick /pɪk/
up /ʌp/, take /teɪk/ up /ʌp/

zvětšit, rozšířit se, vzmáhat se enlarge
/ɪnˈlɑːdʒ/

zvonit ring /rɪŋ/

zvracet, zvracení vomit /ˈvɒm.ɪt/

zvyk, návyk habit /ˈhæb.ɪt/

zvyknout si na get /get/ used /juːst/ to
/tʊ/

**zvýšení, zvednout, vypouknout,
vytáhnout, zřídit, zvýšit** raise /reɪz/

zvyšovat se mount /maʊnt/

Ž

žádný none /nʌn/

žádost, požádání, požadavek, prosba
request /rɪˈkwest/

želatina gelatine /ˈdʒel.ə.tiːn/

žena, ženský, pro ženy female /
ˈfiː.meɪl/

žijící, životní, živoucí living /ˈlɪv.ɪŋ/

život ohrožující life-threatening /
ˈlaɪfˌθret.ᵊn.ɪŋ/

životní styl lifestyle /ˈlaɪf.staɪl/

životní záchrana lifesaver /
ˈlaɪfˌseɪ.vəʳ/

životnost vitality /vaɪˈtæl.ɪ.ti/

živý alive /əˈlaɪv/

žláza gland /glænd/

žláza nadledviny adrenal gland /
əˈdriː.nəlˌglænd/

žloutenka jaundice /ˈdʒɔːn.dɪs/

žvýkat masticate /ˈmæs.tɪ.keɪt/

Bibliography / Literatura

BONEHILL, Jane, ROBERTS, Clare, and WINCOTT, Diana, *Handbook for Dental Nurses* (1st edn, Blackwell Publishing Ltd, 2007) 221 p.

BOTTICELLI, Antonella Toni: *Dentální hygiena. Teorie a praxe.* 1 vyd. Praha, Nakladatelství Quintessenz 2002. 216 s.

Cambridge Advanced Learner's Dictionary http://dictionary.cambridge.org

CAMBRIDGE English Pronouncing Dictionary (17th edn, Cambridge, Cambridge University Press, 2006) 599 p

CHURCHILL's Pocketbook of Clinical Dentistry (2nd edn, Edinborough, Churchill Livingstone, 2002) 544 p

FRAUS. *Ilustrovaný tematický slovník anglicko-český.* 1. vyd. Plzeň, Nakladatelství Fraus 2005. 432 s.

HOLLINS, Carole, *Questions and Answers for Dental Nurses* (2nd edn, Blackwell Publishing Ltd, 2006) 233 p

PAINTIN, Wendy, *A–Z of Dental Nursing* (1st edn, Oxford, Blackwell Publishing Ltd, 2009) 200 p

SEDLÁČEK, Josef: *Anglicko-český stomatologický slovník.* 1. vyd. Praha, Grada Publishing 2007. 204 s.

SEDLÁČEK, Josef: *Česko-anglický stomatologický slovník.* 1. vyd. Praha, Grada Publishing 2007. 188 s.

TOPILOVÁ, Věra: *Anglicko-český, česko-anglický lékařský slovník.* 1. vyd. Praha, Grada Publishing 1999. 878 s.